Functional Exercise Anatomy and Physiology for Physiotherapists

Defne Kaya Utlu
Editor

Functional Exercise Anatomy and Physiology for Physiotherapists

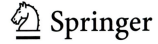

Editor
Defne Kaya Utlu
Physiotherapy and Rehabilitation
Hamidiye Faculty of Health Sciences
University of Health Sciences
Istanbul, Turkey

Section Editors

Cetin Sayaca
Physiotherapy and Rehabilitation
Faculty of Health Sciences
Bursa Uludag University
Bursa, Turkey

Özden Özkal
Physiotherapy and Rehabilitation
Faculty of Health Sciences
Bursa Uludag University
Bursa, Turkey

Abdulhamit Tayfur
School of Physiotherapy and Rehabilitation
Kırşehir Ahi Evran University
Kırsehir, Turkey

Filiz Erdem Eyüboğlu
Physiotherapy and Rehabilitation
Faculty of Health Sciences
Üsküdar University
Istanbul, Turkey

Mahmut Calik
Physiotherapy and Rehabilitation
Faculty of Health Sciences
Haliç University
Istanbul, Turkey

ISBN 978-3-031-27183-0   ISBN 978-3-031-27184-7   (eBook)
https://doi.org/10.1007/978-3-031-27184-7

English translation of the original Turkish edition published by Hippocrates Publishing House, Ankara, 2021

© The Editor(s) (if applicable) and The Author(s), under exclusive license to Springer Nature Switzerland AG 2023

This work is subject to copyright. All rights are solely and exclusively licensed by the Publisher, whether the whole or part of the material is concerned, specifically the rights of reprinting, reuse of illustrations, recitation, broadcasting, reproduction on microfilms or in any other physical way, and transmission or information storage and retrieval, electronic adaptation, computer software, or by similar or dissimilar methodology now known or hereafter developed.

The use of general descriptive names, registered names, trademarks, service marks, etc. in this publication does not imply, even in the absence of a specific statement, that such names are exempt from the relevant protective laws and regulations and therefore free for general use.

The publisher, the authors, and the editors are safe to assume that the advice and information in this book are believed to be true and accurate at the date of publication. Neither the publisher nor the authors or the editors give a warranty, expressed or implied, with respect to the material contained herein or for any errors or omissions that may have been made. The publisher remains neutral with regard to jurisdictional claims in published maps and institutional affiliations.

This Springer imprint is published by the registered company Springer Nature Switzerland AG
The registered company address is: Gewerbestrasse 11, 6330 Cham, Switzerland

We present this book to our beautiful country, Turkey, where we grew up as scientists.

Preface

Dear Colleagues and Students,

As physiotherapists, who add movement and health to life, our greatest weapon in the treatment of diseases and improving health is undoubtedly exercise. Functional exercise approaches enable us to make physical performance and activities of daily living more effective by adapting our exercise prescription according to the movements that individuals make frequently in daily life or during sports.

Functional exercise training aims to improve activities of daily living, from personal care such as showering or dressing to household chores such as cleaning, cooking, or gardening. Although almost all of us have to get out of bed every day and do basic things like getting dressed, eating, and taking care of ourselves regularly, our activities of daily living vary from person to person due to our different habits and lifestyles. Therefore, functional exercise training should be designed differently for everyone.

When designing a functional exercise prescription, physiotherapists should consider previous injuries or surgeries that limit the level of physical activity, general health, muscular strength, endurance, aerobic capacity, and activities that the patient should do in daily life. The functional exercise prescription should be customized according to both the patient's fragility due to injury or surgery and the patient's strengths such as sports/exercise history and healthy eating habits.

The book consists of four different parts: (I) Functional exercise definition, type, and prescription, (II) exercise-specific musculoskeletal anatomy, (III) exercise-specific systems physiology, and (IV) miscellaneous. We explained the concepts of exercise and physical activity, exercise types, and prescription creation within the scope of functional exercise definition, type, and prescription. Under the heading of musculoskeletal system anatomy specific to functional exercise, we have enriched our anatomy knowledge with exercises based on evidence that the function, palpation, and joint movement of the anatomical structures such as fascia, bones, and muscles. The content of functional exercise-specific systems physiology consists of the compliance of each system with exercise, basic exercise physiology information, and the evaluation and treatment of healthy individuals with diseases that affect each system. Additionally, balance, coordination, and proprioception; movement and nutrition principles; nutritional supplements for musculoskeletal health; and exercise-induced anaphylaxis chapters are under the miscellaneous part.

Our aim when designing this book, which consists of subjects that we felt lacking during both our student and academic years, was to create a bedside resource for physiotherapists who solve a defined movement problem and plan and apply functional therapeutic exercises that can be varied according to the patient. We hope that this book will open new horizons for our colleagues and students and that it will be read with pleasure.

Istanbul, Turkey   Defne Kaya Utlu, Professor, PhD, PT

Acknowledgments

I have accumulated great memories, friendships, colleagues, and students in my academic journey, which was challenging but enjoyable at the same time. The stories I have experienced on this journey have often challenged me, and the teachings have always pushed me to do better and better, and have grown and developed me. I have always tried to prepare/tell/write my lectures, articles, speeches, and book/book chapters as I said when I was a student, "I wish it was like this."

It is very meaningful for me to be the chief editor of a work **first** written in Turkish as a native language **and then translated** into English in the 24th year of my academic life and to work with a wonderful team.

With your permission, I would like to list some of my thanks here…

My dear mother **Ayşe Kaya,** who raised me with great sacrifices and in a loving environment to be an honest, hardworking, and good person who loves her country and the world, and my dear father **Zekeriya Kaya,** who is often my mentor guided me to become an academic like him. To my sister **Fatma Duygu Kaya Yertutuanol,** who is both a good doctor and a good academician, the best gift of my life.

To Cetin Sayaca, Ozden Ozkal, Abdulhamit Tayfur, Filiz Eyuboglu, and Mahmut Calik, who are loyal, hardworking, patriotic, and kind-hearted academics and assistant editors of my team, who worked hard from the idea stage to the printing of the book, and I am always proud to be my companions and teachers.

To the authors of the chapters, consisting of young academics, for their efforts in the creation of this bedside book that will shed light on our colleagues and students, who have put incredible effort into the creation of such a difficult book.

To my esteemed professors at Hacettepe University, who have raised me in my education and academic life, shed light on the path I have walked, and have been my icebreaker in my profession.

To all my students who always encourage me to produce with their endless excitement, energy, and desire to learn.

To Springer **Nature Publishing House,** especially **Corinna and Katherine, for their** unwavering support from the first stage of the book to its publication.

To my dear husband **Ceyhan Utlu,** who made me feel that he was with me and proud of me in every step I took, embraced me with his love, and helped me realize most of the changes in my life with his perspective.

I would like to express my endless gratitude to all veterans and martyrs, especially my **Great Leader Mustafa Kemal ATATURK** and his comrades in arms, who risked their lives so that I could become an academician who produced and worked in an independent country as a woman in this land that raised me as a scientist.

With the hope that may science and goodness always illuminate our path……

Defne Kaya Utlu, Professor, PhD, PT

Contents

Part I Introduction to Exercise

1 Description, Types, and Prescription of the Exercise 3
   Defne Kaya Utlu

Part II Exercise-Specific Musculoskeletal Anatomy

2 The Basic Definitions of Anatomy and Anthropometry 21
   Seda Bicici Ulusahin

3 The Bone and Joint Structure 53
   Günseli Usgu and Serkan Usgu

4 The Muscle Structure and Function 77
   Mahmut Calik

5 The Nerve Structure and Function 93
   Cetin Sayaca

6 The Fascia and Movement 111
   Atilla Cagatay Sezik and Ebru Gul Sezik

7 The Axial Skeleton 121
   Kadriye Tombak

8 The Head and Neck Anatomy 153
   Omer Faruk Yasaroglu and Numan Demir

9 The Shoulder 177
   Dilara Kara and Taha Ibrahim Yildiz

10 The Elbow 199
    Seval Tamer

11 The Hand and Wrist................................... 237
    Rabia Tugba Kilic

12 The Pelvis... 261
    Ayca Aklar

13 The Hip 277
    Muharrem Gokhan Beydagi

xi

14	**The Knee**	291
	Abdulhamit Tayfur and Beyza Tayfur	
15	**The Foot and Ankle**	315
	Serdar Demirci and Gurkan Gunaydin	

Part III Exercise-Specific Systems Physiology

16	**Physiological Adaptation**	349
	Manolya Acar	
17	**Cell and Storage**	359
	Buse Ozcan Kahraman	
18	**Adaptation of the Musculoskeletal System to Exercise**	373
	Aslihan Cakmak	
19	**Neural System and Its Adaptation to Exercise**	391
	Cevher Demirci and Saniye Aydogan Arslan	
20	**Bioenergetics and Metabolism**	407
	Ozge Ozalp	
21	**Respiratory System and Its Adaptations to Exercise**	423
	Dilara Saklica	
22	**Circulatory System and Its Adaptation to Exercise**	447
	Filiz Erdem Eyuboglu	
23	**Endocrine System and Its Adaptations to Exercise**	473
	Cemile Bozdemir Ozel	
24	**Renal System, Fluid Balance, and Its Adaptations to Exercise**	489
	Selda Gokcen	
25	**Immune System and Its Adaptation to Exercise**	505
	Ozden Ozkal	

Part IV Miscellaneous

26	**Balance, Coordination, and Proprioception**	521
	Oznur Buyukturan	
27	**Movement and Nutrition Principles**	537
	Metin Guldas, Ozge Yesıldemır, Ozan Gurbuz, Seda Ozder, and Elif Yildiz	
28	**Nutritional Supplements for Musculoskeletal Health**	547
	Aysegul Birlik	
29	**Exercise-Induced Anaphylaxis**	561
	Nurhan Sayaca	

About the Editor

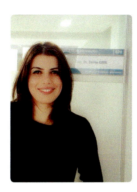

Defne Kaya Utlu, Professor, PhD, PT was born on December 23, 1976, in Turkey. Prof. Kaya Utlu graduated from the Physiotherapy and Rehabilitation at Hacettepe University in 1999. Prof. Kaya Utlu received her master's degree in 2001 by completing her thesis titled "Effectiveness of high voltage pulsed galvanic stimulation accompanying patellar taping on patellofemoral pain syndrome". She worked in the Center for Rehabilitation Science of the University of Manchester on a post-doctoral project entitled "Optimizing Physiotherapy in the Treatment of Patellofemoral Pain Syndrome" as a researcher for 6 months in 2007. In 2008, she completed her thesis entitled "Muscle strength, functional endurance, coordination, and proprioception in patellofemoral pain syndrome" and graduated with her doctoral degree. She worked on all kinds of special orthopedic extremity problems when she worked as a research assistant. She also worked on rehabilitation after medial patellofemoral ligament surgery in "Abteilung und Poliklinik für Sportorthopadie des Klinikum rechts der Isar der TUM" in September 2008. She also worked as a researcher at Manchester University, Centre for Rehabilitation Science, and Arthritis Research UK in November–December 2010 and September to November 2012. In 2010, Prof. Kaya Utlu and her colleagues published a paper titled "The Effect of an Exercise Program in Conjunction With Short-Period Patellar Taping on Pain, Electromyogram Activity, and Muscle Strength in Patellofemoral Pain Syndrome" in journal of Sports Health. It was selected as a suggestion paper by "Australian Sports Commission." In Congress of the 10th Turkish Society of Sports Traumatology Arthroscopy and Knee Surgery, Prof. Kaya Utlu and her colleagues together published a paper titled "Shoulder joint position sense is negatively correlated with the free-throw percentage in professional basketball players" which was awarded the best oral presentation and young researcher. Prof. Kaya Utlu worked as an associate professor in the Department of Sports Medicine, Faculty of Medicine, Hacettepe University. She was the founding head of the Physical Therapy and Rehabilitation department of the Faculty of Health Science and NP Physiotherapy Rehabilitation Clinic at Uskudar University, Istanbul, Turkey. Prof. Kaya Utlu was the founding head of the Physical Therapy and Rehabilitation department of the Faculty of Health Science in Bursa Uludag University, Bursa, Turkey. Prof. Kaya Utlu is a professor at Health Sciences University, Istanbul, Turkey. She became an associate professor in 2013 and a professor in 2018. Prof. Kaya Utlu is a reviewer of many international and national indexed journals. She currently studies the techniques of rehabilitation after ankle injury/surgery, knee injury/surgery, hip injury/surgery, and shoulder injury/surgery. Prof. Kaya Utlu is an associate editor of the *Sports Injuries* published by Springer. She is also an editor of the *Forgotten sixth sense: The Proprioception* which was published by OMICS Groups. She is an editor in chief of the *Proprioception in Orthopaedics, Sports Medicine and Rehabilitation* which was published by Springer. She was on the editorial board of the Turkish Journal of Physiotherapy and Rehabilitation, she was on the editorial board of Muscle Ligament Tendon Journal, and she is an academic editor in Biomed Research International Journal. Prof. Kaya Utlu enjoys squash, plays piano, trekking, fitness, and likes to travel.

Part I

Introduction to Exercise

Description, Types, and Prescription of the Exercise

Defne Kaya Utlu

Abstract

Hippocrates wrote in 1931 that "eating alone will not keep a man well; he must also take exercise." Since then, the impact of these two concepts on healthy life has never changed.

Exercise is a very powerful tool, even medicine, in reducing harmful effects of chronic diseases and mortality rates, as well as in treating and preventing chronic diseases. There is a linear relationship between activity level and health status. People who lead an active and fit lifestyle live longer and healthier. In contrast, physical inactivity has a mind-boggling array of detrimental effects on health. Sedentary people are affected by the chronic disease early and die at a younger age as they do not adapt exercise/sports to their lives. This relationship between illness and a sedentary lifestyle affects all age groups, albeit in varying degrees: children, adults, and the elderly. Current studies show that people with active lifestyles are much healthier. It would not be wrong to say that inactivity, a problem that can be solved by movement, is the biggest public health problem in this era.

D. Kaya Utlu (✉)
Physiotherapy and Rehabilitation, Hamidiye Faculty of Health Sciences, University of Health Sciences, Istanbul, Turkey

In this section, the description, types, and prescription of the exercise that should be done regularly both in illness and health will be explained.

1.1 Exercise and Physical Activity

There is confusion in the definition of physical activity, exercise, physical fitness, and sport. Let us take a look at the differences between these terms.

1.1.1 Physical Activity

It is any movement involving the work of the skeletal muscle(s) that expends energy (calories). Physical activity may include housework, stair climbing, general chores, walking, gardening, or other activities during the day involving movement. Being physically active for at least 150 min a week reduces the risk of disease and improves the quality of life. The term to describe the amount of physical activity is *dosage*. For exercise or physical activity, dose refers to the amount of physical activity performed by a person or participant. Three components determine the total dose or amount of activity: frequency, duration, and intensity. Let us detail the components of physical activity: (1) *Frequency* is usually expressed as sessions, episodes, or bouts on a daily or weekly basis; (2) *Duration* is the amount of time you spend participating in one session of physical activity; and (3) *Intensity* is the rate of energy expenditure required to perform the desired aerobic activity or the magnitude of the force applied during resistance exercise.

1.1.2 Exercise

It is also a type of physical activity. It is planned, structured, and used to improve aspects of physical fitness. The intensity, duration, and frequency of exercise are typically used to measure progress and improvements. In other words, for us to call a physical activity as exercise, it must have a specific purpose or goal, and it must be structured, planned, and repeated. During exercise, you engage in an organized movement for a certain period. This could be running, jogging, jumping rope, lifting weights, swimming, or cycling. Exercise can be planned with many goals such as being healthy; looking beautiful; losing weight; improving body composition; reducing stress; improving blood sugar; lipid or blood pressure control; improving muscular strength, power, and endurance; increasing mental and memory capacity; and improving cardiovascular capacity. Another definition that should be emphasized here is exercise training. "Exercise" and "exercise training" are often used interchangeably and generally refer to physical activity performed in leisure time to improve or maintain physical fitness, physical performance, or health.

1.1.3 Physical Fitness

It refers to the ability of multiple systems in the body to work together to perform certain tasks. The health-related components of physical fitness are collected under five parameters, each of which can be measured by specific tests: muscular strength, muscular endurance, cardiorespiratory fitness, flexibility, and agility.

1.1.4 The Sport

It encompasses a set of physical activities performed within a set of rules and performed as part of leisure or competition. Sports activities often involve physical activity performed by teams or individuals and are supported by an institutional framework such as a sports agency.

1.2 Types of Exercise

Various types of exercise can be used to improve the components of physical activity. These exercises and their effect on physical fitness are summarized in Table 1.1.

1.2.1 Aerobic Exercises

1.2.1.1 Types

Any activity that uses large muscle groups, is sustained, and is rhythmic can be considered aerobic exercise. In general, low-skill aerobic exercises should be included in exercise prescriptions to improve physical fitness. Aerobic exercises that require the least skill and can be easily modified to suit individual physical fitness levels include brisk walking, cycling, swimming, aerobic exercise in water, and slow dancing. Aerobic exercises that are performed at a higher intensity and therefore recommended for people who exercise regularly include jogging, step exercise, fast dancing, and elliptical exercise. Aerobic exercise/activity causes a person's heart to beat faster and breathe more intensely than usual. "*Cardio*" is a

Table 1.1 Exercise types and their effects on physical fitness

Types	Effects
Aerobic	Improves body composition and cardiorespiratory fitness
Strengthening	Improves strength, power, and endurance
Flexibility	Improves flexibility
Neuromuscular	Improves balance, coordination, agility, and proprioception

training ground that offers an unlimited variety of exercises: walking, running, cycling, cross-country skiing, swimming, and dancing. Anything that gets the heart rate above the resting heart rate is *cardio*. However, there are different categories of *cardio*, both aerobic and anaerobic. The most commonly used cardio exercises in clinics are as follows:

Steady-State Exercises (Aerobic)

This type of cardio refers to the pace of the workout and can include any level of intensity. As the name suggests, the goal is to maintain a steady pace and intensity throughout the entire duration of the preferred workout.

Low- and Moderate-Intensity Exercises (Aerobic)

Low-intensity exercise can be defined as any exercise that keeps the heart rate below 50% of the maximum heart rate such as brisk walking or slow cycling. Moderate-intensity exercises keep the heart rate between 50 and 70% of the maximum heart rate. During moderate-intensity exercise, breath control is very important. Thus, care should be taken to ensure that the patient can speak without shortness of breath during exercise.

High-Intensity and Interval Exercises (Anaerobic)

These exercises keep the heart rate at or above 70% of the maximum heart rate. High-intensity exercises include sprinting, some types of resistance training, and high-intensity interval training (HIIT). Intervals are the division of exercises into several segments (i.e., repetitions) and completion as part of the same exercise (i.e., one round). They can be divided into many formats, but the most common is time or distance blocks.

Intervals should usually be designed as lower-intensity movements like walking or resting between high-intensity exercises like sprinting or jumping rope. Here is an example design for the high-intensity training-to-rest ratio: *Initial (ratio: 1/2)*: One unit of high-intensity training interval followed by two more units of low-intensity training interval allows the body to recover before returning to that higher-intensity interval. *Intermediate-to-advanced athlete (ratio: 2/1)*: Twice the time or repetitions are split into high-intensity training intervals, half of which is split into rest intervals: Two units of high-intensity training interval followed by one unit of lower-intensity training interval/rest.

In general, endurance training models designed with HIIT consist of a combination of different training sessions arranged periodically on time scales ranging from micro-cycle (2–7 days) to mid-cycle (3–6 weeks) to macro-cycle (6–12 months; including preparation, competition, and transition periods) (Fig. 1.1).

1.2.1.2 Dosage

The dose of aerobic exercise consists of the frequency (F), intensity (I), duration (time, T), volume (V), and progression (P) of the exercise

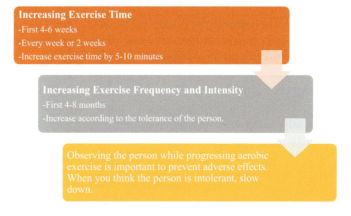

Fig. 1.1 Example of aerobic exercise progress

Table 1.2 Components of FITT-VP

Components	What to have in an exercise prescription?
Frequency, F	How many days per week are reserved for the training session?
Intensity, I	How hard a person works to do the activity? The intensity of exercise can be determined according to objective criteria such as maximal heart rate, heart rate reserve, and maximum oxygen consumption, or it can be adjusted according to the effort perceived by the patient by using some scales. Absolute intensity refers to the amount of energy expended per minute of activity, while relative intensity takes into account a person's exercise capacity or cardiorespiratory fitness level to assess the level of effort. As a general rule, a person doing moderate-intensity aerobic exercise can talk but not sing during the activity. A person doing high-intensity aerobic exercise cannot say more than a few words without pausing for taking a breath (see Table 1.3 for definitions on assessment of aerobic exercise intensity)
Time, T	The length of activity or exercise is performed. Duration is usually expressed in minutes
Type, T	The type of exercise performed
Volume, V	The total amount of training load
Progression, T	The advancement and increase in exercise stimulus over time

Table 1.3 Aerobic exercise intensity measurement methods

Method	Explanation
METs	Metabolic equivalents (METs) are expressed in mL per 1 kg of the person's body weight of oxygen consumed in 1 min. It can be thought of as the energy expended or the amount of oxygen consumed during activity/rest • MET is the rate of energy expended at rest. It is traditionally taken as an oxygen intake of 3.5 mL per kg of body weight per minute • Light-intensity aerobic activity is activity at 1.1–2.9 MET, moderate-intensity activity at 3–5.9 MET, and vigorous activity at 6 and above MET The intensity of aerobic activities can also be measured simply as the speed of the activity (for example, walking at 5 km/h, jogging at 10 km/h)
VO_{2max}/VO_2R	Aerobic intensity as determined by exercise tests can also be expressed as a percentage of a person's maximum oxygen uptake/aerobic capacity (VO_2max) or oxygen uptake reserve (VO_2R)
$\%HR_{max}/\%HRreserve$	Aerobic intensity, which can be measured by maximum exercise tests or estimated by the person's age, can also be expressed as a percentage of a person's maximum heart rate (HRmax)[a] or heart rate reserve (HRreserve)[b]
RPE	Rated perceived exertion (RPE) can score how much difficulty a person feels when exercising

[a] HRmax can be estimated by subtracting age from 220 (classic Karvonen formula) or 206.9 − (0.67 × age) in individuals 19 years and older
[b] HRreserve = HRmax − HRrest, HRtarget = 0.6 HRreserve + HRrest

performed. The exercise type (T) applied together with the other components form the basic principle of the exercise prescription—FITT-VP principle. Definitions related to the FITT-VP principle are summarized in Table 1.2.

The intensity of aerobic exercise can be determined with scales assessing perceived effort by metabolic equivalents, percent of maximum heart rate or heart rate reserve, and percent of maximum oxygen uptake/aerobic capacity or oxygen uptake reserve (Table 1.3).

1.2.1.3 Volume

Volume refers to the total work done at a given stage of training. It includes the duration of the activity, the distance, and the number of times it is repeated during the training period.

1.2.1.4 Progression

Increasing the intensity, duration, frequency, or amount of activity or exercise while the human body adapts to a certain activity pattern is called exercise progression. An example of aerobic exercise progression is given in Fig. 1.1.

1.2.2 Muscular Strengthening Exercises

Muscular strengthening exercises make the muscles do more work than they usually do (overloading the muscles). If an exercise is of medium to high intensity and works major muscle groups of the body, such as legs, hips, back, chest, abdomen, shoulders, and arms, it is considered as a strengthening exercise. Resistance exercises, including weight training, are the best-known example of muscular strengthening exercises that can be prescribed using the FITT framework.

1.2.2.1 Scientific Basis

The force that the muscle can produce is determined by the cross-bridges that form in a sarcomere over some time. The dominant fiber type in the muscle can determine which sport to be successful in; fast-twitch muscle fibers (type 2) produce more force, so training these muscles is of particular importance in power sports. The amount of active motor units at a given time determines the force that the muscle can produce. There are three different motor units in the human body. Type I withstands high fatigue, has a lower activation threshold, contains fewer muscle fibers, and has low force production during contraction. Type IIa is also resistant to fatigue, has a higher activation threshold, and produces a higher force. Type IIb is easily fatigued, has a high activation threshold, innervates the largest number of muscle fibers, and produces the greatest force during contraction.

Maximal force generation is determined by the properties of the contraction. The arrangement of the muscle fibers, the contraction speed, and the traction angle also affect the force generation. The force increases as the cross-sectional area increases.

> **Tips**
>
> Force–velocity relationship: If a muscle changes in length, the force produced by the muscle changes
> As the force increases further, the muscle does not allow shortening and contracts isometrically
> As the shortening rate increases, the force decreases. In other words, to increase the force, it is necessary to slow down the contraction rate
> If the external load on the muscle increases (more than the force the muscle can produce), the velocity becomes negative and the muscle contracts eccentrically (Fig. 1.2)

Likewise, the type of contraction also affects the amount of force generation. For example, in eccentric contraction, the external force applied to the muscle is greater than the muscle can exert. Calculating the difference between the maximum force generated by eccentric and isometric contraction provides the opportunity to design the most appropriate training program. When the force generated by the muscle during eccentric and isometric contraction is equal, we can assume that the muscle produces the best force according to its cross-sectional area. It is clear that the available muscle mass is underutilized when there is a significant difference between the maximum force produced during eccentric and isometric contraction.

Muscular strength training is motor unit training (Fig. 1.3). With muscular strength training, the number of motor units activated, and the firing power and duration of motor units improve. As a result, the resulting force increases. When all motor units are activated, 60–80% of the maximal contraction force occurs, depending on the type of muscle. The threshold for activation of motor units decreases with high-speed contractions.

The force generated in slow-speed contractions is three times greater than in high-speed contractions. Additional power is generated by the synchronization of the motor units. Adaptation to training occurs by agonist–antagonist muscle co-activation. This co-activation depends on the type of contraction, speed, and fatigue. All motor units can be activated at 30% of maximal contraction.

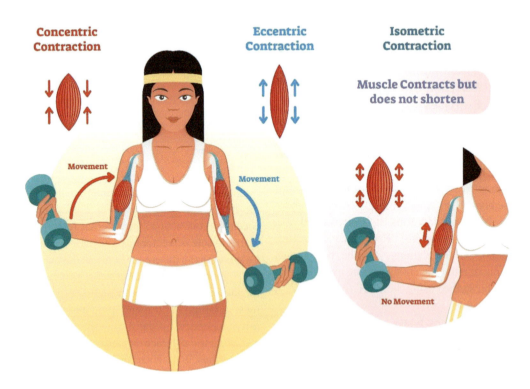

Fig. 1.2 Types of muscle contractions—concentric: visible movement occurs in the joint and the length of the muscle is shortened; isometric: no visible movement occurs in the joint and muscle tone increases, and activation of motor units is preset; eccentric: visible movement occurs in the joint and the muscle lengthens, and additional automatic activation is required (VectorMine/Shutterstock.com)

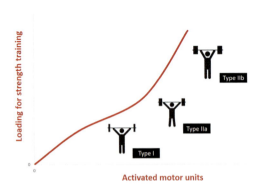

Fig. 1.3 The relationship between loading and motor unit activation (Alex Ghidan/Shutterstock.com)

Anabolic hormone production level also determines strength. Anabolic hormones include: growth hormone (GH), testosterone, and insulin-like growth hormone (IGF-1). (1) *Growth hormone* (GH) is released from the anterior lobe of the pituitary. It is released in the highest dose at night. GH targets organs (including muscle and liver) that stimulate the production of insulin-like growth hormone. After high-intensity physical training, the GH level increases after 10–20 min. The effect on the muscle is in the form of an increase in the cross-sectional area. (2) *Testosterone* is an anabolic hormone produced by the testes and, to a lesser extent, by the adrenal gland. Slow- and fast-twitch muscle fibers differ in testosterone sensitivity. Slow type I fibers show higher sensitivity, while fast IIb is less sensitive to testosterone. Long-term, low-intensity training reduces testosterone levels. Aerobic training provides its cardioprotective effect with a decreased testosterone level. After high-intensity training (over 70%), testosterone level remains high for 30–40 min. (3) *Insulin-like growth hormone (IGF-1)* is an anabolic hormone with a structure similar to insulin. It is generally produced by the liver and can be produced locally in the muscle if needed. IGF-1, like many hormones, works through receptors. Its main function is to promote protein synthesis. Since IGF-1 is a growth stimulant, chronically high levels increase the incidence of different types of cancer. So, a low IGF-1/insulin level means longevity. Long-term aerobic exercise lowers the level of IGF-1, while high-intensity exercise increases the level of IGF-1. IGF-1 level increases in muscle injury, and its anabolic effect increases healing and adaptation processes. Since the level of IGF-1 is closely related to GH production, its level decreases with age, similar to GH.

Before moving on to the prescription principles for muscular strengthening exercises, let us remember the definitions of strength, power, and endurance. The strength, power, or endurance of a muscle is the *ability* of the muscle. (1) *Muscular strength* is the ability to generate force against resistance. It is important to maintain the normal level necessary for a normal healthy life. Muscular weakness or imbalance impairs function. (2) *Muscular endurance* is the ability to produce repetitive muscular contractions against resistance. (3) *Muscular power* is the ability to build force quickly. Combination of force and speed, performance is limited without power.

Whichever is to be developed—muscular strength, power, endurance, and hypertrophy—it is necessary to focus primarily on the predominant criteria.

Tips	
	Predominant parameters (respectively)
Muscle strength and hypertrophy	Loading–repetitions–speed of movement
Muscular power	**Single target:** speed of movement–loading–repetitions **Multi-target:** speed of movement–repetitions–loading
Muscular endurance	Repetitions–speed of movement–loading

1.2.2.2 Dosage
The dose of strengthening exercise is a combination of the frequency, intensity, and volume of the exercise performed. When prescribing resistance exercise to the patient, especially the dosage and type should be determined. Other explanations regarding FITT-VP training principles are summarized in Table 1.4. It is important to remember that every resistance exercise should be done with appropriate techniques. Individuals new to resistance exercises should be trained in all aspects before starting these exercises.

1.2.2.3 Volume
While lowering repetitions with a heavier load develops muscular strength and power, more repetitions with a lighter load improve muscular endurance (Fig. 1.4).

1.2.2.4 Progression
As the patient progresses, the exercise dose may be increased (overload) to improve muscle strength and endurance. Overload can be achieved by regulating several variables: (1) increase the load (or intensity), (2) increase the number of repetitions per set, (3) increase the number of sets per exercise, (4) decrease the rest time between sets or exercises, and (5) increase the frequency of exercise. It is recommended to increase the number of repetitions before increasing the load.

Table 1.4 Principles of strengthening exercise within the framework of FITT-VP

Key component	Details
Frequency, F	1. Number of days per week devoted to exercise specific to each muscle group 2. Depending on the individual's daily schedule, all muscle groups to be trained can be done in the same session (i.e., the whole body), or the body can be "divided" into selected muscle groups during each session so that only a few of them can be trained with the exercise done in any one session. For example: lower body muscles can be worked on Mondays and Thursdays, and upper body muscles on Tuesdays and Fridays (in this case, each muscle group will be worked 2 days a week)
Intensity, I	1. "Load" is the way to express the intensity of the prescribed resistance exercise. "Load" refers to the amount of weight or resistance in an exercise set 2. To estimate the limb-specific weight load for resistance exercise, 1 maximum repetition (1RM) can be determined, and then a certain percentage of that amount (i.e., 1%RM) can be used during each set of the exercise. 1RM: The greatest resistance/weight that can be moved in good posture and in a controlled manner throughout the entire range of motion, that is, the maximum amount of weight that can be lifted once for a given exercise that cannot be lifted a second time
Time, T	1. While a specific amount of time is not recommended for resistance exercise, repetitions and sets are the standard way to refer to the amount of work needed in an exercise prescription 2. "Repetitions" is the performance of a single exercise, like lifting a weight once 3. A "set" consists of non-stop repetitions. A reasonable rest interval between sets is 2–3 min, but a shorter interval may be allowed for low-intensity training (mainly to improve muscular endurance rather than strength and mass). For example: 1 set = 12 times of continuous weight lifting 4. The number of repetitions and resistance performed in each set is inversely proportional to the load of your exercise, meaning the greater the load, the fewer repetitions that need to be completed
Type, T	1. The form of exercise 2. Exercise regimens should include multi-joint or combined exercises. The resistance of multi-joint or combined exercises can be changed with exercise equipment, body weight, or load-bearing
Volume, V	1. Exercise volume or quantity is the product of Frequency, Intensity, and Time. 2. Cardiorespiratory fitness volume can be calculated by how many steps you walked weekly. 3. Resistance exercises volume is calculated by sets and repetitions. . 4. The recommendation for resistance exercise is 2-4 sets with 8-12 repetitions per set with 2-3 minutes rest intervals.

Progression, P	1. It is best to increase intensity first then time/duration.
	2. For cardiovascular training:
	   a. Increasing any of the FITTV categories.
	   b. To reduce the risk of injury, start low and go slow.
	3. For resistance training: It is best to gradually increase the resistance, and/or more repetitions per set, and/or increased the frequency of workouts.
	Progression can be thought of as stairs and the railing of the stairs as the FITT-VP model. If the railing is used as a support, it is safer and faster to reach the top.

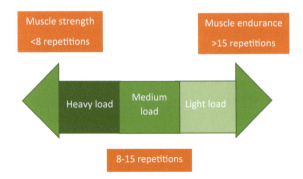

Fig. 1.4 The relationship between repetitions and loading

Training loads can be increased (e.g., ~5%) when the patient can comfortably reach the "upper limit" of the predetermined repetition range, for example, 12–15 repetitions.

1.2.2.5 Strength Training Methods

In training, it needs to be focused on exercises that improve neuromuscular coordination to activate more motor units and synchronize activations. The methods that are frequently used as strength training methods are: *maximal strength training*, *explosive strength training*, and *endurance training*. These methods are described in detail below.

Maximal Strength Training

The maximal strength value is important in all sports because its value affects both explosive power and endurance. Maximum strength reaches its peak at the age of 20–35 in men and 18–30 in women. Maximal strength is developed in two ways: (1) high muscle tension exercises, and (2) high-speed exercises. Maximal strength develops if there are only one to two repetitions in a set. This is the result of adequate motor unit activation and synchronization. The most popular maximal strength development method is high-intensity moderate-resistance exercises (60–70% of 1RM, 6–8 repetitions, 6–8 sets) in the first phase, followed by high-intensity and low-repetition exercises (90–100% of 1RM, 1–3 repetitions, 3–5 sets) (1RM: 1 maximum repetition). If there is more than one goal during a single workout (for example, increasing both maximum strength and endurance), then exercises aimed at developing maximum strength should be planned first.

The following methods are frequently used for maximal strengthening training: (1) *pyramid method*, (2) *isometric training*, (3) *muscle cross-sectional development method*, (4) *eccentric training*, (5) *mid-level submaximal and maximal resistance training*, and (6) *isokinetic training*. (1) *Pyramid method* is based on the principle of continuously increasing the resistance from 60% to the maximum level and then gradually decreasing it. During this training, the large muscle tension necessary for muscle hypertrophy occurs. This method is also suitable for maximum speed exercises (at 60–70% resistance). Activation of fast-twitch motor units is achieved by this method. Due to the high intensity of exercise, anabolic hormone adaptation develops. In this training, mainly concentric contractions occur and 1–3 min of rest is required between sets. (2) *Isometric training* can be performed throughout the joint movement as pain permits. When a true maximal voluntary isometric contraction is performed, it creates more strength gain than a concentric contraction. It provides the opportunity to work within the defined weak joint range of motion, positively affects physical performance, and prevents injuries. Isometric contractions create an acute analgesic effect by changing the excitation/inhibition cycle in corticomotor pathways, thus facilitating dynamic loading. It is a reliable technique for evaluating and monitoring changes in power generation. The tension created by isometric contractions stimulates satellite cells and ensures the formation of new nuclei and muscle growth by splitting muscle fibers. (3) *Muscle cross-sectional development method* is suitable for strength development since there is a close relationship between cross-sectional area and strength. The basic concept consists of working out several repetitions and series with maximal loading (e.g., 70%, 6 × 6 repetitions). Tension stimulates satellite cells and splits muscle fibers, resulting in both the formation of new nuclei and the transverse expansion of the muscle. (4) *Eccentric training* is applied via eccentric contraction occurring when the force produced inside the muscle is less than the force applied externally to the muscle, causing an actively controlled lengthening of the muscle fibers under load. In direct comparison, eccentric muscle contraction can generate more force. Lower levels of neural activation are used for 20–60% higher force compared to concentric contraction. The maximum force is released during maximal eccentric contraction due to high loading. This feature allows for training with light weights. Additional neural gains are achieved during an eccentric contraction, such as greater excitability and influencing a larger brain area. In eccentric training, energy consumption is lower despite the high muscle strength. It creates less fatigue. Muscle damage caused by eccentric training is more in the upper extremity. (5) *Intermediate submaximal and maximal resistance training* is formed by mechanisms activated by high resistance. With eccentric and isometric contractions, it is aimed to increase not only the amount of contracted fiber but also the amount of connective tissue. Tendons connect muscles to bones and store forces produced by sarcomeres. Collagen and elastin have a long life (more than 200 days). The synthesis of connective tissue is slower compared to the contractile structures of the muscle we target in muscle hypertrophy. This training mainly aims to reduce the risk of injury, which is very common at muscle–tendon junctions. Combined eccentric and isometric contractions increase the amount of both contracted fiber and connective tissue. (6) *Isokinetic training* is performed at a constant speed using special machines. Muscle growth occurs thanks to near-maximal tension during exercise.

Clinical Tips

Isometric training	Can change muscle architecture, tendon properties, power generation at significant angles, and metabolic functions
Isometric training	Can be done at different joint angles by varying the contraction duration/intensity

Isometric contractions should be performed in two ways: "push" toward an immovable object and "hold" the joint in position while resisting external force

The maximum isometric force is related to the maximum dynamic force. It should be close to 90–100% of 1RM. If we cannot measure: 8–12 s/6 × 8 repetitions for 100%, should be done

Example formula: 100% of maximal voluntary contraction/8–12 s/6 × 8 repetitions

Important Note

Four techniques are often used in eccentric training

2/1 technique	After concentric movement on both extremities, return is made with eccentric movement with one extremity. The loading should be as fast as possible in the concentric phase and as hard as possible during the eccentric phase. The load in the eccentric phase should be twice that of the concentric phase. Also, 70% of 1RM is enough for a start. Sets of 3–5 repetitions per limb (6–10 total repetitions per set) are performed with a 60-s rest interval
Two-movement technique	It is very technical and difficult to implement. In the two-movement technique, it is recommended that the concentric part be a multi-joint exercise in preparation for the isolated eccentric part. Intensity and load criteria: 5-s eccentric (5 repetitions/4–5 sets) should consist of 90–110% of 1RM. Rest periods should be 1–2 min between sets
Slow/superslow technique	It is a relatively simple technique. The eccentric phase is very slow. The amount of loading is very important in this technique. At low rates of 1RM, long eccentric loading (60%, 10–12 s) gives the same response as 85%, 4 s of eccentric loading. Depending on the amount of load, the type of movement, and the size of the muscle group: 60–85% of 1RM can be done for 2–15 s. A rest period of 60 s is commonly used

Negative (supramaximum) technique	It must be done under the supervision of 1–2 people. In 110–120% of 1RM, 1 concentric contraction is followed by an eccentric contraction for 8–10 s. In 125–130% of 1RM, 1 concentric contraction is followed by an eccentric contraction for 4–5 s

Explosive Strength Training (Plyometrics)

Plyometric exercises aim to activate and synchronize as many motor units as possible. Unlike maximal strength training, which targets muscle growth, the goal in plyometrics is to reach maximum speed. Special situations where the potential rate of contraction of the muscle is higher, such as pre-tension, rapid relaxation contractions, and reactive movements, are beneficial for this type of exercise. A plyometric training consists of three phases: (1) eccentric phase (loading), (2) transition phase (conversion), and (3) concentric phase (no loading).

This training improves the connective tissue of the muscles and, as a result, there are no problems with high-speed movement. Fatigue should not be created in this training. Therefore, rest is very important. With plyometric training, fast-twitch fibers get very tired and are therefore almost impossible to reactivate. Plyometric training is designed to teach more motor units to synchronize when fatigue occurs. Whatever happens during burst strength training, it is necessary to focus on exercising at a maximum speed independent of resistance. In short, speed–strength exercises should be planned at the beginning of the training, right after the warm-up period. Example: 4 s (eccentric phase)—0 s (wait)—2 s (concentric phase)—0 s (wait) or 4 s (eccentric contraction)—0 s (hold in tense position)—1 s (concentric contraction)–0 s (hold in short position).

Important Note

Three techniques are often used in explosive strength training

Dynamic variable resistance method	Goal: Do the exercises at 30–80% of maximum strength. It should be done at a low number of repetitions and maximum speed so that the fast-tiring muscle fibers do not get tired. When we stand up from 90° knee flexion with maximum speed and 60% of body weight with 5 × 3 repetitions, it does not enlarge the muscle but develops neural adaptation against fatigue. Although resistance is added in the future, the level of training that keeps the speed at its maximum and does not cause fatigue should not be surprising
Quick-relax contractions	This method combines isometric and concentric contractions. At the beginning of the exercise, isometric contractions are performed for 3–5 s to increase the tension created by shortening the contractile elements of the muscle and lengthening the elastic elements of the muscle at any angle. Thus, the muscle can contract at maximum speed. This training method perfectly improves neuromuscular control, as a large number of motor units are engaged. Because of the fast-twitch fibers, this exercise should also be given at low resistance and with ample rest intervals
Reactive training	In this training, the eccentric contraction starts from the longest position of the muscle. The muscle accumulates the mechanical energy generated by eccentric contraction, and muscle shortening accelerates even more. This technique can be used in activities such as jumping from a step, jumping the bar, or throwing a ball. Fatigue should be noted during this type of exercise because large muscle contractions and speed carry a higher risk of injury

Endurance Training

It involves prolonged exertion with moderate resistance. It is very important for sports played with the ball, martial arts, middle and long-distance running, cycling, canoeing, and swimming. In designing endurance training, we must be very careful about what sport or activity the person is doing. For example, a tennis player must be given the endurance to hit the ball at 200 km/h even in the fifth hour. Different endurance training programs should be planned for each of the athletes performing wrestling, swimming, and so on.

Important Note	
Two techniques are often used in endurance training	
Low-resistance training	This training is most popular for building endurance (30–50% resistance, 20–50 repetitions, and 8–20 sets). The resistance and the number of sets should be designed individually. Contrary to speed–strength training, exercises in this training should be continued until fatigue develops. During these exercises, fast-twitch fibers may be required as well as slow-twitch fibers. With this technique, intense lactic acid accumulation occurs
Circular training	The targeted muscle can be loaded with the exercise equipment in the station. The ratios to exercises performed with body weight are insufficient in the training of rotational movements. High repetitions and low load (30–50%) should be used. Intense lactic acid accumulation should not be forgotten

1.2.3 Stretching Exercises

It is a therapeutic exercise maneuver that uses physiological principles. It is designed to increase joint range of motion or the extensibility of pathologically shortened connective tissue structures. Stretching exercises increase flexibility, allowing the easier performance of activities that require flexibility. These exercises are a reasonable part of the exercise program and it is not clear whether they reduce the risk of injury. Stretching exercise techniques that are frequently used are given in Table 1.5.

The active stretch of the muscle is determined by alpha and gamma innervation, while the passive stretch is determined by the viscoelasticity of the muscle and the properties of the fascia. Connective tissue exhibits viscoelasticity, which combines flexibility and viscosity properties. Elasticity is the ability of a material to return to its original state (length or shape) after stress or

Table 1.5 Stretching types

Types	Details
Static	It involves voluntary passive relaxation while the muscle is extended
Dynamic	The movement is not held in the final position and involves swinging, bouncing, or rocking during stretching
Active	It involves the active contraction of the agonist's muscle while the antagonist muscle group is stretched
Slow	It involves slow movements of the muscle that are active in situations such as lateral neck flexions, arm rotations, and trunk rotations
Proprioceptive neuromuscular facilitation (PNF)	PNF involves isometric contraction of the muscle after static stretching followed by a greater passive stretch

1 Description, Types, and Prescription of the Exercise

Table 1.6 Some stretching types and application details used in the clinics

Types	Details
Static stretching	• Slow stretching of the muscle up to the range of motion • A moderate tension should be felt • There should be little or no pain • It is applied in two ways: active static and passive static
	1a. Active static stretching: • Should be active • The tension of the agonist should help the antagonist to relax • Same tension-type in Pilates and Yoga
	1b. Passive static stretching: • Should be done in a completely relaxed position • The shortened tissue should be lengthened manually or with other equipment • Before passive stretching, there must be a cool-down phase • Used for post-exercise fatigue and muscle aches
Dynamic stretching	• It is a type of stretching in which springing and swinging movements are also used, within the soft and controlled range of motion limits • Jumping and sudden movements will never happen • It is used for heating purposes • It should be stopped when fatigue occurs • Once every 2 s/15 repetitions/2 sets/day
Ballistic stretching	• It is repetitive, sudden jumping, springing, or forced loading of movement on tensed muscles • It may cause injury • Not suitable for use on injured tissues

load is removed. This changeable property is called *elastic deformation* and is similar to the changes that occur in a rubber band under high strain rates. The rubber band quickly adapts to a new length and can return to its original resting length when the stress is relieved. Stretching types and application details frequently used in clinics are summarized in Table 1.6.

Skeletal muscle adapts acutely and chronically to exercise, stretching, and loading. The acute effects of stretching exercise are an increase in normal joint range of motion and connective tissue mobility. Chronic effects are in the form of a decrease in the motor neuron pool (especially affected by large- and low-amplitude stretching) and moderate sarcomere increase.

Considering the effects of stretching exercise on physical performance, static and proprioceptive neuromuscular facilitation (PNF) stretches performed just before exercise/training (instant effect) affect physical performance negatively (muscular strength decreases), while the instantaneous effect of dynamic stretching is positive (muscular strength increases). The long-term effect of static stretching is to improve performance. Stretching exercises in addition to muscle strengthening exercises are more effective in increasing strength.

Clinical Tips

To get a maximum normal range of motion	Static stretching: 15–30 s
To increase flexibility and lengthen the muscle	2–4 repetitions of static stretching for 10–30 s
Ideal technique for dynamic stretching	15–30 s/2–3 repetitions/2–3 days
The most suitable stretching method used for warming-up in running and jumping	Dynamic
The most suitable stretching method used for warm-up in dance and ballet	Static
Stretches longer than 30 s	Are not recommended as they reduce blood circulation in the tissue

1.2.4 Neuromuscular Exercises

Neuromuscular fitness exercises should be included in the exercise prescription to improve balance, agility, and proprioception. Neuromuscular control is defined as the unconsciously trained response of a muscle to a signal related to dynamic joint stability. Extremity movements are controlled through this system, which should provide the correct information for purposeful movement. Neuromuscular training programs should cover all aspects of sensorimotor function and functional stabilization to improve function and alleviate the patient's symptoms.

Neuromuscular training is based on biomechanical and neuromuscular principles and aims to both improve sensorimotor control and provide compensatory functional stability. Unlike traditional strength training, neuromuscular exercise addresses the quality of movement and aims to achieve joint control in all three planes of motion.

Neuromuscular exercise has many effects such as improving functional performance, biomechanics, and activation of periarticular muscles. Simply, the recovery of mechanical limitations is not sufficient for the functional recovery of a joint, because the coordinated neuromuscular control mechanism required during daily life and sports-specific activities cannot be developed to the desired level in this way.

Exercise programs cannot change mechanical joint instability, but can improve neuromuscular control and dynamic joint stability. Delay in neuromuscular reaction time can cause dynamic joint instability with recurrent joint subluxation/dislocations. Therefore, both mechanical stability and neuromuscular control are critical in achieving a long-term functional outcome, and both aspects should be considered in the design of a neuromuscular rehabilitation program. Sensorimotor control or neuromuscular control is the ability to produce controlled movement through coordinated muscle activity. Functional or dynamic stability is the ability of the joint to remain stable during physical activity.

Neuromuscular training programs are effective in improving function and reducing symptoms in people with joint problems. Neuromuscular exercises involve multiple joint and muscle groups performed in functional weight-bearing positions. Neuromuscular exercises aim to ensure the quality and efficiency of the movement and the proper alignment of the trunk and joints during movement.

Exercises to improve sensorimotor control are performed in different (lying, sitting, standing) closed kinetic chain positions to achieve low, evenly distributed joint surface pressure by muscle co-activation. Sensorimotor functions such as coordination, agility, balance, and proprioception are the components of neuromuscular exercise. The aim is to balance the loaded segments in static and dynamic situations and to provide postural control in activities of daily living or more challenging sports activities. Efficiency and quality of movements should be emphasized during neuromuscular exercise.

Tai Chi, Pilates, Yoga, and Otago exercise programs on balance platforms are frequently used in coordination and balance-focused exercises. Agility exercises are also an important part of neuromuscular training.

1.2.4.1 Coordination Exercises

A coordinated movement has three criteria

1. *Will*: The ability to initiate, maintain, or stop an action.
2. *Perception*: It is the ability to harmonize motor stimulation and sensory feedback in proprioception and subcortical centers. When proprioception is affected, the patient tries to compensate with visual feedback.
3. *Memory*: The putative physical or biochemical change in neural tissue represents a memory. Developing memory should be done with high repetitions of performance. Memory and coordination develop in proportion to the number of repetitions performed just below the maximum level of the individual's ability to perform a movement.

General principles of coordination exercises
1. Several motor activities must be repeated over and over.

2. Sensory stimuli (tactile, visual, proprioceptive) should be used to increase motor performance.
3. The speed of activity should be increased over time.
4. Exercises should initially be broken down into components that are simple enough to perform correctly.
5. Provide support only when needed.
6. Take a short rest after two or three repetitions to avoid patient fatigue.
7. Performance must be done with high repetition for memory formation.
8. When a new movement is trained, various inputs should be given, such as instruction (auditory), sensory stimulation (touch), or positions where the patient can see the movement to improve motor performance (visual stimulation).

1.2.4.2 Balance Exercises

Balance training is use of exercises for the antigravity muscles to increase stability. Most geriatric patients should be included in their treatment plan as it prevents falls, the second cause of accidental or unintentional injury deaths worldwide. Balance exercises are also effective in improving postural and neuromuscular control.

Reactive balance training (RBT) improves control of certain reactions to correct impaired balance and prevent falls. Reactive balance training has the potential to improve many aspects of physical health simultaneously. It can be improved with internal and external perturbation techniques. Internal perturbation occurs when the patient cannot adequately control the center of body mass while performing an expected activity. External perturbation occurs when the force acting on the center of mass causes the center of mass to move and reach or exceed stability limits in the environment outside the patient.

General principles of balance exercises
1. The activity must be at an intensity level that compels patients to react to prevent falls.
2. Exercises should include controlling internal and external perturbations.
3. Exercises should be progressively challenging.
4. The activity needs to be done repeatedly until the patient responds adequately.

1.2.4.3 Agility Exercises

Agility exercises improve the ability to change direction and make position transitions quickly. Agility training should include components such as strength, speed, power, flexibility, and dynamic balance. Agility training provides (a) braking of movement, (b) controlled execution of explosive movements, and (c) sudden and rapid displacement of body weight.

For a better and appropriate agility training
1. *Create explosive moves.* The development of explosive contractions allows an athlete to accelerate and decelerate the movement in a short time in a coordinated manner.
2. *Reduce reaction time.* Response time includes both information processing and the ability to act quickly. When an athlete reacts to an opponent's actions, they must quickly review options, decide on how to react, and then move in the appropriate direction. Mental processing can be accelerated in practice with techniques such as narrowing down choices, learning to anticipate, identifying cues, and visualizing appropriate responses.
3. *Efficient movement mechanics should be used.* Changing direction under control means athletes must quickly break or redirect momentum. It requires the development of dynamic stability to shift the center of gravity in different directions and maintain posture while reversing positions. Agility training teaches improving physical fitness, controlling the center of gravity, shifting the weight in a specified direction, and combining it with mental training to use mechanics-based strategies.
4. *Increase joint stability.* Training should prepare an athlete's joints for the agility of a sport. Injuries inherent in sports can be minimized or prevented with joint training.
5. *Increase trunk strength.* Adequate trunk strength and stability are required when changing weights, reaching, and bending, especially when changing direction quickly.
6. *Increase flexibility.* During agility training, flexibility is required to move easily through long ranges of motion.

Table 1.7 Sets, repetitions, load level, intensity, and rest intervals for muscular endurance, strength, power, hypertrophy, and peak torque gains

	Muscular endurance	Hypertrophy	Muscular strength	Power	Peak torque
Sets	1–3	2–4	2–5	3–5	1–3
Repetitions	12–20	8–12	4–8	3–5	1–3
Loading	Moderate	High	High	High	Low
Intensity	Low	Low	Low–high	Low–moderate	Very high
Rest intervals	30–60 s	60–90 s	150 s–5 min	3–5 min	5–8 min

1.3 Conclusion

Appropriate exercise training, as well as exercise selection, will determine the targeted muscular fitness. At the same time, the rest periods that should be given between exercise sets are also critical (Table 1.7). The movements used by the person in his daily life must be included in the exercise program. Performing the exercise training with the appropriate method, function-specific goal, and generally in the closed kinetic chain position (with body weight) will increase the success and the targeted gains.

Further Reading

Ageberg E, Roos EM. Neuromuscular exercise as treatment of degenerative knee disease. Exerc Sport Sci Rev. 2015;43(1):14–22.

Alsouhibani A, Vaegter HB, Hoeger BM. Systemic exercise-induced hypoalgesia following isometric exercise reduces conditioned pain modulation. Pain Med. 2019;20(1):180–90.

Coffey VG, Hawley JA. Concurrent exercise training: do opposites distract? J Physiol. 2017;595(9):2883–96.

Del Vecchio A, Casolo A, Negro F, Scorcelletti M, Bazzucchi I, Enoka R, Felici F, Farina D. The increase in muscle force after 4 weeks of strength training is mediated by adaptations in motor unit recruitment and rate coding. J Physiol. 2019;597(7):1873–87.

Douglas J, Pearson S, Ross A, McGuigan M. Eccentric exercise: physiological characteristics and acute responses. Sports Med. 2017;47(4):663–75.

Hellsten Y, Nyberg M. Cardiovascular adaptations to exercise training. Compr Physiol. 2015;6(1):1–32.

Hippocrates. Hippocrates. Cambridge: Harvard University Press; 1931. p. 229.

Hughes DC, Ellefsen S, Baar K. Adaptations to endurance and strength training. Cold Spring Harb Perspect Med. 2018;8(6):a029769.

Ketelhut S, Ketelhut RG. Type of exercise training and training methods. Adv Exp Med Biol. 2020;1228:25–43.

Konopka AR, Harber MP. Skeletal muscle hypertrophy after aerobic exercise training. Exerc Sport Sci Rev. 2014;42(2):53–61.

Lepley LK, Lepley AS, Onate JA, Grooms DR. Eccentric exercise to enhance neuromuscular control. Sports Health. 2017;9(4):333–40.

Lundby C, Jacobs RA. Adaptations of skeletal muscle mitochondria to exercise training. Exp Physiol. 2016;101(1):17–22.

Pedersen BK, Saltin B. Exercise as medicine—evidence for prescribing exercise as therapy in 26 different chronic diseases. Scand J Med Sci Sports. 2015;25(Suppl 3):1–72.

Physical Activity Guidelines Advisory Committee. Part C. Background and key physical activity concepts ve Part F. Chapter 1. Physical activity behaviors: steps, bouts, and high-intensity training. In: 2018 Physical Activity Guidelines Advisory Committee, editor. 2018 Physical Activity Guidelines Advisory Committee Scientific Report. Washington, DC: U.S. Department of Health and Human Services; 2018.

Ruegsegger GN, Booth FW. Health benefits of exercise. Cold Spring Harb Perspect Med. 2018;8(7):a029694.

Wewege MA, Thom JM, Rye KA, Parmenter BJ. Aerobic, resistance or combined training: a systematic review and meta-analysis of exercise to reduce cardiovascular risk in adults with metabolic syndrome. Atherosclerosis. 2018;274:162–71.

Part II

Exercise-Specific Musculoskeletal Anatomy

The Basic Definitions of Anatomy and Anthropometry

Seda Bicici Ulusahin

Abstract

An international common terminology is used to clearly explain the human body and its movements. The main reason for using this common terminology is to explain the parts of the human body, their positions, and their movements with respect to each other. Anatomical position is a standard position and as it is the same for everyone, the plane and axis on which the movement occurs can be defined. Joint movements are explained using plane and axis terms. Anthropometric measurements, on the other hand, are employed to classify the physical characteristics of the human body. Anthropometric measurements have been used for many various purposes, such as following growth and development, evaluating performance, as well as monitoring diseases and recovery. Length, diameter, circumference, and fat measurements can be made easily with simple equipment used in a clinic, while more precise measurements can be made thanks to technological devices.

2.1 Anatomy

2.1.1 Anatomical Position

Planes, axes, and movements are depicted through the "anatomical position" so that parts of the human body can be described in a common language when talking about their interrelation, movement, or position. Anatomical position is the position in which the feet are parallel to each other, the legs are close to each other, the palms are facing frontward, and the arms are located next to the body, while the head is facing forward. This position should not be confused with posture. Anatomical position is a position referenced to indicate the movements of the body, its planes, and axes in a terminological way (Fig. 2.1). Imaginary planes are referred to in order to easily understand the relationship and movements of the body parts that cut each other vertically.

2.1.2 Direction Terminology

These are general terms used to describe the positions of the body parts relative to each other. These terms are summarized in Table 2.1 and Fig. 2.2.

S. Bicici Ulusahin (✉)
Gülhane Faculty of Physiotherapy and Rehabilitation, Health Sciences University, Ankara, Turkey
e-mail: seda.ulusahin@sbu.edu.tr

Fig. 2.1 Anatomical position (CLIPAREA/Shutterstock.com)

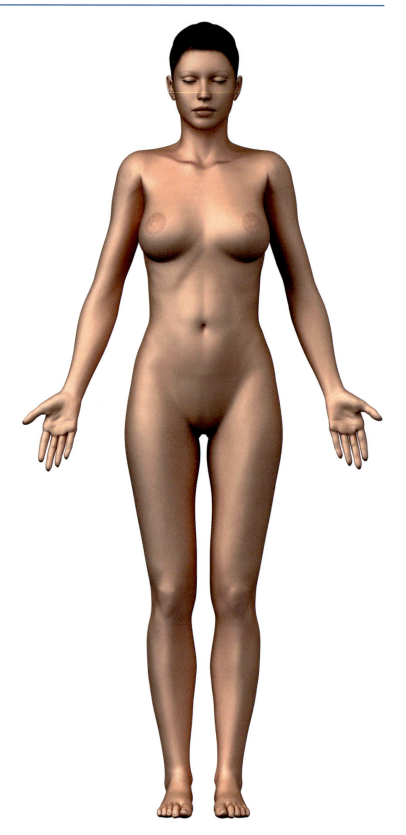

Table 2.1 Anatomical direction terminology

Term	Definition
Anterior/ventral	In front of, front
Posterior/dorsal	Behind, toward, to rear
Superior	Above, over
Inferior	Below, under
Cranial	Closer to the head, the higher
Caudal	Away from the head
Medial	Toward the midline
Lateral	Away from the midline, toward the side
Proximal	Closer to the origin
Distal	Away from, farther from the origin
Superficial	Close to the surface of the body
Profundus	Farther from the surface of the body
Palmar	Palm of hand
Dorsal (of hand)	Posterior surface of hand (dorsum)
Plantar	Sole of the foot
Dorsal (of foot)	Superior surface of foot (dorsum)

2.1.3 Planes and Axes

There are three planes and three axes where angular movements (osteokinematic movements) occur between bones. Planes are two-dimensional like a book page or a photograph. These planes are summarized in Table 2.2.

Sources: Excellent Dream/Shutterstock.com; VectorMine/Shutterstock.com; Auttapon Wongtakeaw/Shutterstock.com; VectorMine/Shutterstock.com

Joint movements occur within the plane and around the axis. Transaction axes are the lines that vertically cut the plane in which the movement occurs, and each plane has an axis. Axes can be thought of as lines that pierce the body like arrows (Fig. 2.3). Joint movement that occurs on any plane is considered to rotate around an

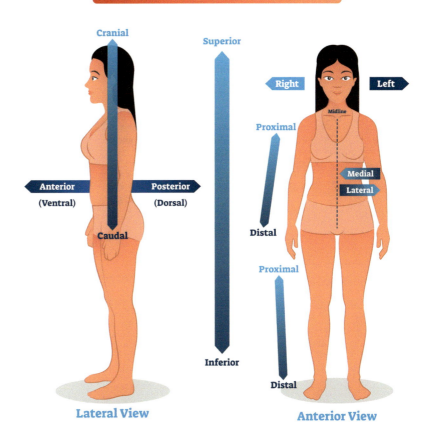

Fig. 2.2 Anatomical direction terminology (VectorMine/Shutterstock.com)

Table 2.2 Anatomical planes and movements

Plane	Definition	Movement Occurring
Sagittal plane	• This is the plane that divides the body in the vertical/upright direction, symmetrically into two halves: right and left • Movements on this plane are seen when the person is observed from the side.	Flexion and extension
Frontal plane	• This divides the body into two, front, and back. • This plane makes a right angle with a sagittal plane. • Movements on this plane are seen when the person is observed from front or behind.	Abduction and adduction
Horizontal/Transverse plane	• This makes right angles with both sagittal and frontal planes. • It divides the body into two parts as the upper and lower parts (superior and inferior). • Movements on this plane are seen when the person is observed from a bird's eye view.	Head rotation Internal-external rotation Supination-pronation movements are movements that occur on this plane. **ARM SUPINATION AND PRONATION**

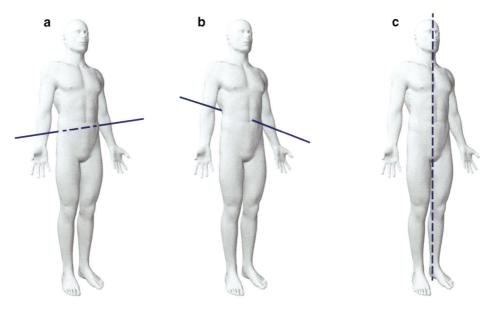

Fig. 2.3 Movement axes: (**a**) frontal axis; (**b**) sagittal axis; (**c**) longitudinal axis (SciePro/Shutterstock.com)

axis. The flexion and extension movement in the sagittal plane occurs around the *transverse/frontal axis* (a side-by-side line). For example, the hip flexion and extension movement that we see when we look at a person from the side, occurs in the sagittal plane, while the pivot point occurs around a line passing through the hip joint, on the frontal axis.

The abduction and adduction movements on the frontal plane occur due to rotation around *the sagittal axis* (a line passing from front to back). For example, the *jumping jack* movement done by opening and closing the arms and legs occurs in the frontal plane, around the sagittal axis.

Practical Animation

Stick a pen through an empty sheet of paper that you hold upright. Consider the paper as the sagittal plane, and the pen you inserted like an arrow as the *transverse/frontal axis* (Ashusha/Shutterstock.com)

Practical Animation
When a compass is held upright and its legs are opened, the connection point of the legs would open by acting as an axis. Consider the connection point of the compass legs as a *sagittal axis* (Rvector/Shutterstock.com)

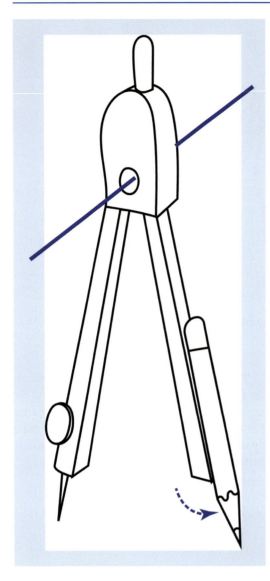

Practical Animation

When playing with a spinning top, remember that it revolves around the line passing through the center. Consider the axis that descends from the top to bottom perpendicularly as the *longitudinal axis* (neural-network/Shutterstock.com)

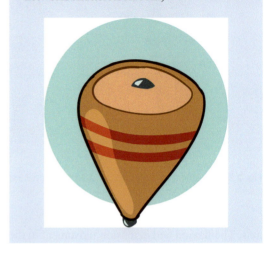

2.1.4 Joint Types

The functional connection or pivot point between two or more bones is called a joint. The joints are divided into two main groups, synarthrosis and diarthrosis joints, according to their movement abilities.

2.1.4.1 Synarthrosis Joints

Fibrous Joints

Rotation movement in the transverse plane occurs around the *longitudinal axis* (a perpendicular line from top to bottom). When a person is observed from above, the movement of the head toward the back occurs in the transverse plane and around the longitudinal axis.

These are the joints that do not have movement ability. There is no gap between the joint surfaces, but they consist of fibrous connective tissue. Examples include joints between skull bones, distal tibiofibular joint syndesmosis, and tooth roots (Fig. 2.4).

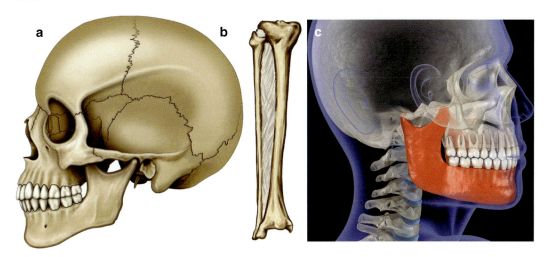

Fig. 2.4 Fibrous joints: (**a**) skull sutures (ilusmedical/Shutterstock.com). (**b**) Syndesmosis structure (stihii/Shutterstock.com); (**c**) tooth roots (Gomphosis) (Alex Mit/Shutterstock.com)

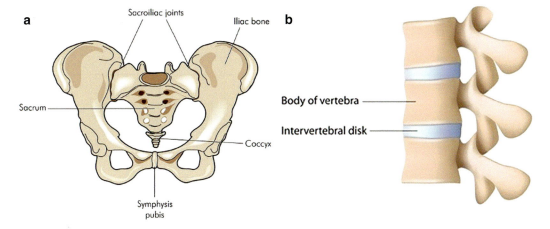

Fig. 2.5 Cartilaginous joints: (**a**) symphysis pubis (Blamb/Shutterstock.com); (**b**) intervertebral joints (Alila Medical Media/Shutterstock.com)

Amphiarthrosis (Cartilaginous) Joints
These are slightly moveable joints. Fibrous cartilage structure is found on bone surfaces. Examples of these joints are the symphysis pubis and intervertebral joints (Fig. 2.5).

2.1.4.2 Diarthrosis Joints (Synovial Joints)

These are the most moveable joints. They comprise the majority of joints in the body. Joint surfaces are covered with cartilage and there is a joint cavity. The structure of the joint capsule that surrounds the joint from the outside consists of fibrous connective tissue. The fibrous joint capsule contributes to the stability of the joint. A synovial membrane covers the inner surface of the joint capsule and produces a joint fluid called synovial fluid. This joint fluid reduces friction by ensuring that the joint surfaces are lubricated and nourishes the joint cartilage. Synovial joints are divided into four types according to the number of axes or six types according to the shape of the joint surfaces. Synovial joint types are summarized in Table 2.3.

2.1.5 Joints and Movements

Joint movements are divided into two categories as osteokinematic and arthrokinematic movements.

2.1.5.1 Osteokinematic Joint Movements

This is a term used to describe angular movements that occur between bones. It can be described as a visible movement of a bone relative to another bone. Osteokinematic movements are named according to planes and axes. Flexion and extension movements occur in the sagittal plane, while abduction and adduction occur in the frontal plane

Table 2.3 Synovial joint types

Joint Type	Number of Axes	Joint Movement
Hinge (Ginglymus) Hinge Joint	Uniaxial The elbow joint	Flexion and extension in the transverse axis Example: Humeroulnar joint
Pivot (Trochoid) Pivot Joint	Uniaxial	Only rotational movement Example: Atlanto-axial joint, radioulnarjoint
Ellipsoid Ellipsoid Joint	Biaxial (sagittal and transverse)	Abduction and adduction on the sagittal axis, flexion, and extension on the transverse axis Example: Radiocarpal joint, metacarpophalangeal joint

Sources: gritsalak karalak/Shutterstock.com; Designua/Shutterstock.com; sciencepics/Shutterstock.com; gritsalak karalak/Shutterstock.com; Natee Jitthammachai/Shutterstock.com; Andrea Danti/Shutterstock.com; Alila Medical Media/Shutterstock.com; Natee Jitthammachai/Shutterstock.com

Table 2.3 (continued)

Joint Type	Number of Axes	Joint Movement
Floods (Saddle) — Saddle Joint	Biaxial (sagittal and transverse)	Abduction and adduction on the sagittal axis, flexion, and extension on thetransverse axis. Example: Sternoclavicular joint, carpometacarpal joint
Spherical (Spheroid/top-socket) — Ball and Socket Joint	Triaxial	Flexion-extension on the transverse axis, abduction- adduction on the sagittal axis and rotation on the longitudinal axis. Example: Glenohumeral joint, coxo-femoral joint
Planar — Plane Joint	No axis	A slight sliding movement. Example: Carpometacarpal joints

and internal–external rotation movements occur in the horizontal plane. These large movements are also called physiological movements.

There are two types of osteokinematic movement: active and passive. Active joint movement occurs during voluntary muscle activation, while passive joint movement occurs passively due to external forces, without voluntary muscle activation. Active joint movement occurs less than passive joint movement, under normal circumstances, because external forces also influence passive joint movement.

2.1.5.2 Arthrokinematic Joint Movements

These are the auxiliary/accessory movements between the joint surfaces that are invisible to the eye and occur involuntarily during osteokinematic movements. A person cannot make these

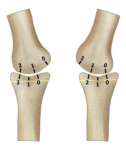

Fig. 2.6 Rolling motion

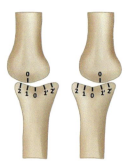

Fig. 2.7 Sliding motion

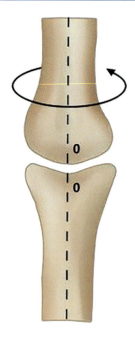

Fig. 2.8 Spinning motion

movements voluntarily in an isolated manner, although the application of external forces (such as mobilization methods) can cause them. There are three basic arthrokinematic movements: *rolling*, *gliding/sliding*, and *spinning*.

Movements occurring in these joints are linear/translatory or rotational. Complete linear movement rarely occurs due to the structure of the joints in the body. Rotational or angular movement is the movement that a segment creates around the axis. Axes change continuously during movements. Those occurring in many joints are the result of a combination of arthrokinematic movements (rolling, sliding, and rotating).

Rolling

This is the rolling motion that one joint surface generates on another joint surface during movement. The contact points between the two joint surfaces continuously change. The direction of the rolling occurs in the direction of the moving joint (Fig. 2.6).

Gliding/Sliding

A fixed contact point of the reference joint surface comes into contact with different points on the other joint surface during sliding movement (Fig. 2.7).

Spinning

Rotational movement occurs on a single axis in the joint. Meanwhile, a point on the surface of one joint touches a point on another joint surface. It can be defined as a rotation movement around an axis (Fig. 2.8).

> **Clinical Information**
> *Convex–concave rule:* Many movements in the body occur through a combination of sliding, rolling, and rotational movements that joint surfaces exert on each other. Most joint surfaces are either concave or convex (Fig. 2.9).
>
> In the case where the concave joint surface is fixed and the convex joint face is moving, the sliding and rolling movements of the convex joint surface exerted on the fixed concave joint are in *opposite directions*. For example, during the abduction movement of the glenohumeral joint in the shoulder abduction, the convex humeral head makes a downward rolling movement on the concave glenoid (Fig. 2.10).
>
> In cases where the convex joint surface is fixed and the concave joint surface is mov-

ing, the sliding and rolling movements are in the *same direction* as the bone movement. For example, when the knee joint (tibiofemoral joint) is in the sitting position, the femur joint surface (convex joint surface) is fixed and the tibia joint surface (concave surface) is moving. When the knee is extended in the sitting position, sliding and rolling movements occur in the same direction, upward, as the tibia (Fig. 2.11).

2.1.5.3 Spine Movements

Spinal movements occur as a result of segmental and local movements. Segmental movement in the spine occurs between two adjacent vertebrae. Osteokinematic movement in the spine can also be defined as rotational movement occurring in three planes (Fig. 2.12 and Table 2.4).

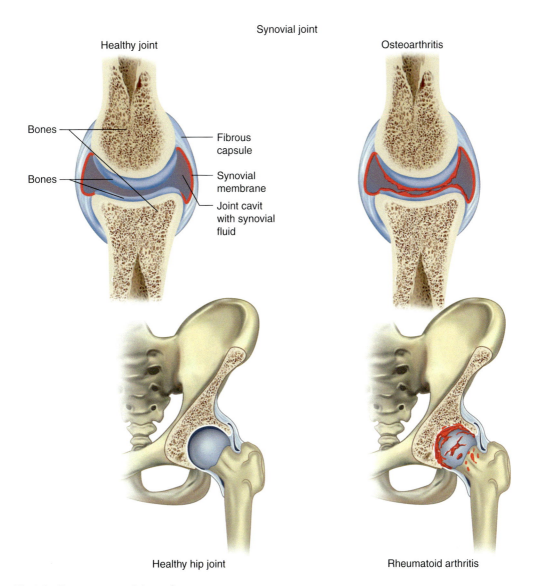

Fig. 2.9 Convex, concave joint surfaces

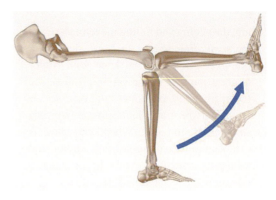

Fig. 2.11 Sliding and rolling movements in the tibiofemoral joint

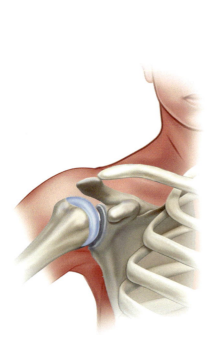

Fig. 2.10 Sliding and rolling movements in the glenohumeral joint (Drp8/Shutterstock.com)

Fig. 2.12 Spinal movement axes (Channarong Pherngjanda/Shutterstock.com)

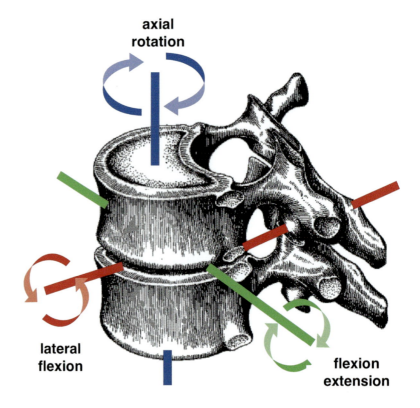

Table 2.4 Spine movement, axes, and planes

Osteokinematic movements	Plane	Axis
Flexion, extension	Sagittal plane	Frontal axis
Right, left lateral rotation	Frontal plane	Sagittal axis
Right, left rotation	Horizontal plane	Longitudinal axis

2.2 Anthropometry

2.2.1 Definition of Anthropometry

Anthropometry is the systematic measurement and classification of the physical characteristics of the human body and its parts. Anthropometry is presented as the basis of physical anthropology, a branch of science that examines the historical development of human physical structure and the differences between races and nationals.

Anthropometric measurements provide objective data. They can be used to track growth, understand diseases, follow-up responses to therapy, evaluate the effects of training on the physical characteristics or structural differences between athletes in various sports, or create source data. Anthropometry is examined in two ways:

- Measurements on living people and cadavers.
  - Somatometry: Body measurements.
  - Cephalometry: Face measurements.
- Measurements on the skeleton.
  - Osteometry: Different measurements of the skeleton.
  - Craniometry: Skull measurements.

Anthropometric measurements are important for the determination of body type and composition. Anthropometric measurements of circumference, length, diameter, and adipose tissue are practical methods that clinicians can easily apply. Thanks to technological developments, devices that can evaluate anatomical structures and organs specifically for individuals are also being developed. In particular, various methods of fat measurement have been developed for determining body composition. In this section, technological devices will be mentioned briefly, while anthropometric measurements that can be easily applied in the clinic will be explained in more detail.

2.2.1.1 Circumference Measurements

- Non-elastic, folding strip tape measures should be used when making circumference measurements. Standard points should be determined in order to ensure reliability in the measurement; whether the tape measure is passed above or under the bottom of these points should be recorded, and the measurements should be repeated by the same person.
- The starting end of the tape measure "0" should be side by side with the measured number, not beneath or on top of it.
- The tape measure should be parallel to the ground on both sides, except for the head measurement. In order to press the hair in the head area, the tape measure should be slightly stretched, but other body parts should not be compressed during measurement.
- The muscles need to be loose during measurement. However, if muscle development is to be monitored, measurements can also be taken during muscle contraction.

Growth curves generated by measuring body weight, height, and head circumference are often used for monitoring growth. Since an increase in head circumference reflects brain growth and development, all children are regularly evaluated up to 2 years of age. When the head circumference is not within the normal value range, the individual should be examined in detail for microcephaly or macrocephaly. The chest circumference measurement value is smaller than the head circumference measurement in a newborn but becomes larger at 1 year of age. How circumference measurements are made is shown in Table 2.5.

Table 2.5 Circumference measurements

Head		The head area is measured from the widest area just above the eyebrows and occipital protrusion. The tape measure must pass over the same level on both sides of the head.
Neck		This measurement is taken from the narrowest area of the neck, just below the thyroid cartilage.
Chest		The person to be measured stands. When the feet are open shoulder-wide, the body weight is evenly distributed on both feet. The arms are kept in slight abduction so as to allow measurement, which is taken while the person is breathing normally. Measurements are taken from the subcostal region, xiphoid protrusion, and just below the axilla.
Waist		While the person is standing in a loose position with feet adjacent to each other, measurements are taken from the narrowest area between the subcostal region and the crista iliaca.

Table 2.5 (continued)

Abdomen		The person stands in a loose position with feet adjacent to each other, measurement is taken from the umbilicus level.
Hip		While the person is standing in a loose position with feet adjacent to each other, the measurement is taken from the widest area of the hip.
Thigh		The person sits with the knee in 90° flexion. The proximal of the patella and the inguinal region is marked and measurement is taken from the midpoint between the two. Different reference points can also be determined for measurement. It can also be measured from 10-15 cm above the patella or from the area where the muscle is most bulging.
Leg		The person to be measured can sit with legs dangling or stand with feet 20 cm open and eight distributed equally on both sides. Measurement is taken from 10-15 cm above the medial malleolus or from the most bulging area between the medial malleolus and the knee.

(continued)

Table 2.5 (continued)

Ankle		Measurement can be taken while the person stands with feet slightly open and weight distributed equally on both lower extremities, or while lying down or sitting with feet hanging down. Measurement is taken from the upper part of the malleolus, where the ankle is thinnest.
Shoulder		This is measured in the standing upright posture position, while the arms are hanging free next to the torso. Measurement is taken from the lower level of the acromion, where the deltoid muscle is most bulging.
Shoulder joint		The person stands with feet open shoulder-wide, and body weight evenly distributed to both feet. The arms are positioned at a slight abduction in order to allow measurement. The tape measure is passed above the acromion so as to enclose the axillary zone
Arm		Measurement can be taken while sitting, standing, or in the lying position. The medial epicondyle of the humerus is taken as a reference point and measurement is taken from 10-15 cm above this point or from the midpoint of the distance between the acromion and the olecranon.

Table 2.5 (continued)

Forearm	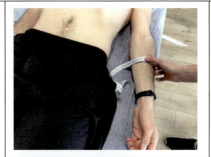	Measurement can be taken while sitting, standing, or in the lying position. The styloid protrusion of the ulna is taken as a reference point and measurement is taken 10-15 cm above this point
Wrist	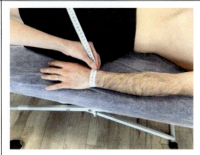	The tape measure is positioned to fully contact the styloid protrusions of the radius and ulna, and the measurement is taken.

2.2.1.2 Length Measurements

Length measurement methods are shown in Table 2.6.

2.2.1.3 Diameter Measurements

The caliper device used for diameter measurement is a tool that is often used to record millimetric measurements in engineering, allowing measurement of length, internal–external diameter, and depth. When the distance between bone protrusions is to be measured, it is necessary to apply a little more pressure to the moving ends of the caliper ruler in order to compress the subcutaneous adipose tissue. Examples for the application of diameter measurements are given in Table 2.7.

2.2.1.4 Skinfold Measurements

Subcutaneous fat measurement of skinfold is a field measurement method commonly used to determine the body fat ratio. Subcutaneous adipose tissue is considered to constitute approximately 40–60% of the total adipose tissue in the body. The person to be measured is to stay upright but in a loose posture. The skinfold in the area to be measured is grasped between the thumb and the index finger and the subcutaneous adipose tissue is lifted so that it is separated from the underlying muscle tissue. The skinfold is held 1 cm away from the grasped area, perpendicular to the folding axis of the skin fold. The value is measured approximately 2 s after the ends of the skinfold are released. If there is a difference of

Table 2.6 Length measurements (ChameleonsEye/Shutterstock.com)

Height		It is recommended to measure height using a stadiometer. The head of the person is oriented in the Frankfurt plane (the plane where the ear hole upper boundary and the eye lower boundary lie on the same plane), the heel, hip, and back of the person come into contact with the vertical axis of the stadiometer. The person stands upright with heels in an adjacent position. The person is asked to take a deep breath and hold it until the measurement is taken.
Total upper extremity		The distance between the acromion and the tip of the longest finger of the hand is measured in the anatomical position.
Arm		The distance between olecranon and acromion is measured while the elbow is in flexion position where the long axis of the forearm is parallel to the ground and the palms are facing each other.
Forearm		When the person is in the same position as the arm length measurement, the distance between the olecranon and the distal of the styloid protrusion of the radius is measured.
Hand		The distance between the distal of the styloid protrusion of the radius and the 3rd fingertip is measured from the dorsal of the hand

Table 2.6 (continued)

Stroke length	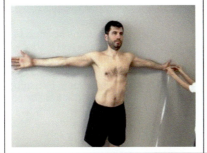	The distance between the middle fingertips of the two hands is measured when the back is against a wall, the arms are opene sideways and the dorsal sides of the hands are in contact with the wall.
Lower extremity length	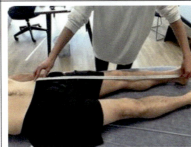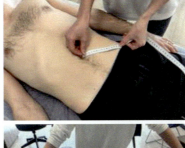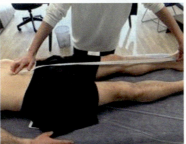	The measurement between anterior superior iliac spine (ASIS) and medial malleolus may not always be accurate. Measurement values may vary as there may be rotation or tilt in case of a problem in the pelvis. Therefore, the length between the umblicus and the ASIS should be measured on the right and left sides, symmetry should be checked and if there is a difference, the pelvic position should be corrected and the measurement should be repeated after symmetry is achieved.
Thigh	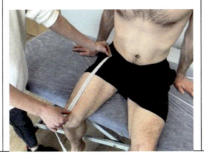	The person sits with legs dangling while the measurement is taken. The length between the midpoint of the inguinal ligament and the proximal edge of the patella is measured.

(continued)

Table 2.6 (continued)

Leg	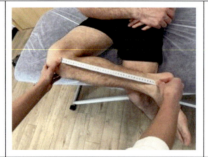	Measurements can be made in two different ways. Either the distance between the tibial plateau and ground is measured while the person is standing, or the distance between the tibial plateau and the medial malleolus is measured while the legs are crossed in a sitting position.
Foot	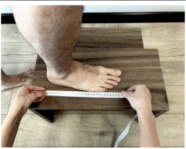	The distance between the heel and the longest fingertip is measured while standing.

Table 2.7 Diameter measurements

Shoulder	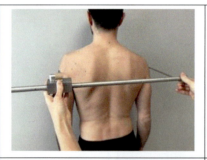	While the person taking the measurement is standing behind and the person to be measured is standing upright, the arms of the caliper are placed on the most bulging place of the deltoid muscle on both sides.
Biiliac	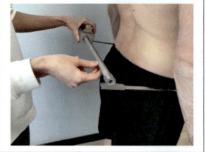	While the person taking the measurement is standing behind the person to be measured stands upright, with feet slightly open and the arms crossed on the chest. The measurement is taken by placing the arms of the caliper on the crista iliaca on both sides at a downward angle of 45°.
Bitrochanteric	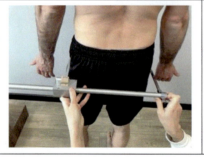	While the person taking the measurement is standing behind, the person to be measured stands upright, the feet slightly open and the arms crossed on the chest. The measurement is taken by placing the arms of the caliper on the trochanter major on both sides.

Table 2.7 (continued)

Knee	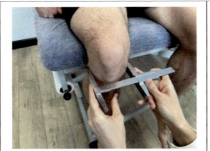	The person to be measured sits with legs hanging down at 90° flexion and the measurement is taken from the front. The distance between the medial and lateral condyles of the femur is measured.
Ankle	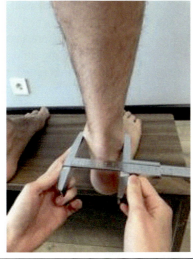	The person to be measured stands on a flat floor with feet open hip-width and weight distributed equally on both sides. The distance between the most protruding points of the medial and lateral malleolus is measured.
Elbow	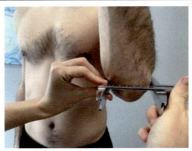	The distance between the medial and lateral epicondyles of the humerus is measured while the elbow is in 90° flexion.
Wrist	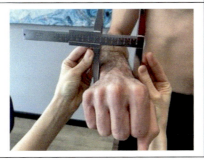	The distance between the styloid protrusions of the radius and ulna is measured.

more than 5% between the two repeated measurement values, it is recommended to take the average value for two repetitive measurements and to take the median value for three repetitive measurements. Skinfold measurement methods are shown in Table 2.8.

2.2.2 Determination of Body Fat Ratio

Methods related to determining the body fat ratio are examined under two headings: direct and indirect. Direct methods can only be applied to cadavers. Indirect methods are divided into two laboratory and field methods. Laboratory methods, which are used as reference or criteria for field methods and formulas, are expensive and difficult to access. The most frequently used laboratory methods are summarized in Table 2.9.

Following the imaging methods (MRI, ultrasound, etc.), advances in technology have allowed the development of optical scanners that can measure body volume. Anthropometric measurement studies and sensor-based research with mobile phone applications are still evolving.

Skinfold measurements and anthropometric methods such as circumference, diameter, weight, and height are field methods that are inexpensive and easy to use. The skinfold measurement method uses mathematical equations formulated specifically for the population evaluated. First of all, the body density (Table 2.10) is calculated by measuring the skin fold thickness of the body parts that are indicated in the mathematical equations created specifically for age and gender. Then the fat content in the body is calculated by a population-specific conversion formula that uses body density data. There are more than a hundred body density and body fat prediction equations that use various combinations of skinfold measurements. The mathematical equations developed by Jackson and Pollock for genders, and Durnin and Womersley for gender and age are the ones most commonly used in the literature for the calculation of body density. The mathematical equation developed by Siri is frequently preferred for body fat percentage. Peterson et al. developed a mathematical equation for estimating body fat percentage in women using skinfold measurements from four places (triceps, subscapular, suprailiac, thighs), along with height, age, and weight data.

Body fat percentage (%) = [(4.95/Body Density) − 4.5] × 100.

In terms of health, it has been stated that the percentage of fat should be at least 3% in men and 12% in women. These are the essential fat percentages that are necessary for the healthy continuation of physiological functions. The reason for the higher ratio in women is thought to be pregnancy and hormonal functions. In general, it is considered normal for young men to have a total (essential and storage) fat content of 12–15% and the norm in young women is 25–28%. The average percentage of body fat determined by gender and age in healthy individuals is indicated in Table 2.11. For athletes, these values can vary according to the sport performed (Table 2.12).

In sports that require explosive power, having extra muscle mass is important for the production of high power. However, the excess fat content in the body increases body weight, and the power produced by the muscle is used to activate the body, hence fat ratio and increased body weight negatively affect performance. This is why it is important to have low-fat content, especially in sports that require speed and strength. For example, swimmers can increase their swimming speed when they can produce maximum force while expending low levels of energy. Among the main factors affecting this efficiency are the stroke technique, the hydrodynamic resistance experienced in stroke movement, body shape, body position, bone density, and fat ratio excluding the amount of contractible muscle. A certain amount of fat positively affects the ability to stay afloat, while the excess fat ratio causes the swimmer to spend more energy to stay on the water and move, and efficiency decreases. While the

Table 2.8 Skinfold measurements

Chest	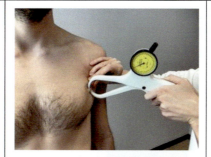	Measurement is taken obliquely on the pectoralis major muscle, from the middle of the distance between the axial line and the nipple in men, and from 1/3 proximal distance in women.
Axilla	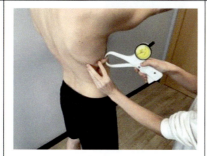	Measurement is taken from the skin which folds parallel to the ground from the point where a parallel line drawn from the xiphoid protrusion of the sternum to the middle axials cuts the axials middle line.
Triceps	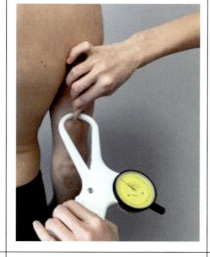	The person to make the measurement stands behind while the arms of the person to be measured are free next to the torso and the hands are in supination. Measurement is taken at a right angle to the ground from the midpoint of the distance between the olecranon and acromion.
Subscapular	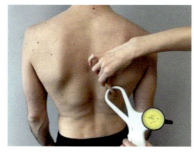	Measurement is taken obliquely at an angle of 45° to the horizontal plane by following the skin fold 1 cm below the inferior angle of the scapula.

(continued)

Table 2.8 (continued)

Biceps		The person stands in front of the person to take the measurement with arms free next to the torso and the hands in the supination position. Measurement is taken from the midpoint of the distance between the olecranon and acromion, above the biceps brachialis, at a right angle to the ground.
Abdominal		Measurement is taken at a right angle to the ground from 2 cm lateral of the umbilicus.
Suprailiac		Diagonal measurement is taken from just above the ilium, over the anterior axillary line.

Table 2.8 (continued)

Thigh	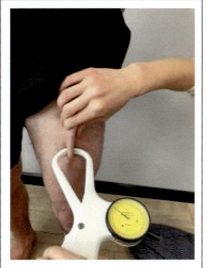	The person stands with the knee of the extremity to be measured is in slight flexion and in a loose position. Measurement is taken at a right angle to the ground from the midpoint of the distance between the hip joint and the proximal of the patella.
Leg	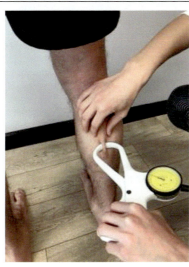	The person stands with the extremity to be measured at slight flexion and in a loose position. Measurement is taken at a right angle to the ground from the midpoint of the distance between the popliteal region and the Achilles tendon (the most bulging part of the gastrocnemius muscle).

Table 2.9 Laboratory methods used to determine body fat

Underwater weight measurement method (Hydrodensitometry)	Using the underwater weight measurement method to measure body density is considered to be the "gold standard" This calculation is made by measuring the weight of the person on the ground, weight in water, body volume, and lung residual volume However, being submerged in water may not be suitable for everyone Errors in the measurement of residual volume can also adversely affect the calculation of body density
Method of air volume and pressure use (plethysmography)	This is a very expensive method that does not require the person to be completely submerged in water or to measure the volume of the lungs Body volume, the total amount of body fat, and lean body weight are measured
Dual-energy X-ray absorptiometer (DEXA)	Total and local body fat percentage, lean tissue mass, and bone mineral density measurements are made This is a measurement method with high accuracy and repeatability It is especially effective in determining the amount of bone and soft tissue It is a very expensive method and the person being measured is exposed to slight radiation
Ultrasonography (US)	The amount of subcutaneous, abdominal, and visceral fat can be measured directly This is a low-cost and easy-to-apply measurement method However, the experience and skill of the person who makes the measurement are important There are no standardized measurement protocols
Magnetic resonance imaging (MRI)	This is a method used for total/local and subcutaneous/visceral fat volume measurement, and for determining the fat content in skeletal muscle, organs, and other internal tissues There is no radiation effect, but it is an expensive method and evaluation takes time
Bioelectric impedance analysis (BIA)	This is an easy, practical, and cost-effective method compared to other laboratory methods. It is used in the calculation of body fat weight and proportions. It gives the fat distribution results for the body and extremities. It cannot be used for the measurement of visceral adipose tissue Weak electrical current impedance is measured in this method. The calculation is made on the assumption that the adipose tissue is a weak conductor for the electric current. Measurement results are influenced by many factors such as length difference in the extremities, nutritional status, resting state, tissue temperature and hydration, electrode placement, and ovulation period. In order for the measurements to be reliable, it is necessary to not eat or drink anything for 4 h prior to the test, not to exercise for 12 h prior to the test, to urinate 30 min before the test, and not to use diuretic drugs within the last week In addition, it is important to use equations specifically developed for the population to be measured

Table 2.10 Equations used in body density calculation

Mathematical Eq. I
Measuring points: Chest, abdomen, thighs (Jackson and Pollock 1978)
Body density for men = $1.10938 - 0.0008267$ (sum of 3 measuring points) + 0.0000016 (sum of 3 measuring points)^2 − 0.0002574 (age)
Body density for women = $1.099421 - 0.0009929$ (sum of 3 measuring points) + 0.0000023 (sum of 3 measuring points)^2 − 0.0001392 (age)

Mathematical Eq. II
Measuring points: Triceps, biceps, subscapular, suprailiac (Durnin and Womersley 1974)
Body density for men = $1.1610 - 0.0632$ log (sum of 4 measuring points)
Body density for women = $1.1581 - 0.0720$ log (sum of 4 measuring points)
Body density for boys = $1.1533 - 0.0643$ log (sum of 4 measuring points)
Body density for girls = $1.1369 - 0.0598$ log (sum of 4 measuring points)

Mathematical Eq. III
Measuring points: subscapular, triceps, thigh, suprailiac (Peterson et al. 2003)
Fat percentage for men % = $20.94878 +$ (age $\times 0.1166$) − (height [cm] $\times 0.11666$) + ([sum of 4 measuring points] $\times 0.42696$) − ([sum of 4 measuring points]$^2 \times 0.00159$)
Fat percentage for women % = $22.18945 +$ (age $\times 0.06368$) + (body mass index $\times 0.60404$) − (height [cm] $\times 0.14520$) + ([sum of 4 measuring points] $\times 0.30919$) − ([sum of 4 measuring points]$^2 \times 0.00099562$)

Table 2.11 Average body fat percentage values in healthy individuals

	<30 years old	30–50 years old	>50 years old
Woman	14–21	15–23	16–25
Man	9–15	11–17	12–19

Table 2.12 Fat percentage for different sports

Sport	Male	Female	Sport	Male	Female
Basketball	6–12	20–27	Rowing	6–14	12–18
Baseball	12–15	12–18	Shot put	16–20	20–28
Bodybuilding	5–8	10–15	Skiing	7–12	16–22
Cycling	5–15	15–20	Short distance running	8–10	12–20
Gymnastics	5–12	10–16	Swimming	9–12	14–24
High and long jump	7–12	10–18	Tennis	12–16	16–24
Marathon	5–11	10–15	Volleyball	11–14	16–25

upper-level elite swimmers have lower fat content and body mass index (BMI), they are taller in height and have more contractible muscle mass.

The fat percentage of athletes playing in different positions in the same sport may vary. For example, there are anthropometric differences between athletes according to the positions they play in soccer. Goalkeepers have been determined to be taller and heavier and have a higher fat ratio than their teammates playing in other positions, while the midfielders have the opposite characteristics.

Table 2.13 Body mass index (BMI) classification

Classification	BMI
Extremely underweight	<16.5 kg/m^2
Underweight	<18.5 kg/m^2
Normal	18.5–24.9 kg/m^2
Overweight	25–29.9 kg/m^2
Class I obese	30–34.9 kg/m^2
Class II obese	35–39.9 kg/m^2
Class III obese (extreme)	≥40 kg/m^2

with waist circumference, body composition, and other measurements.

2.2.3 Body Mass Index (BMI)

Body mass index (BMI) is calculated by dividing the value of body weight in kilograms to the square of the value of height in meters (kg/m^2). The formula "BMI = Weight/Height (kg/m^2)" is used in the calculation. The optimal value range of BMI is suggested to be between 18.5 and 25 kg/m^2. The obesity classification according to BMI values is shown in Table 2.13.

The use of BMI classification may not be appropriate for athletes. Although a bodybuilder with a high BMI appears to be obese according to the classification, he/she will be found to have a high muscle-to-mass ratio with a low percentage of fat when evaluated in terms of body composition. In other words, comparing two individuals with the same BMI rate, one would have a high muscle mass and the other a high fat content. For this reason, BMI should be interpreted together

2.2.4 Waist-to-Hip Ratio

A waist-to-hip ratio can be used to interpret fat distribution in the body and obesity. The waist-to-hip ratio above 0.80 in women and above 0.91 in men is considered a risk factor for heart disease, hypertension, stroke, diabetes, and similar chronic diseases.

2.2.5 Body Types and Analysis

Body type (somatotype) can be defined as the classification of the physical shape and composition of the human body. Today, the *Heath and Carter method* is the most widely applied classification. This method was based on *Sheldon's* somatotype classification according to age, height, weight, and photographs, as well as anthropometric measurements. The terms endomorphy, mesomorphy, and ectomorphy are used when defining the somatotype structure of individuals (Fig. 2.13).

2.2.5.1 Endomorphy

This is characterized by the roundness and softness of the body. This body type is physically fatty and large-bellied, tends to be short, and has quite fatty upper arms and thighs with square shoulders and a round head.

2.2.5.2 Mesomorphy

This body type is characterized by striking muscle and bone structure and a square-looking body. The legs, chest, and arms usually have large bones and are very muscular. The shoulders are wide and the body is lofty.

2.2.5.3 Ectomorphy

This type of body is thin and delicate looking. Bones are small and muscles are thin. The arms

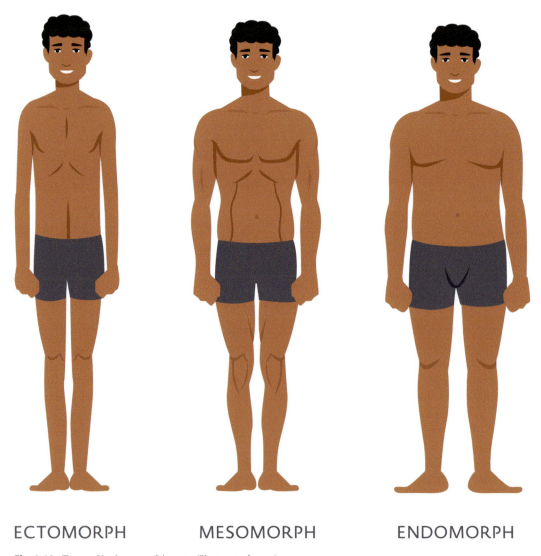

Fig. 2.13 Types of body types (Lio putra/Shutterstock.com)

2 The Basic Definitions of Anatomy and Anthropometry

and legs are long, while the torso is short. The shoulders are narrow and the muscle ratio is low.

Body type is the summation of a person's body constitution as a whole. Lipolysis is associated with endomorphy. Bone strength, muscle strength, and lean body structure are associated with mesomorphy. A slim body structure is associated with ectomorphy and volume and mass are indicated by height.

Body types are also used to identify changes in the body such as growth, aging, training, and physical performance. For example, elite bodybuilders, gymnasts, and long-distance runners may all have the same percentage of body fat. However, the physical characteristics of these athletes are quite different from each other. These differences are clearly revealed by body type classification.

2.2.5.4 Heath and Carter Somatotype Calculation Method

Triceps, subscapular, suprailiac, and leg skinfold values; humerus and femur bicondylar diameter measurements; arm and leg circumference; and height and weight values are among the anthropometric measurements used. Two different methods are used to determine somatotype. In the first method, anthropometric data are processed into the specially prepared evaluation form (Fig. 2.14) and the body type is determined using the somatochart. In the second method, the values obtained from the evaluation form are placed in the mathematical formula and the calculation is made. The manual calculation method is described below.

Manual calculation:

The calculation steps are as follows:

1. Personal information is noted.

Endomorphy Score (2–5)

2. Triceps, subscapular, suprailiac, and leg skinfold measurements are noted.
3. The sum of the triceps, subscapular, and suprailiac skinfold measurement values is written in the box on the left. The total value of these three measurements is equal to the "X" in the form. The resulting X-value is placed in the "height-corrected skinfold" for-

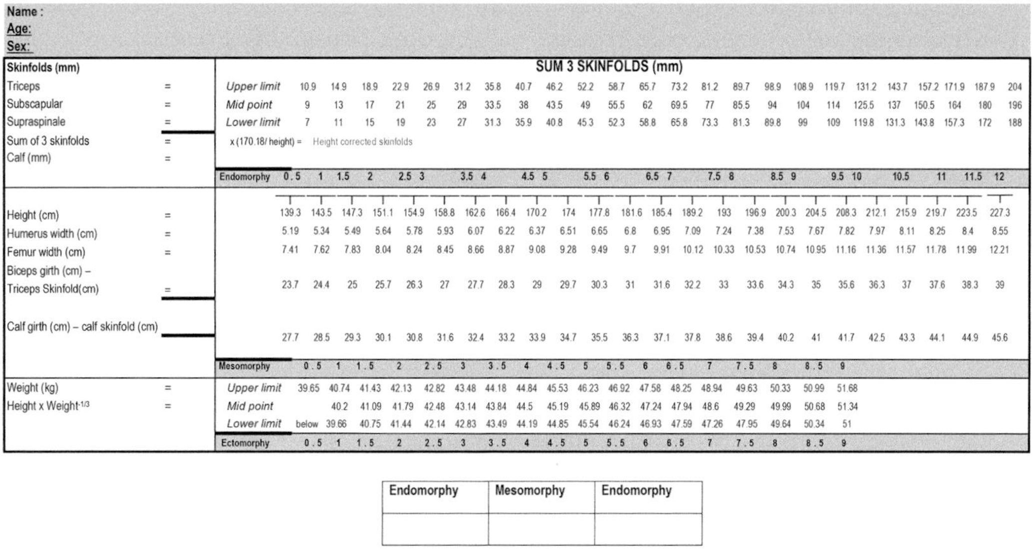

Fig. 2.14 Somatochart

mula [$X \times 170.18$/height (cm)] and calculated.
4. The nearest value in the table to the obtained total value of the three skinfold measurement values is circled. The scale is scanned vertically from bottom to top and horizontally from left to right. The "minimum value" and "maximum value" terms in the table specify the correct limit for each column. This limit is marked if the values are closer to the total value than the median value.
5. The value in the column with the value marked in step 4 is circled in the endomorphy row.

Mesomorphy Score (6–10)

6. The humerus and femur bicondylar diameter measurements and height in centimeter are written in the relevant boxes. Triceps and leg skinfold measurement values should be converted to centimeter. The triceps skinfold measurement (in cm) value is subtracted from the arm circumference measurement. In the same way, the leg skinfold measurement value (in cm) is subtracted from the leg circumference measurement.
7. The height value is scanned for the nearest value in the aligned row and circled.
8. The diameter and circumference measurement values are scanned in the aligned row as in step 7 and the nearest value is circled. If the measurement results correspond to the exact median of the two different values, the smaller value is selected.
9. In this step, the circled values should be considered as units, not as numerical data. The circled values on the left bottom side of the column where the height value was marked are calculated as a negative deviation while the ones on the right bottom side are calculated as positive deviations. The values just below the marked height column are considered to be zero deviations. The mathematical sum of all the deviations (deviation values calculated as units) is indicated by "D." The value obtained from the formula "*Mesomorphy* $= (D/8) + 4$" is rounded up to the nearest half rating unit.
10. The nearest value to the one obtained in the ninth step is circled as a mesomorphy score. If the value obtained is exactly at the middle of two adjacent values, the value closest to 4 is marked as the score. Marking is done this way as a safeguard against false and excessive ratios.

Ectomorphy Score (11–14)

11. Body weight (kg) is written.
12. The formula "*Height-to-weight ratio* $=$ *Height*/$^3\sqrt{weight}$" or *ponderal index (PI)* is used.
13. The nearest value to the height-to-weight ratio is circled in the table.
14. The ectomorphy score is the value below the value marked in the table from the height-to-weight ratio.
15. Calculated endomorphy, mesomorphy, and ectomorphy scores are recorded in the anthropometric somatotype field at the bottom of the form.
16. Somatotype determination is completed by writing the name of the researcher who made the evaluation.

Calculation with Formula:

Endomorphy $= -0.7182 + 0.1451X - 0.00068X^2 + 0.0000014X^3$
$X =$ triceps + subscapular + suprailiac skinfold. X is the height-corrected value of the sum of the values above
Height correction formula >> corrected total skinfold value $= X \times 170.18$/height (cm)
Mesomorphy $= 0.858$ (elbow width [cm]) $+ 0.601$ (knee width [cm]) $+ 0.188$ (corrected arm circumference measurement [cm]) $+ 0.161$ (corrected leg circumference measurement [cm]) $- 0.131$ (height length [m]) $+ 4.5$
Corrected arm circumference measurement = Arm circumference − Triceps skinfold/10
Corrected leg circumference measurement = Leg circumference − Leg skinfold/10

Different equations are used in the calculation of ectomorphy, according to the height-to-weight ratio calculation (height/$^3\sqrt{}$ weight).
If the height-to-weight ratio is >40.75:
  Ectomorphy = 0.732 (height-to-weight ratio) − 28.58 (height-to-weight ratio)
If 38.25< height-to-weight ratio <40.75:
  Ectomorphy = 0.463 (height-to-weight ratio) − 17.63 (height-to-weight ratio)
If the height-to-weight ratio is <38.25:
  Ectomorphy = (0.463 (height-to-weight ratio) − 17.63) + 0.1

2.2.5.5 Determination of the Body Type by Presenting the Results on a Somatochart

The exact position of the body type on the somatochart X–Y coordinate values is calculated using the following formulas. According to the Heath and Carter somatotype calculation method, the intersection point of values on the coordinate plane gives the body type (Fig. 2.15).

  X = Ectomorphy − Endomorphy.
  Y = 2 × Mesomorphy − (Endomorphy + Ectomorphy).

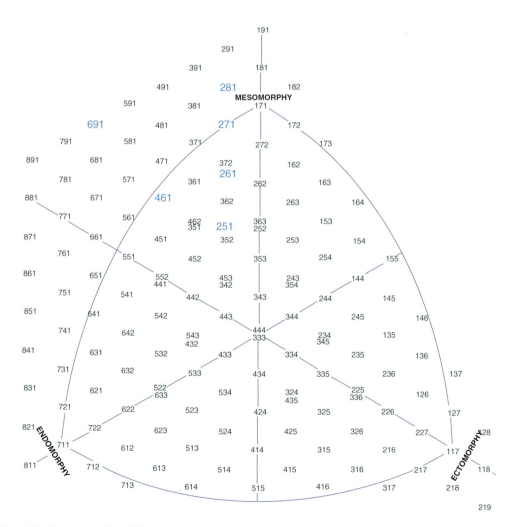

Fig. 2.15 Somatochart for plotting somatotypes

2.3 Conclusion

Knowing the anatomical terms used to indicate the anatomical positions, directions, and movements, and knowing planes, axes, and osteokinematic and arthrokinematic movements of the joints are important for understanding the movements of the body parts using a common language. Flexion, extension, abduction, adduction, and internal and external rotation osteokinematic joint movements are defined in terms of planes and axes. Arthrokinematic movements involving rolling, sliding, and rotating, on the other hand, are accessory movements that accompany osteokinematic movements, allowing joint surfaces to move in harmony and together. The moveable joints in our body are synovial joints, which are classified as ball and socket, hinge, pivot, and ellipsoid according to their shape. Although the human spine shows different characteristics in the cervical, thoracic, and lumbar regions, the spine moves on all planes and axes. Anthropometry is an objective measurement method that provides systematic classification and monitoring. It allows standardized measurement of people's body types, body components, and physical characteristics that must be monitored for various reasons.

Further Reading

Aragon AA, Schoenfeld BJ, Wildman R, Kleiner S, VanDusseldorp T, Taylor L, et al. International society of sports nutrition position stand: diets and body composition. J Int Soc Sports Nutr. 2017;14(1):1–9.

Borga M, West J, Bell JD, Harvey NC, Romu T, Heymsfield SB, et al. Advanced body composition assessment: from body mass index to body composition profiling. J Investig Med. 2018;5:1–9.

Dopsaj M, Zuoziene IJ, Milić R, Cherepov E, Erlikh V, Masiulis N, et al. Body composition in international sprint swimmers: are there any relations with performance? Int J Environ Res Public Health. 2020;17(24):9464.

Duquet W, Caeter Lindsay JE. Somatotyping. In: Eston R, Thomas R, editors. Kinanthropometry and exercise physiology laboratory manual: tests, procedures and data: volume two: physiology. Boca Raton: Routledge; 2013. p. 55–9.

Eston R, Hawes M, Martin A, Thomas R. Human body composition. In: Eston R, Thomas R, editors. Kinanthropometry and exercise physiology laboratory manual: tests, procedures and data: volume two: physiology. Boca Raton: Routledge; 2013. p. 7–29.

Jeukendrup A, Gleeson M. Body composition. In: Jeukendrup A, Gleeson M, editors. Sport nutrition. Champaign: Human Kinetics; 2018. p. 414–30.

Kisner C. Peripheral joint mobilization/manipulation. In: Kisner C, Colby LA, Borstad J, editors. Therapeutic exercise: foundations and techniques. Philadelphia: F.A. Davis Company; 2017. p. 127–38.

Leão C, Camões M, Clemente FM, Nikolaidis PT, Lima R, Bezerra P, et al. Anthropometric profile of soccer players as a determinant of position specificity and methodological issues of body composition estimation. Int J Environ Res Public Health. 2019;16(13):2386.

Moore KL, Dalley AF, Agur M. Clinically oriented anatomy. 8th ed. Philadelphia: Wolters Kluwer; 2018. p. 89–334.

Neumann DA. Axial skeleton: osteology and arthrology. In: Neumann DA, editor. Kinesiology of the musculoskeletal system: foundations for rehabilitation. 3rd ed. Amsterdam: Elsevier Health Sciences; 2017. p. 332–60.

Santos DA, Dawson JA, Matias CN, Rocha PM, Minderico CS, Allison BD, et al. Reference values for body composition and anthropometric measurements in athletes. PLoS One. 2014;9(5):e97846.

Ward LC. Human body composition: yesterday, today, and tomorrow. Eur J Clin Nutr. 2018;72(9):1201–7.

The Bone and Joint Structure

Günseli Usgu and Serkan Usgu

Abstract

The perfect organization between bone structures and joints, muscles, and ligaments in the formation of movement has been investigated for years. Bones are mechanically connected with neighboring structures around them. A joint is defined as the functional connection between different bones of the skeleton. Without bone and articular structures, any motion cannot occur. Bones, which take part in the kinetic chain in terms of transmission and distribution of force, are only one of the tissues that work together with the joints. Gravity, activity, and mechanical stimuli are essential for bone functionality. Bones can adapt very quickly to situations created by internal and external factors. Apart from trauma, they can give different responses to various diseases that cannot be seen as related to bones. Bone tissue, which is indispensable for mobility in our lives, is also related to our other systems that manage essential functions. In this section, the structure and functions of bone tissue and joints are explained.

G. Usgu (✉) · S. Usgu
Physiotherapy and Rehabilitation, Faculty of Health Sciences, Hasan Kalyoncu University, Gaziantep, Turkey
e-mail: gunseli.usgu@hku.edu.tr; serkan.usgu@hku.edu.tr

3.1 Bones

Although bones are often thought of as static structures that offer structural support, they actually function as a complete organ. Bones are a perfect example of the principle: "form follows function." While providing structural support for movement and breathing, it also allows motor movements to be performed. It acts as a reservoir for calcium, phosphate, amino acids, and bicarbonate. Besides its functions such as protection of internal organs, transmission of sound waves, and homeostasis, it is also involved in producing cells necessary for the continuation of life in the bone marrow. Moreover, it affects the bone marrow, brain, kidney, and pancreas with the hormones it secretes, such as osteocalcin and fibroblast growth factor-23. Thanks to the organs it affects, it also undertakes the endocrine organ function by helping regulate bone tissue mineralization, fat metabolism, cognitive functions, and glucose metabolism.

3.1.1 Anatomical Structure of Bones

Bone tissue is divided into primary bone tissue (immature bone) and secondary bone tissue (lamellar, mature bone) according to the arrangement of collagen fibers. Primary bone tissue is an immature bone form that is weak due to the irregular placement of collagen fibers. Secondary bone tissue is the mature (mature) bone form showing regular and parallel collagen arrangement. Adults have only secondary bone tissue.

> **Attention!**
> The transverse growth of bones in childhood and adulthood is the task of the periosteum. A poor bone-healing process in intra-articular femoral neck fractures is due to the absence or very thin structure of the periosteum layer in this region.

Bone consists of two main components: the extracellular matrix, which is organic and inorganic, and cells. The organic component consists of type 1 collagen, noncollagenous glycoproteins, proteoglycans, cytokines, and growth hormones. Type I collagen in the organic structure is responsible for the tensile strength of the bone, while proteoglycans are responsible for the compression. The noncollagenous osteonectin protein is responsible for mineralization and calcium balance. The osteocalcin produced by osteoblasts allows the bone density to be adjusted. Vitamin D stimulates the synthesis of osteocalcin, while parathormone suppresses the synthesis of osteocalcin. Growth factors and cytokines in bone, insulin-like growth factor (IGF), transforming growth factor-beta (TGF-β), bone morphogenic proteins 1–6, and interleukins 1 and 6 are responsible for cell differentiation, activation, growth, and turnover. The inorganic component consists mainly of calcium phosphate organized as hydroxyapatite crystals. It is responsible for the compressive strength of the bone (Fig. 3.1).

The white transparent layer that surrounds all the bones in our body is called the periosteum. The periosteum consists of two layers, fibrous on the outside and osteogenic on the inside. The inner layer of the periosteum, consisting of proliferative bone cells, osteoblasts, and small vessel cells, is located close to the bone. The outer fibrous layer consists of fibroblasts, collagen fibers, and basic material. Collagen fibers in the periosteum are located parallel to the surface. Periosteal collagen fiber bundles called perforating fibers penetrate the bone matrix and connect the periosteum to the bone matrix. These fibers are called *Sharpey's fibers*. *Sharpey's fibers* are found where ligaments and tendons attach to the bones. The direction of collagen fibers is determined by tensile forces. They are located throughout the cortex in areas subject to high tensile forces.

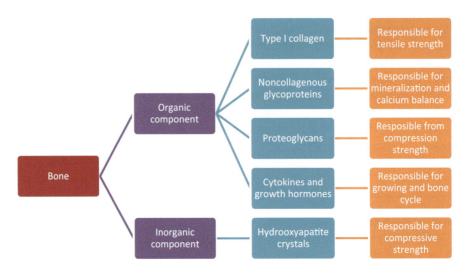

Fig. 3.1 Components and functions of bones

3.1.2 Bone Cells

Four different types of bone cells exist: osteoclasts, osteoblasts, osteocytes, and osteoprogenitor cells. Although these cells have different origins and functions, they work in harmony with each other and in an organized manner to maintain bone homeostasis.

3.1.2.1 Osteoclasts (Catabolic Cells)

A mature osteoclast is a polarized, multinucleated giant cell with a unique morphology. Its main function is to ensure the resorption of the bone matrix. Osteoclasts have receptors sensitive to calcitonin. Interleukin-1 stimulates osteoclastic activity.

3.1.2.2 Osteoblasts (Anabolic Cells)

Osteoblasts are formed from mesenchyme stem cells. It takes part in the production and release of the matrix in the bone structure. Since they are the cells responsible for storing new bones, they play an active role in both skeletal development and fracture healing thanks to this feature. It makes up 6% or less of the total amount of cells in the bones. They accumulate bone matrix around them and eventually become embedded in their own matrix to form osteocytes.

3.1.2.3 Osteoprogenitor Cells

They are mesenchymal cells that can transform into osteoblasts in the Haversian canals, endosteum, and periosteum.

3.1.2.4 Osteocytes

Osteocytes are the most abundant cell type in bones (<90%). It consists of cells as a spider web of interconnected channels, essential for cellular processes. This network-like structure is important for responding to mechanical stimuli and for converting these stimuli into chemical signals that stimulate other bone cells. Cell-to-cell communication is achieved through gap junctions. This also indicates that the osteocyte is not an immobile osteoblast trapped in the bone matrix it has formed. While osteocytes are stimulated by calcitonin, they are suppressed by parathyroid hormone.

Perception of mechanical stimuli directly affects bone formation and resorption by osteocytes. This indicates that osteocytes are the controllers of osteoclast and osteoblast functions. Osteocyte apoptosis has been shown to be a regulatory event for osteoclast formation. In particular, a direct relationship exists between osteocyte apoptosis caused by microfractures and osteoclast formation at the injury site. Osteocytes contribute to increasing osteoclast absorption, re-taking of a high amount of calcium from the bones when it is especially needed by the organism, and regulation of bone mineral homeostasis.

Bones constantly undergo structural and biological changes. In this way, bone remodeling continues throughout life. The skeletal system responds to increased stress, such as resistive strength training, by increasing osteogenesis or causing new bone formation. Bone shape, size, and strength vary depending on the needs in the performance of motor tasks. The bones in the middle ear carry out the transmission of sound waves to the inner ear, although they have minimal strength. Large bones, such as the femur, are extremely strong and can withstand very high stresses before breaking.

Bones have specialized cortical and trabecular structures to perform their functions. The vertebral body, pelvis, and ribs show trabecular bone characteristics, while the femur has both cortical and trabecular bone characteristics. The material properties of bone sections differ. The trabecular bone has less calcium and more water than the cortical bone. The nutrition of the surface of the trabecular bone adjacent to the bone marrow is higher than that of the cortical bone. Absorption occurs along the bony surfaces in the trabecular bone, while in the cortical bone, it occurs in channels that run through the bone. The cortical bone constitutes approximately 80% of the bone mass. Vascular channels are about 30% of this volume. The surface volume ratio of the cortical bone is

Table 3.1 Bone parts and their material properties

Material property	Trabecular bone	Cortical bone
Surface nutrition adjacent to the bone marrow	High	Low
Absorption	Along the bone surface	In channels of bone
Surface-to-volume ratio	High	Low
Amount of calcium	Low	High
Amount of water	High	Low

much lower than that of the trabecular bone. With aging or disease, the cortex becomes more porous, resulting in an increase in surface area and a decrease in bone strength. While 20% of the trabecular bone is bone tissue, the remaining volume is filled with bone marrow and fat. The trabecular bone transfers mechanical loads from the articular surface to the cortical bone and absorbs the shock thanks to its hydraulic feature (Table 3.1).

3.1.3 Histological Structure

The osteon or Haversian system, which is the structural and functional basic unit of the cortical bone, runs parallel to the long axis of the bone. Osteons are important for providing adequate mechanical support and blood supply in the skeletal system. In the center of each osteon is the Haversian canal, which contains blood and lymph vessels, and nerve fibers. The Volkmann canals connecting to the Haversian canals are perpendicular to the major axis of the osteon. The central Haversian canal is surrounded by a concentric layer of mineralized bone "lamella." The small spaces between the lamellae are called lacunae. Lacunae contain osteocytes. Canaliculi are thin channels that connect the lacunae (Fig. 3.2). The canaliculi allow nutrients to reach the osteocytes from the blood vessels in the Haversian canal.

> **Attention!**
> Osteons are dynamic bone structures. Their number, structure, and activity change over time in response to external stimuli acting on the bones.

3.1.4 Bone Types

According to their shape, bones are divided into five categories: long, short, flat, irregular (irregular), and sesamoid bones (Fig. 3.3). Bone types and properties are listed in Table 3.2.

Mechanical or chemical stimuli affect bone sections differently. This process can become more complex with sex, age, and disease.

> **Clinical Information**
> - Trabecular bone loss in the tibial cortex is greater in bed rest immobilization.
> - In patients with chronic kidney disease or those exposed to low-intensity vibration, the strength of the tibia increases due to changes in trabecular bone rather than cortical bone.
> - Parathyroid hormone injections increase trabecular bone mass while decreasing cortical bone mass. The significant increase in bone strength is associated with an increase in the trabecular bone.

The mechanical strength of bones and its resistance to fracture depend on the size, volumetric density, and trabecular structure of the bone. Gonadal hormones affect bone compartments differently depending on sex. While testosterone secreted in men and women supports periosteal bone expansion, estrogen prevents cortical bone loss. Trabecular bone loss is prevented by the secretion of estrogen in women and testosterone in men (Fig. 3.5).

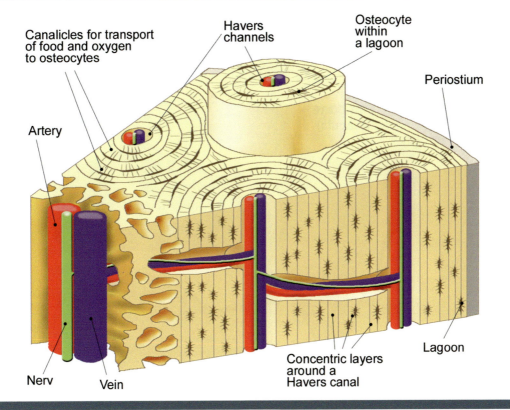
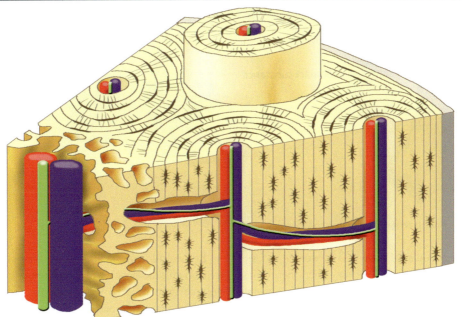

Fig. 3.2 Structure of osteon (Amadeu Blasco/Shutterstock.com)

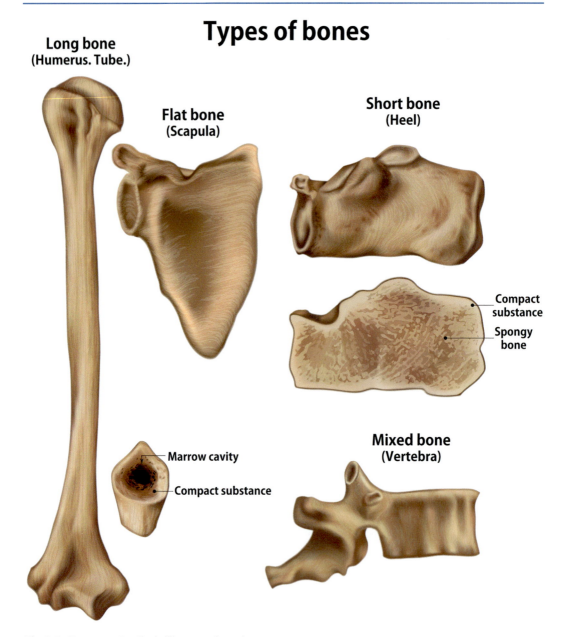

Fig. 3.3 Bone types (studiovin/Shutterstock.com)

Postmenopausal bone loss in women is faster in trabecular bone. However, since the cortical bone makes up 80% of the skeleton, the absolute amount of bone loss from each compartment in the first 10 years is similar.

In the following years, the Haversian canals expand and the bones with an increased surface/volume ratio become weak with the increasing loss of the cortical bone. The loss of regular and dense structures such as the cortical bone affects

Table 3.2 Bone types and properties

Long bones
- They are the main bones of the extremities that are longer than wide
- It consists of the diaphysis (elongated central shaft space), epiphysis (two enlarged end portions), and metaphysis (the part between the diaphysis and the epiphysis)
- The inside of the bones contains a cavity known as the medullary space, which is filled with bone marrow (Fig. 3.4)
- Examples: femur, tibia, and humerus

Short bones
- They are almost equal in length and diameter
- Example: carpal bones

Flat bones
- They are weak bones that look like plates
- Examples: skull bones and sternum

Irregular bones
- They are irregular bones that do not conform in shape to the three bone types mentioned earlier
- Examples: vertebrae

Sesamoid bones
- They are oval-shaped bones located under joints or tendons
- Functions: To protect the joint, to protect the tendon by reducing the pressure on it, to change the force vector of the muscle, and to make the movements faster and with less energy consumption
- Examples: patella and pisiform

the decrease in bone strength more than the trabecular bone losses. With aging, the diameter of long bones increases more in men than in women, which increases the resistance of the bones to bending stresses on the bones.

> **Attention!**
> Since trabecular and cortical bones can be affected differently by hormones and drugs, it is important to evaluate them in each disease process.

3.1.5 Vascularization of the Bones

The mammalian skeleton contains a well-organized vascular network that supplies abundant blood to the bones. Approximately 10–15% of cardiac output at rest is allocated to the nutrition of bone structures. This vascular network in bones ensures the maintenance of bone homeostasis during physiological and pathological conditions (Fig. 3.5). Especially in long bones, vascular anatomy comprises the nutrient arteries; the periosteal, metaphyseal, and epiphyseal arteries; and their venous outflows. After the feeding arteries pierce the periosteum and enter the bones, they pass through the Haversian and Volkmann canals and reach the bone marrow. From here, the bone is fed by giving small branches to the distal and proximal parts of the bones (Fig. 3.6).

The vascular network structure of the bone varies depending on the location of the bone in the skeletal system. For example, arteries in the greater trochanter of the femur enter from the medial, lateral, and superior surfaces of the trochanter and form the vascular network that supplies the trochanteric region. Thanks to this vascular network, the supply of the trochanteric region is separated from the collum femoris, the femoral shaft. The blood supply of long bones changes in line with regional factors such as metabolism, aging, and trauma.

3.1.6 Innervation of the Bones

The bones are stimulated by the muscles and skin nerves (tibial nerve, radial nerve, etc.) overlying them. This is called the *Hilton* rule. The periosteum, mineralized bone, and bone marrow are stimulated by small-diameter myelinated/unmyelinated sensory and autonomic fibers of peripheral nerves. The peripheral nerves innervating the bones travel together with the main artery supplying the bones. The peripheral nerves innervating the bones enter the diaphysis with the artery through the nutrient canal and stimulate the bone marrow cavity. The nerves innervating the articular surfaces enter the bones from both sides of the epiphyses and proceed toward the articular surfaces.

Fig. 3.4 Anatomy of long bones (Designua/Shutterstock.com)

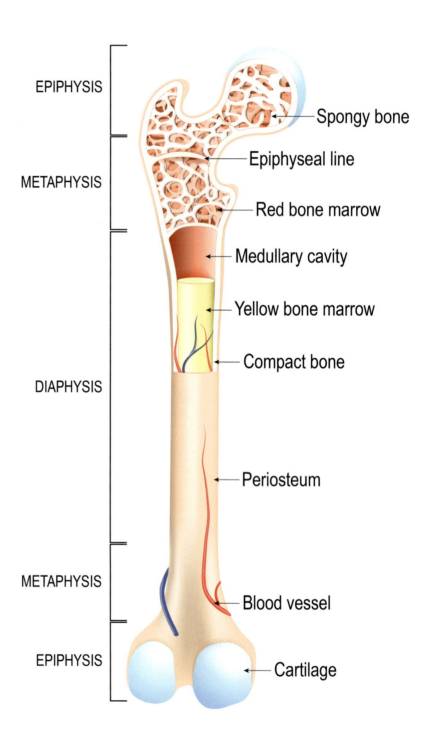

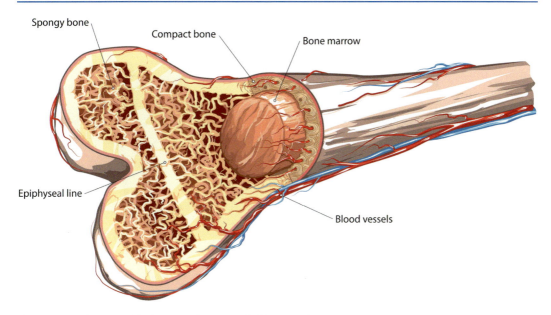

Fig. 3.5 Vascular network in bones (EreborMountain/Shutterstock.com)

3.1.7 Muscular Contribution

Muscle and bone tissue are interrelated in terms of anatomical, mechanical, and metabolic functions. Anatomically, the muscle connects parts of the skeleton through tendinous connections, turning it into a lever system and increasing mobility. Activities such as exercise can create regional adaptations in the bone. Exercises greatly increase the ability of the bone to withstand loads. However, the less change in the mineral content due to loading in bone regions where mechanical loads are high (such as the cortical bone of the collum femoris) causes these regions to be vulnerable to loads.

The mechanical stresses that occur in cortical and trabecular bones with different exercise approaches provide *remodeling* of the bones depending on the amount and direction of the applied force. Long-term, high-intensity exercise increases bone mass in postmenopausal women and women undergoing hormone replacement therapy. Muscle contraction provides severe loads on the bones. Therefore, resistance exercises are recommended to prevent bone loss in situations where there is no gravity, such as prolonged bed rest and space flight. The risk of age-related bone loss and life-threatening fractures in the proximal region of the femur is increased in the geriatric group. Resistance exercise is one way to reduce the effects of age-related bone loss.

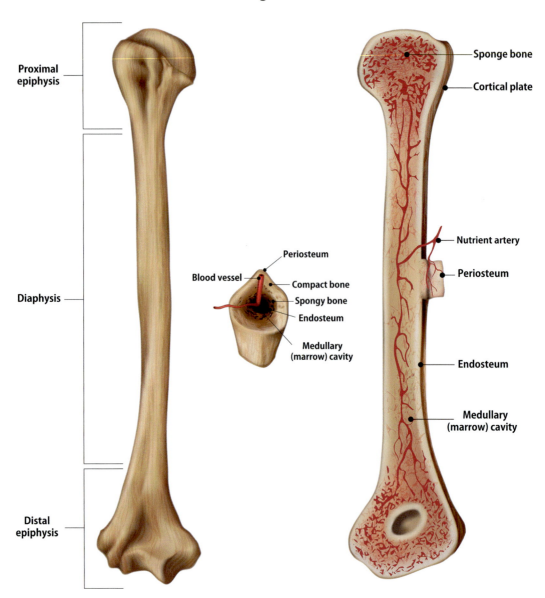

Fig. 3.6 Vascular structure in long bones (studiovin/Shutterstock.com)

3.2 Joints

A joint is defined as the functional connection between different bones of the skeleton. Joints are diverse and versatile skeletal structures. Joints differ not only in anatomical location, architecture, and size but also in the type and degree of movement they allow and in their organic structure. The current and useful classification of joint diversity is largely based on the degree of joint motion. In this section, the joint types, joint nutrition, joint innervation, and anatomical structures within the joint are explained.

3.2.1 Joint Types

Joints can be histologically classified according to the dominant connective tissue type (type) or mobility. Joints are classified histologically as fibrous, cartilaginous, and synovial, and functionally as synarthrosis (immovable joint), amphiarthrosis (semi-movable joint), and diarthrosis (movable joint). Both classifications are related to each other, and synarthrosis joints are fibrous, amphiarthrosis joints are cartilaginous, and diarthrosis joints are synovial (Fig. 3.7).

3.2.1.1 Fibrous Joint

It is an immovable joint composed mainly of collagen, where the fibrous tissue joins the bone ends. Fibrous joints have no mobility (synarthrosis) and joint space. They are divided into three types: sutures, gomphosis, and syndesmosis. Sutures are joints seen in the skull bones, joined in a suture style, and with no mobility feature (Fig. 3.8). During birth, it has a limited range of motion thanks to the connective tissue called fontanelle located between the flat bones in the skull. This allows the skull of the newborn to pass through the birth canal and the development of the brain in parallel with the development of the newborn. As the skull grows, the fontanelles shrink into narrow, fibrous connective tissues called *Sharpey's* fibers. Eventually, the cranial sutures fuse, forming two adjacent plates of the bones. This fusion is called synostosis. Gomphosis is an immovable joint that occurs between the root of the tooth and the socket of the tooth in the mandible and maxilla. A syndesmosis is a small amount of movable

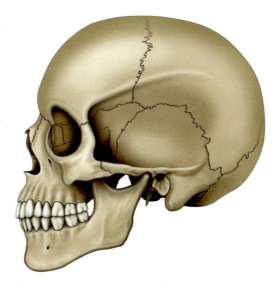

Fig. 3.8 Suture joint (ilusmedical/Shutterstock.com)

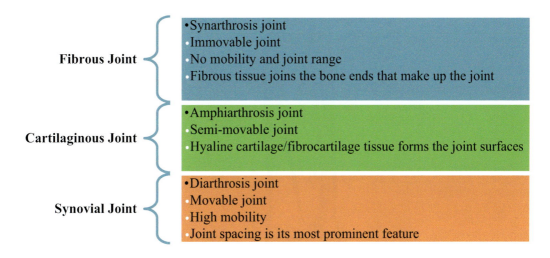

Fig. 3.7 Joint types

joint (amphiarthrosis). In a syndesmosis joint, the two bone surfaces are connected by an interosseous membrane or fibrous tissue. In the upper extremity, the radioulnar joint connects the membrane interossea, the chorda obliqua, and the radius and ulna bones, as an example of a syndesmosis type of joint. In the lower extremity, a syndesmosis joint formed by the distal tibiofibular joint, anterior–posterior tibiofibular ligament, interosseous membrane, and inferior transverse tibiofibular ligament can be given as an example (Fig. 3.9).

Syndesmosis joints vary in their mobility according to their functions. The tibiofibular syndesmosis joint does not allow the movement of the tibia and fibula to provide strength and stability while bearing body weight. The radioulnar syndesmosis joint allows the movement of the radius during the pronation–supination of the forearm.

3.2.1.2 Cartilaginous Joint

In cartilaginous joints, the bony joint surfaces are covered with hyaline cartilage or fibrocartilage tissue. The cartilage on the articular surfaces is divided into *primary* or *secondary cartilaginous joints* according to the type of tissue. The primary cartilaginous joint contains hyaline cartilage. It is found in the joints that occur between the epiphysis and diaphyseal regions of the growing long bones or between the ribs and the sternum. Between the secondary cartilaginous articular surfaces is a hyaline or fibrocartilaginous disk. The symphysis pubis joint is one such joint.

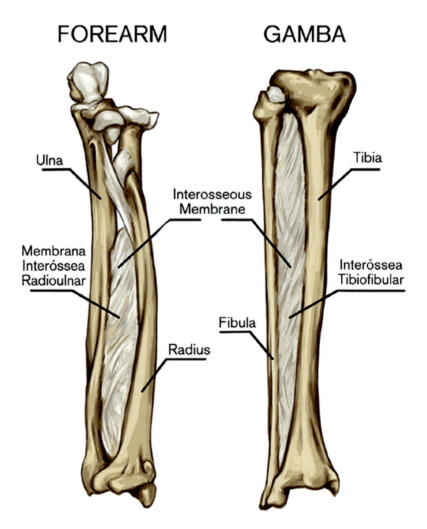

Fig. 3.9 Syndesmosis joint (stihii/Shutterstock.com)

3.2.1.3 Synovial Joint

They are functional joints with high mobility. The joint space is the most prominent feature of the synovial joint. This gap between the joint surfaces has a negative pressure feature (Fig. 3.10). The synovial joint types are listed in Fig. 3.11.

Anatomical Structures Found in the Synovial Joint

Joint Capsule The joint capsule, which is fibrous connective tissue, attaches to the periosteum by enclosing the joint cavity and joint surfaces. It creates negative air pressure by wrapping the joint cavity. The joint capsule consists of two layers: an outer fibrous membrane and an inner synovial membrane (Fig. 3.10). The fibrous membrane is composed of type I collagen, elastin fibers, and nerve fibers containing vessels and mechanoreceptors. The synovial membrane, on the contrary, is a 20- to 40-μm-thick covering layer containing synovial type A and B cells, as well as a subsynovial layer approximately 5 mm thick, consisting of connective tissue, vessels, adipocytes, elastin fibers, and immune cells.

Joint Cavity The joint cavity contains the synovial fluid secreted by the synovial membrane (synovium) surrounding the joint capsule (Fig. 3.10). Thanks to the phospholipids, hyaluronan, and glycoproteins it contains, the synovial fluid reduces the friction force in the joint.

Joint Faces The articular surfaces covered with hyaline cartilage (type II collagen) are avascular. Articular cartilage and synovial membrane are continuous (Fig. 3.10). Type II collagen, aggrecan, and extracellular matrix cells located on the joint surface provide durability to the joint surfaces during movement. Some synovial joints also contain fibrocartilage structures such as the

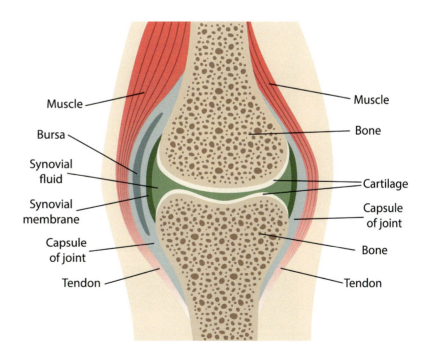

Fig. 3.10 Synovial joint (Olga Bolbot/Shutterstock.com)

meniscus between the articular surfaces. These structures increase the harmony of the joint surfaces, regulate the distribution of the compression forces acting on the joint surface, and help provide joint stability.

Articular Ligaments The structures that connect the bones making up the joint are called ligaments. There are two types of ligaments in synovial joints: internal and external. Articular cartilage and synovial membrane are continuous (Fig. 3.10). Type II collagen, aggrecan, and extracellular matrix cells located on the joint surface provide durability to the joint surfaces during movement. Some synovial joints also contain fibrocartilage structures such as the meniscus between the articular surfaces. These structures increase the harmony of the joint surfaces, regulate the distribution of the compression forces acting on the joint surface, and help provide joint stability.

> **Clinical Information**
> Considering the contribution of elastin fibers to mechanical stability, the content of collagen fibers in the joint capsule and elastin fibers in the joint capsule increases, and the adaptation to this situation is improved to prevent repetitive dislocations in people with shoulder instability.

> **Attention!**
> The muscles are critical in providing support to the synovial joints. The muscles and tendons that cross the joint act as a dynamic ligament against the forces acting on that joint. Therefore, muscular strength is

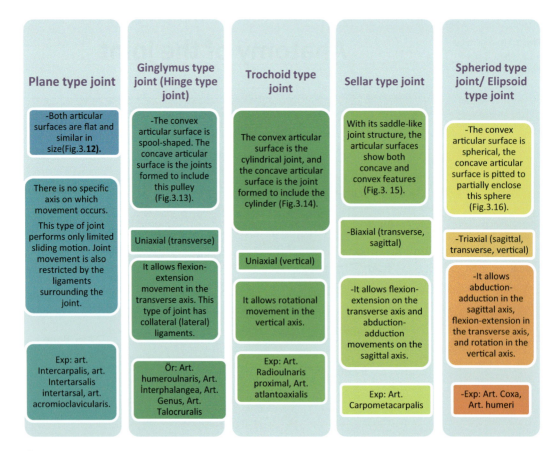

Fig. 3.11 Types of synovial joint

essential for the stability of synovial joints during high-stress activities. It is also very important for joints with weak ligaments (glenohumeral joint, etc.).

Types of Synovial Joints

The main purpose of synovial joints is to prevent the frictional force between the articular surfaces during movement. Synovial joints are classified according to the number of axes (Figs. 3.11, 3.12, 3.13, 3.14, 3.15, and 3.16).

3.2.2 Vascularization of Joints

3.2.2.1 Vascularization of Fibrous Joints

Usually, the perforating branches of the proximal vessels are responsible for the nutrition of the joint. For example, the blood supply to the tibiofibular joint is provided by branches from the anterior tibial artery as well as the peroneal artery.

3.2.2.2 Vascularization of Cartilaginous Joints

Only the peripheral parts of the joint have vascular nutrition because the joint cartilage itself is avascular tissue. For example, the intervertebral disks are supplied by capillaries in the peripheral vertebral body.

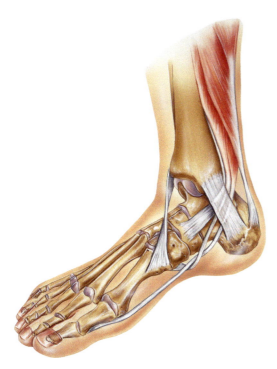

Fig. 3.12 Plane-type joint (Medical Art Inc/Shutterstock.com)

Fig. 3.13 Ginglymus-type joint (Hinge-type joint) (udaix/Shutterstock.com)

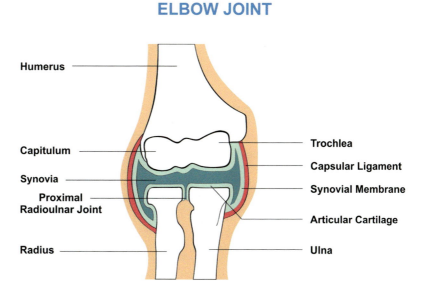

Fig. 3.14 Trochoid-type joint (stihii/Shutterstock.com)

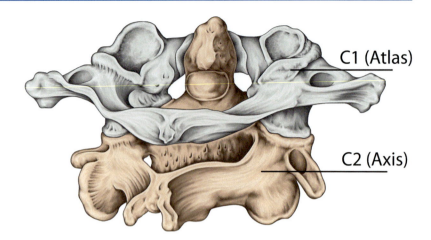

Fig. 3.15 Sellar-type joint (Ira Dvilyuk/Shutterstock.com)

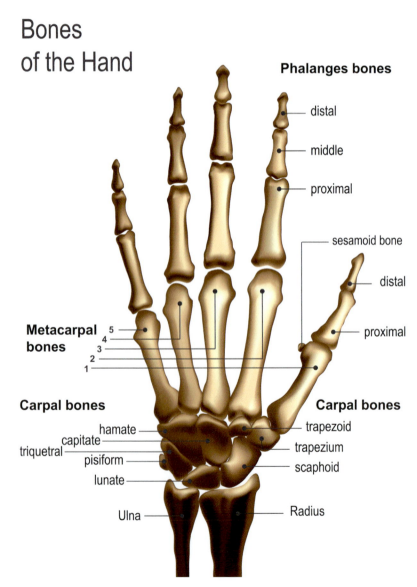

HIP JOINT

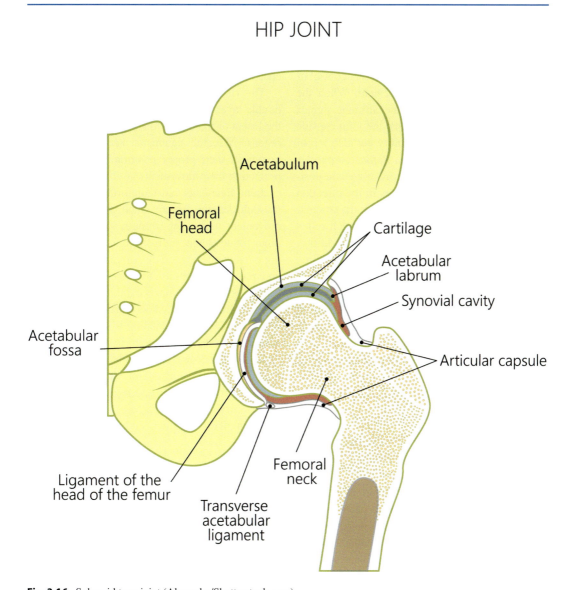

Fig. 3.16 Spheroid type joint (Aksanaku/Shutterstock.com)

3.2.2.3 Vascularization of Synovial Joints

The synovial joints are supplied by a rich arterial network called the periarticular plexus, which extends from both sides of the joint. Some vessels also penetrate the fibrous capsule to form a rich plexus deeper in the synovial membrane. These structures, called the deep plexus, form a ring around the joint margins that supply the joint capsule, synovial membrane, and bones. Articular cartilage, which is avascular hyaline cartilage, is supplied by diffusion from the synovial fluid or subchondral blood vessels.

3.2.3 Innervation of the Joint

Synovial joints have both sensory and autonomic innervation. Autonomic nerves are responsible for controlling vasomotor responses. The sensory nerves of the joint capsule and ligaments provide proprioceptive sensory feedback from the *Ruffini* and *Pacini* mechanoreceptors. The sense of proprioception in the joint allows the reflex control of posture, locomotion, and movement. When the joint is maximally loaded, the afferent signals from the joint area indicate that the joint capsule has not only mechanical stability but also a protective reflexogenic function. *Ruffini* corpuscles are active even when the joint is in a static position and are sensitive to changes in the direction of joint movement, magnitude, and intra-articular pressure. It also helps regulate the stretch reflex and muscle tone under sustained tonic conditions. Any excessive force within the joint resulting from flexion, extension, and rotation movements is reported by *Ruffini* bodies. *Pacini* corpuscles, which adapt quickly, transmit the sensations of rapid joint movement and vibration. *Pacini* corpuscles give a mechanical stimulus when joint movement begins or stops. The free nerve endings transmit widespread pain sensation. The articular cartilage has no nerve innervation.

3.2.4 Intra-Articular Structures

3.2.4.1 Ligaments

Ligaments are fibrous tissues rich in the extracellular matrix, collagen, fibroblast, proteoglycan, and water. Water makes up about 60–70% of the mass of the cytoplasmic matrix. Other components such as elastin and proteoglycan are also incorporated into the cytoplasmic matrix. Collagen constitutes approximately 70–80% of dry weight and is the most important component that carries the load. Type I collagen is the main component of the extracellular matrix of the ligament. In addition, type II, type III, type V, and type XI collagens are also present at a low rate. Type II collagen is usually found at the junction of ligaments and bones. Although the amount of elastin varies according to the properties and function of the ligament, it is usually less than 1% of the dry weight of the ligament. Elastin, together with collagen, gives elasticity and tensile strength to the ligament. Macroscopically, the ligaments can be examined under two headings as visceral ligament and joint ligament. The fact that they are located in different parts of the body is the main reason for the structural difference in the ligaments.

The visceral ligament consists of a single or double layer of peritoneal folds. It is attached to the fascia of the liver, kidneys, and other internal organs. Visceral ligaments keep the internal organs in their proper position, restricting and protecting their movements.

Joint ligaments have important roles in the musculoskeletal system, such as guiding joint movement under low-strength loads, protecting other tissues under high-strength loads, preventing movements beyond the joint range of motion, and providing stability by transmitting tension forces. Articular ligaments exhibit typical nonlinear anisotropic mechanical behavior to perform these tasks. When the loading is small, the collagen fibers in the ligament are in a crimped state. Collagen fibers are compatible with the force applied to the ligament. This situation is represented in the nonlinear end region of the load–strain curve. As the loading increases, the collagen fibers lengthen and the slip between them decreases, increasing the stiffness of the ligament. Collagen fibers maintain their linear elasticity until they reach the stretching threshold. In addition, the mutual sliding effect between the fibrous bundles contributes to the viscoelastic effect of the ligament.

The capillaries in the ligament provide the blood supply necessary for the development of the ligament and its repair after injury. The blood vessels in some ligaments can also provide nourishment to the surrounding bones and other soft tissues.

3.2.4.2 Other Anatomical Structures in the Joint

The meniscus, labrum, and intervertebral disks are located within the joint.

Meniscus

It is a fibrocartilage disk structure that has the ability to transfer the loads acting on the knee joint and to reduce the stress on the articular cartilage like a shock absorber. It increases the harmony of the tibiofemoral joint surfaces. It also has secondary tasks such as increasing stability, lubricity, feeding, and sensing proprioception.

Anatomical Placement of Menisci The menisci are shaped like two crescents located on both the medial and lateral tibial plateaus. The lateral meniscus is C-shaped and covers 75–93% of the lateral tibial plateau, while the medial meniscus is semicircular and covers 51–74% of the medial tibial plateau. The posterior horn of the medial meniscus is firmly attached to the posterior intercondylar fossa (anterior to the attachment of the anterior cruciate ligament [ACL] in the tibia) by bony attachments. Although the anterior horn differs among individuals, the most common location is the flat part of the intercondylar space in front of the ACL. The inferior medial meniscus is attached to the tibia by the medial collateral ligament and coronary ligament. Thanks to these strong connections, the almost immobile medial meniscus becomes more vulnerable to injury. The anterior horn of the lateral meniscus attaches to the anterolateral aspect of the ACL and to the anteromedial aspect of the apex of the lateral tibial eminence. The posterior horn, on the contrary, is located posteromedially of the apex of the lateral tibial eminence, anterior to the tibial attachment region of the posterior cruciate ligament (PCL), and anterolateral to the medial meniscus posterior horn attachment region (Fig. 3.17). Since the lateral meniscus has a more mobile structure than the medial meniscus, it is injured less frequently than the medial meniscus.

Vascular Anatomy of Menisci The fibrous region in the center of the meniscus in adults shows avascular features, and the nourishment of this region takes place by diffusion from the synovial fluid. There is a direct vascular blood supply in 10–30% areas in the periphery of the medial meniscus and 10–25% in the lateral meniscus. The nutrition of these vascular regions is provided by branches of the geniculate and popliteal arteries. When the cross-sectional area of the meniscus is examined, it is divided into

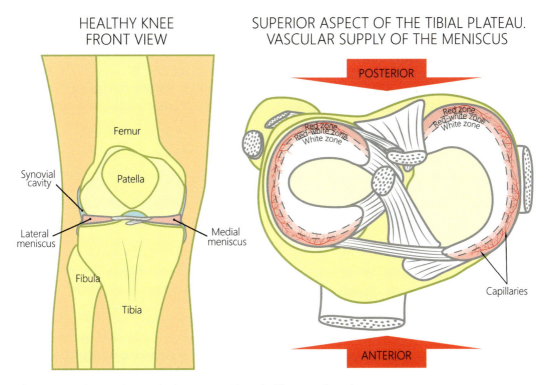

Fig. 3.17 Meniscus and anatomical structures (Aksanaku/Shutterstock.com)

three zones as *red–red*, *red–white*, and *white–white* according to the blood supply feature. The red–red zone in the periphery of the meniscus is fully nourished by the vascular structure, whereas the white–white zone in the center does not have a vascular structure.

> **Attention!**
> The red–red zone on the outer part of the meniscus has excellent vascular structure and healing potential. The red–white zone has a moderate vascular structure and healing potential. Since the inner white–white zone does not contain any vascular structure, the healing potential is minimal. It is thought that the low repair capacity after injury in the inner and middle zones of the meniscus is due to the low vascular structures of these zones.

Innervation of the Menisci There are three different mechanoreceptors (*Ruffini corpuscles*, *Pacini corpuscles*, and Golgi tendon organ) that contribute to proprioception and afferent senses in the peripheral two-thirds of the menisci and in the anterior and posterior horns. *Ruffini* corpuscles are unmyelinated and slowly adapt and transmit pain and joint deformation. *Pacini* corpuscles are myelinated, which are sensitive to tension and pressure changes. There is also a rapidly adapting, myelinated Golgi tendon organ, which contributes to the control of the joint range of motion through neuromuscular inhibition. There is no innervation of the one-third central part of the meniscus.

Labrum

One of the static stabilizers of the joint, the labrum shows morphological changes according to the structural needs of the joint. It is located on both sides of the joint: the glenoid and acetabular labrum.

The glenoid labrum is a fibrocartilage structure that surrounds the edge of the glenoid fossa and also deepens the joint. The labrum continues with the joint capsule and attaches to the medial glenoid and the anatomical neck of the humerus (Fig. 3.18). The anterior and inferior parts of the labrum are smaller and weaker than the superior and inferior parts. The main tasks of the glenoid labrum are to increase the contact area between the humeral head and the scapula by expanding the surface area and depth of the fossa, to protect the intra-articular pressure (especially against traction forces), to keep the joint fluid in the joint space, to provide lubrication, and to increase the lubricity of the long head of the biceps brachii muscle. It provides a place of attachment to the joint capsule with ligaments. The vascular nutrition of the glenoid labrum occurs mainly where it makes a peripheral connection with the joint capsule. The self-repairing ability of the labrum is limited in these regions due to less vascular nutrition in the superior and anterosuperior regions.

The acetabular labrum is a "C"-shaped, complex fibrocartilage structure that connects to the edge of the acetabulum. It consists of the ilium, ischium, and pubis. Between the anterior horn and posterior horn attachment of the labrum is the transverse acetabular ligament. The capsular region of the labrum consists of type I and type III collagens, while the articular region consists of type I, type II, and type III collagens. Where the labrum meets the articular cartilage, the collagen fibers are located perpendicular to the junctional surface, except in the anterosuperior region. The parallel location of the collagen fibers in the anterosuperior region to the junction surface reduces the attachment strength of the labrum and causes labral tear pathologies to occur in this region. Thanks to the anatomical structure of the acetabular labrum: (1) the hip joint socket is deepened to stabilize the hip joint; (2) negative intra-articular pressure is provided; (3) deformation of the joint cartilage is prevented by dissipating the stresses coming from the joint; (4) by keeping the joint fluid in the central compartment between the joint surfaces, the friction force between the joint surfaces is reduced; (5) it plays an important role in the perception of proprioceptive and pain sensation; and (6) it helps in chondral nutrition by keeping the joint fluid in the central compartment.

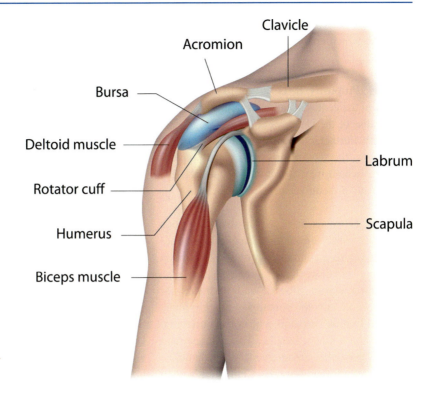

Fig. 3.18 Shoulder joint structures (Alila Medical Media/Shutterstock.com)

The nutrition of the acetabular labrum is provided by the superior and inferior gluteal arteries, the medial and lateral circumflex arteries, and the intrapelvic vascular system. However, its main nutrition is provided by the connective tissue located between the capsule and the capsular part of the labrum. The capsular part of the labrum is better nourished than the articular part. The innervation of the acetabular labrum is provided by branches of the femoral nerve and obturator nerves. The acetabular labrum contains many different mechanoreceptors and free nerve endings. *Krause* corpuscles are cold sensitive, while *Vater-Pacini*, *Golgi-Mazzoni*, and *Ruffini* corpuscles help in proprioception. Free nerve endings are sensitive to pain, temperature, and tactile sensations. Most of the sensory receptors (86%) are located on the articular surface of the labrum, particularly in the anterosuperior part of the chondrolabral junction. The diversity and numerical redundancy of these neural structures indicate that the labrum is important for proprioception and pain sensations.

Clinical Information
The high level of pain in patients with labral tears is attributed to the high density of mechanoreceptors in the anterosuperior and posterosuperior regions of the acetabulum.

Intervertebral Disk
There are 25 intervertebral disks in the human spine, 7 of which are in the cervical, 12 in the thoracic, 5 in the lumbar, and 1 in the sacral region. The inferior surface of the upper vertebral body and the superior surface of the lower vertebral body articulate with the intervertebral disk. The intervertebral disk constitutes approximately 25–30% of the spine length. It allows the vertebral column to be flexible while absorbing the forces acting on the vertebral column and preventing the vertebrae from rubbing against each other during movement. It consists of three main components: the inner *nucleus pulposus (NP)*,

the outer *annulus fibrosus (AP)*, and the *cartilage endplate*, which enable the disk to attach to the vertebrae.

Nucleus Pulposus It is a gel-like structure located in the center of the intervertebral disk. It is the cause of the vertebral column strength and flexibility. Further, 66–86% of the NP consists of water, with the remainder composed of type II collagen (which may also contain types VI, IX, and XI) and proteoglycans.

Annulus Fibrosus It is a ring-shaped fibrous connective tissue surrounding the NP. This structure consists of a combination of 15–25 lamella layers and contains collagen, proteoglycans, glycoproteins, elastin fibers, and extracellular matrix. Each lamella contains collagen fibers arranged in a 60° arrangement in the horizontal plane to the adjacent lamella. This arrangement provides a parallel arrangement of the lamellae and creates a "radial solid." Compared with a fully longitudinally aligned array, this array makes the annulus fibrosus more resistant to compression forces. Products such as automobile tires are inspired by this sequence. The lamellae are connected to each other via translamellar bridges. A balance exists between the number of translamellar bridges per unit area and strength and flexibility. More bridges provide greater resistance to compression forces and limit flexibility, or fewer bridges provide less resistance to compression forces and increase flexibility. The type I collagen content is higher in the outer layer of the annulus fibrosus, whereas the type I collagen content decreases, and the type II collagen content increases as it progresses toward the inner layers. The NP distributes the hydraulic pressure across the intervertebral disk. Thanks to the high water content of the nucleus pulposus, it can distribute the forces acting on the vertebral body in any direction to the entire structure. Considering the general arrangement of the AP fibers in the rostral–caudal direction, it resists the torsional, flexion, and extension movements of the spine. When considered holistically, the intervertebral disks support the spine and keep it flexible. Most intervertebral disks are avascular. The outer part of the AP shows vascular features. The vertebral body is fed by the vessels located at the bony disk junction. Two main ligaments support the intervertebral disk. The anterior longitudinal ligament, which covers the anterolateral surface of the vertebral column from the foramen magnum to the sacrum, prevents hyperextension and anterolateral herniation. Since the posterior longitudinal ligament covering the posterior surfaces of the vertebrae prevents posterior herniation of the intervertebral disks, most of the herniations occur in the posterolateral direction.

3.3 Conclusion

Although bone tissue is thought of as static, it is also dynamic with its soft tissue, endocrine system, and neurophysiological features. It is the key to the musculoskeletal system. Besides providing the functionality and mobility to the humans, it undertakes important tasks for homeostasis together with other important systems. It provides conditions that require mobility and stability by revealing different mechanics in terms of structure together with the joints.

Further Reading

Andrews SH, Adesida AB, Abusara Z, Shrive NG. Current concepts on structure–function relationships in the menisci. Connect Tissue Res. 2017;58(3–4):271–81.

Apostolakos J, Yang JS, Hoberman AR, Shoji M, Weinreb JH, Voss A, et al. Normal and pathological anatomy of the shoulder. In: Gregory İB, Eiji I, Giovanni DG, Hiroyuki S, editors. Glenoid labrum. Cham: Springer International Publishing; 2015. p. 83–91.

Brazill JM, Beeve AT, Craft CS, Ivanusic JJ, Scheller EL. Nerves in bone: evolving concepts in pain and anabolism. J Bone Miner Res. 2019;34(8):1393–406.

Cappariello A, Ponzetti M, Rucci N. The "soft" side of the bone: unveiling its endocrine functions. Horm Mol Biol Clin Investig. 2016;28(1):5–20.

Cervinka T, Sievanen H, Hyttinen J, Rittweger J. Bone loss patterns in cortical, subcortical, and trabecular compartments during simulated microgravity. J Appl Physiol. 2014;117:80–8.

Chen J, Hendriks M, Chatzis A, Ramasamy SK, Kusumbe AP. Bone vasculature and bone marrow vascular niches in health and disease. J Bone Miner Res. 2020;35(11):2103–20.

Hart NH, Nimphius S, Rantalainen T, Ireland A, Siafarikas A, Newton RU. Mechanical basis of bone strength: influence of bone material, bone structure and muscle action. J Musculoskelet Neuronal Interact. 2017;17(3):114–39.

Hartigan DE, Perets I, Meghpara MB, Mohr MR, Close MR, Yuen LC, et al. Biomechanics, anatomy, pathology, imaging and clinical evaluation of the acetabular labrum: current concepts. J ISAKOS. 2018;3(3):148–54.

Hassebrock JD, Gulbrandsen MT, Asprey WL, Makovicka JL, Chhabra A. Knee ligament anatomy and biomechanics. Sports Med Arthrosc Rev. 2020;28(3):80–6.

Haywood L, Walsh DA. Vasculature of the normal and arthritic synovial joint. Histol Histopathol. 2001;16(1):277–84.

Kapiński R, Jaworski L, Czubacka P. The structural and mechanical properties of the bone. J Technol Exploit Mech Eng. 2017;3(1):43–51.

Kraeutler MJ, Wolsky R, Vidal A, Bravman JT. Anatomy and biomechanics of the native and reconstructed anterior cruciate ligament: surgical implications. J Bone Jt Surg Am. 2017;99(5):438–45.

Kubo H, Gatzlik E, Hufeland M, Konieczny M, Latz D, Pilge H, et al. Histologic examination of the shoulder capsule shows new layer of elastic fibres between synovial and fibrous membrane. J Orthop. 2020;22:251–5.

Laumonerie P, Dalmas Y, Tibbo ME, Robert S, Durant T, Caste T, et al. Sensory innervation of the hip joint and referred pain: a systematic review of the literature. Pain Med. 2021;22(5):1149–57.

Markes AR, Hodax JD, Ma CB. Meniscus form and function. Clin Sports Med. 2020;39(1):1–12.

Mostafa HK. Structure and function of periosteum with special reference to its clinical application. Egypt J Histol. 2019;42(1):1–9.

Nilsson M, Sundh D, Mellström D, Lorentzon M. Current physical activity is independently associated with cortical bone size and bone strength in elderly Swedish women. J Bone Miner Res. 2017;32(3):473–85.

Ott SM. Cortical or trabecular bone: what's the difference? Am J Nephrol. 2019;47(6):373–6.

Rux D, Decker RS, Koyama E, Pacifici M. Joints in the appendicular skeleton: developmental mechanisms and evolutionary influences. Curr Top Dev Biol. 2019;133:119–51.

Storaci HW, Utsunomiya H, Kemler BR, Rosenberg SI, Dornan GJ, Brady AW, et al. The hip suction seal, part I: the role of acetabular labral height on hip distractive stability. Am J Sports Med. 2020;48(11):2726–32.

Waxenbaum JA, Reddy V, Futterman B. Anatomy, back, intervertebral discs. Treasure Island (FL): StatPearls Publishing; 2020.

Yao J, Lian Z, Yang B, Fan Y. Frontiers in orthopaedic biomechanics. In: Cheng-Kung C, Savio LYW, editors. Biomechanics of ligaments. Cham: Springer International Publishing; 2020. p. 75–87.

The Muscle Structure and Function

Mahmut Calik

Abstract

Skeletal muscles in the body are specialized structures for both stability and mobility functions. Understanding the function of muscles depends on understanding the structure of the muscle, from the contractile proteins within each muscle fiber to the organization of the fibers in the entire muscle. The important functions of the muscles in the body are as follows: (1) production of force, (2) maintaining posture and body position, (3) joint stabilization, (4) heat production, and (5) protecting internal organs.

Skeletal muscles have important roles in many bodily functions. From a mechanical point of view, the main functions of skeletal muscles are to generate strength and power, maintain posture, and convert chemical energy into mechanical energy for movement production. From a metabolic point of view, skeletal muscles serve as a storage site for important building blocks such as amino acids and carbohydrates. It also contributes to amino acid release from muscles and maintenance of blood glucose levels during fasting.

In this section, skeletal muscles are explained. At the end of the chapter, smooth muscle and cardiac muscle are also briefly mentioned.

M. Calik (✉)
Physiotherapy and Rehabilitation, Faculty of Health Sciences, Halic University, Istanbul, Turkey

4.1 Development of Muscle Tissue

The muscle tissue originates from the mesoderm, which is located between the ectoderm and the endoderm. Myoblasts, which are progenitor muscle cells, migrate to muscle-forming regions in the extremities and chest wall, where they form muscle fibers. The progenitor muscle cells fuse, and new cells are formed from the progenitor cells, containing hundreds of nuclei. Outside the cell membrane, satellite cells (stem cells) attach to myotubes and can transform into myotubes when regeneration is required. The number of satellite cells and the capacity of stem cells to transform into myotubes are limited.

4.2 Anatomy of Skeletal Muscles

4.2.1 Structure of Muscle Tissue

The muscle cell is a long, cylindrical, multinucleated, tubular structure with a length of several centimeters surrounded by a cell membrane called the sarcolemma. The sarcolemma surrounds the cytoplasm called the sarcoplasm. The sarcoplasm contains myofibrils, which are composed of myofilaments such as actin, myosin, troponin, and tropomyosin, and non-filamentous proteins.

Mitochondria are located between the myofibrils. The myofibrils are surrounded by the endoplasmic reticulum, called the sarcoplasmic reticulum, which stores calcium ions necessary for muscle contraction. The sarcoplasmic reticulum terminates in the terminal cisternae. Between the two terminal cisternae, a tubular fold of the sarcolemma called the transverse tubule (T-tubule) is present. Two terminal cisternae and a transverse tubule form a structure called the "triad." T-tubules signal the sarcoplasmic reticulum for the release of calcium ions. The structure of the muscle tissue is shown in Fig. 4.1.

4.2.2 Sarcomere

The sarcomere is the smallest functional unit of the muscle that can contract and is located in the myotubular system. Sarcomeres are attached to the cell membrane called the sarcolemma. A sarcomere consists of actin and myosin filaments. The diameter of myosin is about 15 nm, while the diameter of actin is about 5 nm. Many sarcomeres exist in the myotubular system, which gives the myotubular system a striated appearance. In the striped appearance, the dark-colored filament is myosin (*A* band), and the light-colored filament is actin (*I* band) (Fig. 4.2).

4.2.3 Components of Muscle Tissue

Skeletal muscles consist of contractile muscle tissue and non-contractile connective tissue. Muscle tissue can stretch in response to chemical, electrical, or mechanical stimuli, while connective tissue stretches against passive loading. The properties of these two structures and their relationship with each other form the unique structure of the muscles.

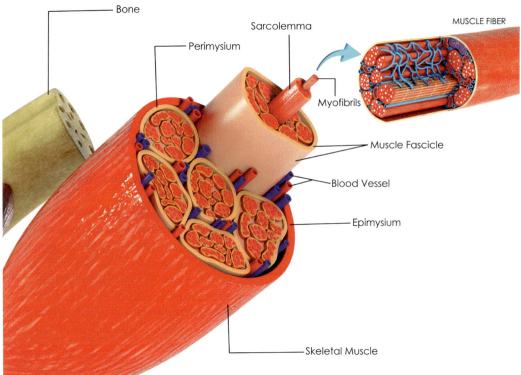

Fig. 4.1 Structure of muscle tissue (stockshoppe/Shutterstock.com)

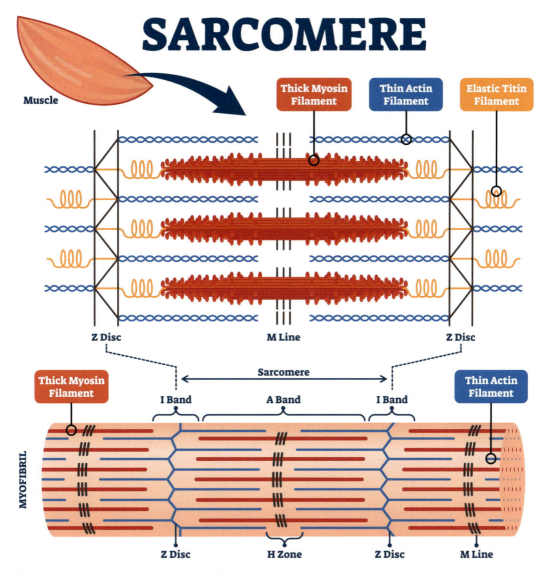

Fig. 4.2 Structure of sarcomere (VectorMine/Shutterstock.com)

4.2.3.1 Contractile Proteins

Skeletal muscle is made up of thousands of muscle fibers, whereas muscle fiber is made up of many tiny filaments called myofibrils. Myofibrils contain the contractile proteins of the muscle fiber and have a distinctive structure. Each myofibril is 1–2 μm in diameter and consists of multiple myofilaments. Myofibrils make up 80–90% of muscle volume. The two most important myofilaments in the myofibril are actin and myosin.

Muscles consist of many fascicles formed by the combination of muscle fibers (cells) surrounded by connective tissue. The arrangement, number, size, and type of these fibers can vary from muscle to muscle. Each muscle fiber consists of a single muscle cell surrounded by a cell membrane called the sarcolemma. Like other cells in the body, the muscle fiber is surrounded by a type of cytoplasm called sarcoplasm. The sarcoplasm consists of contractile myofibrils and non-myofibrillar structures such as ribosomes, glycogen, and mitochondria, which are essential for cell metabolism. The structure of the muscle fiber is shown in Fig. 4.3.

Fig. 4.3 Structure of muscle fiber (Blamb/Shutterstock.com)

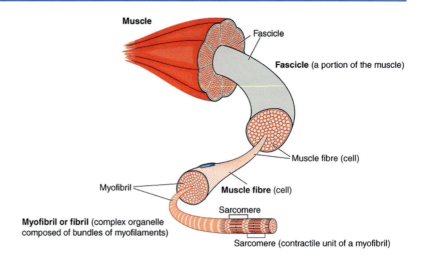

Myofibrils are composed of thick myofilaments called myosin and thin myofilaments called actin. The interaction between these two myofilaments is necessary for muscle contraction to occur. Thin myofilaments consist of two chain-like strings of actin molecules entangled. Troponin molecules are located between two actin strings, and tropomyosin binds to each troponin molecule. Troponin and tropomyosin molecules control the binding of actin and myosin myofilaments.

Each of the myosin molecules has spherical enlargements called myosin heads. The myosin head is the actin-binding site and is important in muscle contraction and relaxation. When viewed under the microscope, the arrangement of thick (myosin) and thin (actin) myofilaments shows a distinctive striated pattern. Therefore, skeletal muscles are often referred to as striated muscles.

The part of the myofibril between the two Z lines is called the sarcomere. Regularly spaced Z lines along the myofibril not only mark the borders of the sarcomere but also connect the thin filaments. The portion of the sarcomere that extends along the length of the thick filaments and a small portion of the thin filaments is called the A band. Areas containing only actin filaments are called I bands. The middle part of the thick filament, which does not overlap with the thin filaments, is called the H band, and the middle part of the H band is called the M line. The appearance of myofilaments during muscle contraction and relaxation is shown in Fig. 4.4.

4.2.3.2 Structural Proteins

Muscle fibers consist of some structural proteins. Some of these proteins provide the structural skeleton for the muscle fibers, while others are involved in the transmission of force along the muscle fibers and to neighboring muscle fibers. Titin, a structural protein, is important in maintaining the position of the thick filament during muscle contraction and providing passive tension. Titin is a large protein that binds along the thick filament and occupies the space from the thick filament to the Z line. The proteins found in skeletal muscles are summarized in Table 4.1.

4.2.4 Connective Tissues of Muscles

The extracellular connective tissues within the muscles are divided into three layers: epimysium, perimysium, and endomysium. The epimysium is a hard structure located in the outermost layer, surrounding the entire surface of the muscle body and separating it from other muscles. The epimysium gives the muscle body its shape and is made up of stretch-resistant collagen fibers. The peri-

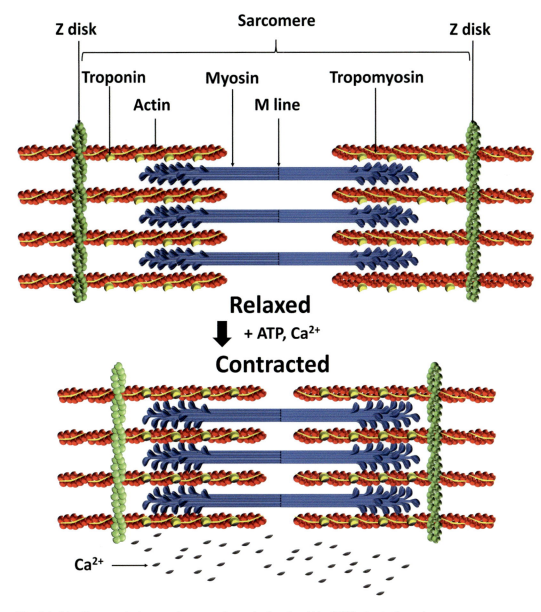

Fig. 4.4 Myofilaments during muscle contraction and relaxation (Akor86/Shutterstock.com)

mysium is located under the epimysium layer and surrounds the fascicles. The fascicles form a canalized structure for the passage of blood vessels and nerves in the perimysium. The connective tissue of the perimysium is hard and thick like the epimysium. Therefore, it is resistant to stretching. The endomysium is the innermost layer that surrounds the individual muscle fibers just outside the sarcolemma (cell membrane). The metabolic exchange between muscle fibers and capillaries takes place in the endomysium. The endomysium consists of dense collagen tissue and transmits some of the contraction force that occurs in the muscle to the tendon. The connective tissue of skeletal muscle is shown in Fig. 4.5.

Table 4.1 Important proteins in skeletal muscles and their functions

Protein	Function
Myosin heavy chain	Binds with actin to create contraction force
Actin	Connects with myosin via the cross-bridge to shorten the sarcomere during muscle contraction
Tropomyosin	Regulates the interaction between actin and myosin, and stabilizes actin myofilament
Troponin	Binds to tropomyosin; tropomyosin prevents myosin from binding with actin in the muscle's resting state, thus preventing contraction
Myosin light chain	Affects the rate of contraction of the sarcomere; regulates the movement of the cross-bridge loop
Nebulin	Runs parallel to actin and connects actin to the Z line
Titin	Titin is one of the largest known proteins; acts as a skeleton that holds the actin and myosin myofilaments in place; provides passive tension within the sarcomere
Desmin	Forms a lattice around the sarcomere at the level of the Z line; they are attached to each other and to the plasma membrane; desmin forms cross-links between neighboring myofibrils
Skelemin	Helps fix the position of the *M* lines
Dystrophin	Provides the structural stability of the cytoskeleton and muscle fibers
Integrins	Stabilizes the cytoskeleton

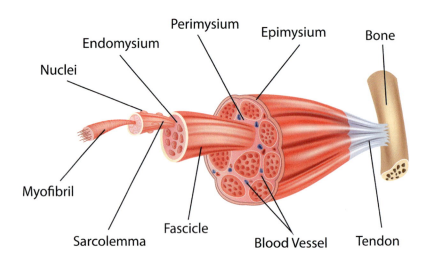

Fig. 4.5 Connective tissue of skeletal muscle (Teguh Mujiono/Shutterstock.com)

4.2.5 Motor Unit

Although the sarcomere is the basic unit of contraction in the muscle, it is actually part of a larger structure called the motor unit. A motor unit consists of an alpha motor neuron and all the muscle fibers innervated by this motor neuron. The stimulus that initiates the contraction process of the muscle fibers is transmitted through the alpha motor neuron. The cell body of the neuron is located in the anterior (ventral) horn of the spinal cord. The axon of the nerve cell extends from the cell body to the muscle, where it divides into many small branches. Each of the minor branches terminates at a motor endplate close to the sarcolemma of a single muscle fiber. All muscle fibers stimulated by a branch of the axon, the cell body of the nerve, and the axon are part of the motor unit.

The contraction of the whole muscle occurs when many motor units fire at different times and again. The magnitude of its contraction depends on the number of motor units activated or the frequency range. The number and structure of motor units in a muscle vary from muscle to muscle.

The motor units vary according to the size of the cell body of the motor neuron, the diameter of the axon, the number of muscle fibers, and the fiber type. Each of these features affects the function of the motor unit. The cell bodies of the motor neuron differ in diameter from each other. The smaller the cell body diameter, the smaller the axon diameter. Therefore, a stimulus reaches the muscle fibers later in a motor neuron with a small axon diameter than in a motor neuron with a larger axon diameter.

The number of muscle fibers within the motor unit is highly variable. Some motor units have only a few muscle fibers, while some motor units have thousands of muscle fibers. Generally, the motor units of the muscles that provide fine motor movements and hence the number of muscle fibers is small. The motor units of the muscles provide gross motor movements and require more force production for movement; therefore, the number of muscle fibers is larger. The motor units of the muscles that control eye movements contain about 10 muscle fibers, while the gastrocnemius muscle has motor units containing about 2000 muscle fibers. In addition, the total number of motor units in a muscle also differs from muscle to muscle. For example, the platysma muscle has small motor units, each consisting of about 25 muscle fibers, but the muscle has about 1000 of these motor units. The gastrocnemius muscle has large motor units, each consisting of about 2000 muscle fibers, but the muscle has about 600 of these motor units.

4.3 Types of Muscle Fibers

The myoblasts develop into myocytes after fusion, which occurs before birth. The muscle cells continue to differentiate and grow into slow-twitch (type I muscle fibers) and fast-twitch fibers (type II muscle fibers). These fibers differ in terms of protein content, energy requirement, and functions. Muscle fibers have three high-energy phosphate sources: creatine phosphate, glycogen, and glucose.

4.3.1 Type I Muscle Fibers (Slow-Twitch Fibers, Slow Oxidative Fibers, and Red Fibers)

Type I muscle fibers have a slower rate of contraction and less developed glycolytic capacity than type II muscle fibers. It uses glycogen as an energy source. Adenosine triphosphatase (ATPase), the enzyme that breaks down adenosine triphosphate (ATP) into phosphate and adenosine diphosphate (ADP), has low activity and a slow cleavage rate. Slow-twitch fibers have many and large mitochondria densities. They are resistant to fatigue because they contain a large amount of myoglobin (bind and store O_2). The slow-twitch fibers are supplied by many capillaries. They are also called red muscle fibers due to their high myoglobin content. Type I fibers can contract 10–30 times per second. The slow-twitch fibers are needed for long-term exercise and endurance activities. Type I fibers are especially found in postural muscles, and the training of these fibers is needed in athletes who do sports that require endurance.

4.3.2 Type II Muscle Fibers (Fast-Twitch Fibers)

The fast-twitch fibers are capable of rapid propagation of action potentials across the sarcolemma. They have the ability to degrade ATP and rapidly use the calcium released from the sarcoplasmic reticulum. The fast-twitch fibers use the short-term glycolytic energy system and can generate two to three times the contraction force of slow-twitch fibers. They can contract 30–70 times per second. Type II muscle fibers are differentiated by the presence of myosin isoforms. Type II muscle fibers in humans are of three subtypes: type IIa, type IIx, and type IIb.

Type IIa muscles fibers (red fibers, rapidly oxidative, fatigue resistant) contain a large number of myoglobin, mitochondria, glycogen, and capillaries. They have a high capacity to produce ATP through oxidation. They break down ATP quickly and have a high contraction rate. They have lower fatigue resistance than slow oxidative fibers. Type IIa fibers move five times faster than type I fibers. Type IIx fibers (fast-twitch, fast-glycolytic, white fibers) have a fast contraction time, low myoglobin and capillary counts, moderate-density mitochondria count, and multiple creatine phosphate stores. Their resistance to fatigue is moderate. The main energy store of type IIb fibers is creatine phosphate. They have few mitochondria and capillaries. Their oxidative capacity is low. Type IIb fibers are innervated by large-diameter motor neurons and therefore contract rapidly. They are activated in anaerobic activities that take less than a minute but require high power. They are very active, especially during ballistic exercises. Type IIb fibers contract ten times faster than type I fibers and are usually activated in athletes who perform sports requiring high speed. The properties of muscle fibers are summarized in Table 4.2.

Clinical Information
Increasing the ratio of type I muscle fibers in a muscle increases the oxygen utilization capacity, that is, aerobic power and endurance. An increase in type II muscle fiber ratio increases anaerobic power, that is, explosive power. Muscles with high type II muscle fiber density are advantageous in sports requiring power and speed, and muscles with high type I muscle fiber density are beneficial in sports requiring endurance. During muscle training in the clinic, the fiber type density of the muscles should be considered.

4.3.3 Muscle Fiber Type and Training

In skeletal muscles, four types of muscle fibers (types I, IIa, IIx, and IIb) coexist in different proportions. In adults and children who do not exercise regularly, the muscle fiber type distribution is approximately 55% type I and 45% type II. Whether a certain type of exercise can change the type of muscle fibers in a muscle is still controversial. It has been shown that after high-intensity endurance training, oxidative capacity in type IIb fibers improves, which is achieved by an increase in the size and number of mitochondria, but with no change in fiber type. Endurance-enhancing activities such as running and swimming cause the gradual conversion of type IIb fibers into type IIa fibers. In type IIb fibers transformed in this way, the muscle fiber diameter shows a slight increase in strength with the number of mitochondria and capillaries.

Clinical Information
Muscle hypertrophy is the increase in the diameter and volume of muscle fibers due to various factors such as nutrition and exercise.
Muscle atrophy is the decrease in the diameter and volume of muscle fibers due to factors such as aging and inactivity.
Muscle hyperplasia is an increased number of muscle fibers and does not occur in a healthy skeletal muscle.
Muscular dystrophies are a progressive, degenerative, and inherited disorder. Duchenne and Becker are the most common types. They are caused by the absence of dystrophin in myofibrils as a result of mutation of the gene responsible for encoding dystrophin. Examples are skeletal muscle atrophy and weakness.

Table 4.2 Structural and functional features of muscle fibers

Feature	Type I	Type IIa	Type IIx	Type IIb
Contraction rate	Slow	Fast	Fast	Very fast
Relaxation time	Slow	Fast	Fast	Very fast
Motor neuron diameter	Small	Medium	Large	Very large
Resistance to fatigue	High	Very high	Moderate	Low
Mitochondrial density	Very high	High	Medium	Low
Capillary density	High	Medium	Low	Low
Oxidative capacity	High	High	Medium	Low
Glycolytic capacity	Low	High	High	High
Storage energy source	Triglyceride	Creatine phosphate and glycogen	ATP, creatine phosphate, and glycogen	ATP and creatine phosphate
Activity	Aerobic	Long-term anaerobic	Short-term anaerobic	Short-term anaerobic
Force generation	Low	Moderate	High	Very high
Energy efficiency	High	Low	Low	Very low
Nerve conduction velocity	Slow	Fast	Fast	Very fast
Muscle fiber diameter	Small	Large	Large	Large
Amount of myoglobin	High	High	Moderate	Low
Motor neuron volume	Small	Large	Large	Very large
Motor neuron threshold	Low	High	High	Very high
Sarcoplasmic reticulum density	Low	High	High	High
Creatine phosphate reservoir	Low	High	High	High
Glycogen store	High	High	High	High
Triglyceride store	High	Moderate	Moderate	Low
Myosin ATPase activity	Low	High	High	High
Glycolytic enzyme activity	Low	High	High	High
Oxidative enzyme activity	High	High	High	Low

4.4 Innervation of Skeletal Muscle

The innervation of skeletal muscles is provided by motor nerves. Basically, the motor nerves emerge from the anterior horn located in the vertebrae. The nerve roots emerging from the cervical and lumbar regions form the brachial plexus in the cervical region and the lumbo-sacral plexus in the lumbo-sacral region. The motor nerves arising from the brachial plexus are the median, ulnar, radial, musculocutaneous, axillary, thoracodorsal, subscapular, and lateral pectoral nerves. These nerves are responsible for the innervation of the muscles around the upper extremity and scapula. The motor nerves emerging from the lumbo-sacral plexus are the iliohypogastric, genitofemoral, femoral, sciatic, and obturator nerves. These nerves provide innervation to the muscles around the lower extremities and pelvis. The trunk muscles are innervated by the nerves originating from the thoracic region. The innervation of skeletal muscles is shown in Fig. 4.6.

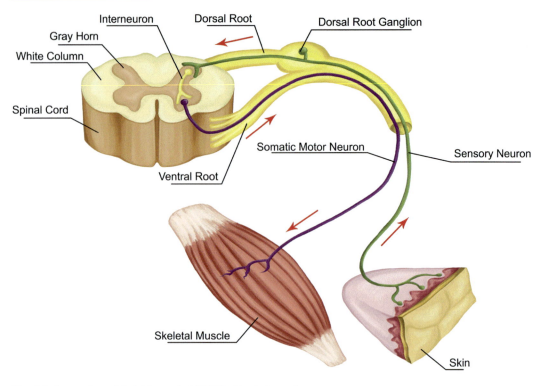

Fig. 4.6 Innervation of skeletal muscle (stihii/Shutterstock.com)

4.5 Blood Supply of Skeletal Muscles

A wide vascular network supplies blood to the skeletal muscles. The main arteries supplying the muscles are distributed along the long axis of the muscles and travel in the epimysium layer of the muscles. The main arteries then branch off into arterioles and enter the perimysium layer of the muscles and run perpendicular to the muscle fibers. The arteriole branches then divide into multiple terminal branches at the endomysium. The terminal branches are the last branches containing vascular smooth muscle. The circulation of skeletal muscle varies according to many factors such as age, sex, race, muscle fiber type, and exercise. The control of blood supply to skeletal muscles is regulated by the autonomic nervous system.

Clinical Information

The sympathetic nervous system (SNS) has an effect on the precapillary sphincters in the vessels entering the muscles. The sympathetic nervous system is active in homeostasis, whereas vasodilation occurs in the precapillary sphincters. Thus, the blood circulation in the muscle tissue increases. However, when the SNS is overactive, vasoconstriction occurs in the precapillary sphincters. In this case, the cardiac output and blood pressure increase, but blood cannot enter the muscle sufficiently through the narrowed vessel. In this case, the circulation of the muscle is adversely affected. If excessive activation of central nervous system (CNS) in the autonomic nervous system continues for a long time, pain (usually burning type) due to circulatory failure and a decrease in the elasticity of the connective tissue may occur.

4.6 Muscle Architecture

Most skeletal muscles have nearly equal proportions of fast-twitch and slow-twitch fiber types. Therefore, the determination of muscle function does not depend only on muscle fiber distribution. In fact, the architecture of the entire muscle may be more important than the fiber type in determining muscle function. The skeletal muscle architecture is related to the angle the fibers make with the force axis (pennation angle), muscle fiber length, muscle length, muscle mass, and physiological cross-sectional area (PCSA). These structural differences affect not only the overall shape and size of the muscles but also the function of the skeletal muscles.

The two most important architectural features that affect muscle function are muscle fiber length and PCSA. The fiber length (or the number of sarcomeres along the fibers) directly determines the amount of muscle fiber shortening or lengthening. A long muscle fiber with more sarcomere can shorten at a greater distance than a short muscle fiber. For example, if muscle fibers can shorten to about 50% of their resting length, a 6-cm-long muscle fiber can shorten by 3 cm. The significance of this is that a muscle with long fibers can move the bone to which it attaches for a longer distance than a muscle with short fibers. However, the relationship between muscle fiber length and the range of motion of the bone to which the muscle attaches is not always directly related. The alignment of the muscle fibers and the length of the moment arm of the muscle affect the length-shortening relationship, and therefore both fiber length and moment arm must be considered.

The PCSA is a measure of the cross-sectional area of the muscle perpendicular to the direction of alignment of the muscle fibers. The amount of force produced by a muscle is directly proportional to the number of sarcomeres lined up side by side or in parallel. Therefore, having a large number of muscle fibers located in a muscle, or increasing the size of the fibers (with the addition of myofibrils), as in pennate muscle, increases its capacity to produce force. A good example of the relationship between muscle structure and function is the comparison between the quadriceps and hamstring muscles. The quadriceps muscle has a larger PCSA, while the hamstring muscle has longer fibers. This architectural structure shows that the quadriceps muscle is designed for force generation and the hamstring muscle is designed for movements requiring a greater range of motion. Since most hamstring muscles span two joints (hip and knee), longer muscle fibers are required during both hip and knee movements.

The arrangement of the fascicles differs between the muscles. The fascicles may be located parallel to the long axis of the muscles as in fusiform muscles or at an angle to the long axis of the muscle as in unipennate, bipennate, and multipennate muscles. Muscles that have a parallel fiber arrangement (parallel to the long axis of the muscle and to each other) are called fusiform muscles. In fusiform muscles such as the sternocleidomastoid or sartorius muscle, the fascicles are long and run along the muscle. In general, fusiform muscles with a parallel fiber arrangement have longer fibers and therefore produce a greater range of motion than muscles with a pennate fiber arrangement.

The muscles whose fiber array connects to the long axis of the muscle at an oblique angle are called pennate muscles. The fibers that make up the fascicles in the pennate muscles are generally shorter and numerous than those in most fusiform muscles. In unipennate muscles such as the flexor pollicis longus, the obliquely located fascicles attach at similar angles to only one side of the central muscle tendon. In bipennate muscles such as the biceps femoris and tibialis anterior, the fascicles are located obliquely on either side of the central tendon. In multipennate muscles such as the soleus or subscapularis, the oblique fascicles converge on several tendons. The angle of pennation of the muscle fibers in the pennate muscle reduces the amount of force produced along the long axis of the muscle. The more obliquely a fiber extends to the long axis of the muscle, the less the force the muscle can exert. This reduction in muscle strength is a function of the cosine of the pennation angle. Many skeletal muscles have a pennation angle of less than 30°. Therefore, the muscle strength in the tendon is reduced by no more than 13% (cos 30° = 0.87). As the muscle shortens during muscle contraction and joint movement, the angle of pennation becomes more oblique, potentially more affecting the force transmitted to the tendon. However, this potentially reduced force in the tendon is offset by an increase in PCSA due to the increased number of muscle fibers in the pennate muscles.

4.7 Types of Muscle Contraction

4.7.1 Isometric Contraction

Isometric contractions are contractions with no visible joint movement. The muscle tone increases, but the length of the muscle does not change. The isometric training can be done at different joint angles by varying the contraction duration/intensity. The isometric contraction is very important in providing joint stabilization.

4.7.2 Concentric Contraction

It is a type of contraction based on the principle of shortening the length of the muscle to create a movement. The sliding of thin filaments over thick filaments and the formation of cross-bridges at each sarcomere create muscle fiber shortening and tension. If enough sarcomeres are actively shortened and one or both ends of the muscle fiber move freely, the muscle fiber shortens. During concentric contraction, the distance between the origin and the insertion decreases. The force released by the muscles is greater than the external force exerted on the muscles.

4.7.3 Eccentric Contraction

It is a type of contraction that occurs with the increasing length of the muscles. During an eccentric contraction, the distance between the origin and the insertion increases. The force applied to the muscles is greater than the internal force generated by the muscles. Eccentric contraction occurs when the force produced inside the muscle is less than the force applied externally to the muscle, causing an actively controlled elongation of the muscle fibers under load. During an eccentric contraction, maximum force is released during a maximal eccentric contraction, since high loading occurs due to the nature of the contraction. This feature allows training with light weights. Eccentric contraction is characterized by high power generation and low energy expenditure compared with concentric and isometric contractions. Eccentric exercise is the best type of exercise for muscle hypertrophy, muscular force generation, and neural activity. However, it is the most commonly used type of exercise in treating tendinopathy.

4.8 Muscle Contraction Theories

4.8.1 Sliding Filament Theory

This theory explains the sliding motion of thin filaments (actin) over thick filaments (myosin). Before the myosin head binds to actin, it cleaves ATP into ADP and inorganic phosphate (Pi). When myosin binds to actin, the actin–myosin–ADP–Pi complex is formed. The myosin heads make a 90° angle at first binding to actin. When the inorganic phosphate is separated from the myosin head, the angle of the myosin head with the neck decreases from 90° to 50°. Cross-bridges are established between actin and myosin filaments, resulting in a power stroke, and the filaments slide over each other. The amount of force produced within the sarcomere depends on the number of simultaneously formed cross-bridges. As the number of cross-bridges increases, the force produced within the sarcomere also increases. When the ADP separates from the myosin head, the angle of the myosin head with the neck decreases to 45° and the sliding process is completed.

4 The Muscle Structure and Function

As the filaments slide over each other, the two Z lines converge and the sarcomere becomes shorter. The length of the *H* and *I* bands becomes shorter, while the length of the *A* band does not change. The actin–myosin complex remains the same at a 45° angle until a new ATP molecule attaches to the myosin head. With ATP rebinding, the myosin head slowly separates from actin. The sliding filament theory is summarized in Fig. 4.7.

4.8.2 Winding Filament Hypothesis

The rotating filament hypothesis assumes that actin undergoes rotation in addition to the sliding motion of actin on myosin. As titin binds to thick filaments in the *A* band and thin filaments in the *Z* lines, the rotation of thin filaments by cross-bridges causes titin to be wound into thin filaments. The rotation of the thin filaments by the

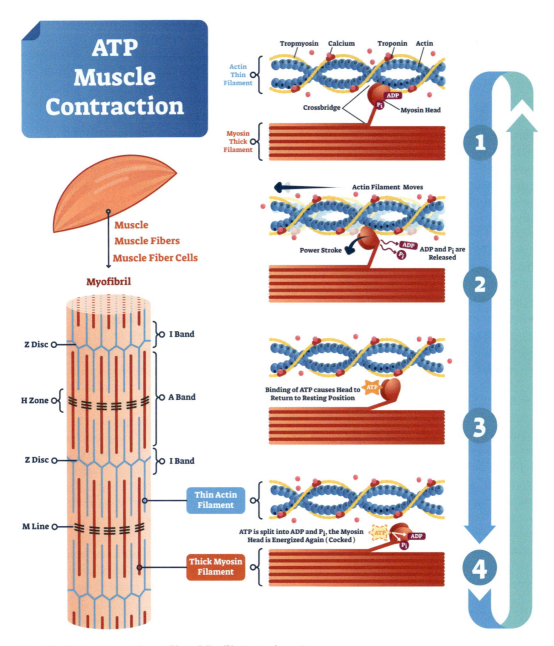

Fig. 4.7 Sliding filament theory (VectorMine/Shutterstock.com)

cross-bridges produces an alpha-actin rotating torque in the Z line. By winding titin on thin filaments, the length and stiffness of the proline–glutamate–valine–lysine (PEVK) region of titin change, and elastic potential energy is stored during isometric muscle contraction and active stretching. This energy can be recovered during active shortening.

The binding of titin to actin abolishes low-strength flattening of immune globulin (Ig) domains proximal to the *I* band caused by the prolonged passive tension of myofibrils. The PEVK segment elongates strongly by stretching the sarcomeres activated by the binding of calcium (Ca^{2+}) to thin filaments. If Ca^{2+} binding between titin and thin filaments can be avoided, active force generation is reduced at short sarcomere lengths. In this case, the contribution of titin to the total active force decreases.

Despite active stretching in the muscles, no movement occurs in the proximal Ig part, and only the PEVK region is stretched. The PEVK segment is stiffer than the proximal immune globulin (Ig) part due to its structure, and the amount of elastic potential energy stored during stretching in the PEVK segment is much higher. In addition, the available evidence shows that the increase in the rotator force during eccentric contraction is due to the activation of titin.

Consequently, the rotating filament hypothesis provides a simple mechanism by which titin contributes to muscle strength development and active shortening of the PEVK segment. This hypothesis is consistent with the structural and viscoelastic properties of the sarcomere in general and titin in particular. The rotating filament hypothesis is important in explaining isometric and eccentric muscle contraction processes, thanks to the function of the titin protein. This hypothesis is based on the sliding filament theory and adds to the explanatory power of this theory. It is not an alternative to the sliding filament theory.

4.9 Other Factors Affecting Muscle Function

4.9.1 Joint Type and Position of the Muscle Relative to the Joint

Since the type of joint directly affects the type of movement (flexion, extension, and rotation) and the range of motion in the joint, it also affects the function of the muscle that produces movement in the joint.

The muscles that make opposite movements to the same joint are called agonist–antagonist muscle pairs. The balance between these muscle pairs is one of the important criteria for the stabilization of the joint. Deviations from normal between agonist–antagonist pairs can create muscle imbalance in the joint. This may cause a risk of injury. For example, weakness of the hip external rotators can lead to excessive internal rotation and strength imbalance in the hip joint during activities such as running and walking. Appropriate strength ratio between agonist–antagonist muscles must be within the treatment goals after joint, muscle, and tendon injuries.

4.9.2 Sensory Receptors

The motor control depends on the coordination of motor pathways descending from the cortex, muscle movements, and a continuous flow of sensory information transmitted to the central nervous system. Many specialized receptors located around the joint are important in providing sensory input. The receptors located in the joint capsule and ligaments around the joint affect muscle activity through the signals they carry to the central nervous system. The injuries to the joint capsule or ligaments cause reflex inhibition of the muscles. The best example of this is reflex inhibition in the quadriceps femoris muscle after anterior cruciate ligament injury. Besides the specialized receptors found in the structures around the joint, two important sensory receptors exist in the muscles: the muscle spindle and the Golgi tendon organ (GTO).

4.9.2.1 Muscle Spindle

They are the largest mechanoreceptors found in the human body. They are a few millimeters (mm) long and about 0.2 mm in diameter. They are sensory proprioceptors that provide information about the length of the muscle. They consist of four to eight specialized intrafusal muscle fibers lying parallel to the extrafusal muscle fibers. They are more in the muscles that provide postural control.

4.9.2.2 Golgi Tendon Organ (GTO)

They are sensory proprioceptors located at the muscle–tendon junction. Approximately 94% of the receptors are located at the muscle–tendon junction, while 6% are located on the tendon. The GTO is sensitive to tension and can be activated by active muscle contraction or by excessive passive stretching of the muscle. When an excessive tension occurs, GTO is stimulated and informs the motor cortex and inhibition occurs. The fast-twitch muscles have more GTOs than slow-twitch muscles.

4.10 Other Muscle Types

4.10.1 Smooth Muscle

They are muscles found in internal organs or blood vessels. The smooth muscles cannot be voluntarily stimulated. Their activation is controlled by the autonomic nervous system (sympathetic and parasympathetic systems). The smooth muscle cells are spindle-shaped and much smaller than striated muscle cells. The smooth muscle does not have sarcomeres. Thin and thick filaments corresponding to actin and myosin filaments in striated muscle are found in bundles. The smooth muscles also lack troponin and tropomyosin. The contraction of smooth muscles occurs by the formation of cross-bridges between thick and thin fibers, as in striated muscle.

4.10.2 Cardiac Muscle

Unlike skeletal muscle cells, cardiac muscle cells contract on their own (autonomously) and continue to contract rhythmically throughout life. Cardiac muscle cells are Y-shaped and shorter and wider than skeletal muscle cells. They are generally mononuclear. The sarcoplasmic reticulum is less developed in cardiac muscle. The calcium ions necessary for the contraction of cardiac muscle fibers are supplied not only from the sarcoplasmic reticulum but also from the extracellular space, as in smooth muscle cells. The cardiac muscle cells cannot be stimulated at high frequencies, thus preventing tetanic contractions. More details on the anatomy and physiology of the heart muscle are covered in the section "Exercise Physiology."

4.11 Conclusion

The muscles are structures having important functions in our body. The concepts such as muscle structural features, anatomy, muscle fiber types, architectural features, and contraction mechanisms must be well understood to understand the function of muscle tissues. In this section, muscle structure and function are explained functionally for physiotherapists.

Further Reading

Celichowski J, Krutki P. Motor units and muscle receptors. In: Zoladz JA, editor. Muscle and exercise physiology. New York: Academic Press; 2019. p. 51–91.

Csapo R, Gumpenberger M, Wessner B. Skeletal muscle extracellular matrix—what do we know about its composition, regulation, and physiological roles? A narrative review. Front Physiol. 2020;11:253.

Finsterer J. Locomotor principles: anatomy and physiology of skeletal muscles. In: Jensen-Jarolim E, editor. Comparative medicine anatomy and physiology. Vienna: Springer; 2014. p. 45–60.

Frontera WR, Ochala J. Skeletal muscle: a brief review of structure and function. Calcif Tissue Int. 2015;96(3):183–95.

Gillies AR, Lieber RL. Structure and function of the skeletal muscle extracellular matrix. Muscle Nerve. 2011;44(3):318–31.

Hunter SK, Brown DA. Muscle: the primary stabilizer and mover of the skeletal system. In: Neumann DA, editor. Kinesiology of the musculoskeletal system: foundations for rehabilitation. 3rd ed. Amsterdam: Elsevier; 2016. p. 47–76.

Monroy JA, Powers KL, Gilomre LA, Uyeno TA, Lindstedt SL, Nishikawa KC. What is the role of titin in active muscle? Exerc Sports Sci Rev. 2012;40:73–8.

Mukund K, Subramaniam S. Skeletal muscle: a review of molecular structure and function, in health and disease. Wiley Interdiscip Rev Syst Biol Med. 2020;12(1):e1462.

Purslow PP. The structure and role of intramuscular connective tissue in muscle function. Front Physiol. 2020;11:495.

Schiaffino S, Reggiani C. Fiber types in mammalian skeletal muscles. Physiol Rev. 2011;91:1447–531.

Trovato FM, Imbesi R, Conway N, Castrogiovanni P. Morphological and functional aspects of human skeletal muscle. J Funct Morphol Kinesiol. 2016;1(3):289–302.

# The Nerve Structure and Function

Cetin Sayaca

Abstract

In this chapter, information is given about the anatomical structure of the nervous system and nerve cells. The nervous system is discussed under two main headings as the central and peripheral nervous system. Under the heading of the central nervous system, information is given about the brain, medulla spinalis, meninges, and the vessels that feed the central nervous system. The peripheral nervous system is investigated separately in terms of anatomical and functional aspects. In addition, the anatomical structure of the nerve cell and other cells of the nervous system are also mentioned.

5.1 Nervous System

The nervous system monitors the changes that occur inside and outside the body, carries the obtained information from one part of the body to another, and creates appropriate responses. It is responsible for perception, behavior, and memory, plans, initiates, and terminates movements. It is divided into the central nervous system (CNS) and the peripheral nervous system (PNS). While the brain and its extension, the medulla spinalis, form the CNS, all nerve structures outside of this system form the PNS. The structures that form the nervous system are given in Fig. 5.1.

5.1.1 Central Nervous System

The main task of the CNS is to integrate all the information that comes to it, to perceive the events that take place, and to conclude with adaptive behavior to all kinds of changes. Information from the peripheral nervous system is transmitted to the coded areas that are associated with them; all obtained information is combined. The final information obtained is transmitted to the appropriate central nervous system area for a response. Finally, from here, a stimulus is sent to the target organ for the formation of the appropriate response, and the most appropriate response is provided against the information obtained.

5.1.1.1 Brain

An adult human brain consists of more than 100 billion nerve cells and neurons. 90% of these cells make up of glial cells. The brain is the common name for six anatomical structures in CNS. These anatomical structures are the medulla oblongata, pons, midbrain, cerebellum, diencephalon, and cerebrum (Fig. 5.2).

C. Sayaca (✉)
Physiotherapy and Rehabilitation, Faculty of Healthy Sciences, Bursa Uludag University, Bursa, Turkey
e-mail: cetinsayaca@uludag.edu.tr

© The Author(s), under exclusive license to Springer Nature Switzerland AG 2023
D. Kaya Utlu (ed.), *Functional Exercise Anatomy and Physiology for Physiotherapists*,
https://doi.org/10.1007/978-3-031-27184-7_5

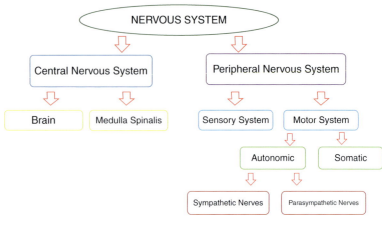

Fig. 5.1 Central nervous system and parts

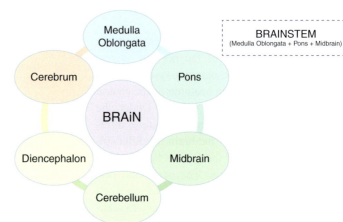

Fig. 5.2 Anatomical structures that make up the brain

Cerebrum

It is the largest structure among that form the brain. It consists of two parts, gray and white matter. The grey matter is formed by neuronal cell bodies while the white matter is formed by the axons. The cerebral cortex is divided into two hemispheres. There are recesses (sulcus) and protrusions (gyrus) formed to expand the surface area in both hemispheres. The hemispheres communicate with each other through the corpus callosum, which is composed of axons (Fig. 5.3). The central sulcus, which is one of the important anatomical structures in the brain, is an important and decisive recess. The lobe in the front of this sulcus is the frontal lobe, and it performs the motor function, which is the main output of the brain. The parietal, temporal, and occipital lobes located behind this sulcus are the structures responsible for the sensory function of the brain. These lobes receive incoming sensory information, process it, and transmit it to the frontal lobe.

Diencephalon

It is the name given to all of the thalamus, hypothalamus, epithalamus, and subthalamus structures located between the cerebrum and midbrain (Fig. 5.3). The thalamus consists of nearly 80% of the diencephalon. The thalamus is the center of call for all senses that go to the cerebrum, except for the sense of smell. The thalamus, which consists of gray matter, is responsible for transmitting sensations to the relevant cerebral areas. The hypothalamus is the structure just anterior–inferior to the thalamus and just above the hypophysis (pituitary gland). The hypothalamus controls body temperature, hunger, thirst, circadian rhythm, and strong emotional responses by

Fig. 5.3 Side view of the structures that make up the central nervous system (Hank Grebe/Shutterstock.com)

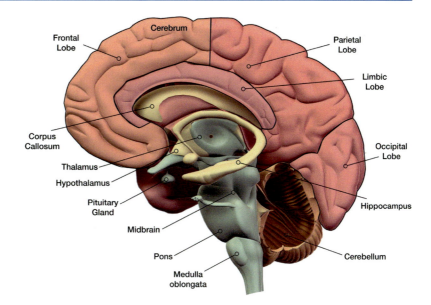

affecting the autonomic nervous system and endocrine system.

Brainstem
The medulla oblongata, pons, and midbrain together are defined as the brainstem. They are responsible for the control of emotional responses given in situations such as circulation, respiration and fear–anxiety, modulation of pain, formation of voice, and regulation of consciousness and sleep cycle. It is directly connected to the cerebrum, basal ganglia, diencephalon, cerebellum, and spinal cord. It is an important structure where the third and 12th cranial nerves (except for a part of the accessory cranial nerve) are located (Fig. 5.3).

Cerebellum
Cerebellum means small brain in Latin. Through the connections it has at different levels, it controls the functions of other anatomical structures of the CNS. The most important function is to control and coordinate the movement by comparing it with purpose. It provides precise control of movement within milliseconds. The cerebellum controls and regulates by making a copy of all motor impulses given from the cerebrum and comparing it with proprioceptive information from the periphery (Fig. 5.3).

> **Clinical Information**
> Not all sensations that pass through the thalamus are transmitted to the sensory cortex. Some of these senses are transmitted to the motor cortex. In this way, it is possible to obtain a motor response from sensory stimulation. The central gyrus is also called the sensorimotor cortex since the motor response can be obtained with the senses.

> **Clinical Information**
> When the control of motor movement is considered at the hierarchical level, the upper centers have inhibition characteristics in order to control the lower centers. After the damage that removes the control of the upper centers, increased excessive activation is seen in the lower centers. The lower centers, which are freed from the control of the upper centers, have a non-functional and increasing uncontrolled activity.

5.1.1.2 Medulla Spinalis

The medulla spinalis (MS) is an extension of the brain. It is responsible for the emergence of rapid and reflexive responses and the continuation of stability in the face of warnings. It also takes part in the transmission of sensory stimuli from the environment to the upper centers and the motor responses from the upper centers to the target organ. While MS has the same length as the spinal canal until the 12th week of intrauterine life, it ends at the level of the third lumbar vertebra at birth and at the level of the first lumbar vertebra in adults. There are several important lines that define MS externally. These are the anteromedian fissure, posteromedian sulcus, anterolateral sulcus, posterior median sulcus, and posterolateral sulcus (from anterior to posterior).

In the cervical region, the transverse diameter of MS is larger than the anteroposterior diameter. Due to this size, it is oval in shape. In the thoracic and lumbar regions, it is round in shape.

The cross-sectional area of MS in the cervical region is greatest due to the density of ascending and descending tracts, while it is smallest in the thoracic region. Ventral and dorsal nerve roots are occurred by the combination of six to eight small nerve fibers. Small nerve fibers that appear from the posterolateral sulcus create the dorsal nerve root. Small nerve fibers that appear from the anterolateral sulcus create the ventral nerve root (Fig. 5.4).

MS is divided into two areas, the white and the gray zone. The white region is an area where the axons of the descending, ascending, and proprioceptive pathways are located. Anatomically, it is divided into three funicles anterior, lateral, and posterior, and functionally, it is divided into three main pathways descending, ascending, and proprioceptive. Axons of the propriospinal tracts originate from nerve cells located in the gray area of the spinal cord. The gray area is an "H" or butterfly-shaped area where the nerve cell bodies are located. It is roughly divided into anterior and posterior horns. There is also a small lateral horn located between T12–L2. The gray area is divided into 10 subregions called the lamina. Laminas and their properties are given in Table 5.1.

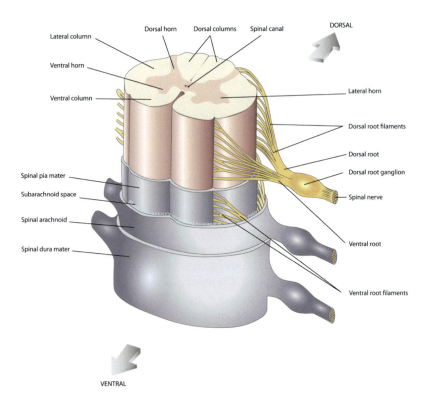

Fig. 5.4 Medulla spinalis (Vasilisa Tsoy/Shutterstock.com)

Table 5.1 Laminas in the gray area of the spinal cord and its features

Lamina area	Features
Lamina I	Pain and heat
Lamina II	Substantia gelatinosa, responsible for all stimuli, sends information to lamina III–IV
Lamina III–IV	Vibration and pressure
Lamina V	Stimuli from the skin, muscle, and skin mechanoreceptors and visceral nociceptors
Lamina VI	Flexor response to painful stimulus
Lamina VII	Numerous interneurons and propriospinal neurons are involved in the movement, reflexes, and autonomic functions
Lamina VIII	Proprioceptive and interneurons, regulation of motor movement
Lamina IX	Motor neurons that excite skeletal muscle
Lamina X	Consists of cells located around the central canal. Axons cross from one side to the other

> **Clinical Information**
>
> While the frontal lobe, located in front of the central sulcus in the cerebrum, is responsible for motor output, the parietal, temporal, and occipital lobes located behind it are nervous system structures that receive and process sensory input and send it to the frontal lobe for motor output. The anterior horn cells in the medulla spinalis have motor character, while the posterior horn has sensory. Similarly, the anterior part of the thalamus is related to motor functions, while the posterior part is related to sensory functions.
>
> While the structures in the anterior part of the central nervous system are responsible for motor movement in general, the structures in the posterior part show a topographic location related to the senses.

5.1.1.3 Meninges

Meninges are the outermost membrane layer that surrounds and protects the central nervous system. The meninges consist of three layers, from the outside to the inside, the dura mater, the arachnoid mater, and the pia mater (Fig. 5.5). The dura mater is the outermost layer of the meninges. There are two layers in the cerebral region, and the outermost layer covers the inner surface of the skull bones and acts as a periosteum. Its inner layer covers the entire CNS, including the spinal cord. The inner layer of the dura mater also forms dense folds that prevent and support the mobility of the brain between both hemispheres (falx cerebri) and between the hemispheres and the cerebellum (tentorium cerebelli). In addition, there are spaces called venous sinuses that provide venous blood flow to the brain within the dura mater. The arachnoid mater is thin and transparent, similar to a spider web. It fuses with the dura mater at the level of the second sacral spine. Between the arachnoid and the pia mater, there is the subarachnoid space that has cerebrospinal fluid. The pia mater is the innermost delicate and thin structure that adheres to the brain and spinal cord structures. It contains many small blood vessels. At the level the spinal cord ends, it forms the filum terminale. The filum terminale extends to the level of the sacral second vertebra.

There are three important gaps between the meninges and the bone tissue. These are (I) the epidural space between the bone tissue and the dura mater, (II) the subdural space between the dura mater and the arachnoid mater, and (III) the subarachnoid space between the arachnoid mater and the pia mater. The subarachnoid space contains cerebrospinal fluid (CSF) and major blood vessels. Anatomical spaces between the meninges are shown in Fig. 5.6.

> **To Learn Easily**
>
> In order to learn the order of the membranes surrounding the CNS, the initials can be combined and coded as DAP, from outside to inside.

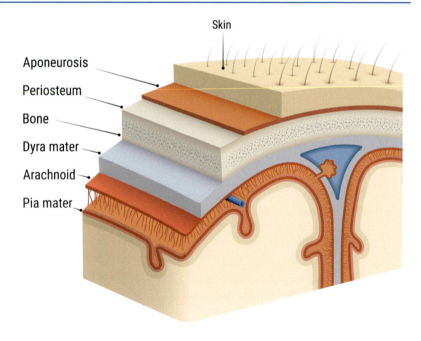

Fig. 5.5 Meninges (Danilina Olga/Shutterstock.com)

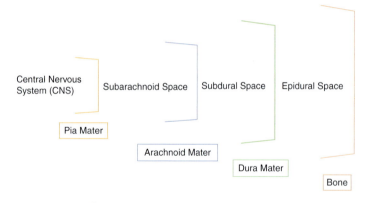

Fig. 5.6 Meninges and spaces between the meninges

5.1.1.4 Vessels Feeding the Central Nervous System

The spinal cord is supplied by branches from the vertebral and segmental arteries. The vertebral artery gives off the anterior and sometimes posterior spinal artery branches. The anterior spinal artery supplies the anterior 2/3 of the spinal cord, including the anterior and lateral funiculus. The remaining 1/3 of the spinal cord (the posterior funiculus) is supplied by the posterior spinal artery. Segmental arteries are the main arteries that provide nutrition in the thoracic and lumbar regions where the spinal arteries begin to become insufficient.

CNS structures other than the medulla spinalis are supplied by the right and left internal carotid and vertebral arteries coming from both sides. Both vertebral arteries join to form the basilar artery. While the posterior cerebral artery is the most important branch of the basilar artery, the anterior and middle cerebral arteries and the anterior and posterior communicating arteries are the most important branches of the internal carotid artery.

The anterior–posterior communicating, anterior–posterior cerebral, and internal carotid arteries anastomose with each other to form Willis Polygon. Willis Polygon gives branches that feed the lower surface of the diencephalon and mesencephalon (Fig. 5.7).

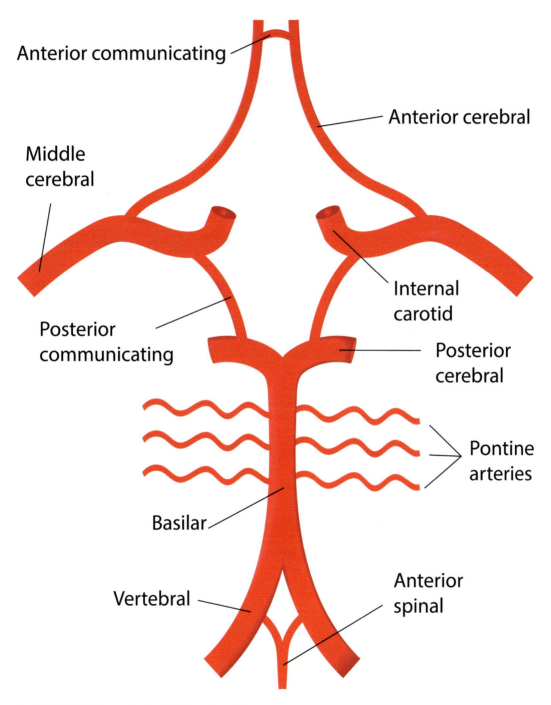

Fig. 5.7 Willis Polygon (joshya/Shutterstock.com)

5.1.2 Peripheral Nervous System

While the PNS consists of three different structures anatomically, cranial nerves, spinal nerves, and autonomic nervous system, it consists of sensory (afferent) and motor (efferent) nerve fibers functionally (Fig. 5.8). While the sensory nerve fibers transmit the impulses from the organs to the CNS, the motor nerve fibers transmit the impulses occurring in the CNS to the skeletal muscle, internal organs, and tissues. Sensory nerve fibers constitute the majority of nerves in the PNS. Motor nerve fibers are divided into somatic and autonomic nerve fibers. Somatic nerve fibers provide contraction of skeletal system muscles, while autonomic nerve fibers provide contraction of cardiac and smooth muscle fibers.

5.1.2.1 Anatomical Peripheral Nervous System

Cranial Nerves
Although it is generally accepted that there are 12 pairs of cranial nerves in the human body, there are also studies that define the terminal cranial nerve as the "0th" or "13th" cranial nerve. This cranial nerve has been described since 1914, especially in the late 1980s called the 0th cranial nerve. It is associated with the gonadotropin-releasing hormone and is thought to play a role in reproductive and behavioral control.

Cranial nerves are named according to their distribution or function. They are located on the inferior surface of the brain and are numbered from top to bottom in the order of attachment to the brain (Fig. 5.9). The names of the cranial nerves, their classification according to their functions, and their functions are given in Table 5.2.

> **To Learn Easily**
> The trochlear nerve (4th) is responsible for the motor stimulation of the oblique superior muscle (SO), the abducens nerve (6th) is responsible for the motor stimulation of the rectus lateralis (RL) muscle, and the oculomotor nerve (3rd) is responsible for the motor stimulation of the remaining eye muscles. It can be formulated as (SO_4-RL_6) $Other_3$.

> **Clinical Information**
> In the cranial nerve examination, it should be noted that while the afferent stimulation of the face is provided by the trigeminal nerve (5th), the efferent stimulation is provided by the facial nerve (7th).

> **Clinical Information**
> The light reflex is evaluated by means of a light source held in the eye. The optic nerve (2nd) is responsible for the afferent stimulation of the light reflex, and the oculomotor nerve (3rd) is responsible for the efferent stimulation. Even if the light is applied to only one eye, constriction occurs in both pupils due to bilateral stimulation.

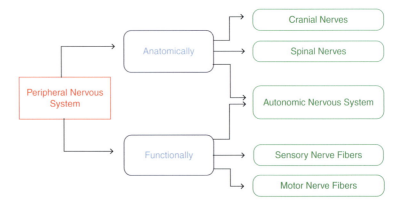

Fig. 5.8 Structures constituting the peripheral nervous system

> **Clinical Information**
> Corneal reflex, the eye is closed when the lateral cornea is touched with the cotton ball while the patient is looking outward and upward. The trigeminal nerve (5th) is responsible for the afferent stimulation of this reflex, and the facial nerve (7th) is responsible for the efferent stimulation.

> **Clinical Information**
> The gag reflex is a motor movement that occurs when the base of the tongue or the pharynx is touched by an abeslang (abaisse langue)-like object. Afferent stimulation is provided by the glossopharyngeal nerve (9th), while the vagus nerve (10th) is responsible for efferent stimulation (motor response). It should be considered that this reflex, which is important in the evaluation of the cranial nerves responsible for swallowing function, may not be present in approximately 40% of even healthy individuals.

Spinal Nerves

They are the nerves that provide communication between the CNS and receptors, muscles, and glands. There are 31 pairs of spinal nerves in the human body, these are 8 cervical, 12 thoracic, 5 lumbar, 5 sacral, and 1 coccygeal. Both ventral and dorsal nerve roots are presented at all levels, with the exception of the first spinal nerve located in the cervical region. In the first spinal nerve, the ventral nerve root is found in everyone, while the dorsal nerve root is found in only 46% of people. Only 28% of individuals with a first dorsal nerve root have a spinal ganglion.

Ventral (motor) and dorsal (sensory) roots emerging from the medulla spinalis unite in the intervertebral canal to form spinal nerves. After the spinal nerves emerge from the intervertebral foramen, they divide into three branches: anterior, posterior, and communicans rami. The posterior branch is responsible for the stimulation of the muscles and skin at the back of the trunk. The anterior branch is responsible for the stimulation of the muscles and skin of the extremities, the anterior-lateral parts of the neck, and the back by forming plexuses. Communicans rami take charge as a part of the autonomic nervous system (Fig. 5.10). The anterior branches of the spinal nerves, with the exception of the thoracic region, expand bilaterally in five regions and mix with each other, and form structures called plexuses. These are cervical (C1–4), brachial (C5–T1), lumbar (T12–L4), sacral (L4–S4), and coccygeal (S3–5) plexuses, from top to bottom.

Autonomic Nervous System

The autonomic nervous system is responsible for body regulatory activities such as blood pressure, heart rate, body temperature, and glandular function. The autonomic nervous system is divided into two subgroups, the sympathetic and parasympathetic nervous systems. While the sympathetic nervous system regulates body functions in a stressful mood, the parasympathetic nervous system regulates body functions in a relaxed mood. The parasympathetic nervous system is the "rest and recovery" system and is distributed throughout the body by the vagus nerve, which is the tenth cranial nerve. The sympathetic nervous system, on the other hand, is described as the "flight, fear, war" system as it distributes to the body from the ganglia located in the anterolateral part of the thoracolumbar spine. The structural differences between the sympathetic and parasympathetic nervous systems are shown in Table 5.3 and their functions are shown in Fig. 5.11. A third autonomic nervous system called the enteric nervous system has been also described to emphasize the strong brain and gut

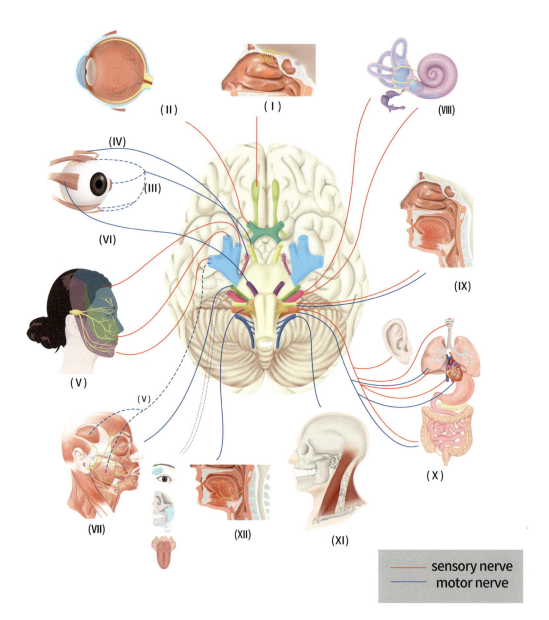

Fig. 5.9 Cranial nerves and target organs (Chu KyungMin/Shutterstock.com)

5 The Nerve Structure and Function

Table 5.2 Classification and functions of cranial nerves

Cranial nerve	Classification according to function	Responsible function
0. Terminal (Nulla) nerve	Sense + Autonomous	• Smell • Transmission of the sense of smell to the limbic areas (amygdala, hypothalamic nuclei) • Secretion of gonadotropin hormones from the hypothalamus
1. Olfactory nerve	Sense	• Smell
2. Optical nerve	Sense	• Vision • Forms the afferent pathway of the pupillary light reflex
3. Oculomotor nerve	Motor + Autonomous	• It stimulates four of the six muscles that move the eyeball (m. rectus medialis, superior, inferior, and obliquus inferior) and the levator palpebrae superior muscle, which lifts the upper eyelid • Parasympathetic fibers form the efferent pathway of the light reflex, constricting the pupil
4. Trochlear nerve	Motor	• Stimulation of the obliquus superior muscle
5. Trigeminal nerve	Sense + Motor	• Stimulation of chewing muscles • Sensory stimulation of the face, anterior scalp, and paranasal sinuses • All sensory stimulation of the anterior two-thirds of the tongue except taste • Afferent innervation of the corneal reflex
6. Abducens nerve	Motor	• Stimulation of the rectus lateralis muscle
7. Facial nerve	Sense + Autonomous + Motor	• Stimulation of all facial muscles • Sense of taste from the anterior two-thirds of the tongue • Motor stimulation of the corneal reflex • Stimulation of parasympathetic fibers, submandibular and sublingual salivary glands from the major salivary glands
8. Vestibulocochlear nerve	Sense	• Responsible for hearing and balance
9. Glossopharyngeal nerve	Sense + Autonomous + Motor	• Sense of taste from the posterior one-third of the tongue • Motor innervation of the stylopharyngeus muscle • Parasympathetic stimulation of the parotid, the largest salivary gland
10. Vagus nerve	Sense + Autonomous + Motor	• Sensory innervation of the supraglottic region • Innervation of the muscles that provide the function of all pharyngeal and vocal cords except the stylopharyngeus muscle • Parasympathetic innervation of all thoracic and abdominal cavity organs
11. Accessory nerve	Motor	• Innervation of the sternocleidomastoid and trapezius muscles
12. Hypoglossal nerve	Motor	• Innervation of tongue muscles

relationship. The ganglia in this nervous system are also called "small brains" because they have a large number and complex organization.

> **Clinical Information**
> When autonomic nerve fibers are injured, the nutritional and metabolic activities of the tissues are disrupted. This disorder is more prominent in the distal tissues (hand and foot). The skin is pale, thin, dry, and shiny. In addition, the nails are brittle and sweating is not observed.

5.1.2.2 Functionally Peripheral Nervous System

Sensory (Afferent) Nerve Fibers

They are responsible for the continuous transmission of the information collected about the current situation to the CNS, both from the environment in which the body is located and through the receptors in the body. Sensory fibers enter the spinal cord from the posterior root and are carried to the upper centers (Fig. 5.12). Receptors are divided into special (photoreceptors on the retina, taste receptors on the tongue,

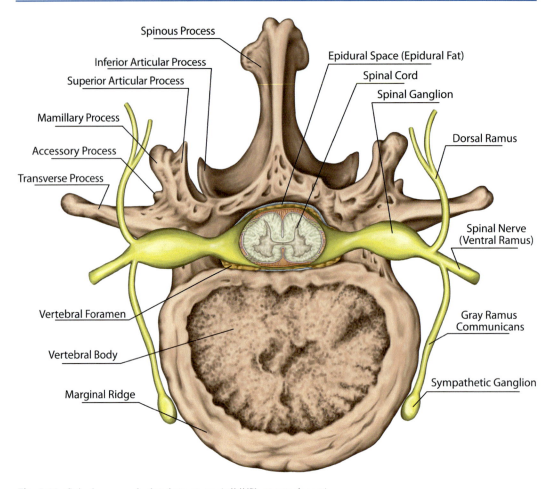

Fig. 5.10 Spinal nerve and related structures (stihii/Shutterstock.com)

Table 5.3 Structural differences between the sympathetic and parasympathetic nervous systems

	Sympathetic nervous system	Parasympathetic nervous system
Exit zones from the CNS	Thoracolumbar region	Craniosacral region
Active state	In stressful situations	In the absence of stress
Neurotransmitter	Acetylcholine norepinephrine	Acetylcholine
Where the ganglia are located	Outside of the CNS but in a nearby area	Near or in the target organ
Length of nerve fibers	Short preganglionic fibers Long postganglionic fibers	Long preganglionic fibers Short postganglionic fibers

etc.) and general receptors scattered throughout the body. The overall receptor density varies according to body regions. For example, cutaneous receptors are more concentrated on the soles of the feet and toes. Since the damage to the receptors will cause a decrease in sensory information, it may also cause a decrease in motor performance. Because the CNS sends appropriate engine commands to the target, thanks to the notification it receives.

Motor (Efferent) Nerve Fibers
Motor nerve fibers are divided into somatic and autonomic nerve fibers. While somatic nerve fibers provide contraction of skeletal system muscles, autonomic nerve fibers provide contrac-

Nervous system

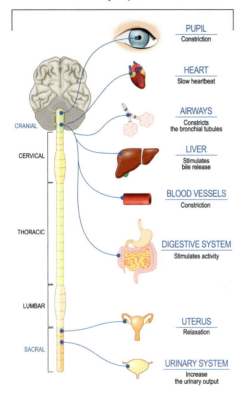
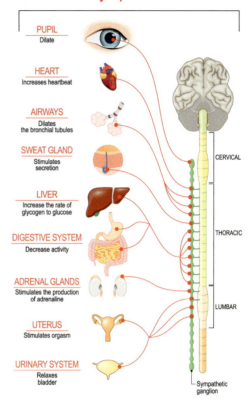

Fig. 5.11 Autonomic nervous system and its functions (Designua/Shutterstock.com)

Fig. 5.12 Sensory (afferent), motor (efferent), and autonomic nerve fibers (stihii/Shutterstock.com)

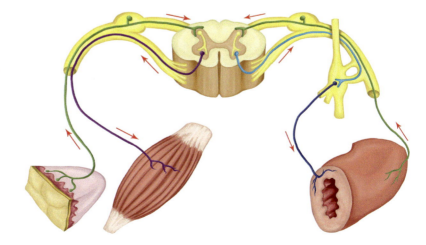

tion of cardiac and smooth muscle fibers. The CNS, by evaluating the feedback it received, transmits the appropriate motor commands it creates to the muscles via the cranial and spinal nerves that form the somatic nerve fibers, thus ensuring that appropriate responses are revealed (Fig. 5.12).

Autonomic Nerve Fibers
Above is mentioned under the title of "*Anatomically Peripheral Nervous System*" (Fig. 5.12).

> **Clinical Information**
> In peripheral nerve injuries, atrophy occurs especially after the first 3 months. Muscle fibers are replaced by fibrous connective tissue. If the nerve is not healed, the fibrous connective tissue covers all the muscle fibers, and the function is irreversibly lost.

> **Clinical Information**
> It contains afferent–efferent, myelinated–unmyelinated, and autonomic–somatic nerve fibers in a peripheral nerve. Autonomic fibers are both afferent and efferent, stimulating organs, blood vessels, and glands. All these structures are mixed in the nerve fiber.

> **Clinical Information**
> The nerve fiber starting from the anterior horn motor cell and the muscle fibers stimulated by this nerve fiber are called motor units. While each muscle fiber is stimulated by one motor neuron, a motor neuron can stimulate more than one muscle fiber. Small motor neurons and a few muscles fiber that are stimulated by these small motor neurons are called *small motor units*. Large motor neurons and a large number of muscle fibers that are stimulated by these large motor neurons are called *large motor units*.

Anterior horn motor cells responsible for fine motor movements stimulate 5–20 muscle fibers, while anterior horn motor cells responsible for gross motor movements, stimulate 100–500 muscle fibers. Not all motor units in a muscle are the same size. In this way, it is possible to gradually increase muscle strength. When a muscle starts to contract with increasing force, small motor units are activated first, and as the stimulation increases, the muscle's contraction force increases by activating large motor units. This situation continues until all the motor units in the muscle are stimulated, and the muscle reaches the highest strength value. Since movements that require fine dexterity require little force–high control, the onset of contraction from the small motor units allows this control to occur correctly.

5.2 Anatomical Structure of Nerve Cell

Nerve cell (neuron) is the smallest functional structure of the nervous system and consists of three parts: cell body, dendrite, and axon. Each nerve cell receives input from another nerve cell or cells and sends output to the other nerve cell or cells. The only exception to this rule is nerve cells that are connected to sensory receptors and muscle fibers.

Dendrites and axons together are called nerve fibers. The cell body consists of the cell nucleus and the cytoplasm. It provides protein synthesis and the healthy functioning of the cell. It is especially concentrated in the gray matter of the CNS. It is responsible for the analysis, consolidation, and storage of information. Dendrites have many branches and have most of the surface area of the nerve. It is responsible for collecting and transmitting information to the cell body. The axon may be less than 1 mm in length or more than 1 m in length and may have many terminal branches. It is responsible for transmitting information directly to the cell body. Axons have different names and conduction rates according to their functions (Table 5.4). Dendrites and axons appear white from myelin and form white matter in the CNS.

Spinal nerves are surrounded by three layers of protective connective tissue. These layers are named as endoneurium, perineurium, and epineurium from the inside out (Fig. 5.13).

Table 5.4 Classification of axons according to their functions

Functionally axon type	Axon type	Transmission speed (m/s)	Function
Sensory (afferent) nerve fibers	Ia	70–120	Deep sense from muscle spindles
	Ib	70–120	Deep sense from the Golgi tendon organ
	II	30–70	Touch, pressure, vibration
	III	12–30	Temperature, touch, pressure, and rapidly transmitted pain
	IV	0.5–2	Slow transmitted pain
Motor (efferent) nerve fibers	Alpha	15–120	Extrafusal muscle fiber
	Gamma	10–45	Intrafusal muscle fiber
	Preganglionic autonomic nerve fiber	3–15	Myelinated preganglionic autonomic nerve fibers, autonomic ganglion
	Postganglionic autonomic nerve fiber	2	Unmyelinated postganglionic autonomic nerve fibers, target organ (organs, blood vessels, glands)

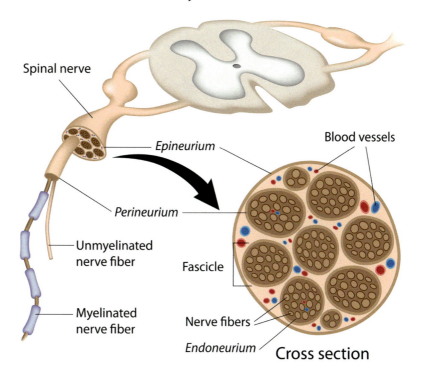

Fig. 5.13 The structure of the spinal nerve fiber (Alila Medical Media/Shutterstock.com)

5.3 Other Cells in the Nervous System

Apart from nerve cells, glia cells are another main cell type found in the CNS. The quantity of glia cells is more than three times the quantity of neuron. There are three types of glia cells: astrocytes, microglia, and oligodendrocytes (Fig. 5.14).

Astrocytes are the most various and numerous cell types in the CNS. They are cells that maintain brain homeostasis, provide physical and metabolic support to the nervous system, and regulate the extracellular space. One of its most important tasks is to regulate synaptic transmission. Microglia cells are the main phagocytic cells of the CNS. Together with astrocytes, they regulate inflammatory processes in the neuroimmune system and undertake a defense function against pathological conditions. Oligodendrocytes, on the other hand, synthesize and form the myelin sheath surrounding axons and increase nerve conduction velocity 10–100 times.

The myelin sheath is produced by Schwann cells in the peripheral nervous system. The myelin sheath surrounds the axon in layers. The greater the thickness of the myelin sheath, the greater the nerve conduction velocity. The myelin sheath is interrupted by structures called the node of Ranvier in every 1–2 mm. In this way, the transmission allows to be transmitted faster by

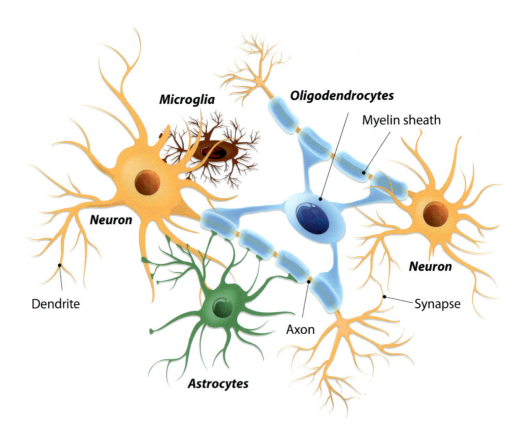

Fig. 5.14 Other cells forming the nervous system (Designua/Shutterstock.com)

jumping. The cells between the two nodes of Ranvier are surrounded with only one Schwann cell. These cells are also surrounded by the endoneurium.

5.4 Hierarchical Structure of Anatomical Structures Responsible for Motor Response in the Nervous System

The upper centers in the nervous system try to keep it under control by inhibiting the lower centers. There are alpha and gamma motor neurons, afferent nerves that carry information from the muscles, and the spinal reflex system at the bottom of the hierarchy in the motor system. These structures can reveal primitive movements independent of the upper centers.

The brainstem is found just above the spinal reflex system. It is essential to regulate the posture in accordance with the changing conditions independently. Posture is kept by spinal and vestibular afferent inputs. In sudden changes in environmental conditions, adaptation to the new situation is achieved with sudden body movements. Here, the main task of the upper centers is to regulate the postural responses of the system in conscious movements and to ensure that the responses given to the suddenly changing environmental conditions emerge in a more controlled manner. If the control of the cerebrum is completely lost, responses such as decortication and decerebration rigidity occur.

The structures that come after the brain stem in the motor hierarchy are the primary motor and sensory cortex. These areas are responsible for basic movements that occur without thought. Above these areas are the premotor, supplementary, and sensory areas located behind the primary sensory cortex. These areas are responsible for the emergence of complex movements that are not as simple as those controlled by the primary motor and sensory cortex but do not require thinking.

The top of the motor hierarchy is consisting of the prefrontal cortex and the parietal, occipital, and temporal association areas. This is the area where the cause–effect relationship is established, which requires reflection before the emergence of the movement. It controls all simple or complex movements made with short or long-term thinking before the motor movement is revealed. The priority is the act of thought to reveal the cause-and-effect relationship (Fig. 5.15).

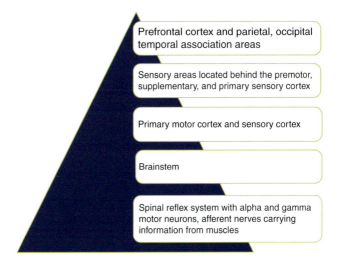

Fig. 5.15 Nervous system structures responsible for the motor hierarchy

5.5 Conclusion

The nervous system differs anatomically and physiologically due to the important functions it undertakes in the human body. The main purpose of all these differences is to perform all the tasks undertaken by the nervous system quickly and completely. In order for the function to occur flawlessly, the entire nervous system must be healthy both anatomically and physiologically. In this chapter, the anatomy of the nervous system has been tried to be organized functionally for physiotherapists.

Further Reading

Abernethy B, Kippers V, Hanrahan S, Pandy M, Mcmanus A, Mackinnon L. Biophysical foundations of human movement. Champaign: Human Kinetics Publishers; 2012. p. 219–23.

Armour JA. Potential clinical relevance of the 'little brain' on the mammalian heart. Exp Physiol. 2008;93:165–76.

Barha CK, Nagamatsu LS, Liu-Ambrose T. Basics of neuroanatomy and neurophysiology. In: Rosano C, Ikram MA, Ganguli M, editors. Handbook of clinical neurology. Amsterdam: Elsevier; 2016. p. 53–68.

D'Angelo E. Physiology of the cerebellum. Handb Clin Neurol. 2018;154:85–108.

Diaz E, Morales H. Spinal cord anatomy and clinical syndromes. Semin Ultrasound CT MR. 2016;37(5):360–71.

Ertan H, Bayram I. Fundamentals of human movement, its control and energetics. In: Angin S, Simsek IB, editors. Comparative kinesiology of the human body. London: Academic Press; 2020. p. 29–45.

Farley A, Johnstone C, Hendry C, McLafferty E. Nervous system: part 1. Nurs Stand. 2014a;28(31):46–51.

Farley A, Johnstone C, Hendry C, McLafferty E. Nervous system: part 3. Nurs Stand. 2014b;28(33):46–50.

Ghannam JY, Al Kharazi KA. Neuroanatomy, cranial meninges. Treasure Island (FL): StatPearls Publishing; 2020.

Halassa MM, Fellin T, Haydon PG. The tripartite synapse: roles for gliotransmission in health and disease. Trends Mol Med. 2007;13:54–63.

Hendry C, Farley A, McLafferty E, Johnstone C. Nervous system: part 2. Nurs Stand. 2014;28(32):45–9.

Karemaker JM. An introduction into autonomic nervous function. Physiol Meas. 2017;38:89–118.

Ruchalski K, Hathout GM. A medley of midbrain maladies: a brief review of midbrain anatomy and syndromology for radiologists. Radiol Res Pract. 2012;2012:1–11.

Sciacca S, Lynch J, Davagnanam I, Barker R. Midbrain, pons, and medulla: anatomy and syndromes. Radiographics. 2019;39:1110–25.

Seira Oriach C, Robertson R, Stanton C, Cryan J, Dinan TG. Food for thought: the role of nutrition in the microbiota–gut–brain axis. Clin Nutr Exp. 2016;6:25–38.

Shafique S, Rayi A. Anatomy, head and neck, subarachnoid space. Treasure Island (FL): StatPearls Publishing; 2020.

Sonne J, Reddy V, Lopez-Ojeda W. Neuroanatomy, cranial nerve 0 (terminal nerve). Treasure Island (FL): StatPearls Publishing; 2020.

Standring S, Gray H. Gray's anatomy: the anatomical basis of clinical practice. Edinburgh: Churchill Livingstone; 2008. p. 1551.

Tubbs RS, Loukas M, Slappey JB, Shoja MM, Oakes WJ, Salter EG. Clinical anatomy of the C1 dorsal root, ganglion, and ramus: a review and anatomical study. Clin Anat. 2007;20(6):624–7.

Waugh A, Grant A. Ross and Wilson anatomy and physiology in health and illness. 13th ed. Edinburgh: Churchill Livingstone; 2018. p. 153–206.

Weber D, Harris J, Bruns T, Mushahwar V. Anatomy and physiology of the central nervous system. In: Horch K, Kipke D, editors. Neuroprosthetics theory and practice. 2nd ed. Singapore: World Scientific Publishing Company; 2017. p. 40–103.

The Fascia and Movement

Atilla Cagatay Sezik and Ebru Gul Sezik

Abstract

Fascia surrounds the whole body without any interruption, divides organs or muscles into compartments, and connects them to each other. It works in coherence with all body systems during movement. Although fascia has been known since ancient times, fascia has been overlooked and ignored among other structures until the last decades. Superficial fascia—which hinders important structures—aponeurotic fascia and epimysium—which hinder access to the muscles—has been considered as structure that needs to be removed or cut. Even though the definition of fascia has conflicted ideas for years, studies are ongoing to determine a common language. Many researchers have defined fascia as only a passive, dense, sheet-like tissue. On the contrary, fascia has a broader scope: both as an anatomical structure and a body system. Currently, fascia is accepted as a mechanically active, highly innervated and dynamic system. In this chapter, fascia and its relationship with movement, the effects of the fascial system on the organization of movements as well as the dysfunctions that occur when fascia loses consistency will be explained.

6.1 Fascia and Fascial System

The definition of fascia has undergone many modifications. The definition currently is made with two different approaches. The anatomical definition states that fascia is a sheet-like connective tissue that forms and determines the histological and topographic structure. The tissue separates, connects and packs the muscles and organs. In the second definition, also called the fascial system is defined as structures that show the functional properties of the fascia at macroscopic levels. The fascial system has three-dimensional continuity and consists of soft, collagen-containing, loose, or dense fibrous connective tissue. The fascial system is composed of adipose tissue, adventitia, neurovascular sheaths, aponeuroses, deep and superficial fascia, epineurium, joint capsules, ligaments, membranes, meninges, myofascial extensions, periosteum, retinaculum, septa, tendons, visceral fascia and all intramuscular and intermuscular endomysium, perimysium and epimysium. These structures bind tissues together by wrapping around organs, muscles, bones and nerves, and filling in between. They form the functional structure that

A. C. Sezik (✉)
Physiotherapy and Rehabilitation, Faculty of Health Sciences, Yuksek Ihtisas University, Ankara, Turkey
e-mail: cagataysezik@yiu.edu.tr

E. G. Sezik
Physiotherapy and Rehabilitation, Faculty of Health Sciences, Ankara Medipol University, Ankara, Turkey
e-mail: ebru.sezik@ankaramedipol.edu.tr

creates an environment for all systems to work together in an organized manner.

6.2 Structure and Types of Fascia

Fascia is examined under three headings from an anatomical point of view: visceral, superficial and deep. Visceral fascia surrounds internal organs and keeps them under tension. Superficial fascia supports surrounding tissues. Deep fascia encloses or compartmentalizes muscles and transmits forces.

Fascia mainly consists of collagen fibres. Collagen types and their fibre arrangements determine the stiffness and tensile strength of the tissue (Fig. 6.1). Fibroblasts produce collagens in response to mechanical loads. Deep fascia transmits forces due to the parallel arrangement of strong collagens. However, superficial fascia shows high flexibility due to disorganized, weak collagen and elastin structure.

6.2.1 Visceral Fascia

There are two distinctly different visceral fascia types that have different properties. The first type shows a close relationship with the internal organs and gives shape to them. Besides being elastic and thin, they contain large numbers of thin, unmyelinated nerve fibres that are thought

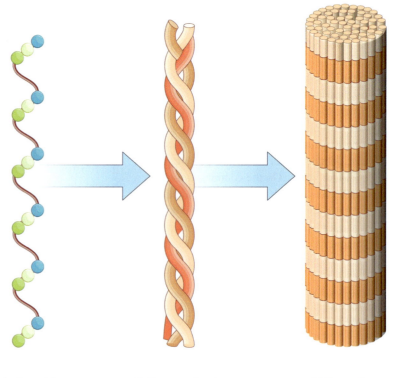

Fig. 6.1 Structure of collagen (Designua/Shutterstock.com)

to be autonomic. The second type is composed of mostly thick and hard fibrous structures that form the organ compartments and connects the organs to the musculoskeletal system. They contain large and myelinated nerve fibres. Thus, the second type has little innervation.

6.2.2 Superficial Fascia

Superficial fascia composed of loose connective tissue is located just under the skin or around organs, glands and neurovascular structures. It is absent on the palms, soles and the face. Superficial fascia is mostly composed of elastin and collagen network. It intertwines with adipose tissue that fills the spaces between the scattered fibres. Superficial fascia also contains blood vessels, lymph and nerves. Superficial fascia affects lymphatic drainage due to these intertwined tissues. Additionally, superficial fascia and adipose tissue provide both thermal insulation and absorption of the forces together.

> **Clinical Information**
> The autonomic nervous system controls blood flow distribution. Increased sympathetic activity reduces the blood flow in the capillaries. Excessive sympathetic activation may decrease the oxygenation of the superficial nerve branches passing through the superficial fascia. Therefore, excessive sympathetic activity may cause several nerve symptoms that can mimic nerve entrapments to emerge.

6.2.3 Deep Fascia

Deep fascia—most of which consists of a parallel array of collagen fibres—is examined as aponeurotic fascia and epimysium. Aponeurotic fascia has two to three layers with different main fibre directions and has a constant tension relationship with other parts of the fascial system such as the epimysium, tendons and ligaments. These structures are composed of thick fibrous tissue rich in type I collagen and transfer forces between distant body parts. Hyaluronic acid exists in the extracellular matrix between the layers of aponeurotic fascia. Hyaluronic acid functions in decreasing friction via improving the sliding of fascial layers. Therefore, it enables the fascial layers to slide over each other. In this case, increasing viscosity affects the sliding function of the fascia and may cause deterioration in the function of the movement.

Hyaluronic acid and lose connective tissue are present between the aponeurotic fascia and epimysium. Epimysium, the outermost layer of fascia that encloses the muscle, acts like a tendon on the surface of the muscle, also separating the muscle from other structures. Epimysium is often thinner than the aponeurotic fascia and also difficult to separate from the muscle. It provides the transfer of forces between the surrounding muscles. Further inside, the perimysium that is connected to epimysium, can be found. Perimysium has a collagen arrangement and types similar to the epimysium, and it encloses the muscle fascicles. The structural properties of the perimysium show that it helps transmit forces alike the epimysium. The perimysium manages the direction of force transmission by coordinating muscle fascicles. Finally, the endomysium surrounds the muscle fibres (Fig. 6.2). The endomysium has a disorganized fibre arrangement and type III collagen fibres constitute its structure. As a result of its properties, material exchanges between capillaries and muscle fibres can easily be achieved. Endomysium can easily deform during contraction and then return to its original state since it is less rigid than perimysium and epimysium. It is almost impossible to separate epimysium from muscle fibre due to this close relationship. Epimysium plays a role in maintaining the sarcomere length.

Structure of Skeletal Muscle

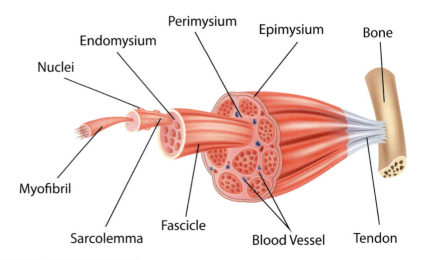

Fig. 6.2 Connective tissues of the muscle (Teguh Mujiono/Shutterstock.com)

6.3 Fascial Functions Related to Movement

Fascia has a wide range of functions from thermoregulation to force transmission. In this part, we will specifically mention its functions related to movement.

6.3.1 Excursion

All tissues slide over each other to a degree with some exceptions. The displacement of tissue in one plane over another is called excursion. A normal movement needs an excursion of tissues. In situations where the excursion is insufficient, there may be a loss of movement or a decrease in quality. For example, muscles slide as they contract. The amount of this excursion varies depending on the muscle's architectural structure and functions. Nerves also slide during joint movements. Fascia that surrounds the tissues plays a role in ensuring excursion. The viscosity of hyaluronic acid, located between fascial layers, is one of the main components of this function. Increased viscosity in the fascia or its layers will adversely affect excursion.

6.3.2 Force Transmission

Aponeurotic fascia maintains a force–tension relationship with its fibres in the line of force. Apart from its line of force, some connections exist and extend from the inner surface toward certain regions of the epimysium and muscle. These extensions ensure fascia stays on optimal tension and stretches selectively during movement. The tension in the fascia helps reduce stress on the surrounding tissues. The constant force–tension relationship must be kept at an optimal level for postural smoothness and well-coordinated movement.

The movement has been considered with the functions of the muscles. It is thought that the muscles contract and create tension on their tendons. Accordingly, this tension creates movement by acting from the point where the tendon attaches to the bone. Deep fascia and components of the fascial system (epimysium, tendon, periosteum), which transmit forces along the main fibre direction can change the forces with their behaviour before they reach the insertion during the transmission of these forces. These structures have active tension control through muscles.

Biotensegrity defines that compression components are connected to each other with pre-stressed tensioned components. For example, in the knee joint, the femur and tibia have no contact with each other. However, structures such as the joint capsule, ligaments and fascia, which are tension components between these two bones, provide force transmission and protect positional relations between the two bones. In other words, bones would not be able to maintain their position without the soft tissues around them. For this reason, bones need connections formed by the myofascial system that are viscoelastic tension components. When a force is applied to the systems based on the tensegrity model, tension components in the system distribute the forces, and the system adapts to the new load by reshaping itself.

At the macroscopic level, a myofascial unit can transfer forces to an adjacent myofascial unit. At the microscopic level, a force in the extracellular matrix can be transferred to the cell membrane and skeleton. Force transmission can happen at macro–macro or micro–micro scales, as well as from macro to micro. In other words, contraction of a muscle or exposure to static tension is thought to affect the apparent structure of the muscle, its effects are not limited to this. Tensegrity behaviour occurs from the tissue to the extracellular matrix until it reaches the cytoskeleton. The cytoskeleton carries this transmission through the cell nucleus. Physical forces, which reach the cell nucleus, may activate biochemical responses. This process is called *mechanotransduction*. Any physical forces applied or created by the tissues also trigger responses at the cellular level.

6.3.3 Energy Storage

Force transmission does not always occur as a tissue-to-tissue transmission. The fascial system can store some transferred forces. They can enable the continuation of force transmission by releasing the stored energy during activities. This occurs especially during activities such as walking and running that involve rhythmic, repetitive movements. Fascia, passive components and tendons surrounding the muscle do not transfer some of the force produced by the muscles. They store the forces as potential energy and turn it into kinetic energy—acting like a spring—to use in different phases of muscle contraction. For example, while rising to the tip of the toe during jumping, the length of the muscle shortens and the tendon lengthens in the first stage. However, the muscle-tendon unit preserves its length. Just before the fingertips lift off the ground, the muscle contracts only isometrically while the length of the tendon suddenly shortens. The muscle-tendon unit length also shortens at this point. The energy stored at the beginning of the movement is used to provide explosiveness in the final step of the movement. In this way, the activity can be done with less energy with the help of the fascia and tendon, without shortening the muscle in rhythmic movements.

6.3.4 Sensorial Organization

The tension perceived through the fascia ensures communication between the tissues. Muscles actively regulate this tension when the body needs to adapt in response to a new load. Tissues correspond to changing conditions by the information, which is obtained via fascial tension. In addition to the communication created by tension, the nervous system also receives information from mechanoreceptors that are densely located in the fascia. Mechanoreceptors are the main structures that perceive alterations in tension. The inputs that come from mechanoreceptors provide information to the nervous system in order to control movement. The fascial system has communication both in tensional and neural ways. Tensional communication occurs faster than the nervous system. Although the mechanical communication provided by tension is fast, the response of the fascial tissues to loading requires quite a long time.

6.4 Myofascial Connections

All tissues work together via the force or tension transmission through the fascia. Contrary to popular belief, this force transfer does not occur only in the traction direction of the muscle toward the tendon. About 30–40% of the forces is transferred to surrounding tissues. However, movements and exercises focus on myofascial connections that provide more linear load transfer. Fascia is acting as a bridge between the muscles that continue in the same direction, establishing myofascial chains. With this approach, the muscles—which were previously thought to act isolated—work as a team in the organization of movement. The preservation of posture or the creation of movements does not only depend on the function of a single muscle but also depend on the effective and coordinated work of myofascial chains. Myofascial chains can transmit, redirect, or absorb the forces.

> **Clinical Information**
> When a volleyball player spikes the ball, the forces do not only derive from the shoulder joint. The forces are transferred from the lower extremity to the upper extremity through myofascial chains. The forces starting from the lower extremity increase like a growing wave on the chain and are transferred from the athlete's hand to the ball at the end of the spike.

Although many researchers have made suggestions for myofascial chains, studies have shown that some of these chains have no structural and mechanical myofascial continuity. In this part, myofascial chains that are proven to be connected anatomically and functionally will be discussed.

Studies suggest that the upper extremity has three different myofascial chains. *The ventral arm chain*, which starts from the pectoralis major muscle, continues with the biceps brachii and joins with the brachial fascia. Then, it forms a lacertus fibrosus that opens distally on both sides in the shape of a fan. After this point, it continues with both brachioradialis and flexor carpi radialis muscles. *The lateral arm chain* starts from the neck and connects the fascia of the upper trapezius and the fibres of the middle deltoid. The lateral arm chain continues with the lateral intermuscular septum and reaches the brachioradialis and extensor carpi radialis brevis muscles. *The dorsal arm chain* starts from the back of the shoulder and the arm and joins triceps brachii through the latissimus dorsi and shoulder external rotator muscles. When it reaches the elbow, it blends with the anconeus muscle. It proceeds toward the extensor carpi ulnaris muscle.

Spiral, anterior and posterior oblique chains, which are thought to be used frequently in daily life or sportive activities, provide force transfer between the lower and upper extremities. Biceps femoris, gluteus maximus, thoracolumbar fascia and latissimus dorsi form *the posterior oblique chain*. It starts from the lower extremity and progresses through both the superficial and deep layers of the thoracolumbar fascia. It crosses the trunk and terminates at the glenohumeral joint on the opposite side via latissimus dorsi. *The anterior oblique chain* terminates at the contralateral glenohumeral joint via the hip adductors, transversus abdominis, internal and external oblique abdominal and pectoralis major muscles. The anterior oblique chain and the posterior oblique chain maintain the balance of forces reciprocally. *The spiral chain* runs distally with peroneus longus and then proximally with the tibialis anterior. It reaches the iliotibial band and tensor fascia latae. From the anterior–superior iliac spine, it reaches the opposite serratus anterior through the oblique abdominal muscles. Serratus anterior blends anteriorly with the rhomboid muscles at the medial edge of the scapula. From this point, splenius capitis and cervicis muscles attach contralateral side.

The superficial posterior chain protects posture against gravity. The eccentric control of this chain must be achieved to have a stable posture. The chain begins with the plantar fascia and continues with achilles tendon and gastrocnemius. It mixes with the fibres of the sacrotuberous ligament at the origin of hamstring muscles. The chain follows the erector spina muscles until the supraorbital region. *The lateral chain* controls the mediolateral stability of the trunk. It starts from the peroneal muscles and reaches the gluteus medius muscle via the iliotibial band. Further, it travels with the oblique abdominal and intercostal muscles until it reaches the sternocleidomastoideus muscle.

Myofascial chains are in constant communication with each other. All these chains have high tensile strength. Parallel fibre arrangements of deep fascia provide high amounts of tensile endurance and force transmission in the direction of the muscle and myofascial chains line of force. They must keep this tension relationship dynamic to use the right movement patterns. In this way, they take part not only in stabilization but also in mobility.

6.5 Fascial Dysfunctions

Pain and dysfunction can occur because of injury to the myofascial system. At the same time, they also can be the result of the adaptations that develop depending on the load. Some responses due to acute or chronic loading may cause the mechanical structure of the tissue to deteriorate or to lose proper function. If the fascia of a muscle that has high excursion skills is not loaded under appropriate conditions or becomes stiff and rigid, this muscle will either experience loss of function or microinjuries. Although the fascia adapts itself according to the load, the adaptations that occur after a certain point will cause the functions to be performed in another way, especially with the increase in muscular activity. That seems like an advantage that allows the body to continue the functions it needs in life-threatening situations; however, it will reduce the efficiency of movement over time.

The increase in stiffness in the muscle is observed not only because of the muscle fibres but also due to the fascia. A movement mismatch between the muscle and fascia will be a disruptive factor. For example, the fascia of a muscle specialized for producing force would have to be stiffer. Otherwise, some of the force produced by the muscle will be absorbed in the fascia. As a result, there may be a loss of force.

Fascia and the fascial system must have excursion skills on the surrounding tissues to create movement. Trauma, immobilization, or improper loading can cause adhesions, scars and densification. These problems limit the excursion ability of fascia. Thus, they limit joint movements or deteriorate their quality. For example, excursion ability is significantly reduced in patients with mechanical low back pain. Disturbances in the coordination or motor control of movement appear as compensations.

Depending on the load, a thickening or densification affects the force transmission in the connective tissue. *Densifications* are reversible problems in which the mobility between the fascial layers decreases (Fig. 6.3). It usually occurs with an increase in the viscosity of hyaluronic acid that is located between these layers. Increasing tissue temperature or performing repetitive movements increase the fluidity of hyaluronic acid. This reduces viscosity and friction between fascial layers. The reason why musculoskeletal injuries are more frequently encountered in exercises performed in cold weather or without warming up may be due to the reduction in viscosity.

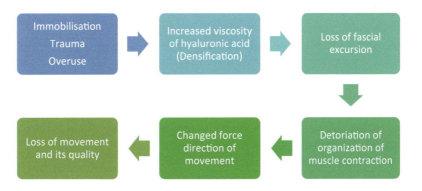

Fig. 6.3 Dysfunction chain caused by densification

The displacement of each fascial system component or fascia layer differs. For example, tendons and ligaments have different degrees of excursions. Even two tendons can show different characteristics in this manner. The displacement of neighbouring structures will also be different. However, after an injury occurs, adhesions bind these adjacent structures together and equalize the displacement. Adhesions—like densifications—limit the excursion abilities of tissues. However, adhesions are more resistive to change compared to densifications. Densification and adhesions can affect the amount or direction of force transmission. Locally, the excursion ability of the tissue may be impaired. The inability of the tissue to fulfil its role in force transmission causes the myofascial chains to develop compensatory mechanisms. Symptoms may occur at distant locations via the myofascial chains. If compensations exceed the level that the tissue can tolerate, pain and dysfunction may appear.

Mechanoreceptors, which receive accurate position and movement information, send signals to the central nervous system. Since the incoming signals are abnormal, the central nervous system interprets these signals as warnings. Pain may be encountered even if there is no active injury to the tissue when trying to create a movement. On the other hand, the intense presence of free nerve endings and pressure receptors in the fascia may cause more pain than expected in a musculoskeletal injury. Fascia, which has the richest sensory innervation after the skin, can aggravate pain. For example, an athlete who has suffered a soleus muscle injury can suddenly have relief in pain after fascial treatments, considering that it takes a long time to heal the muscle tissue.

Myofascial dysfunctions can be the reason for both local and systemic problems. Fascial tissues begin to thicken under prolonged load. Although this seems like a needed adaptation at the beginning, it increases the stiffness of the tissue and decreases its elasticity over time. This situation leads to the gradual limitation of the movement of the fascia, especially in joints where the range of motion is important. Considering a functional activity, the loss of movement in this joint will have to be compensated by another body region. Tissues, where compensation develops, will be subject to injury when they exceed levels they can tolerate. As a result, only a loss of mobility will be observed around fascial thickening where the problem started, while pain and symptoms due to additional injuries will occur around the region of compensation.

6.6 Conclusion

All structures in the body must work in coherence. The formation, smoothness and quality of the movement require the contribution of all tissues such as muscles, tendons and fascia. Fascia and the fascial system provide communication between tissues during movement via continuity without interruption. In doing so, they control and coordinate different tissues associated with movement. These roles make them a unifying system. It will be beneficial to consider this tensional integrity created by the fascial system while planning the movements or exercises.

Further Reading

Adstrum S, Nicholson H. A history of fascia. Clin Anat. 2019;32(7):862–70.

de Bruin M, Smeulders MJ, Kreulen M, Huijing PA, Jaspers RT. Intramuscular connective tissue differences in spastic and control muscle: a mechanical and histological study. PLoS One. 2014;9(6):e101038.

Eng CM, Arnold AS, Biewener AA, Lieberman DE. The human iliotibial band is specialized for elastic energy storage compared with the chimp fascia lata. J Exp Biol. 2015;218(15):2382–93.

Findley T, Chaudhry H, Stecco A, Roman M. Fascia research—a narrative review. J Bodyw Mov Ther. 2012;16(1):67–75.

Huijing PA. Epimuscular myofascial force transmission between antagonistic and synergistic muscles can explain movement limitation in spastic paresis. J Electromyogr Kinesiol. 2007;17(6):708–24.

Ingber DE, Tensegrity I. Cell structure and hierarchical systems biology. J Cell Sci. 2003;116(7):1157–73.

Khan KM, Scott A. Mechanotherapy: how physical therapists' prescription of exercise promotes tissue repair. Br J Sports Med. 2009;43:247–52.

Krause F, Wilke J, Vogt L, Banzer W. Intermuscular force transmission along myofascial chains: a systematic review. J Anat. 2016;228(6):910–8.

Langevin HM, Storch KN, Snapp RR, Bouffard NA, Badger GJ, Howe AK, et al. Tissue stretch induces nuclear remodelling in connective tissue fibroblasts. Histochem Cell Biol. 2010;133(4):405–15.

Langevin HM, Fox JR, Koptiuch C, Badger GJ, Greenan-Naumann AC, Bouffard NA, et al. Reduced thoracolumbar fascia shear strain in human chronic low back pain. BMC Musculoskelet Disord. 2011;12:203.

Masi AT, Nair K, Evans T, Ghandour Y. Clinical, biomechanical, and physiological translational interpretations of human resting myofascial tone or tension. Int J Ther Massage Bodyw. 2010;3(4):16–28.

Purslow PP. Muscle fascia and force transmission. J Bodyw Mov Ther. 2010;14(4):411–7.

Purslow PP. The structure and role of intramuscular connective tissue in muscle function. Front Physiol. 2020;11:495.

Sakuma J, Kanehisa H, Yanai T, Fukunaga T, Kawakami Y. Fascicle-tendon behavior of the gastrocnemius and soleus muscles during ankle bending exercise at different movement frequencies. Eur J Appl Physiol. 2012;112(3):887–98.

Schleip R, Findley T, Chaitow L, Huijing P. Fascia—The tensional network of the human body. London: Churchill Livingstone; 2012.

Schleip R, Hedley G, Yucesoy CA. Fascial nomenclature: update on related consensus process. Clin Anat. 2019;32(7):929–33.

Smith LR, Lee KS, Ward SR, Chambers HG, Lieber RL. Hamstring contractures in children with spastic cerebral palsy result from a stiffer extracellular matrix and increased in vivo sarcomere length. J Physiol. 2011;589(Pt 10):2625–39.

Stecco C, Day JA. The fascial manipulation technique and its biomechanical model: a guide to the human fascial system. Int J Ther Massage Bodyw. 2010;3(1):38.

Stecco C, Gagey O, Belloni A, Pozzuoli A, Porzionato A, Macchi V, et al. Anatomy of the deep fascia of the upper limb. Second part: study of innervation. Morphologie. 2007;91(292):38–43.

Stecco C, Stern R, Porzionato A, Macchi V, Masiero S, Stecco A, et al. Hyaluronan within fascia in the etiology of myofascial pain. Surg Radiol Anat. 2011;33(10):891–6.

Stecco A, Meneghini A, Stern R, Stecco C, Imamura M. Ultrasonography in myofascial neck pain: randomized clinical trial for diagnosis and follow-up. Surg Radiol Anat. 2014;36(3):243–53.

Stecco C, Sfriso MM, Porzionato A, Rambaldo A, Albertin G, Macchi V, et al. Microscopic anatomy of the visceral fasciae. J Anat. 2017;231(1):121–8.

Tesarz J, Hoheisel U, Wiedenhöfer B, Mense S. Sensory innervation of the thoracolumbar fascia in rats and humans. Neuroscience. 2011;194:302–8.

van der Wal J. The architecture of the connective tissue in the musculoskeletal system—an often overlooked functional parameter as to proprioception in the locomotor apparatus. Int J Ther Massage Bodyw. 2009;2(4):9–23.

Wilke J, Krause F. Myofascial chains of the upper limb: a systematic review of anatomical studies. Clin Anat. 2019;32(7):934–40.

Wilke J, Krause F, Vogt L, Banzer W. What is evidence-based about myofascial chains: a systematic review. Arch Phys Med Rehabil. 2016;97(3):454–61.

Yucesoy CA. Epimuscular myofascial force transmission implies novel principles for muscular mechanics. Exerc Sport Sci Rev. 2010;38(3):128–34.

The Axial Skeleton

Kadriye Tombak

Abstract

The skeletal system, which is an essential part of the body movement system, is examined under two headings as the axial and appendicular skeleton. While the axial skeletal system consists of the skull and trunk, which form the vertical axis of the body, the appendicular skeletal system comprises the lower and upper extremities, as well as the pectoral and pelvic girdle to which these extremities are connected (Fig. 7.1).

In this section, the anatomical structures that make up the axial skeleton system, the relations of these structures with each other, the key points to be considered in the observation, the axial skeleton movements, and basic approaches will be explained.

7.1 Noncontractile Structures in the Axial Skeleton

7.1.1 Bone Structures

The axial skeleton is examined under three headings as cranial, vertebral, and trunk bones (Fig. 7.1).

K. Tombak (✉)
Physiotherapy Program, Vocational School of Health Services, Akdeniz University, Antalya, Turkey
e-mail: kadriyetombak@akdeniz.edu.tr

7.1.1.1 Cranial Bones

The cranial bones consist of two parts, the neurocranium and the viscerocranium. The neurocranium is formed by the assembly of eight closed and solid bones that protect the central nervous system structures in the skull. The viscerocranium is formed by the union of 14 irregular bones that make up the face, mouth, nose, and orbit (Fig. 7.2).

Hyoid and ear ossicles can also be included in this group (Fig. 7.2 and Table 7.1).

7.1.1.2 Vertebral Column Bones

Each bone that makes up the vertebral column is called a vertebra. The vertebral column is formed when the vertebrae line up and joint with each other. The vertebral column has three main functions: (1) To support the trunk, (2) to protect the spinal cord and spinal nerve roots, and (3) to ensure the mobility of the trunk. Although the movement of the vertebral column is limited, it has a strong and flexible structure that can combine flexion, extension, lateral flexion and rotation and these movements.

The vertebral column consists of 33 vertebrae and 23 intervertebral discs in the newborn. In childhood, five vertebrae in the sacral region unite to form the sacrum, and 4 vertebrae in the coccygeal region combine to form the coccyx. Therefore, there are 26 vertebrae in the vertebral column of a healthy individual with complete bone development. The length of a healthy verte-

DIVISIONS OF THE SKELETAL SYSTEM

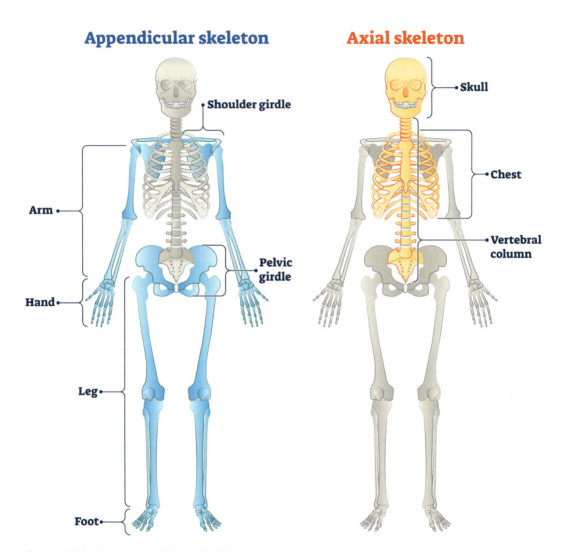

Fig. 7.1 Skeletal system parts (VectorMine/Shutterstock.com)

bral column in adults is 60–70 cm, 75% of which is vertebrae and 25% is intervertebral discs (cartilaginous discs between vertebrae).

> **To Learn Easily**
> The two facet joints made by two adjacent vertebrae and the intervertebral disc between them together form a spinal segment.

The vertebral column has a different structure in terms of anterior, posterior, and lateral aspects. From the anterior and posterior angles, it is observed that the vertical axis of the vertebral column is straight. Laterally, it is seen to have some anatomical curvatures (Fig. 7.3). The vertebral column convexity in late embryological life and at birth has a posterior-facing, kyphotic curvature. Lordotic curves are secondary curves that develop as they begin to bear

7 The Axial Skeleton

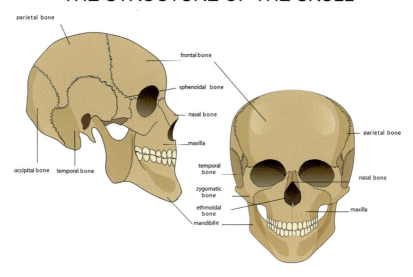

Fig. 7.2 The structure of the cranial bones (front and side view) (Artemida-psy/Shutterstock.com)

Table 7.1 Cranial bones

Neurocranium		Viscerocranium	
Single	Pair	Single	Pair
Frontal bone occipital bone sphenoid bone ethmoid bone	Parietal bone temporal bone	Vomer mandibula	Lacrimal bone zygomatic bone Palatinum bone Nasal bone Maxilla concha nasalis inferior (Hyoid and ear bonelets can also be added)

weight. As the baby gains head control (approximately 4 months), cervical lordosis develops. During motor development, lumbar lordosis, which begins to form as the child begins to sit, occurs as a response of the vertebral column to load bearing and is completed by about one year of age. These anatomical curvatures that occur during the developmental stages of the bipedal period allow the vertebral column to carry more load.

The sum of the cervical and lumbar lordosis angles is equal to the sum of the thoracic and sacral kyphosis angles. Pathological conditions may occur as a result of these anatomical curvatures exceeding their physiological limits. Figure 7.3 shows the physiological curvatures of the vertebral column. The purpose of the secondary curves is to maintain the body balance by providing the necessary muscle strength in the most appropriate way to maintain the upright position of the trunk.

> **Clinical Information**
> C7–T1, T12–L1, and L5–S1 segments, which are the transition points where one of the anatomical curves ends and the other begins, are observed when viewed from the side of the vertebral column. These transition zones are the vertebral segments where injury is most common, as they are the regions with the highest mobility in the vertebral column.

> **Clinical Information**
> Physiological limits and pathological conditions of anatomical curvatures in the vertebral column: cervical area: 30°–35° normal cervical lordosis
> <30° cervical hyperlordosis
> >35° cervical hypolordosis

Thoracic area: 20°–45° normal thoracic kyphosis
  <20° thoracic hypokyphosis
  >45° thoracic hyperkyphosis
Lumbar area: 20°–40° normal lumbar lordosis
  <20° lumbar hyperlordosis
  >40° lumbar hypolordosis

To Learn Easily
An anterior view of the vertebral column shows the vertebral trunks expanding and enlarging from top to bottom. The reason for this is the increase in the amount of load carried on the vertebral corpuscles from the top to bottom.

Spine

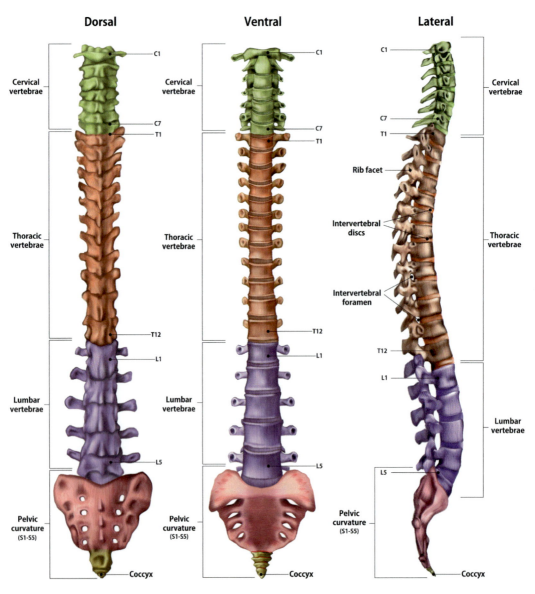

Fig. 7.3 Anterior, posterior, and lateral view of the vertebral column (studiovin/Shutterstock.com)

7 The Axial Skeleton

The vertebral column basically consists of two columns

1. Anterior column: it arises from the vertebral corpuscles.
2. Posterior column: it consists of laminas (of arcus vertebrae, that is, their posterior elements) and spinous, articular, and transverse protrusions (Fig. 7.4).

> **To Learn Easily**
> The thorax resembles an irregularly shaped cylinder with a narrow opening called the aperture thoracic superior above, which is continuous with the neck region, and a wide entrance called the aperture thoracic inferior, which is closed by the diaphragm below.

Spine and structure of segments

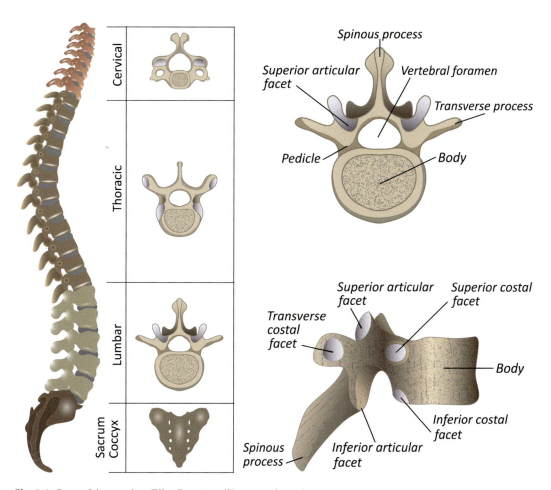

Fig. 7.4 Parts of the vertebra (Ellen Bronstayn/Shutterstock.com)

Table 7.2 Typical features of vertebrae

Cervical vertebrae
- There are 7 vertebrae
- First vertebra is called atlas, second vertebra is called axis
- There is no disc between atlas and axis

Thoracic vertebrae
- There are 12 vertebrae
- Vertebral bodies are larger and heart-shaped than the corpus of cervical vertebrae
- On both sides of the corpus, vertebrae are the superior and inferior fovea costalis and the hood costa

Lumbar vertebrae
- There are 5 vertebrae
- The corpuscles of the vertebrae are large and kidney shaped
- Foramen vertebrae are broad and triangular
- Spinous protrusions are quadrangular in shape

Sacral vertebrae
- It is formed by the union of 5 vertebrae
- It has the appearance of a triangle with the base up and the top down
- It forms the posterosuperior wall of the pelvic cavity
- It creates a joint with the L5 above, with the pelvis on either side, and with the coccyx below

Coccyx
- It is a primitive structure formed by the union of 3–5 vertebrae
- It is a triangular structure with the base above
- It is the attachment site for some muscles that make up the floor of the pelvic cavity

The 7 cervical, 12 thoracic and 5 lumbar vertebrae (usually a total of 24) above the sacrum are called "presacral vertebrae". These vertebrae joint with each other via intervertebral discs (usually 23). However, atlas, which is the first cervical vertebra, and axis, which is the second cervical vertebra, are called atypical vertebrae and there is no disc between them. Atlas is named after the "Atlas" in Greek mythology because it carries the cranium. Atlas and axis are specialized to create a much wider range of motion than other vertebrae. These two atypical vertebrae play an important role in the movements of the head. Typical features of vertebrae by spinal region are summarized in Table 7.2.

7.1.1.3 Trunk Bones

The trunk bones that make up the axial skeleton consist of the costa and sternum. There are 12 pairs of costae on the right and left. The costae are in the flat bone group and consist of two parts, bone and cartilage. The costae are examined in two groups as true and false costae, according to the type of joint they make with the sternum (Table 7.3). Each costa has two ends and a stem. Figure 7.5 shows the combination and structure of the costae with the trunk. Its anterior end, which is close to the sternum, is called "extremitas sternalis," and its posterior end, which is close to the vertebra, is called "extremitas acromialis" (Fig. 7.5). The first, second, 11th, and 12th costae are atypical, while the third and tenth costae are typical. Tables 7.4 and 7.5 show typical and atypical costa features.

In front of the rib cage is the sternum, which is a flat bone. The sternum consists of three parts in adult individuals. These are the broad and superior manubrium sterni, the narrow and longitudinally extending corpus sterni, and the small, inferior xiphoid protrusion. Sternum (Fig. 7.6) and its features are summarized in Table 7.6.

7.1.2 Joints Associated with the Axial Skeleton

Joints of the vertebral column can be arranged from proximal to distal as
- Atlantooccipital joint
- Atlantoaxial joint
- Costovertebral joint
- Costotransverse joint

7 The Axial Skeleton

Table 7.3 Characteristics of true and false costae

True costa (*Costae vera*)	False costa (*Costae spuria*)
• It consists of the first 7 pairs of costae • It is directly attached to the sternum by the cartilage costa anteriorly	• It consists of the last 5 pairs of costae • The 8th, 9th, and 10th costae articulate with each other and then with the seventh costa and attach to the sternum • The 11th and 12th costae (swimmer's ribs) are shorter than the others and have free ends

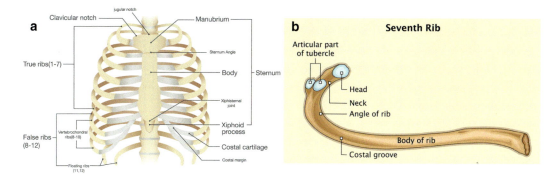

Fig. 7.5 (**a**) Relationship of costae with trunk and spine (solar22/Shutterstock.com), (**b**) the structure of the seventh costa (N.Vinoth Narasingam/Shutterstock.com)

Table 7.4 Common features of typical costae

Common features of typical costae
• It consists of a curved trunk with anterior and posterior ends
• The costa consists of three parts: the hood, the collum, and the corpus
• The hood costa forms a joint with the thoracic vertebrae
• 2.5 cm narrow part after the hood costa is known as collum costa
• The whole part after the collum costa is called the corpus costa. The groove on the inner surface of the corpus costa is called the sulcus costa. The intercostal artery, intercostal vein, and intercostal nerve pass through this groove

Table 7.5 Features of atypical costae

Features of atypical costae			
1st Costa (*Costa Prima*)	2nd Costa (*Costa Secunda*)	11th Costa (*Costa Undecima*)	12th Costa (*Costa Duodecima*)
• It is the shortest and widest costa • It is located under the clavicle • The hood costa has a single articular surface • It has such parts as crista capitis costa, angulus costa, and sulcus costa	• The sulcus costa is more prominent • It has a crista capitis costa structure	• Crista capitis costa and tuberculum costa structures are absent	• Crista capitis costa, angulus costa, tuberculum costa, sulcus costa structures are absent

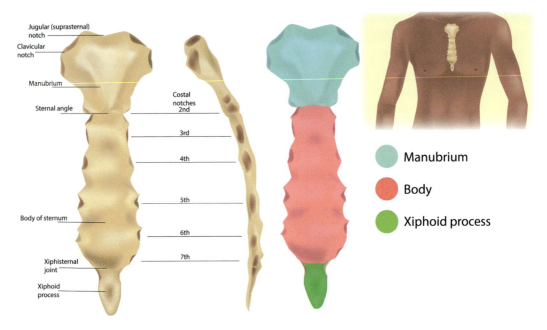

Fig. 7.6 Sternum its parts (Sakurra/Shutterstock.com)

Table 7.6 Parts of the sternum and their features

Manubrium stern	Corpus stern	Xiphoid protrusion
• It forms a joint with the clavicle and the first cartilage articulate with the costa • It has a notch on the upper part called the incisura jugularis • The angle between it and the corpus stern is called the angulus stern (Louis angle)	• It is a long, thin piece in the form of a continuation of the manubrium stern • Its notch structures called incisura costae form a joint with cartilage costae • At the bottom, it forms a joint with the seventh costa	• It is the lowest part of the sternum • It does not form a joint with the costae

Table 7.7 Atlantoaxial joint ligaments

Lateral atlantoaxial ligament	• It occurs between the inferior articular surface on the lower surface of the atlas and the superior articular surface on the upper surface of the axis • It is a plana-type joint and has two pieces, one on the right and the left • Since the joint capsule is loose, it does not restrict head movements
Medial atlantoaxialis mediana	• It occurs between the fovea dentis on the inner surface of the atlas and the dens axis on the axis • It is a trochoid-type joint • Most of the rotational movement on the axis of the atlas takes place at this joint • There are some ligaments specific to this joint that limit the movement of the joint. These are:Lig. Alaria: Limits the rotational movement of the head Lig. Cruciforme Atlantis: Lig. It is a plus-shaped ligament formed by the transversum longitudinalis and the fasciculi longitudinalis Lig. Some fibers leaving the longitudinalis posterius lig in this region. It passes through the middle of the transversum longitudinal. These fibers are called fasciculi longitudinal Lig. Apicis dentis: It is a ligament that goes from the tip of the dens axis to the anterior edge of the foramen magnum and holds the dens axis in its position

- Costosternal joint
- Sacroiliac joint
- Uncovertebral (*Luschka*) joint
- Intervertebral joints
- Zygapophyseal (facet) joints

7.1.2.1 Atlantooccipital Joint
It is the joint that occurs between the occiput condyles and the upper articular surfaces of the atlas. The main movement in this joint is flexion and extension. This movement is accompanied by the sliding movement of the occipital condyles.

7.1.2.2 Atlantoaxial Joint
It is the joint that occurs between the atlas and the axis. It has four articular facets. Two occur between the articular surface of the atlas and the upper articular surface of the axis, and both occur between the anterior ring of the atlas and the odontoid protrusion of the axis. This joint structure allows three-plane movement. The basic movement that occurs is the rotation movement that occurs around the long axis of the odontoid protrusion (DENS).

Atlas and axis make two joints with each other, atlantoaxialis medialis and lateralis (Table 7.7).

> **Clinical Information**
> Membrana tectoria is a structure extending along the faces of all vertebral surfaces facing the vertebral canal and in the form of a continuation of the posterior longitudinal ligament, attaching to the axis above and adhering to the occipital bone, taking the name membrana tectoria from here on. Dens covers the entire axis. It controls the movements of the vertebral column in the direction of extension.

7.1.2.3 Costovertebral Joint
The heads of the 2nd and 9th costae form joints with the upper and lower parts of the adjacent vertebrae with two facets, while the heads of the 1st, 10th, 11th, and 12th costae form joints with a single vertebra.

7.1.2.4 Costotransverse Joint
It is located between the costa tubercle between the 1st and 10th costae and the transverse protrusion of the vertebra. This joint is absent in the 11th and 12th costae.

7.1.2.5 Costosternal Joint
While the first seven costae form joints with the sternum one by one, the 8th, 9th, and 10th costae unite to connect to the 7th costa, while the 11th and 12th costae (floating ribs) are free.

> **Clinical Information**
> Lumbar spinal discs have an avascular structure and fluid flow is provided by passive diffusion. Some researchers report that spinal movements provided with regular exercise increase disc nutrition. At the same time, exercise can slow down the height loss due to fluid loss in the disc.

7.1.2.6 Intervertebral Joints

> **Clinical Information**
> Disc herniations (Fig. 7.7) may develop as a result of damage to the nucleus pulposus or rupture of the annulus fibrosus due to aging, spinal degeneration and traumas.

There are a total of 23 intervertebral discs between the corpuscles of the vertebrae. The intervertebral joint consists of two corpuscles and the intervertebral disc between them. Intervertebral disc thickness increases from cervical to lumbar. Lumbar intervertebral disc thickness is approximately twice the cervical intervertebral disc thickness, with an average thickness of 10 mm. All intervertebral discs consist of the nucleus pulposus in the middle and the annulus fibrosus on the outside. Flexibility in the spinal segment is determined by the size of the intervertebral disc and the resistance to movement of the soft tissue supporting the joint.

Clinical Information

The movements that occur in the thorax during breathing can be explained by analogy with the movements of the pump arm and the bucket handle.

Pump arm movement: The sternal ends of the 2nd and 6th costae rise around the axis passing through the sleeve costa, thereby expanding the anterior–posterior diameter of the costa cage.

Bucket handle movement: The movement of the 7th and 10th costae affects the transverse diameter of the thorax. The costae rise and fall around the Angulus costa. In this movement axis, bucket-handle movement occurs.

7.1.2.7 Sacroiliac Joint

It is a true joint with its synovium, capsule, and ligaments that occurs between the 1st and 3rd sacral vertebrae and the ilium.

7.1.2.8 Uncovertebral (Luschka) Joint

C Lateral edges of C3–C6 vertebral bodies protrude upward. These protrusions are called uncinate, and the joints between them are called uncovertebral joints.

7.1.2.9 Zygapophysial (Facet) Joints

It is a joint formed between the inferior surface of the articular protrusion of the superior vertebra and the superior surface of the articular protrusion of the inferior vertebra. Known as "facet joint" clinically, it is essential in increasing the range of motion. It helps to carry the load on the spine.

Columna vertebralis ligaments: **They are**

Clinical Information

- The anatomical differences of the lumbar facet joints also allow torsional force control and stabilization in these joints.
- Changes in volume and height of the intervertebral disc also cause changes in the facet joints.

analyzed under three headings:
1. Intersegmental ligaments.
2. Intrasegmental ligaments.
3. Articular and capsular structures.

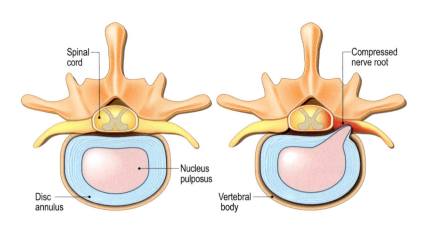

Fig. 7.7 A disc with hernia (Designua/Shutterstock.com)

7 The Axial Skeleton

The intersegmental ligaments consist of the anterior and posterior longitudinal ligaments and supraspinous ligaments that run along the entire spine and run anterior and posterior to the intervertebral discs (Fig. 7.8 and Table 7.8).

Intrasegmental ligaments: They can be listed as interspinous ligament, intertransverse ligament, ligamentum flava, lateral vertebral ligament, and ligaments that strengthen the atlantooccipital/atlantoaxial joints (Table 7.9).

To Learn Easily
- The longitudinal ligaments are viscoelastic and stiffen when loaded rapidly. In this way, it does not store all the energy that stretches it. This property is called hysteresis. With repeated loading, the ligaments become stiffer and the hysteresis decrease
- The most flexible ligament in the trunk is the ligamentum flavum and is the main ligament that restricts flexion.

Fig. 7.8 Spinal ligaments (Designua/Shutterstock.com)

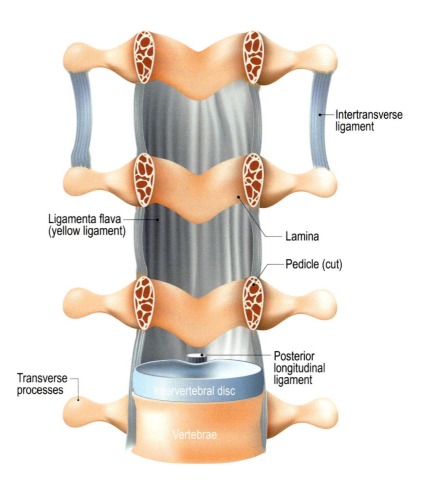

Table 7.8 Intersegmental ligaments and their features

Anterior longitudinal ligament	• The corpus is located on the anterior surface of the vertebrae and intervertebral discs • It restricts excessive extension of the spine
Posterior longitudinal ligament	• It extends along the posterior aspect of the corpus vertebrae between the axis and the sacrum • It extends from the trunk of the axis toward the occiput to the membrane, where it is called tectoria • It restricts excessive flexion of the spine
Supraspinous ligament	• It is a posterior colon ligament • It extends from the outer occipital prominence to the sacrum • This ligament is stretched in flexion and relaxed in extension • It enlarges and thickens in the cervical region and is called the ligamentum nuca. It prevents excessive flexion

Table 7.9 Intrasegmental ligaments and their features

Interspinous ligament	• They are thin ligaments that connect the spinous protrusions • It stretches in flexion and relaxes in extension • It connects two adjacent spinous protrusions • It is the weakest of the spinal ligaments
Intertransverse ligament	• It lies between the transversus protrusions of two adjacent vertebrae • It limits the lateral flexion movement of the spine • During lateral flexion, the convex side ligaments are stretched while those on the concave side relax • It provides spinal stability during lateral flexion and rotation
Ligamentum flava	• It is located between the adjacent arcus vertebrae from the atlas to the first sacral vertebra, connecting all the laminae • It prevents the arcus vertebrae from moving away from each other during forward flexion of the spine • Even in neutral position it is somewhat taut, thus contributing significantly to spinal stability • It is the most stretched ligament in lateral flexion • It plays an important role in providing anterior and posterior stability and preserving the functions of the arches
Lateral vertebral ligament	• It lies between the anterior and posterior longitudinal ligaments. It consists of short fibers firmly attached to the intervertebral discs

7.2 Contractile Structures Associated with the Axial Skeleton

The vertebral column needs strong muscles for movement and stabilization. Anterior group muscle development is superficially and posterior group muscle development is deeply located in terms of embryological development.

Based on the mechanical movements of the axial skeleton, the muscles found here can be examined in four groups as extensor, flexor, lateral flexor and rotator.

In this section, we will examine these muscles according to their anatomical location as back, chest and abdominal muscles.

7.2.1 Back Muscles

Back muscles can be examined under three headings as superficial, medium, and deep muscle groups (Table 7.10). Deep group back muscles start from the dorsal part of myotomes, which are embryological locations, and remain there. These muscles are called "autochthonous back muscles".

Table 7.10 Back muscles

Superficial group muscles	• Trapezium (upper, middle, lower part) • Levator scapula • Rhomboid major • Rhomboid minor • Latissimus dorsi
Middle group muscles	• Serratus posterior superior • Serratus posterior inferior

Deep group muscles	• They are known as autochthonous back muscles
	• They support spine movements and body posture
	   1. Superficial layer
	   2. Middle layer
	   3. Deep layer

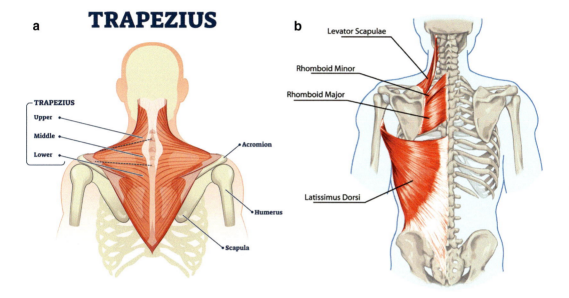

Fig. 7.9 (**a**, **b**) Superficial group of back muscles. (**a**) (VectorMine/Shutterstock.com), (**b**) (stihii/Shutterstock.com)

7.2.1.1 Superficial Group Back Muscles

Known as extrinsic back muscles, they have important functions in upper extremity movements. They are responsible for the synchronized movement of the spine and upper extremities by fixing the upper extremity to the spine (Fig. 7.9).

Trapezius: It consists of three parts, upper, middle, and lower (Table 7.11). This muscle is innervated by the accessory nerve. If the accessory nerve is damaged, the scapula shifts laterally and downward away from the vertebral column (Fig. 7.10).

- It pulls the shoulder back. Thus, the scapula approaches the column vertebralis.
- It helps to pull our body up when we hold on to a high place.
- It pulls shoulder up-in.
- While the clavicle and scapula are fixed, if it contracts unilaterally, it tilts its head to the same side, if it contracts bilaterally, it tilts its head back.
- It prevents/controls the downward (depression) movement of the shoulder while carrying a load.

Table 7.11 Origins and insertions of trapezius muscle parts

Trapezium (upper part)	• Linea nuchae superior starts from protuberancia occipitalis externa, spinous protrusions of all cervical vertebrae, and ligamentum nuchae
Trapezium (middle part)	• It starts from the spinous protrusions of T1–6 vertebrae and the supraspinal ligament
	• The acromion and spina terminate at the upper edges of the scapula
Trapezium (lower part)	• They start from the spinous protrusions of the thoracic 6th–12th vertebrae and the supraspinal ligament
	• They terminate at the medial end of the spina scapula

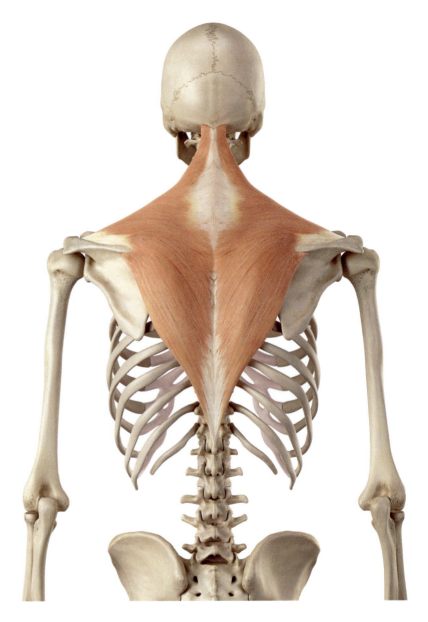

Fig. 7.10 Functions of the trapezius muscle (SciePro/Shutterstock.com)

Levator scapula: It starts from the transverse protrusions of cervical 1–4 vertebrae. It terminates at the superior corner of the scapula and the uppermost part of the margo medialis. It is innervated by the dorsalis scapula nerve. It diverges from the vertebral column of the scapula at the junction of the nerve (Fig. 7.11).

- When it contracts bilaterally, it pulls the head back.
- It pulls the scapula upward and inward.
- When the muscle contracts unilaterally, it pulls the head and neck to its side.

Rhomboid major: It starts from the spinous protrusions of the C7–T5 vertebrae and the supraspinal ligament. It ends in the margin medialis between the inferior corner of the scapula and the spina scapula.

Rhomboid minor: It starts from the spinous protrusions of the C7 and T1 vertebrae and the supraspinal ligament. It ends in the margin medialis between the superior corner of the scapula and the spina scapula (Fig. 7.12). The nerve of the rhomboideus major and minor muscles is the dorsal scapular nerve.

- Both muscles together rotate the scapula up and in.
- One by one, they fix the scapula to the thoracic wall.
- Rhomboideus major rotates the inferior angle of the scapula in the opposite direction to the serratus anterior muscle.

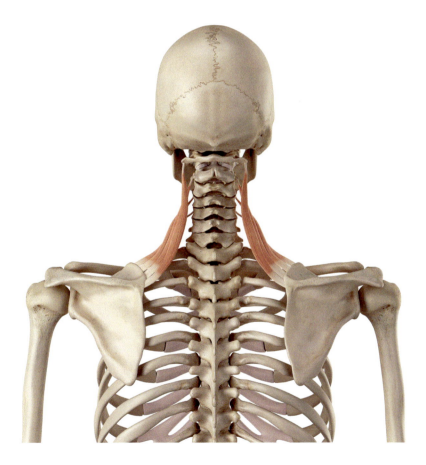

Fig. 7.11 Functions of the levator scapula muscle (SciePro/Shutterstock.com)

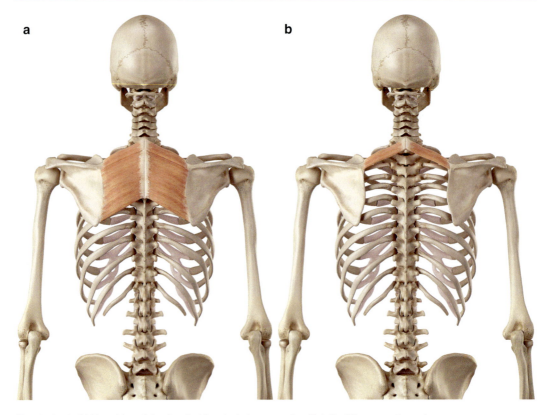

Fig. 7.12 (**a**, **b**) Functions of the rhomboid major/minor muscles (SciePro/Shutterstock.com)

Latissimus dorsi: It starts the spinous protrusions of the thoracic 7–12 and all lumbar vertebrae, the posterior aspect of the iliac crest, and the posterior surface of the 9–12 costae, and insert into the crista tuberculi minora in the humerus. It is innervated by the thoracodorsalis nerve. Adduction and internal rotation of the arm are impaired as a result of damage to the nerve (Fig. 7.13).

- It has a primary task in movements such as rowing, swimming, climbing, pulling up, and chopping wood.
- Coke adduction.
- Internal rotation,
- Extension,
- Help to breathe.

Clinical Information
Petit Triangle: Located just above the iliac crest, this triangular area is bounded below by the iliac crest, posteriorly by the lower outer part of the latissimus dorsi muscle, and anteriorly by the obliquus externus abdominis muscle (Fig. 7.13).

- The obliquus internus abdominis muscle forms the base of the triangle.
- Herniation may occur in this region, which is weaker than other regions

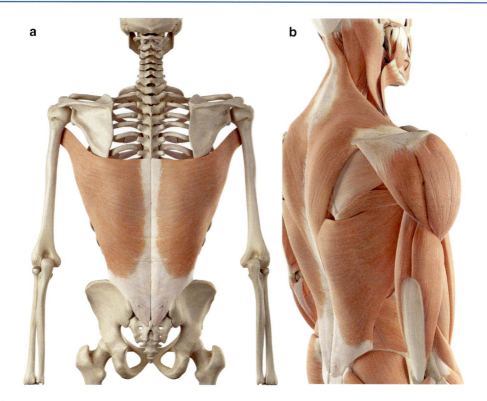

Fig. 7.13 (**a**, **b**) Functions of the latissimus dorsi muscle and the petit triangle (SciePro/Shutterstock.com)

7.2.1.2 Middle Group Back Muscles
It consists of serratus posterior superior and inferior muscles (Fig. 7.14).

- Serratus posterior superior.
  It helps inspiration by pulling the costae up.
- Serratus posterior inferior.
  It helps expiration by pulling down the costae it is attached to.

7.2.1.3 Deep Group Back Muscles
It consists of three groups superficial, middle, and deep layers (Table 7.12).

7.2.2 Chest Muscles

The anterior thoracic wall is called "*regio pectoralis*." This region is bounded by the sternum inside, the plica axillaris anterior externally, the clavicle above, and the lower border of the pectoralis major muscle below.

Here are the muscles and mammary glands connecting the upper extremity and the thoracic

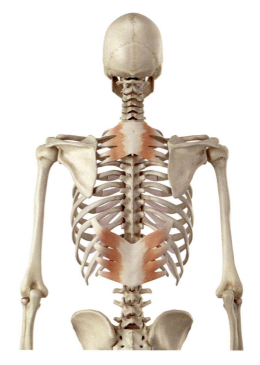

Fig. 7.14 The functions of serratus posterior superior and serratus posterior inferior muscles (SciePro/Shutterstock.com)

Table 7.12 Deep group back muscles and their functions

Superficial layer **Middle layer** **(erector spinae muscles)**	Splenius capitis	• Head extension with bilateral contraction • Head lateral flexion to the same side when contracted unilaterally
	Splenius cervicis	• Head extension with bilateral contraction • Head lateral flexion to the same side when contracted unilaterally
	İliocostalis lumborum	• Extension of the vertebral column when contracted bilaterally • When contracted unilaterally, lateral flexion of the ipsilateral vertebral column • Lumbar and thoracic parts pull down the costae and cause expiration
	Longissimus thoracis cervicis, longissimus thoracis capitis	• M. Longissimus thoracis cervicis tilts the spine posteriorly when contracted bilaterally and to the same side as itself when contracted unilaterally • M. Longissimus capitis causes the face to be turned to the same side by tilting the head back when contracted bilaterally, and tilting the head to the same side when contracting unilaterally
	Spinalis thoracis cervicis, Spinalis thoracis capitis	• They bend the vertebral arm backward in their bilateral contraction • In their unilateral contraction, they tilt the trunk to the same side
Deep layer	Transversospinalis, semispinalis, multifidus, rotators Interspinals Intertransversals Levatores costarum	• They are the muscles in the deepest plane of the back • They provide lateral flexion of the spine to the same side when contracted unilaterally and stabilization of the spine when contracted bilaterally

wall. The nerves of the region are the supraclavicular and intercostal nerves. Between the two leaves of the superficial fascia here are the mammary glands. The fascia pectoralis covers the pectoralis major muscle. It attaches to the sternum on the inside and the clavicle above. Outwardly, the deep fascia of the shoulder and axilla is continued posteriorly by the deep fascia of the cervicodorsal region and below by the rectus sheath on the anterior abdominal wall.

The part called fascia axillaris, which is between the pectoralis major and latissimus dorsi muscles, divides into two on the outer edge of the latissimus dorsi muscle. Later, this fascia wraps around the latissimus dorsi and terminates in the spinous protrusions of the vertebrae.

Pectoralis major: It consists of three parts: clavicular, sternal, and abdominal (Table 7.13, Fig. 7.15).

Function of Pectoralis Major
- It is the strongest adductor of the arm.
- Since it crosses the vertical axis internally, it performs internal rotation.
- It aids inspiration by pulling the costae up.
- If the arm is fixed above, it pulls the body up.

Function of Pectoralis Minor
- It pulls the scapula forward and down. It takes part in the rotation.
- If the shoulder is fixed, it helps the inspiration by pulling up the costae it is attached to.
- It is inactive in normal breathing!
- It pulls the scapula toward the anterior chest wall and stabilizes it.

Subclavius: It is a finger-shaped muscle located between the clavicle and the first costa (Fig. 7.16). It acts as a cushion for the formations located between the clavicle and the first costae.

7 The Axial Skeleton

Table 7.13 The origin and insertions of the pectoralis major muscle

Pectoralis major (clavicular part)	• It starts from the inner half of the clavicle • It attaches to the greater tubercle of the humerus
Pectoralis major (sternocostal part)	• It starts from the anterior surface of the sternum, excluding the xiphoid protrusion, and from the cartilaginous costae attached to it • It attaches to the greater tubercle of the humerus
Pectoralis major (abdominal part)	• It starts from the aponeurosis of the abdominal muscles • It attaches to the greater tubercle of the humerus

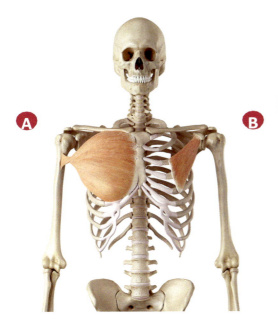

Fig. 7.15 The functions of (**a**) pectoralis major and (**b**) pectoralis minor (SciePro/Shutterstock.com)

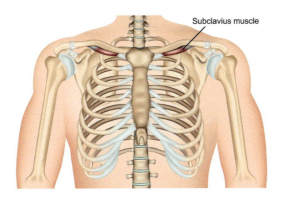

Fig. 7.16 Subclavius muscle (medicalstocks/Shutterstock.com)

It also helps to stabilize the clavicle during shoulder down-forward movement and arm-shoulder belt movements.

Clinical Information
The subclavius muscle prevents injury to the subclavian vessels and brachial plexus (truncus superior) of the broken tip in clavicle fractures.

Serratus anterior: It begins as toothed projections on the outer surface of the first nine costae, leans against the chest wall, wraps around the back, passes through the anterior aspect of the subscapular muscle, and ends at the anterior edge and inferior corner of the scapula (Fig. 7.17).

- It fixes the scapula by pulling it toward the thorax.
- It fixes the scapula on the thoracic wall while pushing against resistance.
- Its upper part is suspensory for the scapula.
- The middle fibers pull the scapula forward.
- It is effective in scapula rotation.
- It is active when the arm is raised more after 90°.
- It is an antagonist of the rhomboid muscles.

Intercostals: They are muscles intercostalis externi, interni, and intima (Table 7.14). They are more commonly known as respiratory muscles.

Clinical Information

It is not only these anatomical structures that affect the spine, but the relationship between these structures and their effects on each other. For example, the interspinous ligament joins the supraspinous ligament and then the thoracolumbal fascia to form the interspinous–supraspinous–thoracolumbal ligamentous junction. This junction connects the lumbar fascia to the lumbar spine. This information is very important in explaining the transmission of tension developed in the extremities to the vertebral column in clinics.

7.2.3 Abdominal Muscles

Abdominal muscles are summarized in Fig. 7.18 and their beginnings and endings are summarized in Table 7.15. Basically, it consists of three flat (external oblique, internal oblique, and transversus abdominus muscles) and two vertical muscle groups (rectus abdominus and pyramidal muscles).

To Learn Easily

Serratus anterior,

- It is one of the strongest muscles that makes the shoulder move, also known as the boxer muscle.
- The strongest part is the inferior part.
- Together with the trapezius muscle, it works in movements of the arm above 90° (such as combing hair, taking off the hat).
- The winged scapula (winged scapula, scapula alata) develops as a result of damage to the thoracic longus nerve, when the medial edge of the scapula becomes dominant by the rhomboid muscles, separating from the thoracic wall and taking on a wing-shaped appearance and hyperabduction of the arm of the person.
- It is an important muscle for healthy scapular rhythm during movements such as pushing, throwing and reaching.

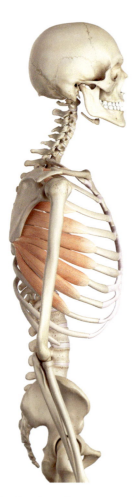

Fig. 7.17 The function of serratus anterior (SciePro/Shutterstock.com)

Clinical Information

- They help the forced expiration that occurs during coughing, sneezing and singing by pulling down the costae and sternum.
- They contribute to micturition, defecation, vomiting, and delivery with the help of increased intra-abdominal pressure with the successive contractions of the diaphragm and closure of the rima glottis.

Table 7.14 Functions of the intercostal muscles

• **Intercostalis external**	• It has 11 pairs • It comes from the level of the costal tubercle in the back to the level of the cartilage costal in the front • It continues into the membrane as intercostalis interni • It makes inspiration by lifting the costae up
• **Intercostalis interni**	• It makes expiration by pulling the costae down
• **Intercostal intima**	• It is part of the intercostalis interni and aids expiration. • The course of the muscle fibers is the same as that of the intercostalis interni • Between it and the intercostalis interni, the intercostal vein and nerve pass

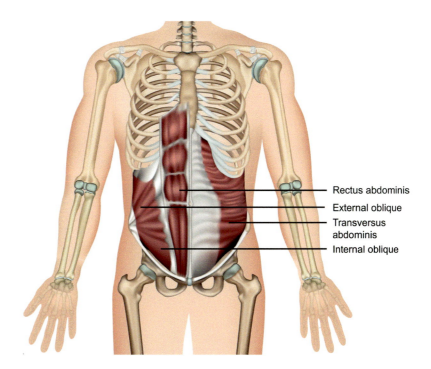

Fig. 7.18 Abdominal muscle (medicalstocks/Shutterstock.com)

Table 7.15 Origo-insertions and functions of the abdominal muscles

External obliques	• It starts from the outer surface of the 5–12 costae • It ends by entering between the serratus anterior above and the latissimus dorsi below
Internal obliques	• It starts from the fascia of the thoracolumba posteriorly, and inferiorly from the outer half of the iliac crest and inguinal ligament • The posterior fibers terminate in the 8–12 costae, and the others ends in the outer lateral edge of the rectus abdominus beaming
• Bilateral contractions of the external and internal abdominal muscles cause flexion of the trunk, and unilateral contractions of the trunk cause lateral flexion and rotation of the trunk	
Transversus abdominus	• It starts from the outer 1/3 of the inguinal ligament, the iliac crest, the deep leaf of the thoracolumbal fascia, and the inner surface of the last 6 cartilaginous costae • It aponeurosis at the outer edge of the rectus abdominus and terminates in the linea alba
Rectus abdominus	• It starts from the symphysis pubis and pubic tubercle • It terminates lateral to the anterior surface of the xiphoid and 5–7 cartilaginous costae in the form of 3 parts above
Pyramidal muscles	• It is a small triangular muscle
• It provides flexion of the trunk and stabilization of the pelvis • They facilitate the placement of the abdominal organs, providing protection and support	

7.3 Palpable Points in the Axial Skeleton

The palpable points in the vertebral column are summarized in Table 7.16.

Table 7.16 Vertebral column palpation points

C7 vertebra	• It is the most protruding, large, and mobile vertebra in neck flexion and extension • It displaces the C7 upper part with neck flexion • It is fixed and immobile to the T1 first costa • It is the most mobile protrusion when the person is doing neck flexion and extension
T2 vertebra	It is at the level of the episternal notch It is at the level of the T2 projection of the upper corner of the scapula
T7 vertebra	It is at the level of the lower corner of the scapula

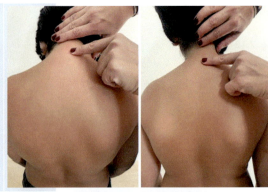

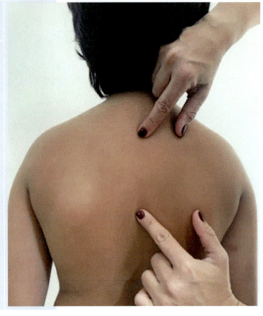

Table 7.16 (continued)

T11-12 vertebrae	The 11th and 12th costae are known as "floating costae" because they are not attached to the costal cartilage	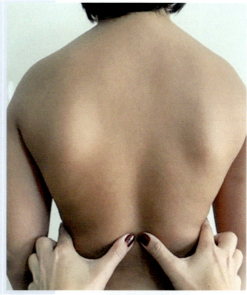
L4 vertebra	It is on the horizontal plane drawn from the iliac crest	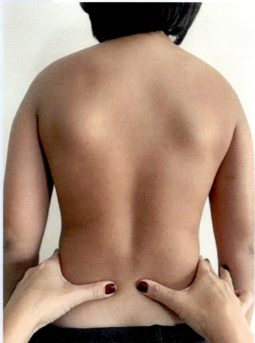

(continued)

Table 7.16 (continued)

11 and 12th costae	It can be felt most comfortably in the prone position	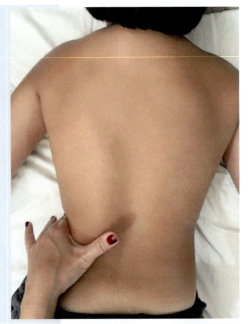
Thoracic transverse protrusions	● The transverse projections of the thoracic vertebrae can be felt in the prone position. The middle finger comes in line with the spinous protrusions, and the two fingers on the sides line up with the transverse protrusions ● Fingers can be moved up and down to feel the muscles and other structures located here	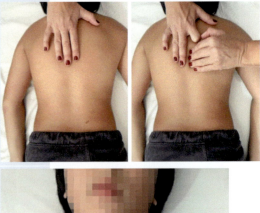
Sternum, 10. costa and xiphoid protrusion	It is felt where the abdominal muscles begin as it travels to the lower part of the sternum Just above here, the lower end of the sternum is the xiphoid protrusion. The 10th costa sticks here	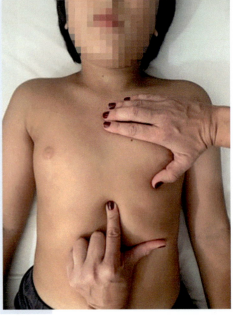

7.4 Vertebral Colon Biomechanics

The vertebral column consists of two columns, the anterior column consisting of the corpus vertebrae, and the posterior column consisting of the arcus vertebrae. The functions of the vertebral column are summarized in Fig. 7.19.

The starting point, which passes through the body center of gravity and is formed by the intersection of the horizontal, sagittal, and frontal planes, is called the primary reference plane (Fig. 7.20). Movements occurring in these planes are:

Sagittal plane: It is the plane perpendicular to the horizontal and frontal planes, which is assumed to divide the body into two equal parts, right and left, passing through the center of gravity from the anteroposterior direction. Flexion and extension movements occur in this plane.

Frontal plane: It is the plane perpendicular to the horizontal and sagittal planes, which is assumed to divide the body into two equal parts passing through the center of gravity from one side to the other. In this plane, the trunk performs lateral flexion and right-left sliding movements.

Sagittal plane
Coronal plane
Transverse plane

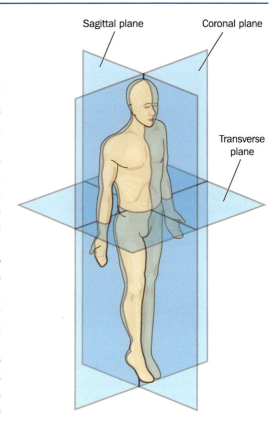

Fig. 7.20 Movement planes (Blamb/Shutterstock.com)

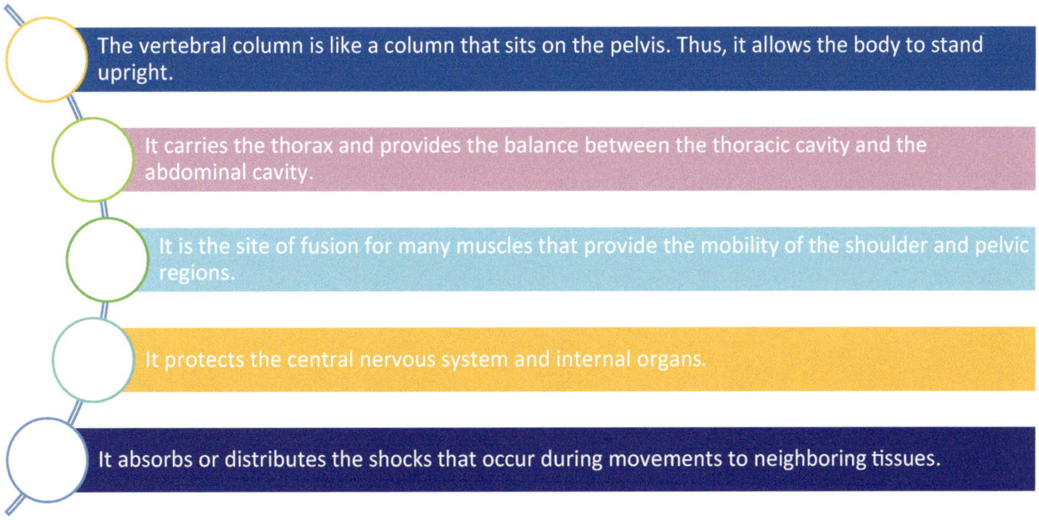

The vertebral column is like a column that sits on the pelvis. Thus, it allows the body to stand upright.
It carries the thorax and provides the balance between the thoracic cavity and the abdominal cavity.
It is the site of fusion for many muscles that provide the mobility of the shoulder and pelvic regions.
It protects the central nervous system and internal organs.
It absorbs or distributes the shocks that occur during movements to neighboring tissues.

Fig. 7.19 Functions of the vertebral column

Horizontal plane: It is the plane that divides the trunk into two parts, upper and lower, passing through the center of gravity.

Rotational movements occur in this plane.

The movements that occur in the spine and the biomechanical changes that occur during these movements are summarized in Figs. 7.21, 7.22, and 7.23.

> **Clinical Information**
> Movements that occur in the vertebral column very rarely occur in isolation. The movements that occur are usually in interaction with each other. It is necessary to pay attention to these interactions, especially in postural or positional problems that occur in the spine.

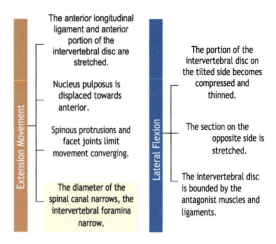

Fig. 7.22 Biomechanical changes during vertebra extension and lateral flexion movements

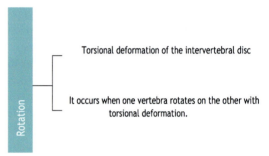

Fig. 7.23 Biomechanical changes that occur during rotational movement in the vertebra

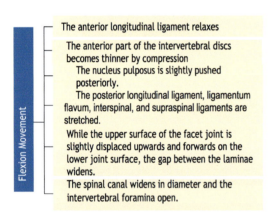

Fig. 7.21 Biomechanical changes that occur during flexion movement in the vertebra

7.5 Basic Exercise Examples for the Axial Skeleton

Basic exercises for the axial skeleton are shown in Table 7.17.

Table 7.17 Basic exercises for the axial skeleton

Muscle Group	Exercise Position
Trapezius	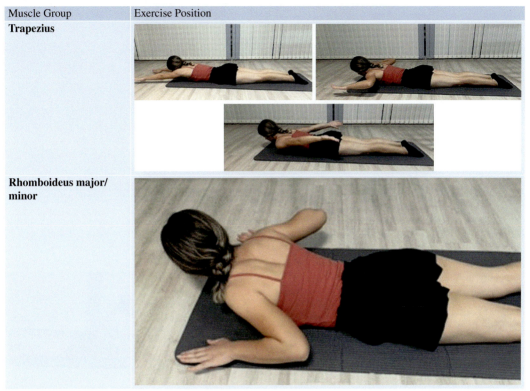
Rhomboideus major/ minor	

Muscle Group	Exercise Position
Latissimus dorsi	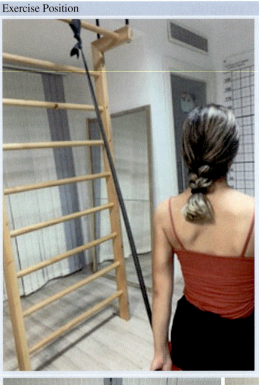
Erectors/Multifidus/Rotators	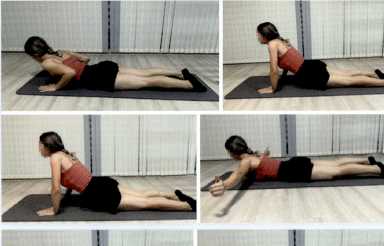
Multifidus	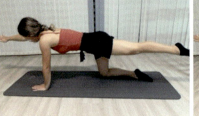

7 The Axial Skeleton

Muscle Group	Exercise Position
Pectoralis major/minor	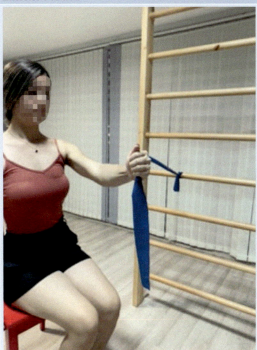
Rectus abdominus/ External -internal oblique	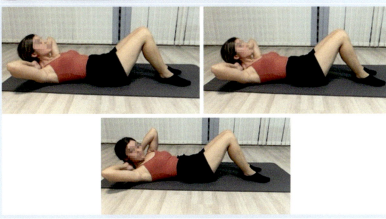
Transversus abdominus	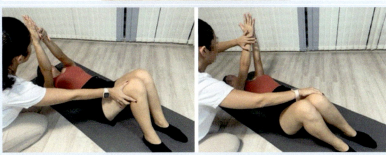

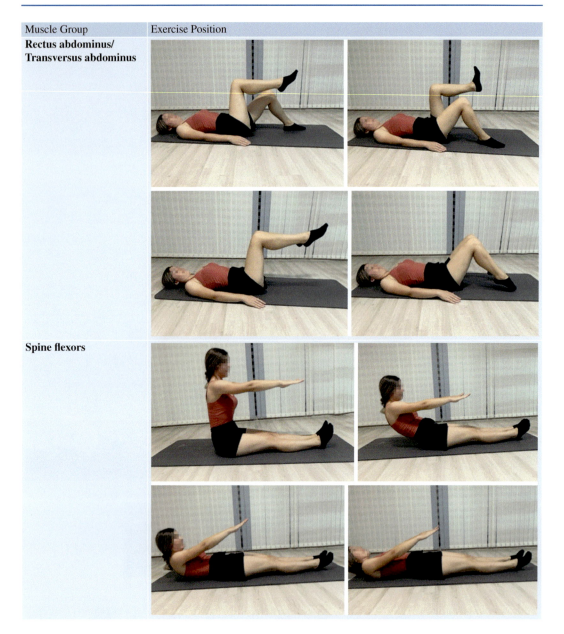

7.6 Conclusion

The axial skeleton, which is summarized in general terms, is in contact with all body structures. There are two features that distinguish humans from other living things. The first is to be able to think, and the second is to be able to walk in an upright posture. In order to fulfill these two important features, the axial skeleton described in this section must be able to move in sync with other body parts and provide the necessary and sufficient support. These synchronized movements are greatly affected in problems in the musculoskeletal system or in diseases or injuries affecting this system. Therefore, it is necessary to pay attention and give importance to holistic approaches for treatment processes in clinics.

- The vertebral column is like a column that sits on the pelvis. Thus, it allows the body to stand upright.
- It carries the thorax and provides the balance between the thoracic cavity and the abdominal cavity.
- It is the site of fusion for many muscles that provide the mobility of the shoulder and pelvic regions.
- It protects the central nervous system and internal organs.
- It absorbs or distributes the shocks that occur during movements to neighboring tissues.

Further Reading

Biel A. Spine and thorax. In: Biel A, editor. Trail guide to the body: how to locate muscles, bones, and more. Boulder: Books of Discovery; 2017. p. 165–223.

Bonnel F, Dimeglio A. Vertebral column: muscles, aponeurosis, and fascia. In: Vital JM, Cawley DT, editors. Spinal anatomy. New York: Springer; 2020. p. 279–320.

DeSai C, Reddy V, Agarwal A. Anatomy, back, vertebral column. Treasure Island (FL): StatPearls; 2020.

Farrell C, Kiel J. Anatomy, back, rhomboid muscles. Treasure Island (FL): StatPearls; 2020.

Franz A, Klaas J, Schumann M, Frankewitsch T, Filler TJ, Behringer M. Anatomical versus functional motor points of selected upper body muscles. Muscle Nerve. 2018;57(3):460–5.

Jaworski Ł, Karpiński R. Biomechanics of the human spine. J Technol Exploit Mech Eng. 2017;3(1):8–12.

Mahadevan V. Anatomy of the vertebral column. Surgery (Oxford). 2018;36(7):327–32.

Mallo M. Chapter 13—The axial musculoskeletal system. In: Baldock R, Bard J, Davidson DR, Morriss-Kay G, editors. Kaufman's atlas of mouse development supplement. New York: Academic Press; 2016. p. 165–75.

Muto M, Muto G, Giurazza F, Tecame M, Fabio Z, Izzo R. Anatomy and biomechanics of the spine. In: Marcia S, Saba L, editors. Radiofrequency treatments on the spine. New York: Springer; 2017. p. 1–10.

Newell N, Little JP, Christou A, Adams MA, Adam CJ, Masouros SD. Biomechanics of the human intervertebral disc: a review of testing techniques and results. J Mech Behav Biomed Mater. 2017;69:420–34.

Nikita E. Chapter 1—The human skeleton. In: Nikita E, editor. Osteoarchaeology. New York: Academic Press; 2017. p. 1–75.

Rehnke RD, Groening RM, Buskirk ERV, Clarke JM. Anatomy of the superficial fascia system of the breast: a comprehensive theory of breast fascial anatomy. Plast Reconstr Surg. 2018;142(5):1135–44.

Sénégas J. Comparative anatomy of the axial skeleton of vertebrates. In: Vital JM, Cawley DT, editors. Spinal anatomy. New York: Springer; 2020. p. 3–18.

Seth A, Dong M, Matias R, Delp SL. Muscle contributions to upper-extremity movement and work from a musculoskeletal model of the human shoulder. Front Neurorobot. 2019;13:90.

Waxenbaum JA, Futterman B. Anatomy, back, thoracic vertebrae. Treasure Island (FL): StatPearls; 2017.

Waxenbaum JA, Reddy V, Williams C, Futterman B. Anatomy, back, lumbar vertebrae. Treasure Island (FL): StatPearls; 2020.

Williams S, Alkhatib B, Serra R. Chapter 3—Development of the axial skeleton and intervertebral disc. In: Olsen BR, editor. Current topics in developmental biology. New York: Academic Press; 2019. p. 49–90.

The Head and Neck Anatomy

Omer Faruk Yasaroglu and Numan Demir

Abstract

The head consists of skull bones, mimic muscles, brain and many nerves, and blood vessels. All the functions we perform with our five senses such as sight, hearing, smell, touch, and taste take place in the head region. In addition, emotions are expressed thanks to the facial muscles. One of the most essential functions performed in the head area is speech. Speech is a fundamental human characteristic that enables communication and social engagement. The only movable bone in the head is the mandible. The movement of the head is mostly owing to its articulation with the neck. It acts as a bridge between the body and the head. Due to their proximity and directly linked functions, the head and neck regions are mentioned together. The head and neck areas are crucial to swallowing function. Therefore, the head provides the realization of many intertwined vital functions with both the contractile and noncontractile structures it contains in the head and neck region. In this chapter, the anatomy of the head and neck region, the muscles it contains, and evidence-based exercises for these muscles will be explained.

O. F. Yasaroglu (✉) · N. Demir
Faculty of Physical Therapy and Rehabilitation, Hacettepe University, Ankara, Turkey
e-mail: farukyasaroglu@hacettepe.edu.tr; numan@hacettepe.edu.tr

8.1 Noncontractile Structures in the Head and Neck Region

8.1.1 Head Bones

The skeletal system consists of bones, joints, and cartilage structures associated with them. Bone structures not only provide the body structure but also form a support surface for the soft tissue. The bones of the skull consist of cranial bones and facial bones. The cranial bones protect the brain by surrounding it. Through the cavities in the skull, blood vessels and nerves can pass. The facial bones form the face and provide support for functions such as chewing, speaking, and breathing. The head bones are given in the table (Table 8.1).

There are 22 bones in the human skull, excluding the middle ear bones. Except for the mandible, all other bones are immobile. Thanks to the temporomandibular joint it forms with the tempo-

Table 8.1 Head bones

Cranial bones	Facial bones
• Occipital (single)	• Vomer (single)
• Frontal (single)	• Mandible (single)
• Sphenoid (single)	• Lacrimal (paired)
• Ethmoid (single)	• Nasal (paired)
• Parietal (paired)	• Inferior nasal conchal (paired)
• Temporal (paired)	• Zygomatic bones (paired)
	• Maxillae (paired)

ral and the mandible bones are mobile. The skull also articulates with the vertebral column in the neck region. When viewed from above, the skull displays a single piece of the frontal bone in the front, two connected pieces of parietal bone on the sides, and a single piece of the temporal bone in the back. The junction of bone structures is called a suture. Laterally, the sphenoid and ethmoid bones can be seen. In the anterior part of the skull are the facial bones, including the maxilla, mandible, and zygomatic bone (Fig. 8.1). The maxillary bone comprises the upper jaw. The mandible is the lower jaw. Several facial bones are shared by one or more soft tissues. An anomaly in the facial bone also affects many soft tissues.

In the lower part of the skull are the foramen and the hard palate. The hard palate forms the floor of the nasal cavity and the roof of the mouth. The foramen provides a passageway for the cranial nerves that innervate the blood vessels supplying the head and neck. The mandibular branch of the nervus trigeminalis (V) passes through the foramen ovale. The internal carotid artery and the sympathetic carotid plexus pass through the carotid canal. Just behind the styloid process is the stylomastoid foramen, where the N. facialis (VII) emerges from the skull to the face. The jugular foramen, placed medial to the styloid process, allows the internal jugular vein, the N. glossopharyngeus (IX), the N. vagus (X), and the N. accessorius to pass through (XI). The spinal cord, vertebral arteries, and nerve accessory (XI) go via the foramen magnum, the largest clearance in the lower view (Fig. 8.2).

8.1.2 Temporomandibular Joint (TMJ)

Ginglymoarthrodial diarthrosis formed between the mandible and the temporal bone is a joint. The

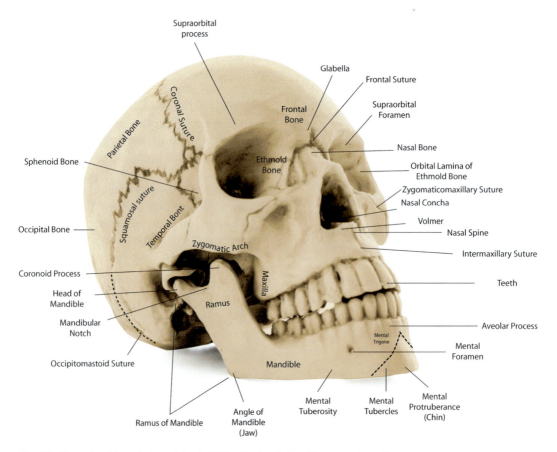

Fig. 8.1 Frontal and lateral view of the skull (Quality Stock Arts/Shutterstock.com)

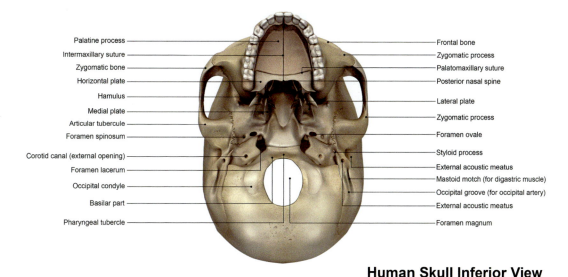

Fig. 8.2 Inferior view of the skull (sciencepics/Shutterstock.com)

TMJ consists of the joint capsule, articular disc, synovial fluid, and several ligaments. The temporal bone forms the cranial surface of the TMJ. The area of temporal bone where the condyle of the mandible articulates is known as the glenoid fossa. The articular disc is placed slightly below the glenoid fossa and covers the condyle of the mandible. It has a biconcave or oval shape. The anterior part of the disc contacts the joint capsule, articular eminence, condyle, and lateral pterygoid muscle. The margins of the cartilaginous disc surround the joint and partially fuse with the fibrous capsule. The joint disc facilitates and regulates the joint's mobility during movement.

Three main ligaments connect the joint to the cranium: the temporomandibular, stylomandibular, and sphenomandibular ligaments. The temporomandibular ligament supports the lateral joint capsule and is regarded as the main connector for the joint. This ligament prevents the mandible from moving backward excessively. The stylomandibular ligament prevents excessive protrusion of the mandibula. The primary function of the sphenomandibular ligament is to hinder excessive translation of the TMJ condyle after the mouth is opened 10°. The other two ligaments tighten when the mandible protrudes, preventing excessive movement (Fig. 8.3). These bonds direct the forces on the TMJ and form proprioceptive afferents. Furthermore, joint capsule receptors, masticatory muscles, skin receptors, and periodontal ligaments contribute to joint proprioception.

During the opening of the mandible, the joint undergoes two fundamental motions: rotation and translation. The first movement of the joint, a 20–25 mm rotation, is followed by translation, which refers to the forward sliding of the joint. A mouth opening of 40–50 mm is considered normal. Trismus refers to the pathology of opening fewer than 35 mm. The TMJ is involved in many functions such as sucking, chewing, swallowing, speaking, breathing, and facial expressions.

8.1.3 Neck Bones

The cervical vertebrae consist of 7 vertebrae located between the skull and the thoracic vertebrae. There are transverse foramens on either side of the vertebral foramen. The vertebral artery passes through these transverse foramens. The first (atlas) and second (axis) cervical vertebrae are specifically defined because of their proximity to the skull and their unusual anatomy. The

TMJ DISORDER

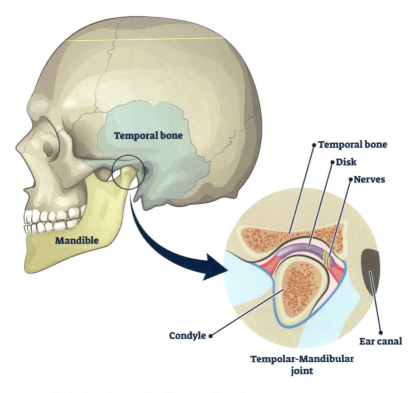

Fig. 8.3 Temporomandibular joint (VectorMine/Shutterstock.com)

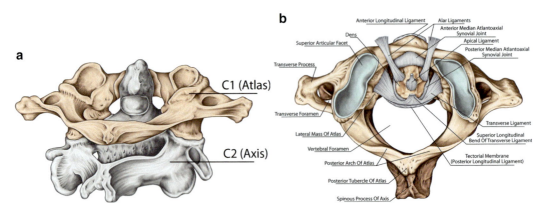

Fig. 8.4 (**a**, **b**) Atlantoaxial joint (stihii for both/Shutterstock.com)

atlas is in the form of an irregular ring connected by a short anterior arch and a longer posterior arch. The axis has a vertical projection called the dens anteriorly. The dens articulates with the anterior arch of the atlas (Fig. 8.4).

Located at the level of the third cervical vertebral, anterior–superior to the thyroid cartilage, the hyoid bone does not articulate with any structure. Many muscles such as the suprahyoid and infrahyoid muscles connect to the hyoid. The

Fig. 8.5 Larynx (Alila Medical Media/Shutterstock.com)

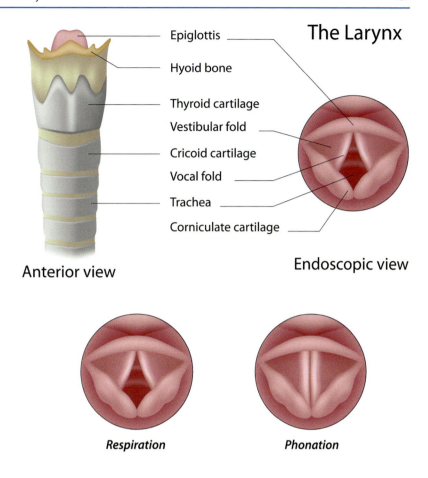

hyoid bone with its connected muscles forms the base of the tongue. It takes part in functions such as swallowing, chewing, speaking, and breathing. The hyoid bone may rise and fall in response to muscle contraction and function. The epiglottis is the cartilage structure at the base of the tongue. This structure forms the root of the tongue and the anatomical cavity called the vallecula. It undergoes retroflexion with the effect of gravity during swallowing. The movement of the epiglottis is facilitated by the elevation of the larynx, its contact with the base of the tongue, and the weight and movement of food passing over it. Epiglottis movement helps to close the airway during swallowing. Vocal cords are responsible for primary phonation. During swallowing, it abducts and closes the airway (Fig. 8.5).

8.2 Contractile Structures in the Head and Neck Region

Muscles contract and relax by innervation of the corresponding nerves. They cause movement of soft tissue or bones along with contraction. It is essential to understand where the muscle starts and where it ends. Origin is often connected to the structure that moves the least. The opposite end of the muscle, the insertion, is the more movable part. Generally, when the muscle contracts, it moves from the insertion to the origin. The head and neck region are divided into six main groups based on their functions: mimic muscles, chewing muscles, tongue muscles, hyoid muscles and pharynx muscles, and cervical muscles. The muscles of the ear, eye, and nose are not included.

8.2.1 Mimic Muscles

Mimic muscles are the muscles humans use to express themselves and their emotions (Fig. 8.6). These muscles also contribute to the functions of speaking, chewing, and swallowing. Innervation of all mimic muscles is provided by N. facialis (VII). Both halves of the face are innervated separately. Mimic muscles are given in the table (Table 8.2). The sensation of the face is received by the branches of the trigeminal nerve and cervical plexus.

8.2.2 Chewing Muscles

The chewing muscles consist of four muscles attached to the mandible: M. masseter, M. temporalis, M. pterygoideus medialis, and M. pterygoideus lateralis (Fig. 8.7). The masseter is the strongest of the chewing muscles. The temporomandibular joint enables mandibular movements while chewing (TMJ). Therefore, pathologies of these muscles may be related to TMJ dysfunctions. The table below lists the chewing muscles (Table 8.3).

8.2.3 Hyoid Muscles

The hyoid muscles attach to the hyoid bone and assist functions such as chewing, swallowing, and speaking. The muscles are divided into two based on the way they are attached to the hyoid bone from above or below: suprahyoid and infrahyoid. During swallowing, the suprahyoid muscles are primarily responsible for elevating the hyolarynx. By closing the airway in this manner, safe swallowing is maintained. The infrahyoid muscles, on the other hand, operate as a suspension during hyoid movement, ensuring smooth and fluent movement. Additionally, when the hyoid bone is fixed, the suprahyoid muscles also act as mouth opening. The hyoid muscles and their innervations are given in the table (Table 8.4).

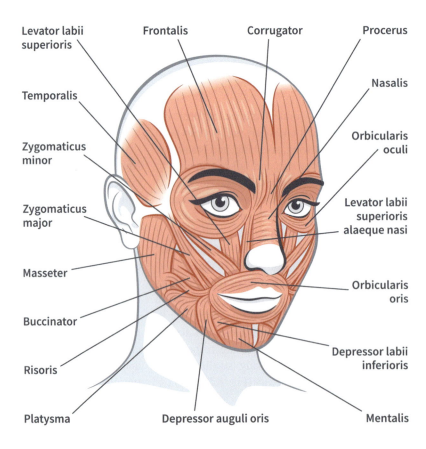

Fig. 8.6 Mimic muscles (ORLY Design/Shutterstock.com)

Table 8.2 Mimic muscles

Muscle	Function	Sensation
Mentalis	Depression and outward movement of the lower lip, wrinkling of chin skin	It expresses emotions such as sadness and doubt
Platysma	It depresses the mandible and the rim of the mouth It stretches the lower face and anterior neck area	It helps to express many emotions such as fear and surprise
Frontalis	Primary eyebrow elevation	It serves to raise an eyebrow during the confusion. It works vertically and creates horizontal lines on the forehead
Corrugator	It pulls eyebrows down and inward	It is the main muscle that expresses pain. It creates vertical ridges on the nose when the eyebrows are frowned upon (vertical ridges)
Procerus	It pulls eyebrows down	It creates horizontal wrinkles on the nose as it ends in the skin on the nasal bridge
Buccinator	It pushes the cheeks into the oral cavity	It enables blowing. It helps regulate intraoral pressure
Orbicularis oris	It closes and shrinks lips	It allows moving the lips, blowing, and kissing while speaking
Orbicularis oculi	It consists of three parts. The largest part is responsible for eye closure. Its upper part is called the depressor supercilii. It helps to pull the eyebrows down	It is used for voluntary tight eye closure, bringing the eyebrows slightly closer together and pulling them down
Risorius	It pulls the corner of the mouth laterally	It helps with expressions such as smiles and grins
Levator labii superioris	It elevates the upper lip	It allows the emergence of maxillary teeth. It is used to express emotions such as smiling and arrogance
Levator anguli oris	It elevates the corner of the mouth	It helps to smile
Depressor anguli oris	It depresses the corner of the mouth	It allows the expression of emotions such as sadness and anger
Depressor labii inferioris	It depresses the lower lip	It allows the expression of emotions such as sadness
Zygomaticus major	It elevates the corner of the mouth posterior-superiorly	It helps to smile
Zygomaticus minor	It elevates the upper lip	It allows the emergence of maxillary teeth. It is used to express emotions such as smiling and arrogance

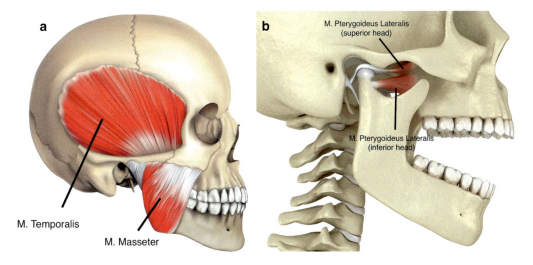

Fig. 8.7 (**a**, **b**) Chewing muscles (RuMax/Shutterstock.com) (**a**), (Alex Mit/Shutterstock.com) (**b**)

Table 8.3 Chewing muscles

Muscle	Origin-insertion	Function
Masseter	**Origin:** Maxilla, inferior zygomatic arch **Insertion:** Lateral surface of mandibular ramus	Elevation of the mandible Superficial fibers: Mandible protrusion
Temporalis	**Origin:** Temporal fossa **Insertion:** Coronoid process of the mandible	Anterior and middle fibers: Mandible elevation Posterior fibers: Mandible retraction
Pterygoideus lateralis	**Origin:** Superior part: Infratemporal part of the greater wing of the sphenoid bone Inferior part: Lateral surface of the sphenoid bone **Insertion:** Superior part: Temporomandibular joint capsule Inferior part: Mandibular condyle	Mandible depression Superior part: Stabilizing the condyle and disc during elevation
Pterygoideus medialis	**Origin:** Medial surface of the maxilla and sphenoid bone **Insertion:** Medial aspect of mandibular ramus	Mandible elevation and protrusion

Table 8.4 Hyoid muscles

Muscle		Origin	Insertion	Innervation
Suprahyoid muscles	Mylohyoid	Mandibula	Hyoid bone	By the mylohyoid nerve of the mandibular branch of the trigeminal nerve
	Digastric	**Anterior belly:** Intermediate tendon **Posterior belly:** Mastoid notch of the temporal bone	**Anterior belly:** Medial surface of the mandible **Posterior belly:** Intermediate tendon	**Anterior belly:** By the mylohyoid nerve of the mandibular branch of the trigeminal nerve **Posterior belly:** By the posterior digastric nerve, a branch of the facial nerve
	Geniohyoid	Mandibula	Hyoid bone	First cervical nerve, led by the hypoglossal nerve
	Stylohyoid	Styloid process of the temporal bone	Hyoid bone	By the stylohyoid, a branch of the facial nerve
Infrahyoid muscles	Omohyoid	Scapula	Hyoid bone	Second and third cervical nerve
	Sternohyoid	Posterior and superior aspects of the sternum	Hyoid bone	Second and third cervical nerve
	Thyrohyoid	Thyroid cartilage	Hyoid bone	Second and third cervical nerve
	Sternothyroid	Posterior aspect of the sternum	Thyroid cartilage	Second and third cervical nerve

8.2.4 Tongue Muscles

The tongue is a thick mass of voluntary muscles coated by a mucosal membrane and attached to the floor of the mouth by the lingual frenum. It performs intricate functions during speech, chewing, and swallowing. Two types of muscles make up the tongue: the extrinsic and intrinsic tongue muscles. Intrinsic muscles are placed inside the tongue, whereas extrinsic muscles are located outside. The insertions of the extrinsic muscles are located inside the tongue. In terms of their direction, intrinsic tongue muscles are classified as superior longitudinal, inferior longitudinal, vertical, and transverse. The contraction of these muscles changes the shape of the tongue. Extrinsic muscles attach the tongue to bony structures and move the tongue (Table 8.5). All tongue muscles are innervated by the hypoglossal nerve.

Table 8.5 Tongue muscles

Extrinsic muscles	Function
Styloglossus muscle	It pulls the tongue back, moves it up and back
Genioglossus muscle	Different parts of the muscle can protrude the tongue from the oral cavity or press parts of the tongue surface
Hyoglossus muscle	It depresses the tongue

8.2.5 Pharyngeal Muscles

The pharynx is the region bounded by the oral cavity anteriorly and the nasal cavity superiorly, extending to the upper sphincter of the esophagus. It establishes a passageway for both breathing and swallowing. It has three components: the nasopharynx, oropharynx, and laryngopharynx. The pharynx consists of the stylopharyngeus, salpingopharyngeus, soft palate muscles, and pharyngeal structures. Stylopharyngeus, salpingopharyngeus, and palatopharyngeus are laryngopharyngeal elevators. The stylopharyngeus begins from the styloid portion of the temporal bone and extends longitudinally and terminates at the pharyngeal wall. It is innervated by the glossopharyngeal nerve.

Pharyngeal structures compose the posterior and lateral pharyngeal walls. These structures consist of three parts upper, middle, and lower parts. Pharyngeal structures elevate the pharynx and larynx and create pharyngeal pressure to deliver nutrients to the esophagus. They are innervated by the pharyngeal plexus. As a continuation of the hard palate, the roof of the mouth is formed by the five pairs of soft palate muscles. Additionally, these structures are connected to the tongue. All muscles are involved in speaking and swallowing. The tensor veli palatini muscle is innervated by the mandibular branch of the trigeminal nerve, while all other soft palate muscles are innervated by the pharyngeal plexus (Fig. 8.8). Soft palate muscles are given in the table (Table 8.6). The pharyngeal plexus innervates the pharyngeal muscles. These muscles are formed by the pharyngeal plexus vagus and glossopharyngeal nerve branches. The glossopharyngeal nerve receives the sensation in the plexus, while the vagus performs its motor innervation. Only the stylopharyngeus is innervated by the glossopharyngeal nerve.

8.2.6 Cervical Muscles

The cervical muscles are responsible for the mobility and stability of the neck. M. trapezius and M. sternocleidomasteideus are the largest and most superficial muscles (Fig. 8.9). Cervical muscles are given in the table (Table 8.7).

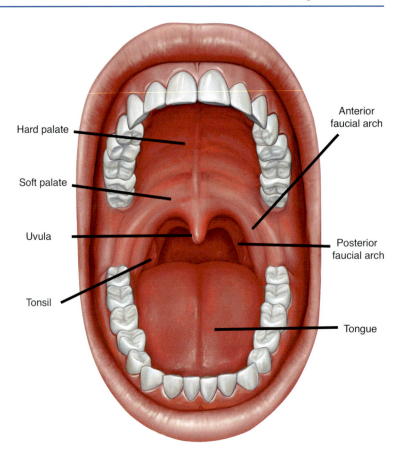

Fig. 8.8 Anterior faucial arch (Andrea Danti/Shutterstock.com)

Table 8.6 Soft palate muscles

Muscle	Function
Palatoglossus (it forms the anterior faucial arch)	It elevates and angles the tongue towards the soft palate, and depresses the soft palate towards the tongue, forming the sphincter that separates the oral cavity from the pharynx
Palatopharyngeus (it forms the posterior faucial arch)	It moves the palate posterior-inferiorly and the posterior pharyngeal wall anterior-superiorly to close the nasopharynx
Levator veli palatini	It elevates the soft palate
Tensor veli palatini	It slightly depresses the soft palate
Muscle of the uvula	It closes the nasopharynx

Fig. 8.9 Cervical muscles (Mister_X/Shutterstock.com)

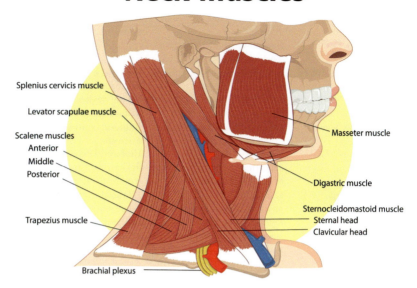

Table 8.7 Cervical muscles

Muscle	Origin-insertion	Function	Innervation
Sternocleidomastoideus (SCM)	**Origin:** The medial part of the clavicle and the superior-lateral surface of the sternum **Insertion:** Mastoid process of the temporal bone	When contracted unilaterally, the head lateral flexes to the same side and rotates to the opposite side	XI. Cranial nerve
Trapezius	**Origin:** External surface of the occipital bone and the posterior midline of the cervical and thoracic regions **Insertion:** Lateral third of clavicle and scapula	Cervical fibers elevate the shoulder.	XI. Cranial nerve C3–C4
Scalene muscles	**Origin:** Transverse protrusion of cervical vertebrae (process) **Insertion:** The superior surface of the first and second costae	Neck flexion with bilateral contraction Lateral flexion (ipsilateral) and rotation (contralateral) with unilateral contraction Neck lateral flexion Elevation of costae	C4–C8
Longus colli	**Origin:** C3–C5 transverse tubercle Anterior of C5–T3 body **Insertion:** Anterior of C2–C6 body	Neck flexion when contracted bilaterally Neck lateral flexion and neck rotation when contracted unilaterally (contralateral)	C2–C7
Longus capitis	**Origin:** C3–C6 transverse processes **Insertion:** Basilar part of the occipital bone	Neck flexion when contracted bilaterally Neck rotation when contracted unilaterally (ipsilateral)	C1–3
Rectus capitis anterior	**Origin:** Anterior surface of the atlas bone **Insertion:** Basilar part of the occipital bone	Neck flexion when contracted bilaterally Neck rotation when contracted unilaterally (ipsilateral)	C1–2

(continued)

Table 8.7 (continued)

Muscle	Origin-insertion	Function	Innervation
Rectus capitis lateralis	**Origin:** Superior surface of the atlas bone **Insertion:** Jugular process of the occipital bone	Lateral flexion of the neck when contracted unilaterally (ipsilateral)	C1–2
Semispinalis capitis	**Origin:** Transverse processes of the upper thoracic vertebrae **Insertion:** Occipital bone	**Bilateral contraction:** Head neck extension **unilateral contraction:** Lateral flexion, head and neck rotation (contralateral)	Cervical and thoracic spinal nerves
Semispinalis cervicis	**Origin:** Transverse processes of the upper thoracic vertebrae **Insertion:** Spinous processes of C2–C4 vertebrae	**Bilateral contraction:** Head neck extension **Unilateral contraction:** Lateral flexion, head and neck rotation (contralateral)	Cervical and thoracic spinal nerves
Splenius capitis	**Origin:** C7–T3 spinous process, inferior part of the ligamentum nuchae **Insertion:** Temporal bone mastoid process and lateral part of the nuchal line of the occiput	**Bilateral contraction:** Neck extension **Unilateral contraction:** Head and neck lateral flexion and rotation	Cervical spinal nerve
Splenius cervicis	**Origin:** T3–T6 spinous processes **Insertion:** C1–C3 transverse processes	**Bilateral contraction:** Head neck extension **Unilateral contraction:** Head and neck lateral flexion and rotation	Cervical spinal nerve
Levator scapula	**Origin:** C1–C4 transverse processes **Insertion:** Superior of the medial scapula	**Bilateral contraction:** Neck extension with fixed scapula elevation, adduction, rotation, insertion **Unilateral contraction:** Neck lateral flexion and rotation (ipsilateral) while insertion is fixed	N. dorsalis scapula (C5), cervical spinal nerves (C3–C4)
Rectus capitis posterior major	**Origin:** Spinous process of atlas **Insertion:** Inferior lateral part of the nuchal line of the occiput	**Bilateral contraction:** Head extension **Unilateral contraction:** Head rotation (ipsilateral)	Suboccipital nerve (C1 posterior ramus)
Rectus capitis posterior minor	**Origin:** Tubercle of the posterior arch of the atlas **Insertion:** Inferior medial part of occiput nuchal line	**Bilateral contraction:** Head extension	Suboccipital nerve (C1 posterior ramus)
Obliquus capitis superior	**Origin:** Transverse process of atlas **Insertion:** Occiput	**Bilateral contraction:** Head extension **Unilateral contraction:** Head lateral flexion (ipsilateral)	Suboccipital nerve (C1 posterior ramus)
Obliquus capitis inferior	**Origin:** Spinous process of the axis **Insertion:** Transverse process of atlas	**Bilateral contraction:** Head extension **Unilateral contraction:** Head rotation (ipsilateral)	Suboccipital nerve (C1 posterior ramus)

8.3 Neural Structures in Head and Neck Region

There are 12 separately defined cranial nerve pairs in the head and neck region. They innervate all striated and smooth muscles of the head and receive sensation. In addition, they are responsible for the sensations of sight, smell, and hearing, as well as structures such as the salivary and lacrimal glands. Cranial nerves and their functions are given in Chap. 5.

8.4 Movements in the Head and Neck Region

Knowing the movements of the head and neck region enables clinicians in the evaluation and treatment of very common diseases such as cervical disc herniation, headache, temporomandibular joint problems, and swallowing disorders.

8.4.1 Movements of the Head

Movements of the head are shown in Table 8.8.

8.4.2 Movements of the Temporomandibular Joint (TMJ)

The temporomandibular joint (TMJ) slides and rotates in front of each ear and consists of the mandible and the temporal bone. The TMJs along with several muscles allow the mandible to move up and down, side to side, and forward and back. When the mandible and the joints are properly aligned, smooth muscle actions, such as chewing, talking, and swallowing, can take place. When muscles, ligaments, the disk of the TMJ, and jaw and temporal bones are not aligned, several problems may occur. Movements of the temporomandibular joint are shown in Table 8.9.

Table 8.8 Movements of the head

MOVEMENT	
Cervical neutral position (anterior view): The gravity line passes through the midline of the head. There is no lateral flexion or rotation.	
Cervical neutral position (lateral view): The gravity line passes through the earlobe. 20-35° cervical lordosis (C2-C7 Cobb Angle) is regarded normal.	
Cervical rotation (left): The head turns to the left	

Table 8.8 (continued)

Cervical rotation (right): The head turns to the right	
Cervical lateral flexion (right): The head tips to the right side or touches an ear to the right shoulder	
Cervical lateral flexion (left): The head tips to the left side or touches an ear to the left shoulder	
Cervical flexion: The head bends forward towards the chest	
Cervical extension: The head bends forward-backward with the face towards the sky	

Table 8.9 Movements of the temporomandibular joint

MOVEMENT	
Mandible depression: Mouth opens with downward movement of the mandible.	
Mandible lateral deviation (right): The mandible is shifted to the right.	
Mandible lateral deviation (left): The mandible is shifted to the left.	
Mandible protrusion: The mandible is pushed forward.	
Mandible Retrusion: The mandible is pulled back.	

8.5 Head and Neck Palpation

The explanations of the anatomic structures of the head and neck and their palpation techniques are given in Table 8.10. In order not to cause/trigger pain, no more than 1.5 kg of pressure should be applied during palpation [painful range (2.0 kg of palpation); pain-free range (0.5 kg and 1.0 kg of palpation)]. Palpation should be performed bilaterally, in a relaxed and seated facing position, with the tip of the finger or by pincer palpation, when no underline bone support is present.

Table 8.10 Palpations of head and neck anatomic structures

ANATOMIC STRUCTURE	PALPATION
Temporalis muscle: The borders of the temporalis muscle were identified by palpation during repetitive clenching. One or two fingers are gently placed on the temple area of the head and the patient/client is asked to clench their teeth.	
Masseter muscle: During palpation, the limits of the muscle are determined by asking the patient to clench their teeth. 2-3 fingers are placed on the patient's/client's cheek and the patient is asked to clench their teeth.	
Digastric muscle: Fingers are placed slightly diagonally under the patient's chin. Attention should be paid to submental lymph nodes.	
Medial pterygoid muscle: After pressing with the fingers from the medial of the patient's mandible ramus to the cranial, the fingers are shifted laterally. It should be ensured that the submandibular lymph nodes are not compressed.	

Table 8.10 (continued)

Lateral pterygoid muscle: The index finger is brought forward between the cheek and teeth of the patient and palpated by applying light pressure in the carinal direction just behind the zygomatic arch. This point can be sensitive and heavy in general. Palpation should be applied gently.	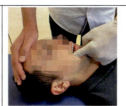
Sternocleidomastoid muscle (SCM): The patient/client is asked to rotate the head to the opposite side and to make slight lateral flexion, and the muscle is highlighted. The muscle body is palpated lightly by touching it with two fingers or by taking it between the thumb and index fingers.	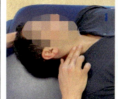 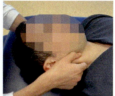
Suboccipital muscles: With the patient lying on his back, the fingers are placed just below the occiput.	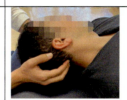
Infrahyoid muscles: 2-3 fingers are placed under the hyoid bone, on the edge of the thyroid and cricoid cartilages, and the patient/client is asked to swallow.	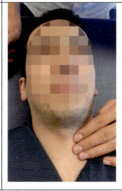

Table 8.10 (continued)

Hyoid bone: The hyoid bone is located in the midline of the neck, at the base of the mandible, and at the level of the fourth cervical vertebra. The greater cornua on both sides of the hyoid bone are palpated with the thumb and index finger.	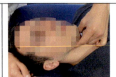
Thyroid cartilage: It is easily palpated just below the hyoid bone. It is shield-shaped and has prominent laryngeal prominence in males (known as Adam's apple)	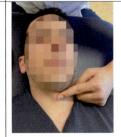
Thyroid (up) and cricoid (down) cartilage: After the thyroid cartilage is palpated, cricoid cartilage just below it can be palpated. It surrounds the trachea with its ring-shaped shape.	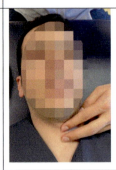

8.6 Evidence-Based Exercises for the Head and Neck Region

Head and neck problems are common among people. It is often confused with the vertebral column and shoulder–arm complex problems, and so, neglected. The head/neck, one of the five kinetic chain checkpoints (head/neck, shoulders, lumbo–pelvic–hip complex, knees, and feet/ankles) is affected by and influences all movements of the other kinetic chain points. Evidence-based exercises for the head and neck region are shown in Table 8.11. Hyoid and hyolaryngeal mobilizations, Masako maneuver, and head lift exercises should be performed while lying on the back, while others should be performed in a sitting position.

8 The Head and Neck Anatomy

Table 8.11 Evidence-based exercises for the head and neck region

EXERCISE	
Cervical extensors stretch: One hand is placed behind the head. The head is tilted forward until you feel a stretch in the back of the neck. After the head is held at the endpoint for 15-30 seconds, it is taken to the starting position. This is repeated for the other side.	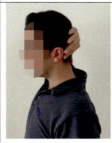 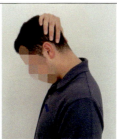
Cervical lateral flexors stretch: The right hand is placed on the left side of the head. The head is tilted to the right until tension is felt on the left side of the neck. After holding the head for 15-30 seconds at the endpoint, it is taken to the starting position. This is repeated for the other side.	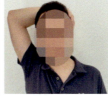 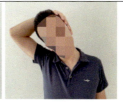
Sternocleidomastoid (SCM) muscle stretch: The right hand is placed on the left side of the head. The head is brought into left rotation-right lateral flexion until tension is felt in the SCM muscle. After holding the head for 15-30 seconds at the endpoint, it is taken to the starting position. This is repeated for the other side.	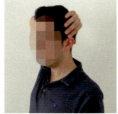 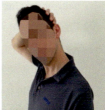
Isometric extension: One hand is placed behind the head. While holding the hand steady, press the head towards the palm for 10-30 seconds. It is repeated 3-5 times.	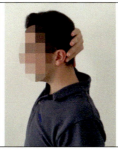

Table 8.11 (continued)

Isometric flexion: A hand is placed on the forehead. While holding the hand steady, press the head towards the palm for 10-30 seconds. It is repeated 3-5 times.	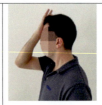
Isometric lateral flexion: The right hand is placed on the left side of the head. While holding the hand steady, press the head towards the palm for 10-30 seconds. It is repeated 3-5 times.	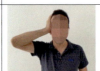
Masako maneuver: The patient/client swallows while the tongue is positioned between the teeth. The degree of difficulty can be increased by asking the patient to protrude the tongue more. It is applied by the patient for 3 sets, 8-12 repetitions.	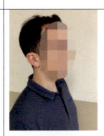
Proprioceptive neuromuscular facilitation (PNF): The patient is asked to bring his head diagonally against resistance and from left rotation to flexion-right rotation while his mouth is open (concentric contraction). At the end of the movement, the patient maintains the position for 6 seconds (stabilizing contractions). Then, while the patient tries to maintain the head and mouth position, the therapist brings the head back to the starting position (eccentric contraction). 1 set (30 repetitions) every day is repeated 3 days a week. **Head lift exercise:** The patient raises the head in the supine position, looks at the toes, holds the head for 60 seconds, and rests for 60 seconds. It repeats this 3 times (isotonic). Then the patient raises his head 30 times and leaves without holding it (isometric).	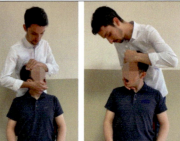 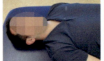

Table 8.11 (continued)

Chin tuck with a towel: A rolled towel is placed under the neck. The patient is asked to press the towel by making a chin tuck. Three sets are repeated 8-12 times.	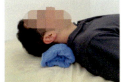 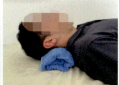
Chin tuck against resistance exercise (CTAR) with a ball: The ball is placed under the chin, and the chin tuck is done towards the ball.	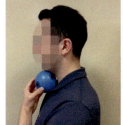 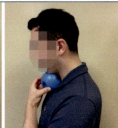
Elastic band row with chin tuck: The elastic band is attached to a door handle or similar, and the patient grasps the ends. While maintaining the chin tuck, the theraband is pulled by bringing the shoulder from flexion to extension.	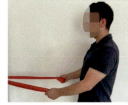 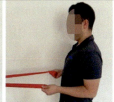
Chin tuck against resistance exercise (CTAR) with an elastic band: The elastic band is placed on the forehead of the patient and the back of the patient is passed. While holding the elastic band taut, the patient is asked to chin tuck.	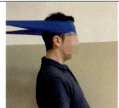 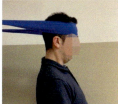

Tab. 8.11 (continued)

Hyoid mobilization: palpated the greater cornua on both sides of the hyoid bone with the thumb and index finger. When grabbing hyoid bone, care should be taken not to disturb breathing and compress the carotid arteries. Mobilize left and right at a speed that allows you to move from the end of each side in one second, with a range and intensity of some resistance. This is repeated 4 times for 30 seconds to relax the muscles around the hyoid bone.	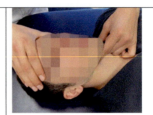
Hyolaryngeal mobilization: The distal phalanges are placed in the submental area and slowly pulled in the superior-anterior direction. Never apply pressure in the posterior direction. It is constantly checked whether there is an uncomfortable situation by looking at the face of the patient. It is applied 15-20 repetitions for 3-5 minutes.	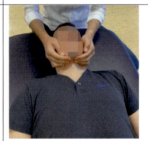

8.7 Conclusion

All body functions are either directly or indirectly connected to the head and neck. This region is responsible for vital tasks such as feeding, breathing, hearing, speaking, seeing, and smelling. This region is frequently impacted by neurological diseases, head and neck cancers, and head traumas. All other systems are affected by the deterioration of nutrition and respiratory functions in particular. Due to the fact that the physiological actions that occur during swallowing are so distinct, this subject must be studied separately. The head and neck region is highly intricate owing to the presence of hundreds of muscles of different sizes and the connections between the brain and cranial nerves. Thorough knowledge of the anatomy and physiology of this region is essential for the development of a correct and effective rehabilitation program.

Further Reading

Bordoni B, Varacallo M. Anatomy, head and neck, temporomandibular joint. Treasure Island (FL): StatPearls Publishing; 2022.

Brennan PA, Mahadevan V, Evans BT. Clinical head and neck anatomy for surgeons. In: "Chapter 1: The Scalp" and "Chapter 2: Anatomy of the ageing face" and "Chapter 6: Temporal bone, middle ear and mastoid" and "Chapter 9: Oral cavity" and "Chapter 14: Mandible" and "Chapter 16: Infratemporal fossa, pterygopalatine fossa and muscles of mastication" and "Chapter 17: Temporomandibular joint" "Chapter 18: Pharynx" and "Chapter 21: Larynx, trachea and tracheobronchial tree" and "Chapter 24: The Neck" and "Chapter 27: Cervical spine" and "Chapter 31: Overview of the cranial nerves". Boca Raton: CRC Press; 2015. p. 3–23.

Fehrenbach MJ, Herring SW. Illustrated anatomy of the head and neck. In: "Chapter 2: Surface Anatomy" "Chapter 3: Skeletal System" and "Chapter 4: Muscular System" and "Chapter 5: Temporomandibular Joint" and "Chapter 8: Nervous System". Amsterdam: Elsevier Health Sciences; 2015. p. 11–126.

Gross AR, Paquin JP, Dupont G, Blanchette S, Lalonde P, Cristie T, et al. Exercises for mechanical neck disorders: a Cochrane review update. Manual Ther. 2016;24:25–45.

Kılınç HE, Arslan SS, Demir N, Karaduman A. The effects of different exercise trainings on suprahyoid muscle activation, tongue pressure force and dysphagia limit in healthy subjects. Dysphagia. 2020;35(4):717–24.

Krekeler BN, Rowe LM, Connor NP. Dose in exercise-based dysphagia therapies: a scoping review. Dysphagia. 2021;36(1):1–32.

Martini ML, Neifert SN, Chapman EK, Mroz TE, Rasouli JJ. Cervical spine alignment in the sagittal axis: a review of the best validated measures in clinical practice. Glob Spine J. 2021;11(8):1307–12.

Sayaca C, Arslan SS, Sayaca N, Demir N, Somay G, Kaya D, et al. Is the proprioceptive neuromuscular facilitation technique superior to shaker exercises in swallowing rehabilitation? Eur Arch OtorhinoLaryngol. 2020;277(2):497–504.

The Shoulder

Dilara Kara and Taha Ibrahim Yildiz

Abstract

The shoulder joint is anatomically the glenohumeral joint formed between the humeral head and the glenoid fossa of the scapula. However, functionally, it consists of a complex of four joints formed by the humerus, scapula, clavicle, and sternum bones. The shoulder functions are performed by the coordinated movements of the glenohumeral, scapulothoracic, sternoclavicular, and acromioclavicular joints and their associated contractile and noncontractile structures. In this section, the contractile and noncontractile structures of the shoulder joint and their palpation, the joints that generate the shoulder complex and these joint motions, and evidence-based exercises for the muscles responsible for shoulder function are explained.

D. Kara (✉)
Faculty of Physical Therapy and Rehabilitation, Hacettepe University, Ankara, Turkey

T. İ. Yildiz
Faculty of Physical Therapy and Rehabilitation, Hacettepe University, Ankara, Turkey

Physiotherapy and Rehabilitation, Faculty of Health Sciences, Afyonkarahisar Health Sciences University, Afyonkarahisar, Turkey

9.1 Noncontractile Structures in the Shoulder Joint

9.1.1 Bone Structures

The shoulder complex consists of the humerus, scapula, clavicle, and sternum. These bones and bony prominences are attachment points for the muscles around the shoulder and scapula. Table 9.1 shows the muscles located on special bones and bony prominences according to the starting (origo) and ending (insertio) points.

9.1.2 Shoulder Girdle Joints

The shoulder joint is anatomically the glenohumeral joint. However, functionally, it is a complex structure consisting of four joints. The glenohumeral, acromioclavicular, and sternoclavicular joints are true synovial articulation, while the scapulothoracic joint is a functional joint. In other words, structures such as joint capsule, ligaments, synovial fluid, and cartilage are absent in the scapulothoracic joint.

9.1.2.1 Glenohumeral Joint
It is a ball-and-socket joint formed between the humeral head and the glenoid fossa. Flexion–extension, abduction–adduction, and internal–external rotation movements occur in this joint in three different axes.

Table 9.1 Shoulder muscles by their origo and insersio

Starting from bony prominences	Muscles
Scapula	• Supraspinatus • Infraspinatus • Subscapularis • Teres major • Teres minor • Triceps brachii (long head) • Biceps brachii (long head)
Coracoid process	• Biceps brachii (short head) • Coracobrachialis
Spina scapula	• Deltoid
Clavicle	• Deltoid • Pectoralis major (clavicular portion)
Ribs	• Serratus anterior • Pectoralis major • Pectoralis minor
Sternum	• Pectoralis major (sternocostal portion)

Ending on bony prominences	Muscles
Greater tubercle of the humerus	• Supraspinatus • Infraspinatus • Teres minor
Lesser tubercle of the humerus	• Subscapularis
Upper-mid shaft of the humerus	• Deltoid • Pectoralis major • Latissimus dorsi • Teres major • Coracobrachialis
Scapula	• Serratus anterior • Rhomboid muscles • Levator scapula
Coracoid process	• Pectoralis minor
Spina scapula	• Trapezius
Clavicle	• Trapezius

9.1.2.2 Acromioclavicular Joint

It is a planar joint formed between the distal end of the clavicle and the acromion. Clavicular rotation is the main movement in this joint. In addition, rotation in the longitudinal axis, protraction and retraction in the vertical axis, and elevation and depression in the horizontal axis occur.

9.1.2.3 Sternoclavicular Joint

It is a sellar-type joint formed between the sternal portion of the clavicle and the articular surfaces of the manubrium sterni and the upper surface of the first rib. A disk is present between the articular surfaces, which ensures the harmony of the surfaces with each other. Elevation–depression, protraction–retraction, and rotation movements occur in three different axes.

9.1.2.4 Scapulothoracic Joint

It occurs between the anterior surface of the scapula and the posterolateral wall of the thorax. It is not a true joint (synovial joint) but is expressed as a functional joint. The connection of the scapula with the thorax is provided by the clavicle and various muscles. The scapula carries out its movement on the thorax through the sternoclavicular and acromioclavicular joints. Three rotations (up–down rotation, anterior–posterior tilt, and internal–external rotation) and two translational movements (elevation–depression and protraction–retraction) occur in the scapulothoracic joint. Through these wide movements in the scapulothoracic joint during arm elevation, normal shoulder functions are maintained.

9.1.3 Joint Capsule and Ligaments

The glenohumeral joint capsule consists of a thin fibrous structure in the outer layer and a synovial membrane in the inner layer. It attaches just outside the glenoid labrum medially, around the glenoid cavity, and laterally on the anatomical neck of the humerus. Most of the fibrous fibers of the capsule run horizontally, but oblique fibers are also present. It contributes little to static joint stabilization due to its thin and loose fibrous structure.

It is possible to divide the glenohumeral joint capsule into three regions: anterior, posterior, and inferior (axillary). Since the anterior surface of the capsule is surrounded by glenohumeral ligaments, the anterior capsule is significantly thicker than the posterior joint capsule. When the arm is free on the side, the superior surface of the joint capsule is tense and the inferior (axillary) surface is loose. With arm abduction, the inferior surface of the capsule is tightened and the superior surface is relaxed.

The relationship of the rotator cuff tendons with the joint capsule is important. These tendons attach to the tubercles of the humerus, and hence they completely mix with the fibrous capsule of the glenohumeral joint. Therefore, an increase in tension occurs in the joint capsule with the contraction of the rotator cuff

Clinical Information

The limitation of passive joint movement in the shoulder may be due to two different factors: (1) fibrous adhesions and adaptive shortening in the joint capsule, and (2) an increase in the resting contraction due to protective spasm in the rotator cuff muscles. Therefore, both static and dynamic structures need to be evaluated.

muscles, and an increase in joint stabilization is achieved.

Many of the ligaments in the shoulder joints mix with the joint capsule of the involved joint, supporting the capsule and increasing stabilization. In particular, all ligaments of the glenohumeral joint strengthen the joint capsule, which is a thin fibrous structure. Therefore, these ligaments are also known as capsular ligaments. Table 9.2 presents the ligaments associated with the synovial shoulder joints, the anatomical locations, and the functions of these ligaments.

Table 9.2 Shoulder ligaments, anatomical locations, and functions

Glenohumeral ligaments		
Ligaments	Anatomical locations	Functions
Superior glenohumeral ligament	Originates from the supraglenoid tubercle and attaches to the beginning of the long head of the biceps and to the lesser tubercle of the humerus	Limits the inferior translation of the adducted arm. Also, it limits the external rotation of the abducted arm with the coracohumeral ligament
Middle glenohumeral ligament	Originates from the supraglenoid tubercle and the anterosuperior part of the labrum and attaches to the lesser tubercle by mixing with the fibers of the subscapularis tendon	Limits anterior translation of the humeral head when the arm is in full adduction and abduction up to 30°–45°
Inferior glenohumeral ligament	Originates from the anterior and posterior glenoid margins and attaches to a large area at the head and neck junction of the humerus Supports the humeral head from the inferior like a hammock. It has three parts: anterior band, posterior band, and axillary pouch	Limits the anteroinferior motion of the humeral head, especially when the arm is in external rotation, abduction, and extension Anterior band: stretches with shoulder abduction and external rotation. It is the main stabilizer of the glenohumeral joint, especially when the arm is in the 90° abduction and external rotation Posterior band: it is the primary static stabilizer when the arm is in flexion and internal rotation. Provides posterior stability
Coracohumeral ligament	Originates from the lateral edge of the coracoid process and mixed with the supraspinatus tendon fibers and attaches to the anterior surface of the greater tubercle of the humerus	Limits the posterior and inferior translation of the humeral head when the arm is free at the side Provides inferior stabilization while the arm is in adduction. Stretches with external rotation
Acromioclavicular ligaments		
Ligaments	Anatomical locations	Functions
Acromioclavicular ligament	Connects the lateral part of the acromion and the clavicle It consists of two parts, superior and inferior	Strengthens the acromioclavicular joint capsule and stabilizes the clavicle
Coracoacromial ligament	Connects the upper lateral aspect of the coracoid process and the inferior aspect of the acromion It does not cross the acromioclavicular joint directly, it forms a "V" shaped roof over the humeral head	Acts as a protective belt over the humeral head and limits the superior translation of the humeral head

(continued)

Table 9.2 (continued)

Acromioclavicular ligaments		
Ligaments	Anatomical locations	Functions
Coracoclavicular ligament	It does not directly cross the acromioclavicular joint. Connects the coracoid process and the clavicle. It consists of two parts, the trapezoid and conoid ligament The trapezoid ligament extends from the superior of the coracoid process to the superolateral and attaches to the clavicle The conoid ligament is located posterior and medial to the trapezoid ligament. It extends vertically from the proximal of the coracoid process and attaches to the clavicle	It is the strongest stabilizer of the acromioclavicular joint Limits the vertical translation and rotation of the scapula relative to the clavicle

Sternoclavicular ligaments		
Ligaments	Anatomical locations	Functions
Sternoclavicular ligament	Connects the sternal end of the clavicle to the manubrium sterni anteriorly and posteriorly. It has two parts, anterior and posterior sternoclavicular ligaments	Limits the movement of the medial part of the clavicle in the anterior–posterior direction The anterior sternoclavicular ligament limits posterior movement, and the posterior sternoclavicular ligament limits the anterior movement of the clavicle
Costoclavicular ligament	Connects the inferior surface of the clavicle to the superior surface of the first costal cartilage. It is a short, flat, rhombic-shaped ligament	Limits excessive elevation of the clavicle
Interclavicular ligament	Lies on the jugular notch above the manubrium sterni and connects the sternal ends of both clavicles	Limits excessive depression of the clavicle

9.1.4 Other Structures (Glenoid Labrum and Bursae)

9.1.4.1 Glenoid Labrum

It is a fibrocartilaginous ring that surrounds the glenoid cavity and increases the depth and surface area of the glenoid cavity. The labrum contributes to approximately 50% of the shoulder joint depth. Therefore, it is one of the important structures that contribute to shoulder stabilization. The labrum is also the attachment site for the glenohumeral ligaments. The long head of the biceps muscle tendon attaches to the upper point of the labrum and contributes to shoulder stabilization.

Clinical Information

In glenoid labrum pathologies, shoulder stabilization is impaired and instability occurs. When the glenoid labrum is considered as a clock dial, the long head of the biceps brachii attaches to the upper point of the labrum at the 12 o'clock position. In superior labral tears (SLAP), this tendon can also be separated from its attachment. In the Bankart lesion, the labrum is separated from the anteroinferior (3–6 o'clock position) and anterior shoulder instability occurs.

9.1.4.2 Bursae

They are small fluid-filled vesicles that act as gliding surfaces to reduce friction between body tissues. All of the bursae are located in body regions where friction forces are high between tendons, joint capsules, ligaments, or two muscles. Six bursae are present in the shoulder. The three most important of these, clinical problems are frequently encountered.

Subacromial Bursa

It is located below the acromion and above the supraspinatus muscle in the subacromial space. It protects the supraspinatus tendon from the inferior aspect of the acromion.

Subdeltoid Bursa

It is the lateral extension of the subacromial bursa. It reduces the friction force between the deltoid and the underlying supraspinatus tendon and the humeral head.

Subscapular Bursa

It lies between the tendon of the subscapularis muscle and the shoulder joint capsule.

> **Clinical Information**
> Bursae are rich in nerve supply. For example, the subacromial bursa has suprascapular and axillary nerve endings. Nociceptors transmit the painful stimuli, receive from the bursae to the central nervous system. Therefore, in cases of bursal inflammation in the shoulder, the patient reports severe pain. There is local tenderness on palpation. Suppression of this inflammation should be given priority in treatment.

9.2 Contractile Structures Associated with the Shoulder Joint

The muscles associated with the shoulder joint are located in a large area extending to the humerus, scapula, ribs, vertebrae, and even the sacrum. Table 9.3 illustrates the muscles separated by regions and the functions of these muscles. Table 9.4 shows the nerves responsible for the innervation of these muscles.

The humeral head must maintain its relationship with the glenoid cavity for proper shoulder functions. The rotator cuff, scapulothoracic joint muscles, and other shoulder muscles work in agonist, antagonist, and synergistic relationships for the positioning of the glenoid cavity on the scapula and the movement of the humeral head. The muscles responsible for the superior–inferior movement of the humeral head are listed in Table 9.5, and the muscles that provide the scapular movements are shown in Table 9.6.

> **Clinical Information**
> The increase in the movements of the humeral head in the superior direction causes an increase in the compressive loads in the subacromial space. This initiates a process that starts with subacromial pain syndrome and extends to partial or full-thickness rotator cuff tears in the later stages. Therefore, the balance between the muscles pulling the humeral head in the superior and inferior directions should be maintained in the prevention and treatment of shoulder pain.

Table 9.3 Muscles associated with the shoulder joint and their functions

Rotator cuff muscles		
Muscle	Action	Function
Supraspinatus	Shoulder abduction	Initiation of arm elevation and stabilization of the humeral head within the glenoid fossa during arm elevation
Infraspinatus	Shoulder external rotation and horizontal abduction	Rotating the arm backward during throwing and striking movements, stabilization of the humeral head within the glenoid fossa during arm elevation
Subscapularis	Shoulder internal rotation	Rotating the arm inward during throwing and striking movements, bringing the hand behind the body, swinging the arm back during walking, and stabilization of the humeral head within the glenoid fossa during arm elevation
Teres minor	Shoulder external rotation and horizontal abduction	Rotating the arm backward during throwing and striking movements, lowering the arm from the overhead position, and stabilization of the humeral head within the glenoid fossa during arm elevation
Scapulothoracic muscles		
Muscle	Action	Function
Upper trapezius	Scapular elevation and upward rotation	Shoulder shrug, carrying, lifting, and positioning of the scapula during overhead activities
Middle trapezius	Scapular retraction	Stabilization of the scapula on the rib cage, performing strong pushing and pulling activities, and transferring body weight to the arms
Lower trapezius	Scapular depression and upward rotation	Stabilization of the scapula on the rib cage, performing strong pushing and pulling activities, transferring body weight to the arms, and positioning of the scapula during overhead activities
Serratus anterior	Scapular protraction and upward rotation	Stabilization of the scapula when bodyweight is transferred to the arms, positioning the scapula during overhead activities, pushing, throwing, reaching, and assisting with thoracic expansion
Rhomboid major and minor	Scapular retraction, elevation, and downward rotation	Transferring body weight to the arm, strong pulling activities, stabilization, and positioning of the scapula during arm lowering
Pectoralis minor	Scapular depression, protraction, downward rotation, and tilt	Pushing, performing push-ups, using a racket, swimming strokes, and assisting with thoracic expansion
Other muscles		
Muscle	Action	Function
Levator scapula	Scapular elevation and downward rotation	Carrying, lifting, and positioning of the scapula during reaching, and the arm lowering
Pectoralis major	Shoulder adduction and internal rotation	Strong throwing, striking, swimming at the overhead level, lowering the arm from the overhead or pulling objects at this level, pushing an object, and performing push-ups
Teres major	Shoulder internal rotation, adduction, and extension	Pulling the trunk by transferring body weight on the arms during climbing, overhead striking, swimming, and throwing
Latissimus dorsi	Shoulder internal rotation, adduction, and extension	Lowering the arm from the overhead after activities such as throwing, striking, and swimming, lifting the trunk by transferring body weight to the arms (lifting oneself from the chair, walking with crutches, parallel bar, and ring exercises in gymnastics, climbing activities)
Deltoid	Shoulder abduction, flexion, and extension	It is the primer mover muscle in almost all activities in the shoulder. Performing all overhead and shoulder-level movements, such as pushing, pulling, throwing, and striking
Biceps brachii	Elbow flexion and forearm supination	Carrying, raising the arm overhead, turning the forearm and hand into the drinking position, throwing, and controlling the racket in sports such as badminton and tennis
Coracobrachialis	Shoulder adduction and flexion	Sportive activities involve arm adduction, such as swinging the arm in front of the body (hitting the golf club), grasping the parallel bar and ring exercises in gymnastics, and stabilization of the arm during walking
Triceps brachii	Elbow extension	Bringing the arm back during activities such as pulling and wearing clothes and straightening the elbow when pushing

9.3 Palpation of Bone Structures and Muscles in the Shoulder Joint

The explanations about the bone structures in the shoulder joint and their palpation are given in Table 9.7, and the images of these palpation points are illustrated in Fig. 9.1. Table 9.8 depicts the explanations of the muscles associated with the shoulder joint and their palpation, and Fig. 9.2 shows the images of these palpation points.

> **Attention!**
> Palpation positions given in the images are examples. Palpation of a muscle or bony prominence can be performed in multiple positions (sitting, supine, prone, or standing). The most appropriate palpation position should be selected, taking into account the functional status of the patient and the ergonomics of the therapist.

Table 9.4 Innervation of the muscles associated with the shoulder joint

Nerves	Nerve roots	Muscles
Accessory (cranial nerve XI) and cervical plexus	C2–C4	• Trapezius
Dorsal scapular	C3–C5	• Rhomboids • Levator scapula
Suprascapular	C4–C6	• Supraspinatus • Infraspinatus
Axillary	C5–C6	• Teres minor • Deltoid
Musculocutaneous	C5–C7	• Coracobrachialis • Biceps brachii • Brachialis
Upper subscapular	C5–C6	• Subscapularis
Lower subscapular	C5–C7	• Teres major • Subscapularis
Lateral pectoral	C5–C7	• Pectoralis major • Pectoralis minor
Medial pectoral	C8–T1	• Pectoralis minor
Long thoracic	C5–C7	• Serratus anterior
Thoracodorsal	C6–C8	• Latissimus dorsi

Table 9.5 Muscles that move the humeral head

Superior movers	Inferior movers
Deltoid	Infraspinatus–teres minor
Pectoralis major (clavicular portion)	Subscapularis
Biceps brachii (short head)	Pectoralis major (sternocostal portion)
Triceps brachii (long head)	Teres major
Coracobrachialis	Latissimus dorsi

Table 9.6 Muscles providing scapular movements

Scapular movements	Muscles
Retraction	• Middle trapezius • Rhomboids
Protraction	• Serratus anterior • Pectoralis minor
Elevation	• Upper trapezius • Levator scapula • Rhomboids
Depression	• Lower trapezius • Pectoralis minor
Upward rotation	• Upper trapezius • Lower trapezius • Serratus anterior (lower fibers)
Downward rotation	• Rhomboids • Levator scapula • Pectoralis minor
Scapular tilt	• Pectoralis minor

Table 9.7 Palpations of bone structures of the shoulder joint

Bone structures	Palpation
Acromion	The fingers are moved forward by palpating along the clavicle toward the lateral (distal) side. This bony extension is felt at the most distal point (Fig. 9.1a)
Coracoid process	The concave surface at the lateral (distal) end of the clavicle is found. It is palpated on one finger inferior to this surface, deep in the pectoralis major muscle (Fig. 9.1b) *For easy palpation:* The person's arm is moved between 15° and 30° abduction–adduction. At this time, the movement in the bony prominence is felt by palpation Another method is to hyperextend the arm backward while it is on the side of the body. Since the scapula tilts anteriorly during hyperextension, the coracoid process is clearly felt and disappears when the arm is brought to the neutral position
Acromioclavicular joint	After palpating the acromion, the fingers are moved medially toward the clavicle. This joint is palpated at the point where the smoothness is impaired at the lateral end of the clavicle (Fig. 9.1c) *For easy palpation:* The person is asked to move the arm in the flexion–extension direction. At this time, the movement in the joint is felt by palpation
Sternoclavicular joint	After palpating the jugular notch on the manubrium sterni, the fingers are moved laterally. It is felt at the junction of the medial (proximal) end of the clavicle and the sternum (Fig. 9.1d) *For easy palpation:* The person is asked to move the arm at different angles. At this time, the movement in the joint is felt by palpation
Spina scapula	The spina scapula is the posterior continuation of the acromion. Therefore, after palpating the acromion, the fingers are moved posteriorly. Proceeding posteriorly medially (to the T3 vertebra), the spina scapula is found (Fig. 9.1e) *For easy palpation:* As the spina progresses on the scapula from the posterior of the acromion to the medial region, when the clinician moves his fingers up and down, he can feel the sharp areas of the bony prominence
Spina scapula root	The fingers are moved until the soft tissue starts medially (to the vertebral column) on the spina scapula. Just before the soft tissue, the spina scapula root is palpated at the medial edge of the scapula (Fig. 9.1f) *For easy palpation:* The person is asked to do protraction–retraction. During retraction, this point becomes more prominent
Medial border of the scapula	After palpating the spina scapula, the fingers are moved from the medial edge of the scapula in a superior–inferior direction and palpated vertically at the most medial point (Fig. 9.1g) *For easy palpation:* The person is asked to do protraction–retraction. During retraction, this edge becomes more prominent
Inferior angle of the scapula	The fingers are moved inferiorly along the medial edge of the scapula while palpating. The bony prominence is palpated at the most distal point just before the soft tissue initiation (Fig. 9.1h)
Greater tubercle (*tuberculum majus*)	The anterolateral round point of the proximal humerus is palpated just below the anterolateral edge of the acromion. It is located lateral to the bicipital groove (Fig. 9.1i) *For easy palpation:* The person's arm is rotated internally and externally. The greater tubercle is felt when the arm is in neutral/internal rotation, and the lesser tubercle is felt as it is externally rotated When the person abducts the arm during palpation, the greater tubercle moves below the acromion and cannot be palpated. This can be used to test the accuracy of the palpated location
Lesser tubercle (*tuberculum minus*)	After palpating the greater tubercle, the person's arm is rotated externally without interrupting finger contact. In the meantime, the fingers first enter into the bicipital groove. As the rotation continues, the lesser tubercle is felt as a bump. It is located medial to the bicipital groove (Fig. 9.1j) *For easy palpation:* The person's arm is rotated internally and externally. The greater tubercle is felt when the arm is in neutral/internal rotation, and the lesser tubercle is felt as it is externally rotated
Bicipital groove	After palpating the greater tubercle, the person's arm is rotated externally without interrupting finger contact. At this time, the fingers first enter the bicipital groove (Fig. 9.1k) *For easy palpation:* The person's arm is rotated internally and externally. The bicipital groove is felt as the arm moves from neutral to external rotation

9 The Shoulder

Table 9.7 (continued)

Bone structures	Palpation
Posterior capsule[a]	When lying on the side, with the shoulder in a 90° abduction position, the capsule is palpated deep into the infraspinatus muscle when the fingers are moved approximately two fingers down from the posterior aspect of the acromion on the posterior surface of the glenohumeral joint (Fig. 9.1l)

[a] The posterior capsule of the glenohumeral joint gets sensitive in many shoulder problems. It is often palpated in clinical evaluations. Therefore, despite no bony prominence, given in this table

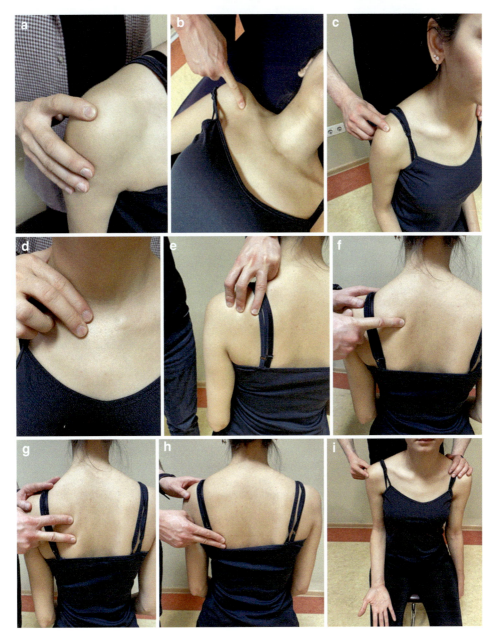

Fig. 9.1 Palpations of bone structures of the shoulder joint (**a**) acromion, (**b**) coracoid process, (**c**) acromioclavicular joint, (**d**) sternoclavicular joint, (**e**) spina scapula, (**f**) spina scapula root, (**g**) medial border of the scapula, (**h**) inferior angle of the scapula, (**i**) greater tubercle, (**j**) lesser tubercle, (**k**) bicipital groove, (**l**) posterior capsule

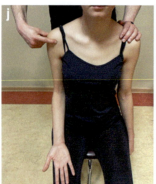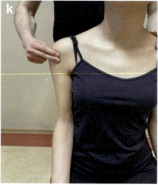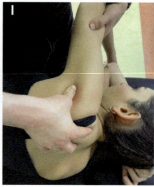

Fig. 9.1 (continued)

Table 9.8 Palpations of the muscles associated with the shoulder joint

Muscles	Palpation
Supraspinatus	After detecting the spina scapula, the supraspinatus muscle body is palpated in the fossa just above it (Fig. 9.2a). The supraspinatus tendon can be palpated in two different ways. First, the line extending from the spina scapula to the greater tubercle of the humerus is determined. At the end of this line, the tendon is palpated on the anterior surface, just below the acromion. Second, after detecting the bicipital groove, the tendon is palpated at the point just posterior to this groove toward the greater tubercle of the humerus (Fig. 9.2b) *For easy palpation:* The person is asked to perform resistive shoulder abduction with very small angles (10°–20°) to feel the fibers of the muscle In another method, the person is asked to place the dorsal side of the hand on the waist and the greater tubercle is positioned anteriorly. The tendon is palpated over the greater tubercle that becomes prominent anteriorly
Infraspinatus–teres minor	After detecting the spina scapula, the infraspinatus muscle body is palpated in the fossa just below it. The teres minor muscle body can be palpated along the upper lining of the lateral border of the scapula. The common tendon of these two muscles is palpated posteriorly at the end of the spina scapula by moving the fingers toward the greater tubercle of the humerus (Fig. 9.2c) *For easy palpation:* The fibers of the muscles are felt by resistive external rotation
Subscapularis	In the supine position, the person's shoulder is flexed and the axilla is exposed. After palpating the lateral edge of the scapula, the body of this muscle is palpated on the axilla by moving fingers anteriorly. The fingers are slowly moved superolaterally in the subscapular fossa to reach the tendon of this muscle. The tendon is palpated here when the lesser tubercle of the humerus is felt (Fig. 9.2d) Palpation of this muscle can be uncomfortable for the person. For this reason, the person should be asked to take deep breaths, and palpation should be done with clear and slow touches *For easy palpation:* The fibers of the muscle are felt by resistive internal rotation
Levator scapula	Transverse processes of C1–C4 cervical vertebrae are detected. The superior angle of the scapula is found just above the root of the spina scapula. The muscle body lies between these two points. The part near the end of the muscle is palpated above the superior edge of the scapula, deep into the trapezius muscle. For palpation of the muscle body, the fingers are moved superiorly and medially (toward the vertebrae) (Fig. 9.2e) *For easy palpation:* The fibers of the muscle are felt by resistive scapular elevation In another method, the muscle fibers can be palpated by asking the person to place the dorsal side of the hand on the waist while the person is in the prone or sitting position
Upper trapezius	The muscle body between the spina scapula and the clavicle is palpated at the most bulging part at the level of the lower cervical vertebrae (Fig. 9.2f) *For easy palpation:* The fibers of the muscle are felt by resistive scapular elevation (shoulder shrug)

Table 9.8 (continued)

Muscles	Palpation
Middle trapezius	The fibers of the middle trapezius lie horizontally. Therefore, after the root of the spina scapula is felt, it is palpated by placing the fingers horizontally at the level of the T1–T5 vertebrae (Fig. 9.2g) *For easy palpation:* The person is asked to bring his arm to 90° abduction like an airplane while bringing the scapulae closer. Light resistance can also be applied to the abducted arm over the elbow
Lower trapezius	The fibers of the lower trapezius lie diagonally. Therefore, after the root of the spina scapula is felt, it is palpated by placing the fingers diagonally at the level of the T6–T12 vertebrae (Fig. 9.2h) *For easy palpation:* The person is asked to raise the arm to the overhead level at approximately 120°–135° abduction (parallel to the muscle fibers of the lower trapezius) while bringing the scapulae closer. Light resistance can also be applied to the abducted arm over the elbow
Rhomboids	Spinous processes of C7–T5 vertebrae are detected. Then the medial edge of the scapula is palpated. Between these two points, the fibers of these muscles are felt deep in the trapezius muscle (Fig. 9.2i) *For easy palpation:* The person is asked to bring the scapulae closer. At this time, the fibers of the muscle are felt In another method, the muscle fibers can be palpated by asking the person to place the dorsal side of the hand on the waist
Serratus anterior	The lateral wall of the chest is exposed by flexing the person's shoulder. After palpating the lateral edge of the scapula, the muscle fibers are palpated on the ribs, on the lateral wall of the trunk, by moving anteriorly and inferiorly (Fig. 9.2j) *For easy palpation:* The fibers of the muscle are felt by resistive scapular protraction (like punching upward or forward)
Teres major	The lateral edge of the scapula is palpated. The muscle body can be palpated at the posterior edge of the axilla in the direction extending from the inferior of this edge to the humerus. Muscle fibers can also be grasped as soft tissue at the posterior axillary edge with the latissimus dorsi (Fig. 9.2k) *For easy palpation:* The fibers of the muscle are felt by resistive internal rotation or extension of the shoulder
Latissimus dorsi	All the fibers of this muscle, which is located superficially in a wide region extending to the inferior angle of the scapula, the spinous processes of the T7–L5 vertebrae, the posterior of the iliac crest, and the sacrum, are palpated by placing the palmar side of the hand on the posterior of the trunk. In addition, since the lateral fibers of this muscle shape the posterior edge of the axilla, the muscle body can be grasped (together with teres major) from the posterior of the axilla with the thumb and other fingers. The endpoint of the muscle can be palpated on the anterior surface of the humerus medial to the bicipital groove (Fig. 9.2l) *For easy palpation:* Muscle fibers are felt by resistive shoulder extension
Pectoralis major	Starting from the inferior of the clavicle, all fibers of the muscle located superficially in a large area between the axilla and the sternum are palpated by placing the palmar side of the hand. In addition, the muscle can be grasped with the fingers from its lateral edge, just medial to the axilla. The sternocostal portion can be palpated horizontally over the ribs toward the sternum, and the clavicular portion can be palpated obliquely toward the humeral attachment just below the clavicle (Fig. 9.2m) *For easy palpation:* All fibers can be felt with resistive internal rotation of the shoulder. The fibers of the sternocostal portion are felt clearly by resistive shoulder adduction, and the fibers of the clavicular portion by the combination of resistive shoulder flexion–adduction movement
Pectoralis minor	First, the coracoid process is palpated. From here, the fingers are placed obliquely on the 3–4—fifth rib toward the inferior and medial surfaces. The muscle body is palpated deep into the pectoralis major muscle (Fig. 9.2n) *For easy palpation:* While the person is in the supine position, the dorsal side of the hand is placed below the waist. The fibers of this muscle are clearly felt when he pushes the bed with his hand and forearm

(continued)

Table 9.8 (continued)

Muscles	Palpation
Deltoid (anterior-middle fibers)	The lateral border of the clavicle and the acromion are palpated. When the fingers are moved from here toward the deltoid tubercle, the anterior fibers of the muscle are palpated on the clavicular side and the middle fibers on the acromion side on the humerus (Fig. 9.2o) *For easy palpation: The fibers of the muscle are felt by resistive shoulder flexion or abduction*
Deltoid (posterior fibers)	In the prone or sitting position, the muscle body is palpated posterior to the humerus, in the direction of the spina scapula, with the shoulder at 90° abduction (Fig. 9.2p) *For easy palpation: The fibers of the muscle can be felt by resistive horizontal extension*
Biceps brachii	The muscle body of the biceps brachii is held between the shoulder and forearm medial to the humerus (Fig. 9.2q). For the long head of the biceps brachii tendon, the bicipital groove is found on the anterior surface of the humerus. The tendon in this groove is palpated by placing the finger in the direction of the glenoid (Fig. 9.2r) *For easy palpation: Muscle fibers or tendons are felt by resistive elbow flexion. In addition, the sliding tendon can be felt by moving the finger placed on the bicipital groove in the medial and lateral directions*
Coracobrachialis	With the shoulder abducted at 90° and the elbow flexed at 90°, the fingers are moved from the anterior edge of the axilla to the medial shaft of the humerus. The muscle body is palpated deep (posterior) into the biceps brachii (Fig. 9.2s) *For easy palpation: The muscle fibers are felt by resistive horizontal adduction* *Resistive elbow flexion can be performed to separate this muscle from the short head of the biceps brachii. While contraction is felt at the short head of the biceps brachii, no contraction occurs in the coracobrachialis muscle with elbow flexion*
Triceps brachii	The body of the muscle is palpated by grasping with the fingers along the humerus, from the olecranon superiorly (Fig. 9.2t) *For easy palpation: Muscle fibers are felt by resistive shoulder or elbow extension*

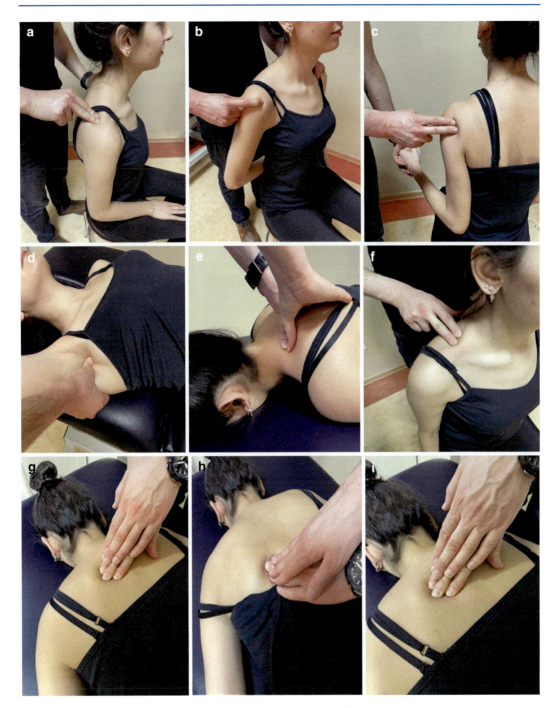

Fig. 9.2 Palpations of the muscles of the shoulder joint (**a**). Supraspinatus muscle body, (**b**). Supraspinatus, (**c**). Infraspinatus-teres minor common tendon (**d**). Subscapularis, (**e**). Levator scapula, (**f**). Upper trapezius, (**g**). Middle trapezius, (**h**). Lower trapezius, (**i**). Rhomboids, (**j**). Serratus anterior, (**k**). Teres major, (**l**). Latissimus dorsi, (**m**). Pectoralis major, (**n**). Pectoralis minor, (**o**). Deltoid (anterior-middle fibers), (**p**). Deltoid (posterior fibers), (**q**). Biceps brachii muscle body, (**r**). long head of the biceps brachii, (**s**). Coracobrachialis, (**t**) triceps brachii

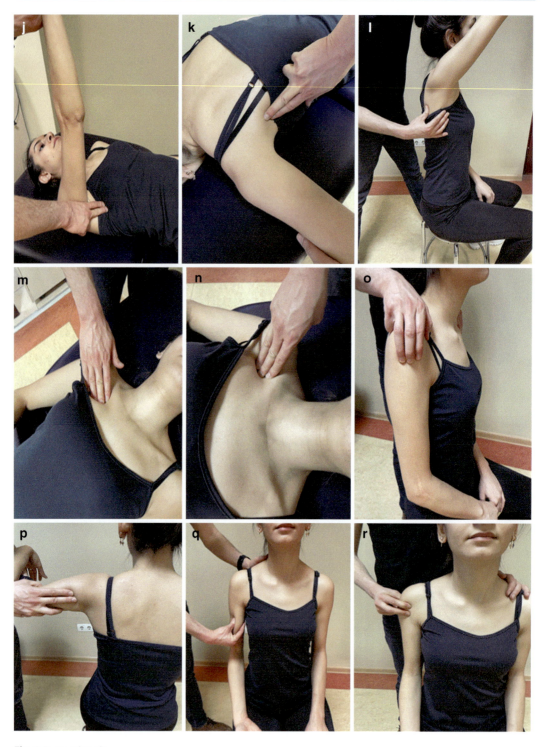

Fig. 9.2 (continued)

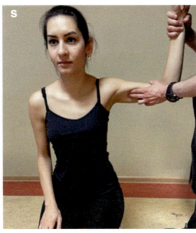
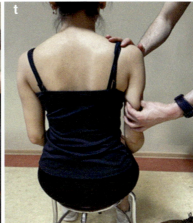

Fig. 9.2 (continued)

9.4 Shoulder Joint Motions

The glenohumeral joint has the widest range of motion in the body, with flexion–extension, abduction–adduction, and internal–external rotation movements in three planes. During these joint motions, the convex humeral head makes glide, spin, and roll movements to maintain its relationship with the concave glenoid cavity. The humeral head rolls upward along the glenoid and slides downward during glenohumeral abduction. The humeral head only rotates around itself during glenohumeral flexion. Sliding and rolling movements are not required. During glenohumeral external rotation, the humeral head rolls back and slides forward.

> **Clinical Information**
> These movements of the humeral head guide the physiotherapist during shoulder joint mobilizations. For example, the patient with passive abduction limitation in the shoulder joint may benefit from inferior humeral head mobilization. However, this approach relies on the traditional convex–concave theory. Recent studies indicate that, regardless of the direction of movement, multidirectional mobilizations stretch different parts of the capsuloligamentous complex. Therefore, appropriate mechanics and joint range of motion can be gained by improving flexibility in multiple directions.

In the shoulder, the term "*elevation*" can be expressed as bringing the humerus to the overhead position in three different planes: frontal plane (abduction), sagittal plane (flexion), and scapular plane (scaption). Shoulder elevation occurs with simultaneous movements of the glenohumeral, scapulothoracic, sternoclavicular, and acromioclavicular joints. When arm elevation is considered as 0°–90° and 90°–180° as two phases, the movements occurring in these joints and their average degrees are shown in Table 9.9.

> **Attention!**
> The degrees given in the table are approximate values obtained as a result of the studies. The degree of movement in the joints varies according to the plane of elevation, characteristics of the movement (passive, active, and resistive), type of muscle contraction (concentric and eccentric), and body positions.

Table 9.9 Movements in shoulder joints during shoulder elevation

Elevation degree	Glenohumeral joint	Scapulothoracic joint	Sternoclavicular joint	Acromioclavicular joint
0°–90°	60° abduction	30° upward rotation	20°–25° elevation	5°–10° upward rotation
90°–180°	60° abduction	30° upward rotation	5° elevation, 40° posterior rotation	20°–25° upward rotation
0°–180° (in total)	120° abduction	60° upward rotation	30° elevation, 40° posterior rotation	30° upward rotation

Clinical Information

The scapula is positioned at an angle of 30°–45° with the frontal plane at rest. This position is called the "scapular plane." during the scapular plane elevation, the glenohumeral joint surfaces are fully compatible, the rotator cuff tendons and the fibers of the capsuloligamentous complex are properly aligned, and the supraspinatus-deltoid muscles are in an optimal length–tension relationship. Many functional activities are performed on this plane.

These features specific to the scapular plane are frequently used in shoulder rehabilitation. Exercises are started in the scapular plane to keep the passive tension on the rotator cuff and capsuloligamentous complex at the lowest level, especially in the early painful period or after surgery. Potential anterior–posterior translations of the humeral head can be reduced by exercises performed in the scapular plane in individuals with shoulder instability.

9.4.1 Scapulohumeral Rhythm

The harmonious movement between the scapulothoracic joint and the glenohumeral joint during shoulder joint motions is called the scapulohumeral rhythm. The ratio between glenohumeral and scapulothoracic joint motion is approximately 2:1. Only glenohumeral joint movement occurs in the first 30° of shoulder elevation. Beyond this degree, for every 2° of glenohumeral movement, 1° of scapulothoracic joint upward rotation occurs. However, this ratio varies according to the plane of the shoulder elevation, angle of elevation, amount of resistance, and characteristics of the movement (active or passive). For example, during passive joint movement, scapular motion occurs later, because it does not require scapulothoracic muscle contraction.

The scapulohumeral rhythm serves three functional purposes
- Allows for wider (over 120°) shoulder elevation degree.
- Maintains optimal contact between the humeral head and the glenoid fossa.
- Maintains the optimal length–tension relationship of the glenohumeral muscles.

Clinical Information

Kinematic analysis studies have shown scapulohumeral rhythm changes in many shoulder pathologies. However, whether this movement problem is a cause or a consequence of shoulder pathology has not been proven. For this reason, problems in contractile and noncontractile structures should be determined with a good clinical evaluation. Exercise approaches to provide the correct scapulohumeral rhythm are an important part of shoulder rehabilitation.

9.5 Evidence-Based Exercises for the Shoulder Muscles

Shoulder problems are one of the most common musculoskeletal injuries. A motion that occurs in one joint of the shoulder complex also affects the other joints. During shoulder movements, the muscles associated with the shoulder joint act as agonists, antagonists, or stabilizers.

9.5.1 Supraspinatus

The supraspinatus muscle compresses the humeral head during shoulder elevation, preventing abnormal displacement of the humeral head superiorly. In addition, it abducts the glenohumeral joint and helps to a certain amount of external rotation. The supraspinatus muscle, which is one of the four rotator cuff muscles, and responsible for the dynamic stabilization of the shoulder joint, generally shows high activation during shoulder movements. Therefore, it is possible to increase the control of the supraspinatus muscle during plenty of shoulder exercise. It is also possible to strengthen the supraspinatus in isolation using several exercises.

The "*full-can*," "*empty-can*," and prone horizontal abduction (135° abduction and external rotation) are three of the most important exercises to train the supraspinatus muscle (Fig. 9.3). The supraspinatus muscle shows high electromyographic activity during all three exercises. However, during the "*empty-can*" exercise, the greater tubercle narrows the subacromial space due to internal rotation in the humerus and the deltoid muscle also shows high activity. Therefore, care should be taken especially in individuals with shoulder impingement syndrome during the "*empty-can*" exercise. Both the concentric and eccentric phases of exercises are important in strengthening the supraspinatus muscle. The increase in the number of serial sarcomeres in the muscle with eccentric exercise is also of clinical importance.

9.5.2 Infraspinatus–Teres Minor

The infraspinatus and teres minor muscles form the posterior rotator cuff group. During shoulder movements, they pull the humeral head inferiorly and compress it to the glenoid fossa. By doing so, they prevent abnormal upward and forward displacement of the humeral head. In addition, they are primarily responsible for the external rotation of the shoulder joint. The infraspinatus muscle also assists in shoulder abduction.

The infraspinatus and teres minor muscles demonstrate electromyographic activity, especially during the exercises involving shoulder external rotation. However, the shoulder elevation degree affects the force-generating capacity of the infraspinatus muscle considerably. The infraspinatus is more effective in lower shoulder elevation degrees; however, the lever arm of the muscle fibers decreases significantly at higher elevation degrees. This causes decreased efficiency of the infraspinatus muscle at higher shoulder elevation degrees. In contrast to the infraspinatus muscle, teres minor is

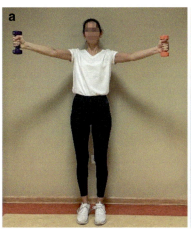 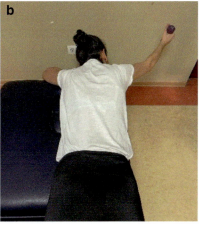

Fig. 9.3 (**a**) Full-can, (**b**) prone horizontal abduction

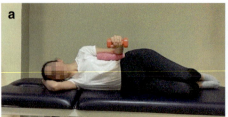
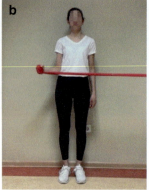
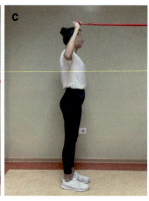

Fig. 9.4 (**a**) Side-lying external rotation, (**b**) external rotation at 0° shoulder abduction, (**c**) external rotation at 90° shoulder abduction

less affected by the degree of shoulder elevation. The lever arm of the infraspinatus muscle remains almost constant during different shoulder elevation degrees. In general, side-lying external rotation and resistive external rotation exercises at 0° abduction (Fig. 9.4a, b) are the most efficient exercise for the posterior rotator cuff muscles. Besides, horizontal abduction in a prone position and external rotation at 90° abduction (Fig. 9.4c) also show increased posterior rotator cuff activity.

In patients with shoulder injuries, it is important to generate decreased deltoid muscle activation during the exercise not to negatively affect dynamic shoulder stabilization. Therefore, this should be one of the factors affecting exercise selection and execution. During the exercise for the posterior rotator cuff, the activation of the deltoid muscle can be minimized by performing the exercise in the 0° shoulder abduction and at moderate intensity. As the intensity of the exercise increase, the activation level of the deltoid also increases. Therefore, training at lower shoulder elevation degrees and low to moderate intensities provide more isolated infraspinatus and teres minor activations.

9.5.3 Subscapularis

The subscapularis muscle surrounds the shoulder joint anteriorly and forms the anterior portion of the rotator cuff musculature. It provides stabilization by compressing the humeral head to the glenoid fossa and pulling it downward. It also acts as an anterior hammock for the humeral head and prevents abnormal anterior displacement. In addition, the subscapularis has a role in the shoulder internal rotation and abduction.

Subscapularis activation level is higher during the exercises that involve shoulder internal rotation. It also shows significant muscle activation during shoulder external rotation due to its stabilizing role. Internal rotation performed at 0° shoulder abduction and at 90° abduction is the most effective way of strengthening the subscapularis muscle (Fig. 9.5a, b). Among these two exercises, the force-generating capacity of the muscle is higher when the shoulder is in 0° abduction, compared to 90° abduction. However, the pectoralis major muscle also shows increased activity during the internal rotation performed at 0° abduction. Therefore, internal rotation at the 90° abduction provides more isolated subscapularis muscle activity. Lastly, proprioceptive neuromuscular facilitation (PNF) technique (horizontal adduction–extension), side-lying shoulder abduction (0°–90°), and "*push-up plus*" (Fig. 9.5c) exercises are other exercises that induce increased subscapularis activity.

9.5.4 Deltoid

The deltoid muscle is the uppermost muscle of the shoulder girdle and constitutes the appearance of the shoulder. It consists of three parts that

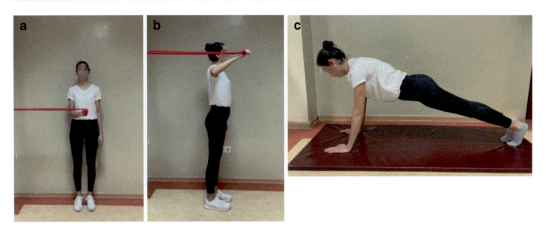

Fig. 9.5 (**a**) Internal rotation at 0° shoulder abduction, (**b**) internal rotation at 90° shoulder abduction, (**c**) push-up plus

Fig. 9.6 (**a**) Shoulder abduction, (**b**) military-press

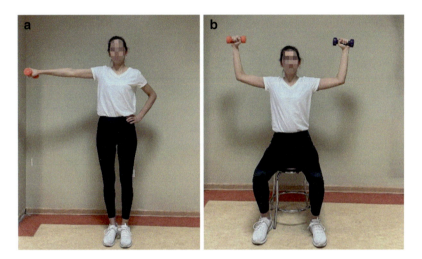

have different functions. The anterior deltoid is responsible for flexion, abduction, and some internal rotation, whereas the posterior deltoid is involved in extension, adduction, and external rotation movements. The middle deltoid is the largest part of all and is responsible for shoulder abduction. Abduction movement is also the most basic task of the deltoid muscle. Moreover, the deltoid muscle helps the stabilization of the glenohumeral joint.

The deltoid muscle is primarily responsible for shoulder abduction. It shows high activity, especially during abduction performed with shoulder external rotation (*full-can*). In the abduction during shoulder internal rotation (*empty-can*), the deltoid muscle also shows increased activity. However, the deltoid has decreased mechanical advantage during empty-can exercise, hence the efficiency of the muscle is decreased. The activity of the deltoid muscle is greatest between 60° and 90° of shoulder abduction (Fig. 9.6a). Besides the shoulder abduction, "*military-press*" exercise induces increased activity in the deltoid muscle (Fig. 9.6b).

9.5.5 Serratus Anterior

The serratus anterior is mainly responsible for shoulder protraction and, together with the trapezius muscle, performs the scapular upward rotation. It shows high activity in situations where

Fig. 9.7 (a) Dynamic hug, (b) serratus anterior-punch

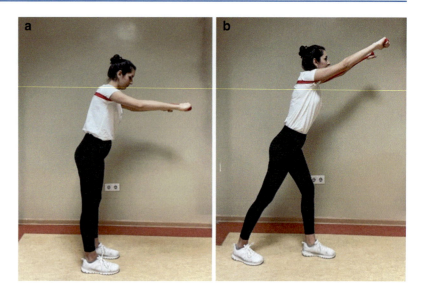

these two movements are combined. The push-up exercise is one of the primary exercises with the highest activation of the serratus anterior. Serratus anterior activation can be increased with shoulder protraction (*push-up plus*) at the end of the push-up movement (Fig. 9.5c). Hence, the protraction movement should be added to the push-up exercise. Performing the push-up exercise on a stable surface helps focus on the serratus anterior muscle and positively affects the serratus anterior/upper trapezius muscle activation ratio. Besides the push-up exercise, dynamic hug and serratus anterior-punching (punch with 120° shoulder elevation) are also effective ways of strengthening the serratus anterior (Fig. 9.7). In addition, increased serratus anterior activation can also be achieved with shoulder abduction in the scapular plane above 120°. However, caution should be taken during this exercise, especially after shoulder injuries since it may narrow the subacromial space.

9.5.6 Trapezius

The upper, middle, and lower trapezius muscles are mainly involved in scapular stabilization. The upper trapezius muscle is particularly active during the shrug (Fig. 9.8a), prone to retraction and horizontal abduction. The middle trapezius muscle, similar to the upper trapezius, has increased muscular activation during shrug and horizontal abduction movements combined with prone retraction and external rotation. The lower trapezius muscle is more active during prone horizontal abduction (especially at 135° shoulder abduction) (Fig. 9.3b), external rotation at 90° abduction (Fig. 9.4c), and high scapular retraction (Fig. 9.8b). Another important point in the exercises for the trapezius muscle is the activation rates of the lower and upper trapezius muscles. The lower trapezius/upper trapezius ratio is particularly higher during prone horizontal abduction (at 135° shoulder abduction) and scapular retraction with bilateral external rotation (Fig. 9.8c). Therefore, these exercises are suggested in individuals with shoulder problems, especially in the early period.

Examples of evidence-based exercises that can specifically train the muscles involved in shoulder joint movements are summarized in Table 9.10.

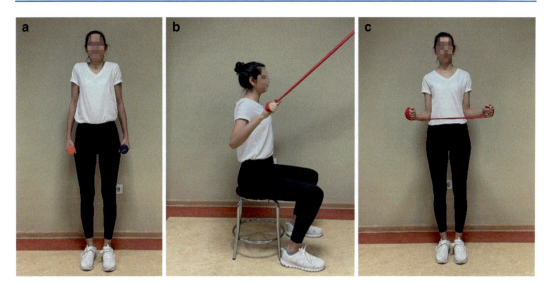

Fig. 9.8 (a) Shrug, (b) high scapular retraction, (c) scapular retraction with bilateral external rotation

Table 9.10 Evidence-based exercises for the shoulder muscles

Muscle	Type of muscle contraction	Exercise
Supraspinatus	Concentric	• Full-can • Prone horizontal abduction
Infraspinatus Teres minor	Concentric	• External rotation at 0° shoulder abduction • Side lying external rotation • External rotation at 90° shoulder abduction
Subscapularis	Concentric	• Internal rotation at 90° shoulder abduction • Internal rotation at 0° shoulder abduction • Push-up plus
Deltoid	Concentric	• Shoulder abduction • Military-press
Serratus anterior	Concentric	• Push-up plus • Dynamic hug • Serratus anterior-punch
Upper trapezius	Concentric	• Shrug • Prone retraction • Prone horizontal abduction
Middle trapezius	Concentric	• Shrug • Prone retraction • Prone horizontal abduction
Lower trapezius	Concentric	• Prone horizontal abduction at 135° shoulder abduction • High scapular retraction • External rotation at 90° shoulder abduction

9.6 Conclusion

The contractile structures are responsible for the stabilization of the shoulder joint since its' static stabilization is insufficient. Harmonious motions of these structures provide appropriate joint kinematics and normal shoulder functions. These structures should be evaluated within the kinetic chain principle in the prevention and treatment of shoulder injuries. The proper training regime should focus on both selecting the proper exercise selection for the isolated training and the kinetic chain as a whole.

Further Reading

Boettcher CE, Gınn KA, Cathers I. Which is the optimal exercise to strengthen supraspinatus? Med Sci Sports Exerc. 2009;41(11):1979–83.

Camargo PR, Neumann DA. Kinesiologic considerations for targeting activation of scapulothoracic muscles—part 2: trapezius. Braz J Phys Ther. 2019;23(6):467–75.

Castelein B, Cagnie B, Parlevliet T, Danneels L, Cools A. Optimal normalization tests for muscle activation of the levator scapulae, pectoralis minor, and rhomboid major: an electromyography study using maximum voluntary isometric contractions. Arch Phys Med Rehabil. 2015;96(10):1820–7.

Cleland J, Koppenhaver S, Su J. Shoulder. In: Cleland J, Koppenhaver S, Su J, editors. Netter's orthopaedic clinical examination: an evidence-based approach. Amsterdam: Elsevier Health Sciences; 2015. p. 449–526.

Cricchio M, Frazer C. Scapulothoracic and scapulohumeral exercises: a narrative review of electromyographic studies. J Hand Ther. 2011;24(4):322–33.

Escamilla RF, Yamashiro K, Paulos L, Andrews JR. Shoulder muscle activity and function in common shoulder rehabilitation exercises. Sports Med. 2009;39(8):663–85.

Ha SM, Kwon OY, Cynn HS, Lee WH, Kim SJ, Park KN. Selective activation of the infraspinatus muscle. J Athl Train. 2013;48(3):346–52.

Kang FJ, Ou HL, Lin KY, Lin JJ. Serratus anterior and upper trapezius electromyographic analysis of the push-up plus exercise: a systematic review and meta-analysis. J Athl Train. 2019;54(11):1156–64.

Kara D, Harput G, Duzgun I. Trapezius muscle activation levels and ratios during scapular retraction exercises: a comparative study between patients with subacromial impingement syndrome and healthy controls. Clin Biomech (Bristol, Avon). 2019;67:119–26.

Lippert LS. Clinical kinesiology and anatomy of the upper extremities. In: Lippert LS, editor. Clinical kinesiology and anatomy. Philadelphia: FA Davis Company; 2011. p. 113–94.

Lugo R, Kung P, Ma CB. Shoulder biomechanics. Eur J Radiol. 2008;68(1):16–24.

Muscolino JE. Palpation of the muscles of the shoulder girdle. In: Muscolino JE, editor. The muscle and bone palpation manual with trigger points, referral patterns and stretching. Amsterdam: Elsevier Health Sciences; 2009a. p. 137–80.

Muscolino JE. Upper extremity bone palpation and ligaments. In: Muscolino JE, editor. The muscle and bone palpation manual with trigger points, referral patterns and stretching. Amsterdam: Elsevier Health Sciences; 2009b. p. 69–92.

Neumann DA. Upper extremity. In: Neumann DA, editor. Kinesiology of the musculoskeletal system-e-book: foundations for rehabilitation. Amsterdam: Elsevier Health Sciences; 2013. p. 119–304.

Neumann DA, Camargo PR. Kinesiologic considerations for targeting activation of scapulothoracic muscles—part 1: serratus anterior. Braz J Phys Ther. 2019;23(6):459–66.

Reinold MM, Macrina LC, Wilk KE, Fleisig GS, Dun S, Barrentine SW, et al. Electromyographic analysis of the supraspinatus and deltoid muscles during 3 common rehabilitation exercises. J Athl Train. 2007;42(4):464–9.

Reinold MM, Escamilla RF, Wilk KE. Current concepts in the scientific and clinical rationale behind exercises for glenohumeral and scapulothoracic musculature. J Orthop Sports Phys Ther. 2009;39(2):105–17.

The Elbow

Seval Tamer

Abstract

The elbow joint plays an essential role in positioning the hand during daily life and self-care activities. This hinge-type joint between the distal humerus and the proximal articular surfaces of the radius and ulna bones acts as a support point for bearing weight and the forearm. The elbow joint has complex biomechanical properties for stability and function. The complexity of the joint, due to the important surrounding ligaments and neurovascular structures, makes surgical interventions very difficult. The elbow is often injured during sports such as shooting, tennis, golf, weightlifting, bowling, and other professional activities requiring frequent joint use. Rehabilitation requires a detailed understanding of elbow joint anatomy and biomechanics. The bone structures that comprise the elbow joint, as well as the joint capsule, ligaments, muscles, biomechanical properties, palpation of the adjacent anatomical structures, and exercises specific to the elbow joint are all defined in this chapter.

10.1 Non-contractile Structures in the Elbow Joint

10.1.1 Bone Structures

10.1.1.1 Distal Humerus

The humerus is a long bone in the upper arm. The humeral shafts terminate distally, the larger one medial to the epicondyle and the smaller one lateral to it.

The lateral collateral ligament (LCL) and the extensor and supinator muscle groups attach to the lateral epicondyle, while the flexor and pronator muscle groups and the medial collateral ligament (MCL) attach to the medial epicondyle. The ulnar nerve runs behind the medial epicondyle through the ulnar groove. The trochlear groove, which is spool-shaped medially, and the capitulum humeri are articular surfaces on the anterior side of the distal humerus between the two epicondyles.

The condyle of the humerus is formed by the trochlea and capitulum of the humerus. The articular surface of the trochlea and capitulum humeri are internally rotated 5°–7° in relation to the transepicondylar axis. Moreover, the medial projection of the trochlea is 6°–8° larger than the lateral projection. Physiologically, the elbow valgus angle results from these two conditions. The humeral articular surface is 30° anterior in the sagittal plane. The coronoid fossa is located above the trochlea on the anterior aspect of the distal

S. Tamer (✉)
Physiotherapy and Rehabilitation, Faculty of Health Sciences, Kütahya Health Sciences University, Kütahya, Turkey
e-mail: seval.tamer@ksbu.edu.tr

humerus, and the radial fossa is situated above the capitulum. The coronoid process of the ulna and the radial head are in sync with these fossae when the elbow is fully flexed. When the elbow is fully extended, the fossae align with the olecranon of the ulna. The trochlea humerus's 30° angular articular surface is covered with cartilage tissue. The capitulum of the humerus is spherical in shape and covered in 2-mm thick hyaline cartilage. A projection known as the supracondylar process can be found 5–7 cm proximal to the medial epicondyle in 1–3% of people. Starting from this prominence, a fibrous band called Struthers' ligament may extend to the medial epicondyle. This band abnormally attaches to the coracobrachialis and pronator teres muscles. It is thought that there is a connection between this abnormal protrusion and the incidence of ulnar and median nerve compression syndrome (Fig. 10.1).

10.1.1.2 Proximal Ulna

This bone, distal to and medial to the elbow joint, is comprised of two parts: the olecranon process and

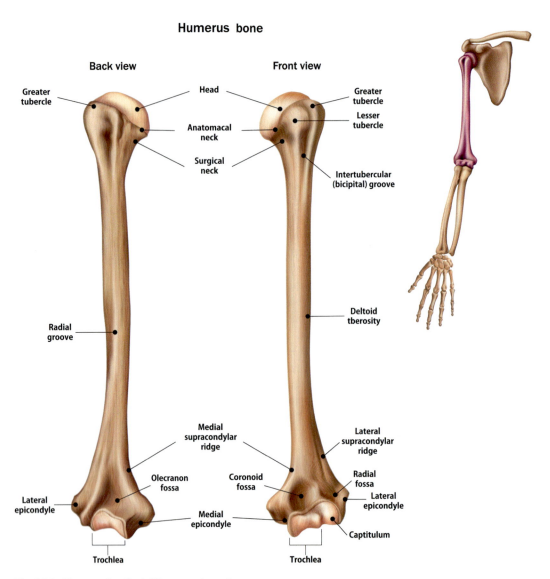

Fig. 10.1 Humerus (studiovin/Shutterstock.com)

the coronoid process. These two structures join to create the large elliptical sigmoid notch (trochlear notch) anteriorly, which is perfectly aligned with the humeral trochlea and forms the humeroulnar joint. To accommodate the anterior angulation of the distal humerus, this notch forms a 30° posterior angle to the long axis of the ulna. The coronoid process also serves as a connection point for the brachialis muscle and the oblique cord. The small sigmoid notch (radial notch) is located lateral to the coronoid process and distal to the greater sigmoid notch, forming the proximal radioulnar joint with the radial head. This depression in the form of an approximately 70° arc articulates with the radial head to form the proximal radioulnar joint just below the lateral aspect of the coronoid process. The supinator prominence is proximal to the lesser sigmoid notch where the supinator muscle originates and the LCL attaches. The sublime tubercle is located medial to the coronoid process, which is attached to the anterior bundle of the MCL. The ulnar tuberosity is distal to and anterior to the ulna neck. When viewed from the front, the body of the ulna forms an angle of 1°–6° laterally. The *"carrier angle"* is formed as a result of this angulation (Fig. 10.2).

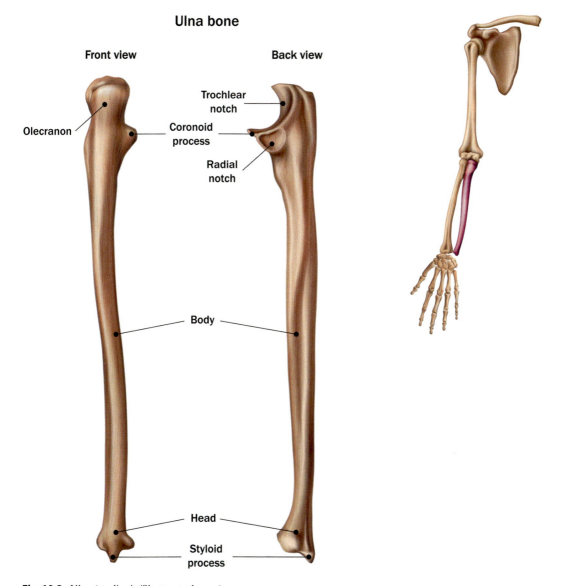

Fig. 10.2 Ulna (studiovin/Shutterstock.com)

10.1.1.3 Proximal Radius

Distal to and lateral to the elbow joint, the concave exterior of the radial head, which articulates with the capitulum, is covered with cartilage. The annular ligament stabilizes and covers the disc-shaped radial head's 240° angular surface, which articulates with the small sigmoid notch. The radial head's anterolateral one-third lacks cartilage and subchondral bone. As a result, joint fractures are common in the bone that does not connect to the joint. Because of its weakness, this region is the most frequently broken area. The radial head tapers distally and forms the radial neck. The radial head is 15° anterior to the long axis of the radius. The insertion site of the biceps tendon, attached to the radius tuberosity, is located on the radial neck distal and anterior-medial surfaces. The radial head acts as a secondary stabilizer of the joint and the muscles surrounding it (Fig. 10.3).

> **Clinical Information**
>
> The '*carrying angle*' is the angle formed by the long axis of the humerus and the long axis of the ulna. Men have a 11°–14° range, while women have a 13°–16° range. It results from the inclination of the long axis of the top of the humeral body, the bottom of the ulna body, and the humerus of the trochlea relative to each other.

10.1.2 Joint Capsule and Ligaments

10.1.2.1 Joint Capsule

The synovial elbow joint is surrounded by the joint capsule. Folds form on the anterior side of the joint capsule in flexion and on the posterior side in extension. Some brachialis fibers anteriorly and anconeus and triceps brachialis fibers posteriorly adhere to the joint capsule preventing these folds from entering the joint space. The role of the capsule in passive stability is debatable. Although studies show that stabilization does not change after the capsule is removed (capsulotomy), it has been reported that the anterior capsule covers 15% of the varus–valgus stress when the elbow is fully extended. The radial, median, and ulnar nerves widely innervate the elbow capsule. Clinically, the elbow joint capsule is responsible for the development of elbow contracture following trauma. The joint capsule is examined in two parts: anterior and posterior.

Anterior Capsule

Located near the coronoid and the radial fossa, the anterior capsule attaches medially to the anterior surface of the coronoid and laterally to the annular ligament. The anterior joint capsule has three fibrous bands: (I) The anterolateral band extends distally and anteriorly to the superior annular ligament, beginning at the lateral supracondylar process and ending at the anterolateral aspect of the humerus, (II) the anteromedial oblique band arises from the superior medial trochlear process anterior to the elbow. It connects to the annular ligament anteriorly, centrally, and medially, (III) the anterior transverse band begins below the medial trochlear process and attaches mediolateral to the annular ligament. The anterior capsule is thin and reinforced with bands that help to stabilize the annular and lateral collateral ligaments.

Posterior Capsule

Attached to the medial and lateral margins of the greater sigmoid notch proximal to the olecranon fossa, the posterior capsule has three fibrous bands: (I) The transverse band begins at the medial and lateral posterior trochlear processes and extends below the olecranon fossa in a mediolateral direction, (II) the posterior medial oblique band originates from the medial posterior trochlear process, (III) the posterior lateral oblique band arises from the lateral posterior trochlear process. All extend to the posterior-superior end of the olecranon. Posterior bands are tight in flexion and prevent dislocation of the trochlear joint in hyperflexion.

10.1.2.2 Ligaments

The medial and lateral thickening of the joint capsule forms the collateral ligaments of the elbow joint.

RIGHT RADIUS

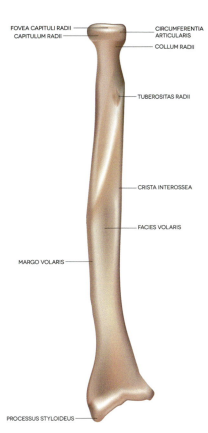
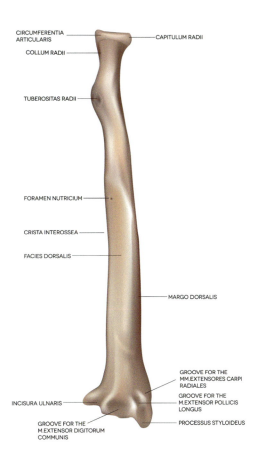

FROM IN FRONT   FROM BEHIND

Fig. 10.3 Radius (TimeLineArtist/Shutterstock.com)

Medial Collateral Ligament (MCL)

The MCL is comprised of three bundles: anterior, posterior, and transverse. The anterior bundle is the most important structure responsible for MCL complex stabilization. It runs from the anteroinferior to the medial epicondyle to the sublime tubercle in the coronoid process of the ulna. This ligament primarily compensates for valgus and internal rotation stress. It is taut during elbow extension and provides valgus stabilization during elbow flexion. Regardless of forearm position, it provides stability against varus and valgus stresses. The posterior bundle extends medially to the middle of the greater sigmoid notch from the anterior bundle. It stabilizes the elbow in a 120° flexion position. Its damage causes posteromedial instability. The transverse bundle, also known as Cooper's ligament, runs obliquely from the medial epicondyle to the olecranon and coronoid processes and has little impact on stabilization (Fig. 10.4).

Lateral Collateral Ligament (LCL)

The LCL is divided into four sections: the radial collateral ligament (RCL), the annular ligament (AL), the accessory lateral collateral ligament (ALCL), and the lateral ulnar collateral ligament (LUCL). This ligament is the primary stabilizer

Ulnar Collateral Ligament

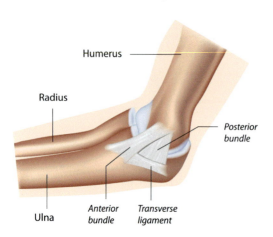

Fig. 10.4 Medial collateral ligament (Alila Medical Media/Shutterstock.com)

against varus and external rotation stresses. It stretches during full flexion.

Located between the lateral epicondyle and the supinator ridge, distal to the lesser sigmoid tubercle, the LUCL is the primary lateral stabilizer of the elbow. It stretches in both flexion and extension. It is the primary lateral stabilizer against varus and posterolateral rotator stress. The anconeus muscle provides similar stress support. The RCL is located anterior to the LCL between the lateral epicondyle and the AL. Its average length is 20 mm, and its width is 8 mm. The RCL originates near the joint's transverse axis. As a result, it stretches in flexion and extension. The tension is nearly constant throughout the normal joint range of motion, providing stability against varus stress. It is joined to the supinator and extensor carpi radialis brevis muscles. The AL is a strong ligament that forms a ring around the radial head to prevent it from protruding. This ligament, which protects the radioulnar joint, attaches to the anterior and posterior edges of the small sigmoid notch. It narrows distally to form a funnel. To reduce friction, the inner periphery of the AL is covered with cartilage. Because the radial head is not a complete circular disc, the anterior part of the AL is stretched in supination and the posterior part in pronation. The ALCL runs from the AL to the inside of the radial neck. It helps stabilize the proximal radioulnar joint during forearm pronation and supination, increasing the AL's ability to stabilize under varus stress.

> **Clinical Information**
>
> The lateral collateral ligament is roughly shaped like a "Y." Its two short ends extend anteriorly to the radius and ulna.

Oblique Cord

A small fibrous tissue bundle located between the ulna and the radius tuberosities is the oblique cord. Although its morphological and functional significance is debatable, it is thought to control supination.

The Interosseous Membrane

As the starting point for the intrinsic muscles of the forearm and hand, the interosseous membrane joins the radius and ulna, enabling force transfer between the bones. It is loose during full pronation and supination of the forearm and stretched from the mid-angle of pronation and supination.

10.1.3 Other Structures

10.1.3.1 Bursae

Joint structures that aid in protecting soft tissues during movement are called bursae. Although there are different opinions on the number of bursae in the elbow region, it is generally agreed that there are seven.

Olecranon Bursae

The most common bursa at the back of the elbow, the olecranon bursae, develops after age seven. It is visible between the olecranon and the subcutaneous tissue.

Subtendinous Bursae
This bursa is located where the triceps tendon attaches to the olecranon.

Subanconeus Bursae
This bursa, located under the anconeus muscle, is found in approximately 12% of the population.

Medial and Lateral Epicondylar Subcutaneous Bursae
Located both medial and lateral to the elbow joint, the medial subcutaneous epicondylar bursa is more common than the lateral subcutaneous epicondylar bursa.

Radiohumeral Bursae
Located between the radiohumeral articular surface and the extensor carpi radialis brevis muscle (deep in the common extensor tendon), the radiohumeral bursa is thought to play a role in the etiology of lateral epicondylitis.

Bicipitoradial Bursae
Positioned to separate the biceps tendon from its attachment, the bicipitoradial bursa is reportedly present in approximately 20% of individuals and protects the biceps tendon during full pronation.

10.1.3.2 Nerve Structures
The musculocutaneous, radial, median, and ulnar nerves provide sensory and motor innervation to the elbow and forearm. These nerves emerge from the C5–T1 roots of the spinal cord. Table 10.1 lists the nerves that control elbow joint movements and the muscles they innervate.

Musculocutaneous Nerve
Derived from C5–C7, the musculocutaneous nerve is a lateral fascicle branch. After passing through the coracobrachialis muscle, it moves between the biceps brachii and brachialis muscles and innervates them. The cutaneous antebrachial is the lateral branch of this nerve that receives sensations from the lateral half of the forearm (Fig. 10.5).

Table 10.1 Nerves innervating muscles in the elbow joint

Nerves	Muscles
Musculocutaneous nerve	• Biceps brachii • Brachialis
Radial nerve	• Triceps brachii • Anconeus • Brachioradialis • Supinator • Extensor carpi radialis longus • Extensor carpi radialis brevis • Extensor digitorum • Extensor carpi ulnaris
Median nerve	• Pronator teres • Flexor carpi radialis • Palmaris longus • Flexor digitorum superficialis
Ulnar nerve	• Flexor carpi ulnaris

Radial Nerve
The largest branch of the brachial plexus is the radial nerve. It is the continuation of the posterior fasciculus and stems from C5–C8 and T1. It is divided into the posterior cutaneous, inferior lateral cutaneous, and posterior antebrachial cutaneous sensory branches. It innervates the skin of the lateral and posterior regions of the posterior upper elbow, forearm, and wrist. The radial nerve crosses the triceps brachii muscle from medial to lateral at the elbow and posterior to the humerus, then travels through the lateral intermuscular septum to the anterior of the arm. Located between the brachialis and brachioradialis muscles, it travels posteriorly from the capitulum under the extensor carpi radialis longus and brevis, which is known as the radial tunnel. It divides into superficial and deep interosseous branches at the level of the radiocapitellar joint and separates into the triceps, anconeus, brachialis, brachioradialis, extensor carpi radialis longus, and the periosteum of the lateral epicondyle before branching. Its superficial branch continues to the wrist through the brachioradialis muscle. The deep limb of the radial nerve branches into the supinator and extensor carpi radialis brevis

muscles before passing from the supinator muscle to the back of the forearm. At the level of the radiocapitellar joint, it becomes the posterior interosseous. The extensor digitorum, extensor digiti minimi, extensor carpi ulnaris, abductor pollicis longus, extensor pollicis brevis, extensor pollicis longus, and extensor indicis are all innervated by it. The proximal part at the level of the radial head is stretched in full supination and relaxed in pronation (Fig. 10.5).

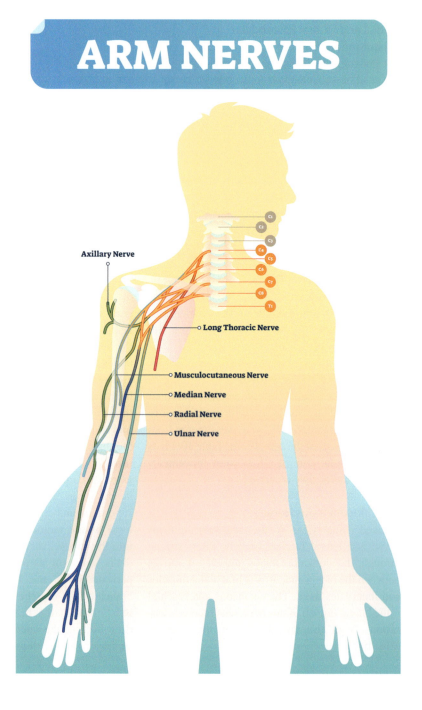

Fig. 10.5 Nerve structures (VectorMine/Shutterstock.com)

> **Clinical Information**
>
> The deep branch of the radial nerve may be damaged in proximal radius fractures because it travels close to the radius as it passes through the supinator muscle. It may also be exposed to pressure from the supinator muscle. Lesions of the radial nerve's posterior interosseous branch in the radial tunnel can mimic the general symptoms of lateral epicondylitis.

Ulnar Nerve

Stemming from C7, C8, and T1, the ulnar nerve continues to the forearm without branching. It passes between the medial intermuscular septum and the medial triceps head at the elbow to reach the sulcus behind the medial epicondyle of the humerus. It then travels through the cubital tunnel, innervating the medial half of the flexor carpi ulnaris and flexor digitorum profundus muscles anterior to the forearm. Many of the intrinsic muscles of the hand and the skin on the medial side of the hand are innervated by it (Fig. 10.5).

> **Clinical Information**
>
> The fibrous band (Osborne's ligament) between the two heads of the flexor carpi ulnaris muscle passes over the ulnar nerve and can result in band nerve compression.

Median Nerve

Formed in the brachial plexus by the medial and lateral fascicles, the median nerve crosses the brachial artery between the biceps brachii and brachialis muscles at the elbow. It runs deep into the bicipital aponeurosis, medial to the biceps brachial tendon, and in front of the brachialis muscle in the elbow joint with the artery. The median nerve then passes beneath the pronator teres muscle, between the humeroulnar and radial heads of the flexor digitorum superficialis muscle and enters the forearm. It gives off an anterior interosseous branch 5–8 cm distal to the lateral epicondyle. It innervates the forearm flexor muscles (pronator teres, flexor carpi radialis, palmaris longus, flexor digitorum superficialis, lateral flexor digitorum profundus, flexor pollicis longus, pronator quadratus), lateral lumbrical muscles, and thenar muscles of the hand (Fig. 10.5).

10.1.3.3 Arteriovenous Structures

Arteries

The brachial, radial, and ulnar arteries, as well as their recurrent branches, supply the elbow joint. The brachial artery runs through the center of the elbow between the median and ulnar nerves. It enters the cubital fossa from the biceps brachial tendon's medial side and the median nerve's lateral side, dividing into the radial and ulnar arteries at the radial neck. The posterior ulnar recurrent branch of the ulnar artery anastomoses with the upper and lower ulnar collateral branches of the brachial artery and supplies the medial epicondyle, trochlea medial, and olecranon posteromedial aspect. The radial and middle collateral arteries (originating from the profunda brachial) anastomose with the interosseous and radial recurrent arteries on the posterior aspect of the lateral epicondyle to supply the lateral epicondyle and capitellum. Radial recurrent branches also supply the radial head and neck. The superior ulnar, radial, and middle collateral arteries anastomose proximally posterior to the elbow, while the interosseous recurrent arteries distally supply the lateral trochlea, supracondylar region, and olecranon.

Veins

Deep veins share the same names as all artery branches. The superficial veins are dense on the back of the hand and run as the basilic vein medially and the cephalic vein laterally. They connect with the median cubital vein to form the axillary vein in the cubital fossa.

10.1.4 Joints Associated with the Elbow

10.1.4.1 Humeroulnar Joint

A simple hinge-type joint that forms between the humeral trochlea and the ulnar trochlear prominence, the humeroulnar joint allows for flexion and extension movements in the transverse axis. The coronoid tip enters the coronoid fossa in extreme flexion to prevent posterior dislocation. In full extension, because of the structure of the trochlea, the ulna is positioned laterally relative to the humerus, thereby forming the carrying angle. In full flexion, the lateral olecranon does not make complete contact with the trochlea allowing for the formation of supination and pronation movements. The slight rotational movement of the ulna during flexion and extension, the sliding movement of the radial head on the humerus and ulna, and the abduction and adduction sliding movements are also due to this asymmetry. The elbow joint is stable in full extension.

10.1.4.2 Humeroradial Joint

A trochoid joint formed between the radius's concave surface and the capitellum on the humerus's convex surface, the humeroradial joint allows for forearm supination and pronation. The radial head is larger than the capitellum. This inequity allows for less stability and a greater range of motion. In full extension, there is little or no physical contact at the humeroradial joint. The joint is stable at 90° elbow flexion and 5° forearm supination.

10.1.4.3 Proximal Radioulnar Joint

A trochoid joint that occurs between the head of the radius and the small sigmoid notch of the ulna, the proximal radioulnar joint is stable at 5° supination. The AL provides stability to the joint. The articular axis connects the radial head and the capitellum. It provides the rotation required for supination and pronation movements.

10.1.4.4 Distal Radioulnar Joint

Together with the proximal radioulnar joint, the distal radioulnar joint provides pronation and supination movements of the forearm. It is a trochoid-type joint. During pronation and supination, the concave surface of the radius rolls and slides in the same direction on the ulna. While the radius is parallel to the ulna during supination, it crosses from above in pronation. Joint stability is provided by joint geometry, radioulnar ligaments, and the triangular fibrocartilage complex.

10.2 Contractile Structures Associated with the Elbow Joint

The muscles surrounding the elbow joint are examined in four groups. Elbow extensors are triceps brachii and anconeus subanconeus (Figs. 10.6 and 10.7). Elbow flexors are biceps brachii, bra-

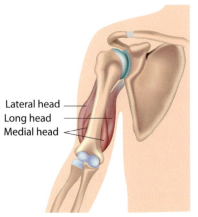
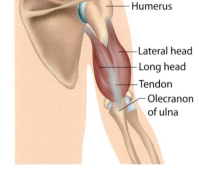

Fig. 10.6 Triceps muscle (Alila Medical Media/Shutterstock.com)

Muscles of the Forearm
(right arm, posterior compartment)

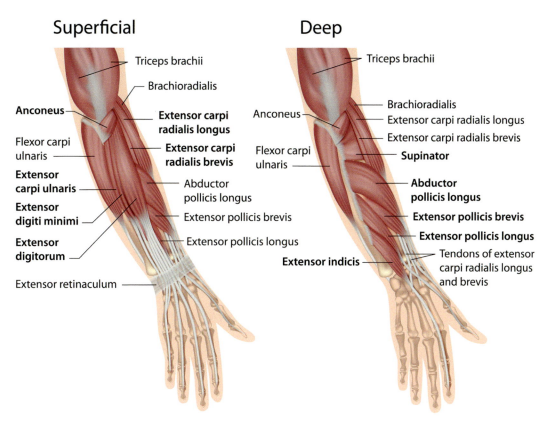

Fig. 10.7 Elbow extensor, forearm supinator, and wrist extensor muscles (Alila Medical Media/Shutterstock.com)

chialis, and brachioradialis (Fig. 10.8). Forearm supinator and wrist extensor muscles are supinator, extensor carpi radialis longus, extensor carpi radialis brevis, extensor digitorum, and extensor carpi ulnaris (Fig. 10.7). Forearm pronator and wrist flexor muscles are pronator teres, flexor carpi radialis, palmaris longus, flexor carpi ulnaris, and flexor digitorum superficialis (Fig. 10.9). Table 10.2 describes origins and insertions of the muscles associated with the elbow joint, Table 10.3 describes functions and roles of muscles in elbow joint movement.

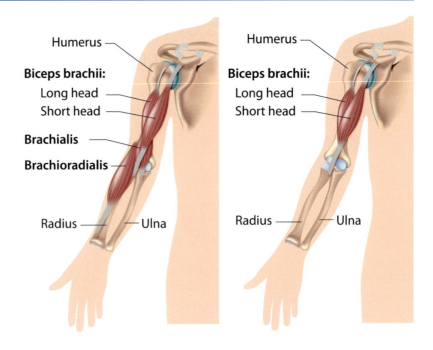

Fig. 10.8 Elbow flexor muscles (Alila Medical Media/Shutterstock.com)

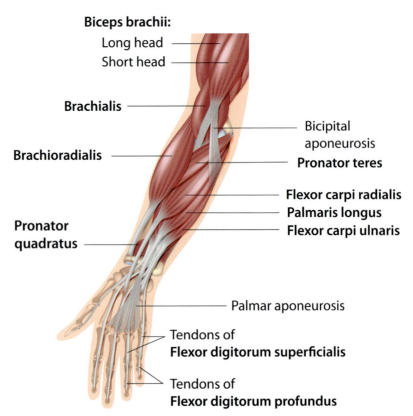

Fig. 10.9 Forearm pronator and wrist flexor muscles (Alila Medical Media/Shutterstock.com)

Table 10.2 Origins and insertions of the muscles associated with the elbow joint

Muscles	Attachment points Origin	Insertion
Triceps brachii	• The scapula's infraglenoid tubercle (long head) • The proximal half of the posterior humeral shaft (lateral head) • The distal half of the posterior shaft of the humerus (medial head)	• Proximal olecranon
Anconeus	• Humerus lateral epicondyle	• Dorsal and lateral ulna
Biceps brachii	• Tubercle of the scapula supraglenoid (long head) • The coracoid process (short head)	• Tuberositas radii • Bicipital aponeurosis • Antebrachial fascia
Brachialis	• Distal half of the anterior humerus	• Tuberositas ulna
Brachioradialis	• Proximal two-thirds of the lateral supracondylar of the humerus	• Radius styloid process
Supinator	• Humerus lateral epicondyle • Radial and ulnar collateral ligaments • Ulna supinator crest	• The dorsal third of the proximal radius
Extensor carpi radialis longus	• Lateral of the humerus's supracondylar process	• Dorsal base of the second metacarpal
Extensor carpi radialis brevis	• Humerus lateral epicondyle	• Dorsal base of the third metacarpal
Extensor digitorum	• Humerus lateral epicondyle	• Dorsal aponeurosis of the second-fifth fingers
Extensor carpi ulnaris	• Humerus lateral epicondyle • Anconeus aponeurosis of the ulna	• Dorsal base of the fifth metacarpal
Pronator teres	• Humerus medial epicondyle • Ulna coronoid process	• Center of the lateral radius
Flexor carpi radialis	• Humerus medial epicondyle	• Base of the second metacarpal
Palmaris longus	• Humerus medial epicondyle	• Palmar aponeurosis
Flexor carpi ulnaris	• Humerus medial epicondyle (humeral head) • Coronoid process of the medial ulna (ulnar head)	• Pisiform • Hamatum • Fifth metacarpal
Flexor digitorum superficialis	• Humerus medial epicondyle • Ulnar collateral ligament • Medial of the ulna coronoid process (medial head) • Proximal two-thirds of the radius	• Middle phalange corpus of the second-fifth fingers

Table 10.3 Functions and roles of muscles in elbow joint movement

Muscles	Functions	Roles
Triceps brachii	• Elbow extension • Arm extension and abduction (long head)	To extend the shoulder while rowing, interact with the latissimus dorsi, posterior deltoid, and teres major
Anconeus	• Elbow extension • Thought to provide abduction of the ulna during pronation	Provides stabilization during supination and pronation
Subanconeus	• Thought to aid in stabilizing the fat pad during elbow extension	–
Biceps brachii	• Supination • Flexion of the forearm in supination	Helpful in situations requiring strong supination, such as screwing and cork unwinding

(continued)

Table 10.3 (continued)

Muscles	Functions	Roles
Brachialis	• Flexion of the elbow at all angles	Provides a lift function in the independent forearm position, especially in pronation traction
Brachioradialis	• Elbow flexion • Supination of the forearm in pronation • Pronation of the forearm in supination	Enables flexion in a neutral forearm position
Supinator	• Supination	Employed while using a wrench and screwdriver
Extensor carpi radialis longus	• Wrist extension • Radial deviation	Strong wrist extension and radial deviation during backhand and rowing in tennis
Extensor carpi radialis brevis	• Wrist extension • Radial deviation.	Functions during backhand strokes in tennis
Extensor digitorum	• Wrist extension • Second-fifth metacarpophalangeal joint extension • Helps elbow flexion while the forearm is pronated	–
Extensor carpi ulnaris	• Wrist extension • Ulnar deviation	Used in conditions that require wrist extension and ulnar deviation, such as hammering and throwing
Pronator teres	• Pronation • Strong pronation to the forearm (after pronator quadratus) • Weak elbow flexion	Functions during activities that require vigorous rotation, such as using a screwdriver
Flexor carpi radialis	• Wrist flexion • Radial deviation	Provides strong flexion during throwing and radial deviation during rowing
Palmaris longus	• Wrist flexion • Stretches the palmar aponeurosis	Maintains force continuity during gripping and catching and provides stability in throwing sports that require strong wrist flexion with full elbow extension
Flexor carpi ulnaris	• Wrist flexion • Ulnar deviation	Functions in a firm grip, hammering, and backhand in tennis
Flexor digitorum superficialis	• Flexion of proximal interphalangeal joints and wrist	Functions when playing or grasping the piano or similar instruments

10.3 Palpation of Bones and Muscles in the Elbow Joint

10.3.1 Palpation of Bone Structures

Table 10.4 describes the palpation of bone structures in the elbow joint.

10.3.2 Palpation of Muscle Structures

Figure 10.11 describes the palpation of muscle structures at the elbow joint

Table 10.4 Elbow joint bone structure and muscle palpation

Structure	Position	Palpation	Test
Olecranon	Elbow flexed	Locate the round, rigid structure with the most protruding back of the elbow using the tip of your finger (Fig. 10.10a)	Passive elbow flexion and extension should not affect it
Olecranon fossa	Elbow flexed	Use your fingertip to locate the olecranon. Proceed to the pit area from the back and the top (Fig. 10.10b)	Elbow extension should be used to reduce the area
Medial epicondyle	Elbow flexed, forearm in supination	Use your fingertip to locate the olecranon. Feel for the rounded protrusion of the epicondyle, medial and slightly anterior to the olecranon (Fig. 10.10c) The ulnar nerve can be easily palpated in the cubital tunnel, medial to the olecranon, without reaching the medial epicondyle	Elbow movements should not affect it
Lateral epicondyle	Elbow flexed, forearm in supination	Use your fingertip to locate the olecranon. Feel the large round protrusion of the epicondyle by moving laterally and slightly anteriorly (Fig. 10.10d)	Elbow movements should not affect it
Radial head	Elbow flexed, forearm in a neutral position	Use your fingertip to locate the lateral epicondyle. Move your finger distally while remaining lateral to the olecranon (Fig. 10.10e)	It is localized and tested during forearm passive pronation and supination
Cubital fossa topography	It is the area between the brachioradialis and pronator teres muscles anterior to the elbow. The musculocutaneous nerve, biceps tendon, brachial artery, and median nerve pass through the fossa from lateral to median. The musculocutaneous nerve is difficult to palpate and is located deep between the brachioradialis and the biceps brachial tendon. The brachial artery is detected by a pulse located medial to the biceps below the biceps aponeurosis (Fig. 10.10f)		
Triceps brachii	Prone position, forearm in pronation	Use your fingertip to locate the olecranon. Thumb and fingers grip the pincer-shaped muscular body towards the humerus (Fig. 10.11a)	Resist shoulder and elbow extension
Anconeus	Elbow flexed, forearm in a neutral position	The thumb is placed between the lateral epicondyle, the lateral ulna, and the humeroradial articular surface (Fig. 10.11b)	Resist elbow extension
Biceps brachii	Elbow slightly flexed, forearm in supination	Grip the muscular body in a pincer shape with the thumb and other fingers, between the shoulder and forearm, at the anterior of the forearm. Palpate the muscle-tendon in the same position by sliding your fingertips towards the cubital fossa (Fig. 10.11c)	Resist elbow flexion
Brachialis	Elbow slightly flexed, forearm in pronation	Form a clamping grip on the medial epicondyle and palpate the borders under the biceps (Fig. 10.11d)	Resist elbow flexion
Brachioradialis	Elbow flexed, forearm in a neutral position	The muscle is clamped on the lateral biceps tendon (the distal third of the humerus towards the lateral epicondyle) (Fig. 10.11e)	Resist elbow flexion
Supinator	Elbow flexed, forearm in a neutral position	With the thumb in line with the radial head, palpate the muscle body anteriorly (Fig. 10.11f)	Resist forearm supination
Extensor carpi radialis longus	Elbow flexed, forearm in a neutral position	Put your thumb on the radial head. The fingers should glide over the crista supracondylaris and palpate the muscular body anteriorly (Fig. 10.11g)	Resist wrist extension and radial deviation

(continued)

Table 10.4 (continued)

Structure	Position	Palpation	Test
Extensor carpi radialis brevis	Elbow flexed, forearm in a neutral position	Palpate the lateral epicondyle. Using your thumb, locate the extensor carpi radialis longus, then palpate the muscle medially and distally (Fig. 10.11h)	Resist wrist extension and radial deviation
Extensor digitorum	Elbow flexed, forearm in pronation	Use your fingertip to locate the olecranon. With your thumb, move distally along the ulna's lateral edge. Palpate between the extensor carpi radialis brevis and extensor carpi ulnaris muscles (Fig. 10.11i)	Confirm by asking the participant to move their fingers as if playing the piano
Extensor carpi ulnaris	Elbow flexed, forearm in pronation	Use your fingertip to locate the olecranon. With your thumb, move distally along the lateral aspect of the ulna. Palpate lateral to the extensor digitorum, parallel to the ulna's bone line (Fig. 10.11j)	Resist wrist extension and ulnar deviation
Pronator teres	Elbow flexed, forearm in supination	Palpate the medial epicondyle. With the thumb, the muscle trunk is palpated distally and laterally (in the cubital fossa) (Fig. 10.11k)	Resist forearm pronation
Flexor carpi radialis	Elbow and wrist flexed, forearm in supination	Palpate the lateral epicondyle. With your thumb, palpate the muscle medial to the brachioradialis (Fig. 10.11l)	Resist wrist flexion and radial deviation
Palmaris longus	Elbow and wrist flexed, forearm in supination	Palpate the flexor carpi radialis using your thumb. Palpate the muscle by shifting your finger medially (Fig. 10.11m)	Resist elbow flexion
Flexor carpi ulnaris	Elbow and wrist flexed, forearm in supination	With your thumb, locate the palmaris longus. Palpate the muscle by sliding your finger medially (Fig. 10.11n)	Resist wrist flexion and ulnar deviation
Topography of flexor muscles	Topography of the thumb pronator teres, index finger flexor carpi radialis, middle finger palmaris longus, and ring finger flexor carpi ulnaris when placed parallel to the anterior of the forearm with the little finger of one hand out (Fig. 10.11o)		

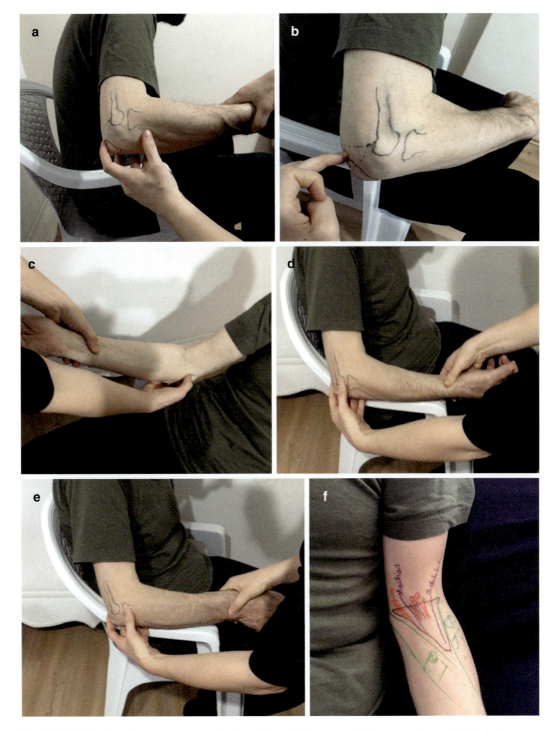

Fig. 10.10 Palpation of bone structures in the elbow joint (**a**) Olecranon. (**b**) Olecranon fossa. (**c**) Medial epicondyle. (**d**) Lateral epicondyle. (**e**) Radial head. (**f**) Cubital fossa topography

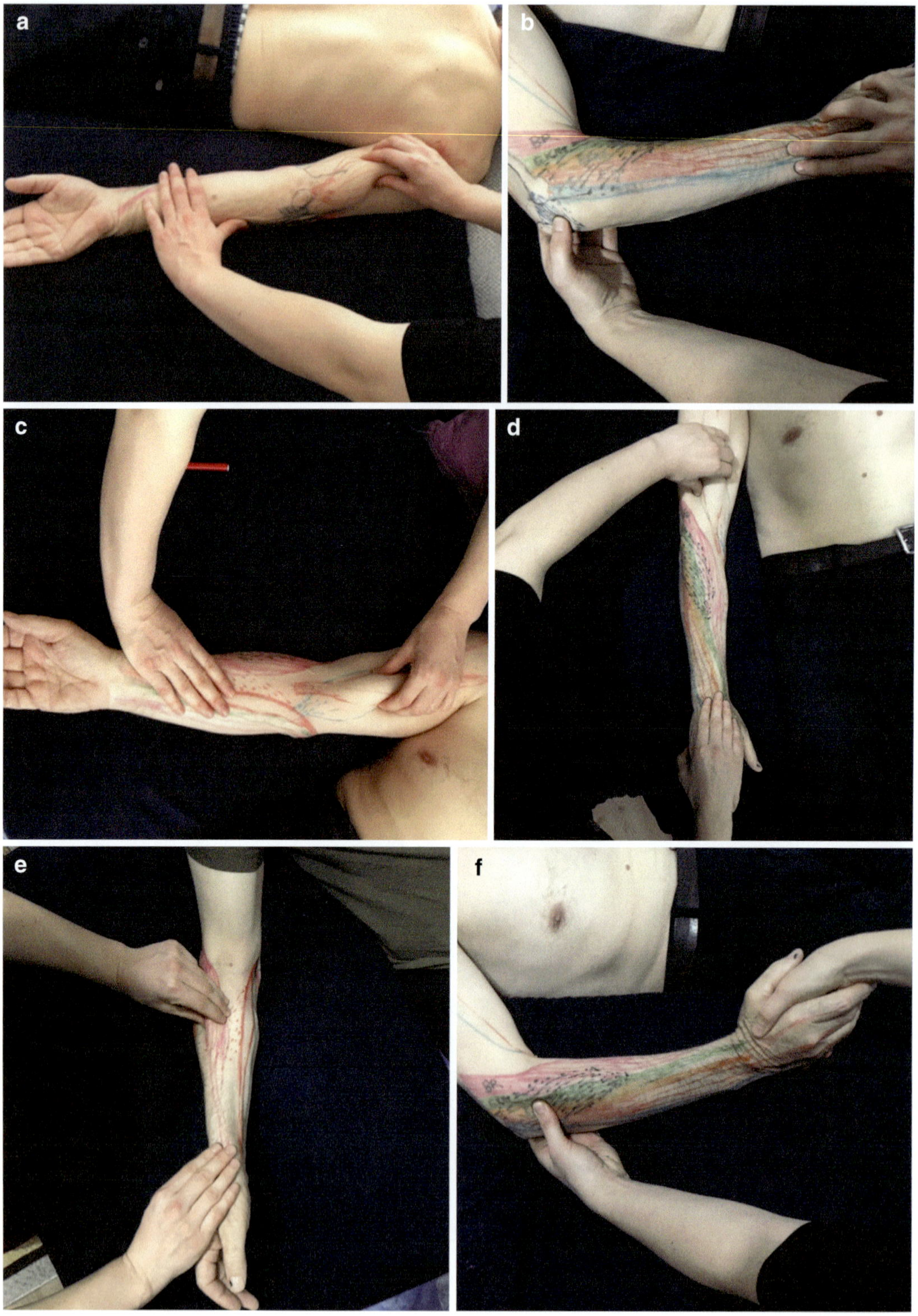

Fig. 10.11 Muscle palpation at the elbow joint. (**a**) Triceps brachii, (**b**) anconeus, (**c**) biceps brachii, (**d**) brachialis, (**e**) brachioradialis, (**f**) supinator, (**g**) extensor carpi radialis longus, (**h**) extensor carpi radialis brevis, (**i**) extensor digitorum, (**j**) extensor carpi ulnaris, (**k**) pronator teres, (**l**) flexor carpi radialis, (**m**) palmaris longus, (**n**) flexor carpi ulnaris, (**o**) topography of flexor muscles

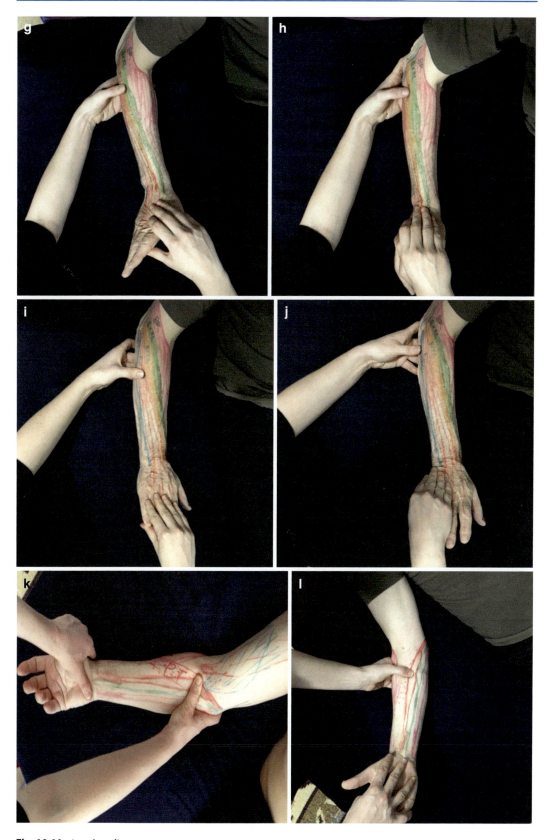

Fig. 10.11 (continued)

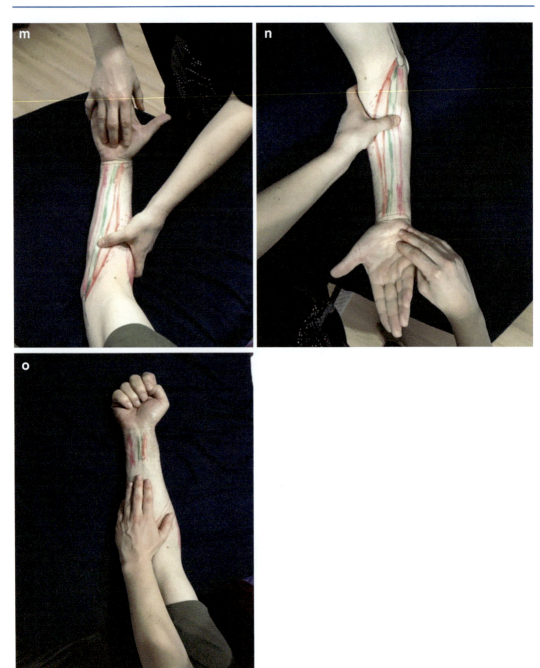

Fig. 10.11 (continued)

10.4 Elbow Joint Movements

10.4.1 Normal Joint Movement

The elbow joint has a range of motion between 0°–140° flexion and extension, 15° hyperextension, 85° supination, and 75° pronation. Functionally, 30°–130° flexion and 50° supination and pronation are sufficient.

10.4.1.1 Flexion and Extension

Rotational and sliding movements occur concurrently in the humeroulnar and humeroradial joints during flexion–extension. The joint has approximately 3°–4° varus–valgus laxity during all elbow flexion. The axis of rotation is a line that runs from the center of the capitellum to the anteroinferior aspect of the medial epicondyle and provides a 2–3 mm offset during movement. The humeroulnar joint is thus assumed to be a uniaxial joint (except for extreme degrees of flexion and extension). The extension is restricted by the olecranon, stretching anterior capsule, and flexor muscles. Active flexion is limited by the volume of the flexor muscles and contraction of the triceps muscle. Passive flexion is limited by contact of the coronoid with the radial head fossa.

10.4.1.2 Pronation and Supination

The radius rotates around the ulna when the forearm rotates. Although shoulder abduction can help compensate for supination loss, there are no effective mechanisms to compensate for pronation. The longitudinal axis of forearm rotation extends from the center of the radial head and capitellum to the base of the ulna's styloid process. The axis of rotation shifts slightly in the ulnar and volar directions during supination and slightly in the radial and dorsal directions during pronation. The joint reaction force increases as the radius moves 1–2 mm proximally in pronation. Muscles and ligaments limit the range of motion.

10.4.2 Stabilization

Because of its compatible joint structure, the elbow joint is one of the most stable joints in the human body. The humeroulnar joint structure provides primary stability, with the anterior portion of the MCL and LCL providing secondary stability. Dynamic stabilization is provided by the muscles that pass through the elbow joint.

10.4.2.1 Bone and Joint Stabilization

The olecranon's geometric structure and articulation with the humerus (30° anterior angulation) provide passive bone stabilization of the humeroulnar joint. The greater sigmoid process encompasses 75–85% of the valgus during flexion and extension. The small sigmoid process provides varus stress at 60% in flexion and 67% in extension. The coronoid process prevents posterior translation and stabilizes the humeroulnar joint by approximately 50%. The radiohumeral joint provides valgus and posterior control, especially when the MCL is insufficient. When there is no problem with the MCL, it is thought to contribute approximately 30% to stabilization.

10.4.2.2 Ligament-Based Stabilization

Ligaments are the most basic structures that provide stability. As movement in the elbow joint occurs along an axis passing through the center of the capitulum humeri and the trochlea humerus, different bands of the MCL are stretched to varying degrees of elbow flexion. The anterior oblique band of the MCL complex primarily provides valgus stabilization and is stretched in extension and relaxed in flexion. The posterior oblique band, which stretches in flexion and relaxes in extension, forms the floor of the cubital tunnel. The transverse (*Cooper's*) ligament does not play a significant role in stabilizing the coronoid and olecranon. When the MCL is intact, the radial head does not create a significant additional limitation against valgus stress. In contrast, it contributes as a secondary stabilizer against valgus stress when the MCL is cut. The anterior band of the MCL is also divided into sections based on functions. The anterior fibers of the anterior band are taut in extension, while the posterior fibers are taut in flexion.

> **Clinical Information**
>
> The MCL and radial head contribute to elbow stability in the same way that the anterior cruciate ligament and menisci do to knee stability. The MCL is injured as a result of valgus stress in full extension. Throwing movements that are repeated are also more likely to cause its injury.

The LUCL is an important structure for stabilizing the elbow joint against varus and rotational stresses. Because the LCL works with all of its parts, it is as the primary stabilizer of the elbow joint. While the AL stabilizes the proximal radial ulnar joint, the ALCL also provides lateral elbow stability. The LUCL is the primary lateral stabilizer that provides posterolateral rotational stability to the elbow. Because the RCL is located near the rotational axis of motion, it offers equal resistance during flexion and extension.

> **Clinical Information**
>
> LCL injuries are uncommon on their own but are frequently associated with radial head fracture, LUCL tear, and coronoid tip fracture, a condition known as the "terrible triad of elbow dislocation." LUCL injuries are most common at the end of the deceleration phase in throwing sports.

10.4.2.3 Bone and Ligament Interaction

Varus stress is carried by the joint 55% of the time, the anterior capsule 32% of the time, and the RCL 14% of the time when the elbow is fully extended. When the elbow is in 90° flexion, the anatomical structure of the joint contributes 75% to varus stability. Valgus stability is equally compensated by the MCL, anterior capsule, and bony-joint structure at elbow full extension. When the elbow is in 90° flexion, the bone-joint structure provides 55% and MCL 35% stabilization, respectively. In the extension position, the anterior capsule provides 85% of the distraction resistance, while in the 90° flexion position, the MCL provides 78% of the distraction resistance. If the MCL is not damaged, the radial head does not affect valgus stress; however, it contributes significantly to valgus stabilization with MCL damage. Recent research has found that the forearm's rotational position helps stabilize the elbow. If the MCL is insufficient, the elbow is more stable in supination, and if the LCL is insufficient, the elbow is more stable in pronation. With a coronoid fracture, the elbow is more stable in supination than in pronation. These conditions are critical for placing the elbow in the best position during rehabilitation.

> **Clinical Information**
>
> After shoulder dislocations, elbow dislocations are the most common. In 80% of cases, posterolateral rotational instabilities are observed. Falling on the hand causes external rotation of the ulna and radius relative to the distal humerus and posterior displacement of the radius relative to the capitulum. Typically, the LCL is torn, and depending on the severity of the injury, the MCL may also be damaged.

10.4.2.4 Muscular Stabilization

The muscles surrounding the joint control dynamic stabilization. When the joint is fully extended, the load on it is greatest. Muscles allow movement not only of the elbow but also of the wrist and fingers. The roles of common extensor tendons and flexor/pronator muscles (especially flexor carpi ulnaris and flexor digitorum superficialis) in elbow joint stabilization are currently unclear. These tendinous structures are likely important secondary elbow stabilizers and are frequently ruptured during dislocations. Furthermore, it is extremely difficult to dislocate the elbow experimentally without cutting these structures. However, studies have shown no increase in activation of these muscles against valgus and varus stress or after MCL failure, and they do not contribute to stabilization.

Functional insufficiency of the biceps brachii, triceps brachii, and brachialis muscles increases varus-valgus instability in all flexion positions. The flexor and pronator muscles are important secondary stabilizers against valgus force, and their stabilizing role is most prominent in the forearm supination position. It has been reported that the flexor carpi ulnaris can be especially effective in providing medial support. The common extensor muscles have the most tension in full pronation and function most effectively as a varus stabilizer. The anconeus muscle is thought to provide dynamic stabilization to varus and posterolateral instability. In general, any muscle crossing the elbow can reportedly protect ligaments and other anatomical structures by applying compressive pressure.

10.4.3 Force Transmission

When the elbow is extended, the humeroulnar joint carries about 40% of the total axial load, while the humeroradial joint carries 60%. The force passing through the proximal ulna is 93% in varus stress and 12% in valgus stress. The radius head carries the greatest load during pronation and 0°–30° flexion.

10.5 Evidence-Based Exercises for Elbow Muscles

Muscles' maximal voluntary isometric contraction (MVIC) is expressed as low at 0–20%, moderate at 21–40%, high at 41–60%, and very high at 60% and above in electromyographic measurements (EMG). Endurance and strength training should be preferred according to these ratios (for strength training, exercises with higher activation are chosen).

10.5.1 Evidence-Based Exercises for Elbow Extensor Muscles

The triceps brachii is the primary muscle responsible for elbow extension. As a result, numerous studies examine triceps brachii muscle activation during elbow extension. All triceps brachial muscle fibers are activated when the elbow is extended from a 90° flexion position. The medial head is active throughout the entire elbow extension. The long and lateral heads are activated when the elbow is extended, and resistance is applied against the extension. Furthermore, the triceps brachii aid shoulder extension, prevent humeral head downward displacement and stabilize the glenohumeral joint when the shoulder is abducted. However, due to its poor function on the shoulder joint, the triceps brachii is often neglected in clinical evaluations of the shoulder. It has been shown that the effect of the triceps brachii on shoulder extension torque increases to 0°–80° with a maximum of 0°–40° shoulder flexion and decreases in 80°–120° flexion.

Table 10.5 lists evidence-based exercises for elbow extension. The MVIC of the triceps brachii was activated 60% of the time during lateral pulldowns (LPD), 59% during bench presses (BP), and 78% during triceps lying (TL). Furthermore, the pull-over (PO) activated the triceps 62.5% more than the BP.

In the study in which the triceps brachii was examined during TL, BP, LPD, and PO exercises, during concentric contraction, the highest activation was with TL at 67.7%, then BP at 49.2%, PO at 34.3%, and LPD at 12.4% and during an eccentric contraction, 37.6, 23.8, 20.5, and 9.7%, respectively. Also, activation was similar during PO and BP exercises.

In the BP exercise, the lateral part of the triceps brachii was examined at different inclinations (−15°, 0°, 30°, 45°). Significantly more activation was observed during the concentric phase than in the eccentric phase. During concentric contraction, a 45° incline resulted in greater muscle activation than a 0° incline (MVIC 102.2% at −15°, 106.0% at 0°, 114.3% at 30°, 117.8% at 45°). During an eccentric contraction, muscle activation is similar between slopes. When triceps brachial activation was examined by holding bars of different widths (100, 150, and 200% of the biacromial width) during the BP movement, it was observed that activation decreased significantly as the width increased. Maximum activation was at a width of 100%. When BP and push-up movements (under similar loads) were compared, it was found that they had similar kinematics and muscle activation (biceps brachii, triceps brachii, both parts of the pectoral muscle, and the anterior part of the deltoid were examined).

Table 10.5 Evidence-based exercises for elbow muscles

Muscles	Exercise type	Exercise name/position
Elbow extensor muscles	Concentric and eccentric	• Triceps lying • Pull-over • Bench press • Lateral pull-down • Push-up • Elbow extension (*Thrower's ten*)
Elbow flexor muscles	Concentric and eccentric	• Dumbbell curl • Barbell curl • Incline curl • Pull-up • Chin-up • Perfect pull-up • Elbow flexion (*Thrower's ten*)
Wrist extensor and forearm supinator muscles	Concentric and eccentric	• Eccentric exercises with flexible bar • Supination (*Thrower's ten*) • Wrist flexion (*Thrower's ten*) • Wrist extension at full elbow extension or 70° and 90° flexion
	Stretching	• Stretching with elbow extension, forearm pronation, and wrist flexion (especially with flexion of the second and third fingers)
Wrist flexor and forearm pronator muscles	Concentric and eccentric	• Eccentric exercises with flexible bar • Pronation (*Thrower's ten*) • Wrist extension (*Thrower's ten*) • Wrist flexion at full extension of the elbow or 70°–90° flexion positions
	Stretching	• Stretching with finger extension, elbow extension, anterior supination, and wrist extension

In the TL exercise, the person lies supine on a horizontal bench and holds the bar 87% of the biacromial distance with the hand pronated and the elbow extended. The person flexes the bar to bring it 2 cm closer to the face, then completes the exercise by fully extending the elbow (Fig. 10.12).

In the BP exercise, the person lies on their back on a horizontal bench holding the bar twice as wide as the biacromial distance, with their feet touching the ground and their wrist pronated. The exercise begins with the person touching their chest and ends with the elbows fully extended (Fig. 10.13).

In the LPD exercise, the person is in a sitting position holding a bar twice the width of the biacromial space with the wrist in pronation and the elbow in full extension. The person pulls the shoulder blades back and lowers the bar to the bottom of the chin while keeping the trunk and hips fixed (Fig. 10.14).

In the PO exercise, the person lies supine on a horizontal bench. When the hand is pronated, and the elbow is fully extended, the person holds the bar with a width of 87% of the biacromial distance. The person performs full shoulder flexion (a maximum of 40° flexion at the elbow is permitted), then extends the shoulder at about 90° (Fig. 10.15).

In the push-up exercise, the person lies face down on the floor and then stands on the tips of the feet and hands (at shoulder width) with the whole trunk and lower extremities straight. Then the person raises the entire body straight on the arms, lowering it again so that the chest does not touch the ground (Fig. 10.16).

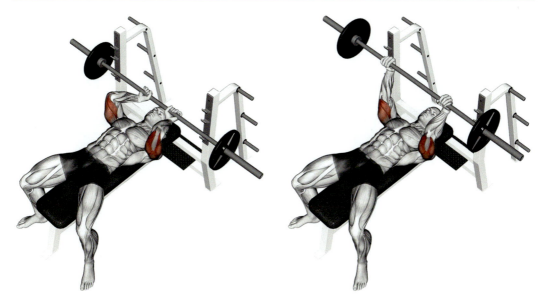

Fig. 10.12 Triceps lying (Makatserchyk/Shutterstock.com)

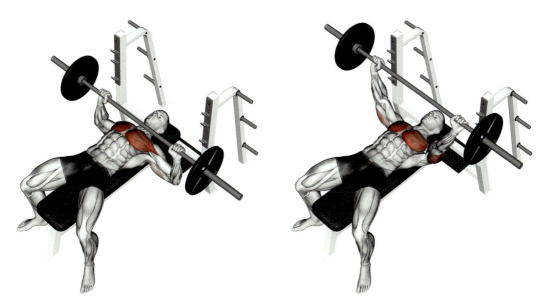

Fig. 10.13 Bench press (Makatserchyk/Shutterstock.com)

10.5.2 Evidence-Based Exercises for Elbow Flexor Muscles

The brachialis muscle contributes the most to elbow flexion torque (47%) of all elbow flexor muscles. The maximum isometric flexion force at the elbow occurs at a 90°–110° flexion angle.

The biceps brachii long head is the shoulder flexor and abductor. It also aids in the upward and anterior stability of the humeral head. The activation of both heads of the biceps brachii (measured by keeping the forearm neutral) is unchanged by different elbow flexion angles, but it increases with increasing shoulder elevation.

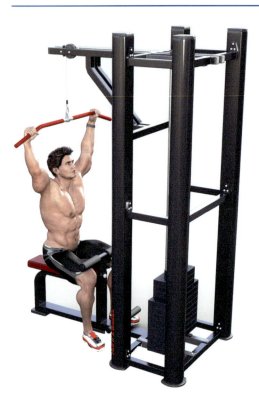 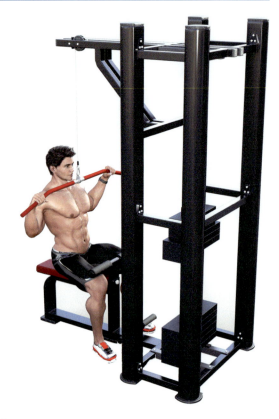

Fig. 10.14 Lateral pull-down (Sport08/Shutterstock.com)

External shoulder rotation with elevation produces more muscle activation than internal rotation. The biceps brachii is especially important in athletes during dynamic upper extremity activities that require elbow flexion. Table 10.5 lists evidence-based exercises for these muscles.

According to studies on biceps brachii activation, the muscle has a maximum isometric contraction of 33.6% in rock climbers (during the pull-up movement with forearm pronation), 44% in baseball pitchers (during the acceleration phase of the throw), and 86% in tennis players (in the acceleration phase of the forehand stroke).

The biceps brachii has a larger physiological cross-sectional area and a higher pennation angle than the brachioradialis, but the brachioradialis has a longer fiber/muscle length. The brachioradialis fiber type has a faster contraction feature than the biceps brachii. Both muscles produce torque in the same direction, but their functions are thought to differ due to differences in muscle structure and fiber type.

A study looked at the coordination of the biceps brachii and brachioradialis in supination, pronation, and neutral forearm positions with elbow flexion. As a result, the forearm position did not affect biceps brachii activation, and the brachioradialis had higher muscle activation with pronation than neutral or supination positions. The biomechanical disadvantage of the biceps brachii in pronation results in increased brachioradialis activation.

Dumbbell curls (DC) and barbell curls (BC) are two common exercises for the elbow flexors.

DC can be performed in two ways: incline curl (IC) and hammer curl (HC).

The HC is an exercise in which the arms are at the side of the trunk (close to the body), and the palms are facing each other (wrist in neutral) while using dumbbells and bending the elbows (Fig. 10.17).

Fig. 10.15 Pull-over (Lio putra/Shutterstock.com)

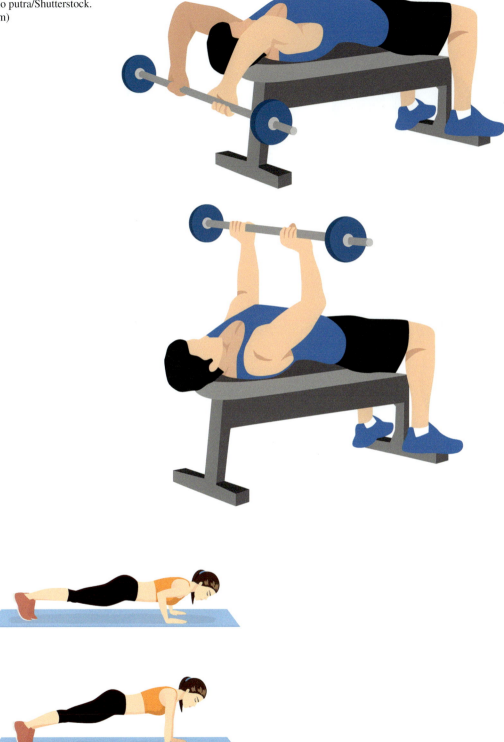

Fig. 10.16 Push-up (solar22/Shutterstock.com)

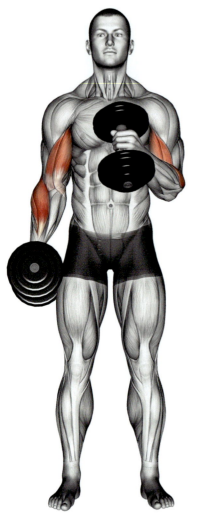

Fig. 10.17 Dumbbell curl (Makatserchyk/Shutterstock.com)

On the other hand, the IC is a variation of the HC done on a bench lying in an inclined position. Studies on the effects of IC and HC exercises on the biceps brachii and brachialis muscles show that these exercises activate the brachialis muscle more effectively because they stretch the long head of the biceps brachii (Fig. 10.18).

For BC exercises, the person holds the weight bar while standing upright, arms shoulder width apart, wrist in supination. The weight is then lifted from the shoulders (Fig. 10.19). The BC has been shown to increase activation of the short head of the biceps brachii muscle while not loading the long head. When the bar is grasped with the pronated hand, the brachioradialis muscle is activated more (Fig. 10.19).

A study on the effects of BC and DC exercises (in supination position) on the biceps brachii and brachioradialis found that both muscles were more active during concentric phases than eccentric phases. The BC was found to activate the muscles more than the DC. Compared to the DC, the BC only induced higher muscle activation in the biceps brachii during the eccentric phase.

Pull-up exercises for elbow flexion are quite common. The bars used during these exercises with the individual's body weight can be of various widths and the wrists in different positions.

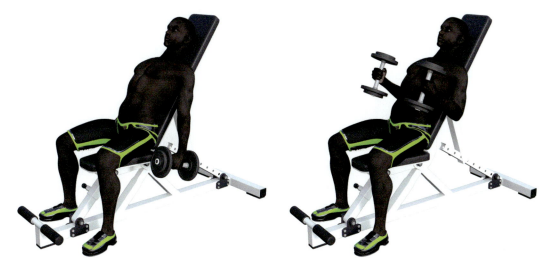

Fig. 10.18 Incline curl (Sport08/Shutterstock.com)

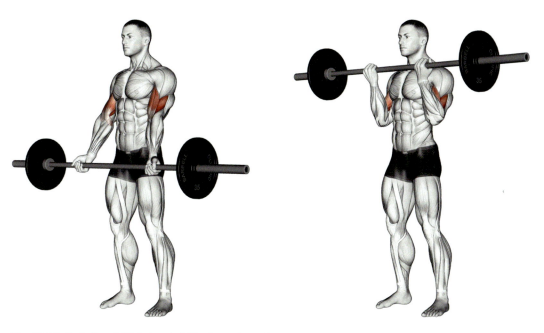

Fig. 10.19 Barbell curl (Makatserchyk/Shutterstock.com)

During a pull-up, the person raises their entire body towards the bar (Fig. 10.20). Performing the pull-up by holding the bar in the wrist supination is called a chin-up (Fig. 10.21).

In the "*Perfect Pull-Up*," the person holds the pull-up bar through a sling that allows dynamic movement. The person raises their entire body above the bar, as in arm pull-ups.

In a published study, pull-up exercises were evaluated by holding different wrist positions with a dynamic rope (pronation, supination, and neutral grip). With two bars placed parallel at 0.24 m intervals in a neutral grip, the biceps brachii was activated at 81.3, 92.9, 93.0, and 91.1%, and the brachioradialis at 97.4, 89.8, 93.5, and 96.2% MVIC, respectively. While the

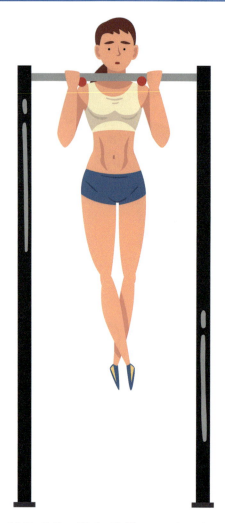

Fig. 10.20 Pull-up (NotionPic/Shutterstock.com)

biceps brachii and brachioradialis are the primary muscles responsible for movement, the middle trapezius, latissimus dorsi, and infraspinatus control both concentric and eccentric phases.

> **Clinical Information**
>
> According to the literature, the biceps brachii (80–100% MVIC) is activated during the concentric phase of the chin-up, perfect pull-up, and pull-up movements, following the latissimus dorsi. Because of the high EMG activation, these exercises should be used for strengthening.

10.5.3 Evidence-Based Exercises for Forearm Supinator-Pronator Muscles

During supination, the biceps brachii and supinator muscles are active. During pronation, the pronator quadratus and pronator teres are active. The biceps brachii is the primary supination muscle.

Pronation is stronger at the middle and full flexion values of the elbow. The pronator teres is an accessory muscle to the pronator quadratus. When supination and pronation movements are performed while holding a strong grip, the primary supinator and pronator muscles are active at 45–68% MVIC (elbow in 90° flexion position). Pronation increases the activity of the brachialis, brachioradialis, flexor carpi radialis, palmaris longus, pronator quadratus, and pronator teres muscles. In contrast, supination increases the activity of the forearm abductor pollicis longus, biceps brachii, and supinator muscles. Both the deep and superficial parts of the pronator quadratus are active during supination and pronation, suggesting that the pronator quadratus is an important distal radioulnar joint stabilizer.

Supination is stronger than pronation. Biceps brachii elbow flexion activity decreases by 50% when the forearm is pronated. When the forearm is supinated, it is active at 35–68% MVIC. Activation is greater at 90° and 135° flexion (65–68% MVIC) than at 0° and 45° flexion.

The brachioradialis acts as a supinator for the pronated arm and a pronator for the supinated arm. According to research, while maintaining the 135° flexion position of the elbow, the forearm from neutral to pronation is activated by 40–58% MVIC and supination by 27–37% MVIC. As a result, the brachioradialis acts as a stabilizer or synergist.

The extensor carpi radialis brevis has high muscle activation during both supination (26–43% MVIC) and pronation (17–55% MVIC) movements. This shows that the muscle is the forearm flexor stabilizer for gripping in pronation and the main mover of wrist extension in supination. The increased muscle activity during supination and pronation movements may result in injuries due to stress on the musculoskeletal system in the forearm.

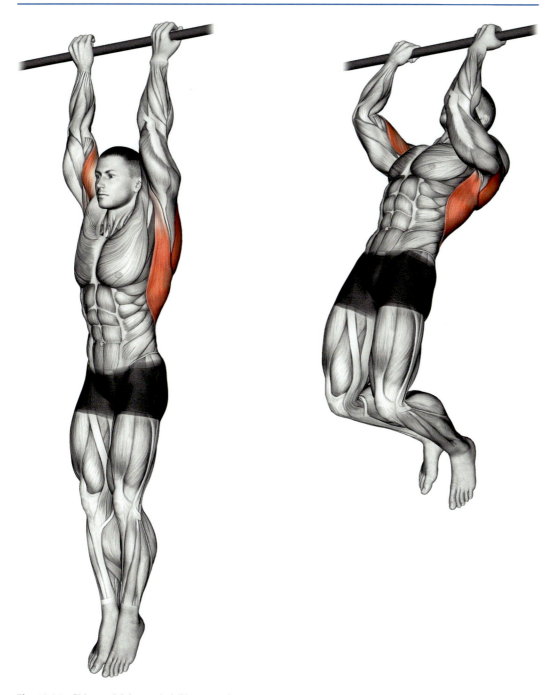

Fig. 10.21 Chin-up (Makatserchyk/Shutterstock.com)

10.5.4 Evidence-Based Exercises for the Forearm Supinator and Wrist Extensor Muscles

In wrist movements, the muscles associated with the elbow joint and attached to the lateral and medial epicondyles are more effective. However, the exercises in the elbow joint must be mentioned because they cause problems (such as tendinitis) in the elbow joint. These muscles are exercised in conjunction with wrist extension and supination, wrist flexors, and pronation in the literature. Table 10.5 lists evidence-based exercises for these muscles.

Elbow ligament and muscle injuries are common in athletes that throw. Most wrist and elbow muscles show low to moderate activity during the cocking phase of the throw. In contrast, the extensors (extensor carpi radialis longus, extensor carpi radialis brevis, and extensor digitorum) show moderate to high muscle activity (59 and 75% MVIC, respectively). The triceps brachii has extremely high activation during acceleration with wrist flexors (flexor carpi radialis, flexor carpi ulnaris, flexor digitorum superficialis, such as (120, 112, 80% MVIC, respectively). At this stage, the pronator teres muscle is also active (85% MVIC). Muscle activity decreases with the transition from the deceleration phase to the follow-through phase. At that time, the biceps brachii and brachioradialis muscles are active and provide elbow extension control.

Thrower's ten exercises are frequently used for patient rehabilitation. For this purpose, "press-up" (when the person is in a sitting position, the hands hold the edge of the chair at shoulder width and the person lifts himself), push-up, elbow flexion (Fig. 10.22), elbow extension (Fig. 10.23), forearm pronation (Fig. 10.24) (weight and/or exercise band pronated from neutral forearm position), forearm supination (weight and/or exercise band supinated from neutral forearm position) (Fig. 10.25), wrist flexion (Fig. 10.26) (wrist flexed while the forearm is supinated in elbow flexion), and wrist extension (Fig. 10.27) (wrist extended while the forearm is pronated in elbow flexion) exercises are used.

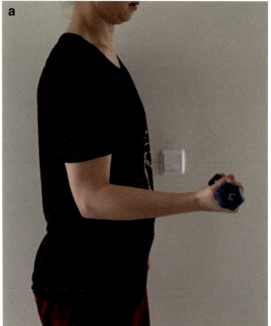 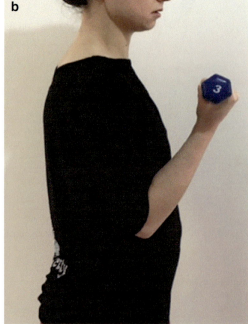

Fig. 10.22 Elbow flexion. (**a**) Start position. (**b**) End position (Makatserchyk/Shutterstock.com)

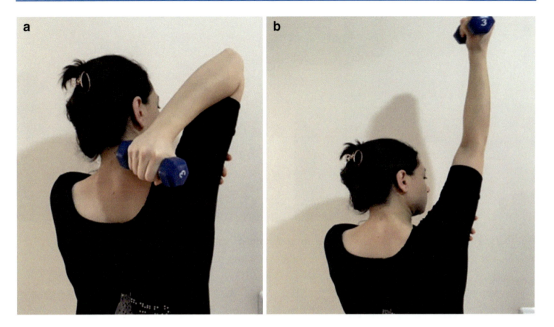

Fig. 10.23 Elbow extension. (**a**) Start position. (**b**) End position

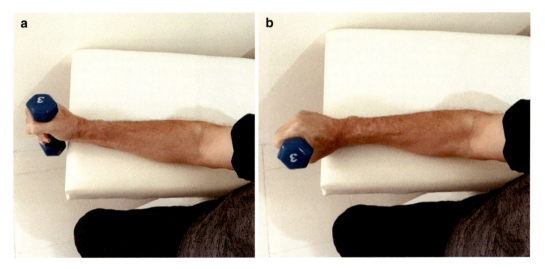

Fig. 10.24 Forearm pronation. (**a**) Start position. (**b**) End position

Stretching in the elbow extension, forearm pronation, wrist flexion, and ulnar deviation positions is the most effective method for stretching the extensor carpi radialis longus and extensor carpi radialis brevis (17.8 and 13.8% tension, respectively). The extensor carpi radialis brevis is commonly associated with lateral epicondylitis pathology. Anatomical studies have revealed that the index finger segment of the extensor digitorum derives from the extensor carpi radialis brevis tendon. In contrast, the middle finger segment derives from the extensor carpi radialis brevis tendon and the lateral epicondyle. Recent cadaver studies have shown that index and middle finger flexion, wrist flexion and ulnar deviation,

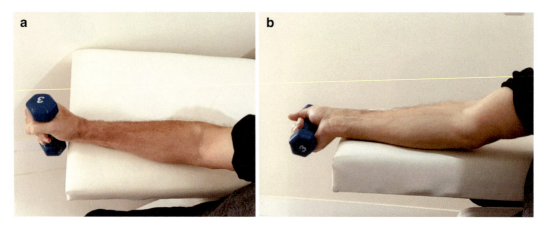

Fig. 10.25 Forearm supination. (**a**) Start position. (**b**) End position

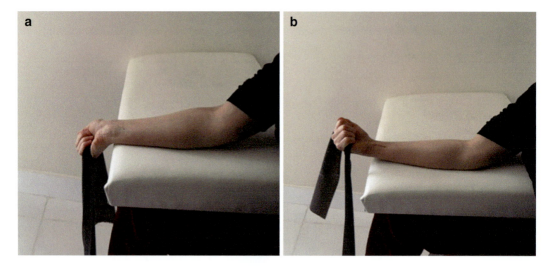

Fig. 10.26 Wrist flexion. (**a**) Start position. (**b**) End position

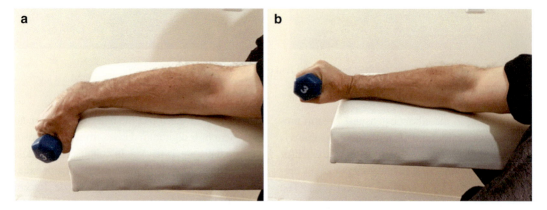

Fig. 10.27 Wrist extension. (**a**) Start position. (**b**) End position

forearm pronation, 15° elbow flexion, and elbow varus stress create the most tension in the extensor carpi radialis brevis tendon to stretch the wrist extensors. As a result, this stretching position should be preferred during rehabilitation. In static stretching applications, 30 s, 3–4 repetitions, and 30 s of rest are frequently preferred because they produce the most effective results (Fig. 10.28).

It has been reported that full elbow extension and forearm pronation have the greatest effect on strengthening the wrist extensor muscles. For concentric wrist extensor exercises, the person actively extends the wrist to full extension in the bed or sitting position, with the elbow in full extension or 70°–90° flexion, the forearm in pronation, and the wrist in full flexion. When resisting with an exercise band, the band should be tight in extension and loose in flexion (Fig. 10.29). For eccentric wrist extensor exercises, the person is asked to slowly lower the wrists in the flexion direction while on the bed or sitting, with the elbow in full extension or 70°–90° flexion positions, the forearm in pronation, the wrist in extension, and the hand hanging from the side of the bed. The person then passively returns the hand to the starting position with the other hand. In addition to *Therabands* and weights, exercises with flexible rubber bars are an alternative method that provides eccentric work. Eccentric exercises performed with a flexible rubber bar were found to reduce pain by 81% and increase strength by 79%. This method is frequently used, especially in the treatment of lateral epicondylitis. The lower end of the rubber bar is held perpendicular to the floor, with the wrist extended and the elbow flexed at 90°. The other end of the bar is held by the healthy hand. The elbows are extended with the patient's healthy hand, bar, and arm in front of the trunk. The patient slowly flexes the wrist with the healthy hand by rotating the bar in the flexion direction. As a result, an eccentric contraction is performed on the patient's wrist extensors. Eccentric wrist contraction can last up to 4 s. It is recommended to perform 3 sets of 15 repetitions with 30 s of rest in between. Progress is achieved by increasing the bar hardness (Fig. 10.30).

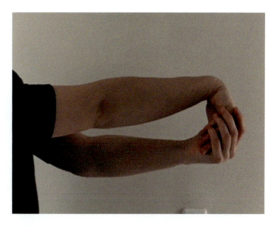

Fig. 10.28 Stretching for wrist extensor muscles

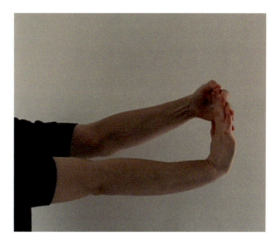

Fig. 10.29 Stretching for wrist flexor muscles

Clinical Information

Supination strengthening exercises (performed with full elbow extension, forearm pronation, and therapeutic tape) combined with eccentric and concentric exercises were found to be more effective than stretching exercises combined with eccentric and concentric exercises in individuals with lateral epicondylitis. As a result, including supinator muscle strengthening during rehabilitation would be beneficial.

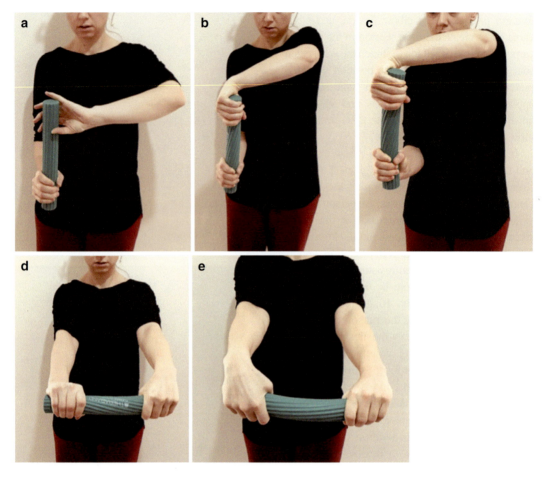

Fig. 10.30 eccentric exercise for wrist extensors with flexbar (right side affected). (**a**) Start position, (**b**) 2nd position, (**c**) 3rd position, (**d**) 4th position, (**e**) end position

10.5.5 Evidence-Based Exercises for the Forearm Pronator and Wrist Flexor Muscles

The common flexor tendon is 3 cm long and is formed by the pronator teres, flexor carpi radialis, palmaris longus, flexor carpi ulnaris, and flexor digitorum superficialis. One of the most common injuries to this tendon is medial epicondylitis, which occurs due to repetitive wrist flexion and forearm pronation. Table 10.5 lists evidence-based exercises for these muscles.

Because of their positive effects on recovery, eccentric exercises are frequently recommended in the literature for medial epicondylitis. For eccentric exercises of the wrist flexor and pronator muscles, one end of a rubber bar is held parallel to the ground with the wrist positioned in flexion, the forearm in supination, and the elbow in flexion. The other end of the bar is grasped in pronation with the healthy hand and turned in the flexion direction (anterior to the patient). The elbows are extended at the same time as the arms are in front of the body. After both arms are in front of the body, the wrist is slowly extended with the tension of the bar (Fig. 10.31).

Eccentric wrist flexor exercises involve slowly lowering the wrist in the direction of extension while lying or sitting, with the elbow in full extension or 70°–90° flexion, the forearm in supination, the wrist in flexion, and the hand hanging from the side of the bed. The person then passively returns the hand to its starting position with the other hand. The exercise progresses by using an exercise band or weight (Fig. 10.26).

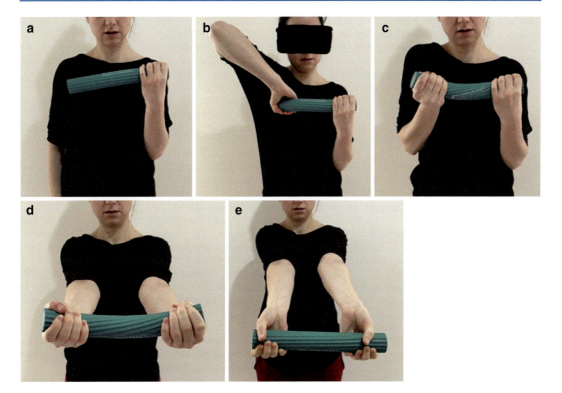

Fig. 10.31 Eccentric exercise for wrist flexors with flexbar (left side affected). (**a**) Start position, (**b**) 2nd position, (**c**) 3rd position, (**d**) 4th position, (**e**) end position

Stretching exercises for the wrist flexor muscles are performed with the wrist and fingers extended and the elbow fully extended (Fig. 10.29).

Although they do not significantly contribute to elbow joint movements, different exercise methods (radial and ulnar deviation, wrist flexion or extension together or separately, with finger participation) and forearm muscle exercise types are important in elbow joint injuries (according to the related muscle activity). Depending on the individual's needs and clinical conditions, isometric exercises, proprioceptive neuromuscular facilitation, various stretching and strengthening techniques and perturbation exercises may be preferred.

10.6 Conclusion

In this chapter, the precise anatomy and biomechanics of the elbow joint, palpation information that physiotherapists need in evaluation and therapy, and detailed information about evidence-based exercises used in elbow rehabilitation are explained in detail with clinical information. In addition, basic information for elbow joint therapy can be found in this section.

Further Reading

An K, Zobitz M, Morrey B. Biomechanics of the elbow. In: Morrey B, Sotelo J, Morrey M, editors. Morrey's the elbow and its disorders. Amsterdam: Elsevier; 2018. p. 39–63.

Avcı Ş, Un Yıldırım N, Bakar Y. Elbow, forearm, wrist and hand. In: Ergun N, editor. Functional anatomy: musculoskeletal anatomy, kinesiology and palpation for manual therapists. Ankara: Nobel Medicine Bookstore; 2017. p. 125–82.

Badre A, Axford DT, Banayan S, Johnson JA, King GJW. The effect of torsional moments on the posterolateral rotatory stability of a lateral ligament deficient elbow: an in vitro biomechanical investigation. Clin Biomech (Bristol, Avon). 2019;67:85–9.

Calatayud J, Vinstrup J, Jakobsen MD, Sundstrup E, Carlos Colado J, Andersen LL. Attentional focus and grip width influences on bench press resistance training. Percept Mot Skills. 2018;125(2):265–77.

Cavalheiro CS, Filho MR, Rozas J, Wey J, de Andrade AM, Caetano EB. Anatomical study on the innervation of the elbow capsule. Rev Bras Ortop. 2015;50(6):673–9.

Day JM, Lucado AM, Uhl TL. A comprehensive rehabilitation program for treating lateral elbow tendinopathy. Int J Sports Phys Ther. 2019;14(5):818–29.

Dickie JA, Faulkner JA, Barnes MJ, Lark SD. Electromyographic analysis of muscle activation during pull-up variations. J Electromyogr Kinesiol. 2017;32:30–6.

Felstead AJ, Ricketts D. Biomechanics of the shoulder and elbow. Orthop Trauma. 2017;31(5):300–5.

Islam SU, Glover A, MacFarlane RJ, Mehta N, Waseem M. The anatomy and biomechanics of the elbow. Open Orthop J. 2020;14(1):95–9.

Kholinne E, Zulkarnain RF, Sun YC, Lim S, Chun J-M, Jeon IH. The different role of each head of the triceps brachii muscle in elbow extension. Acta Orthop Traumatol Turc. 2018;52(3):201–5.

Landin D, Thompson M, Jackson M. Functions of the triceps brachii in humans: a review. J Clin Med Res. 2018;10(4):290–3.

Lauver JD, Cayot TE, Scheuermann BW. Influence of bench angle on upper extremity muscular activation during bench press exercise. Eur J Sport Sci. 2016;16(3):309–16.

Marcolin G, Panizzolo FA, Petrone N, Moro T, Grigoletto D, Piccolo D, et al. Differences in electromyographic activity of biceps brachii and brachioradialis while performing three variants of curl. Peer J. 2018;6:5165.

Padasala M, Sharmila B, Bhatt H, D'Onofrio R. Comparison of efficacy of the eccentric concentric training of wrist extensors with static stretching versus eccentric concentric training with supinatör strengthening in patients with tennis elbow: a randomized clinical trial. Ita J Sports Reh Po. 2020;7(3):1597–623.

Reichel LM, Morales OA. Gross anatomy of the elbow capsule: a cadaveric study. J Hand Surg Am. 2013;38(1):110–6.

Reichert B. Elbow complex. In: Reichert B, editor. Palpation techniques surface anatomy for physical therapists. Stuttgart: Thieme; 2015. p. 47–68.

Rooker JC, Smith JR, Amirfeyz R. Anatomy, surgical approaches and biomechanics of the elbow. Orthop Trauma. 2016;30(4):283–90.

Ruangchaijatuporn T, Gaetke-Udager K, Jacobson JA, Yablon CM, Morag Y. Ultrasound evaluation of bursae: anatomy and pathological appearances. Skelet Radiol. 2017;46(4):445–62.

Saeterbakken AH, Solstad TEJ, Stien N, Shaw MP, Pedersen H, Andersen V. Muscle activation with swinging loads in bench press. PLoS One. 2020;15(9):0239202.

Shirato R, Aoki M, Iba K, Wada T, Hidaka E, Fujimiya M, et al. Effect of wrist and finger flexion in relation to strain on the tendon origin of the extensor carpi radialis brevis: a cadaveric study simulating stretching exercises. Clin Biomech. 2017;49:1–7.

van den Tillaar R. Comparison of kinematics and muscle activation between push-up and bench press. Sports Med Int Open. 2019;3(3):74.

Wilk KE, Arrigo CA, Hooks TR, Andrews JR. Rehabilitation of the overhead throwing athlete: there is more to it than just external rotation/internal rotation strengthening. PM R. 2016;8(3):78–90.

Youdas JW, Amundson CL, Cicero KS, Hahn JJ, Harezlak DT, Hollman JH. Surface electromyographic activation patterns and elbow joint motion during a pull-up, chin-up, or perfect-pullup™ rotational exercise. J Strength Cond Res. 2010;24(12):3404–14.

The Hand and Wrist

11

Rabia Tugba Kilic

Abstract

The hand (*manus*), the most distal part of the upper extremity, has the most complex movements in the upper extremity. The wrist joint is located between the carpal bones and the radius. A good understanding of the anatomical structure, functions, palpation, and exercises of the hand is of primary importance in hand treatment and rehabilitation. In this section, we have tried to present all the information about the hand and wrist from a holistic and clinical perspective.

11.1 Hand and Wrist

The bony skeleton of the hand and wrist consists of the carpal, metacarpal, and phalanx bones, respectively. These bones are important in the formation of hand movements and are interconnected through joints, ligaments, and muscles. Fingers are named as the thumb (*pollex*), index finger (*index, digitus demonstratus*), middle finger (*medio, digitus medius*), ring finger (*annular, ring, digitus annularis, digitus medicinalis*), and little finger (*digitus minimus*). The palm of the hand is called the *palma manus*, and the back of the hand is called the *dorsum manus*. In terms of direction, the palm is also expressed as the palmar or volar aspect, and the back of the hand as the dorsal aspect. The little finger is located on the ulnar side, while the thumb is located on the radial side.

By means of its fine motor skills thanks to its anatomy, the hand is a structure responsible for various activities that it has mastered in daily life and many specialized fields (sports, music, art, etc.). Therefore, a good understanding of the anatomical structure and functions of the hand is important in the interpretation of these activities. The grasping/grip functions of the hand are divided into two groups: the gross (coarse) and fine grip. The gross grip is divided into three groups: cylindrical, spherical, and hook grips; the fine grip is divided into three groups: the pinch, lateral and triple grips (Fig. 11.1). In the resting position, the hand is passive/inactive. During grasping, the fingers move towards the palmar surface of the hand. In this way, an object between the fingers and the palm or an object between the fingers can be grasped easily. Depending on the size of the grasped object, grip depends on the harmonious functioning of the long flexor muscles leading to the fingers, the intrinsic muscles located on the palmar surface of the hand, and the extensor muscles of the wrist.

This chapter explains the noncontractile and contractile structures of the hand/wrist, the

R. T. Kilic (✉)
Physiotherapy and Rehabilitation, Faculty of Health Sciences, Ankara Yıldırım Beyazit University, Ankara, Turkey

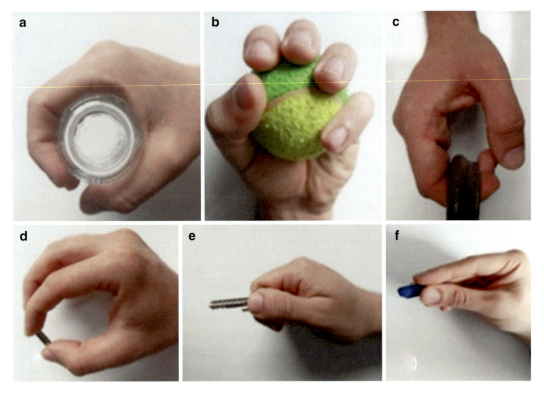

Fig. 11.1 (**a**) Cylindrical grip, (**b**) Spherical grip, (**c**) Hook grip, (**d**) Pinch grip, (**e**) Lateral grip, (**f**) Triple grip

movements occurring in the joints, palpation of the bones and muscles, and evidence-based exercises.

11.2 Noncontractile Structures in the Hand/Wrist Joint

11.2.1 Bone Structures of the Hand

The skeleton of the hand consists of eight carpals located in the wrist, five metacarpals in the hand, and 14 phalanx bones in the fingers (Fig. 11.2). The carpal bones are examined from lateral to medial, and in anatomical stance, from the thumb to the fifth finger. The carpal bones are composed of the scaphoid, lunate, triquetrum, and pisiform, respectively, from lateral to medial in the proximal row, while in the distal row, they consist of the trapezium, trapezoid, capitate, and hamate, from lateral to medial.

The *scaphoid* is located as the most lateral of the carpal bones in the proximal row. It

Clinical Information
Each of the carpal bones begins to ossify at different ages. Because of this characteristic, information about the bone age and growth potential of the person can be obtained with wrist radiographs taken. Hand/wrist radiographs are generally used to determine bone age. Children's bone ages can be determined by comparing with serial sections in radiography atlases.

Clinical Information
Because the epiphyseal plates are not fully closed in young children, epiphyseal fractures are more common than in adolescents. The distal epiphyseal plates of the radius and ulna radiologically close at the age of 18 in boys and the age of 16 in girls.

The Skeletal System
Hand Anatomy

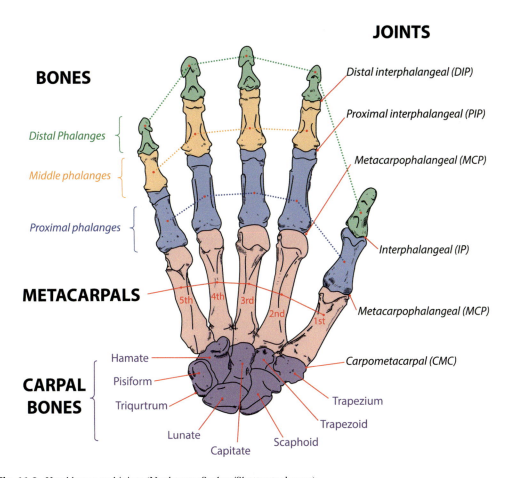

Fig. 11.2 Hand bones and joints (NatthapongSachan/Shutterstock.com)

articulates with the radius, lunate, capitate, trapezium, and trapezoid. The retinaculum flexorum, formed as a result of the thickening of the deep fascia of the forearm, attaches to the scaphoid tubercle of this bone. The scaphoid bone lies inferior to the anatomical snuffbox (*fovea radialis*). The supply of this bone is provided by the palmar branch of the radial artery, which runs through the anatomical snuffbox.

This artery enters from the distal part of the bone and divides into branches. Fracture in this area and the fracture line being located more proximal than the entry point of the artery to the bone results in avascular/aseptic necrosis of the proximal part of the bone after the fracture.

The *lunate* is located between the triquetrum and the scaphoid bones in the proximal row.

> **Clinical Information**
> The scaphoid bone is the most frequently broken bone among the carpal bones. The scaphoid bone may be fractured as a result of falling on the wrist, while the wrist is in the extension and the fingers are in the abduction position. Post-fracture pain occurs on the radial side of the wrist, in the anatomical snuffbox (*fovea radialis*) region (Fig. 11.3), and especially during extension and abduction of the wrist. It is very difficult to detect a fracture immediately. Since the destruction (breaking up) of the broken bone pieces will take 2–3 weeks, the fracture line may not be observed in the X-ray taken immediately after the fracture. X-rays taken from the lateral are valuable for diagnosis.

Among the carpal bones, the most dislocations occur in the lunate. It articulates with the radius, capitate, hamate, scaphoid, and triquetrum.

The *triquetrum* lies between the lunate and pisiform bones in the proximal row. It articulates with the lunate, pisiform, hamate, and also with ulna via a disc.

The *pisiform* is located as the most medial of the carpal bones in the proximal row. It is the last bone to develop and is the smallest bone among the carpal bones. It has a single articular surface that articulates with the triquetrum. The flexor carpi ulnaris, abductor digiti minimi tendons, and the retinaculum flexorum, which is formed by the thickening of the deep fascia of the forearm, attach to this bone. The carpi transversum, which forms the basis of the retinaculum flexorum, divides into two parts and forms *Guyon's canal*. The ulnar nerve bundle passes through this canal (Fig. 11.4).

The *trapezium* is located as the most lateral of the carpal bones in the distal row. The retinaculum flexorum, which is formed as a result of the thickening of the deep fascia of the forearm, attaches to this bone. It articulates with the scaphoid, trapezoid, and the first and second metacarpal bones.

The *trapezoid*, located in the distal row, is the smallest of the carpal bones. It is between the capitate and trapezium bones. It articulates with the scaphoid, trapezium, capitate, and the second metacarpal bone.

The *capitate* lies between the hamate and trapezoid bones in the distal row. It is the largest of the carpal bones and the first to develop. Some fibers of the adductor pollicis muscle attach to this bone. It articulates with the trapezoid, lunate, scaphoid, hamate, and the second and fourth metacarpal bones.

The *hamate* is located as the most medial of the carpal bones in the distal row. It articulates with the lunate, triquetrum, capitate, and the fourth and fifth metacarpal bones. The retinaculum flexorum, which is formed as a result of the thickening of the deep fascia of the forearm, attaches to the hook of the hamate, called the *hamulus ossis hamati*.

The *metacarpal bones* have a long bone structure, and there are five. Like the carpal bones, they are named with Roman numerals from lateral to medial. The proximal ends of the metacarpal bones where they articulate with the carpal bones are called *basis ossis metacarpalis*, their body is called *corpus ossis metacarpalis*, and the

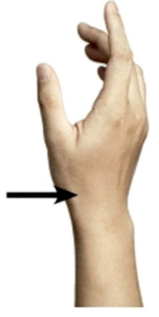

Fig. 11.3 Anatomical snuffbox (Neo Tribbiani/Shutterstock.com)

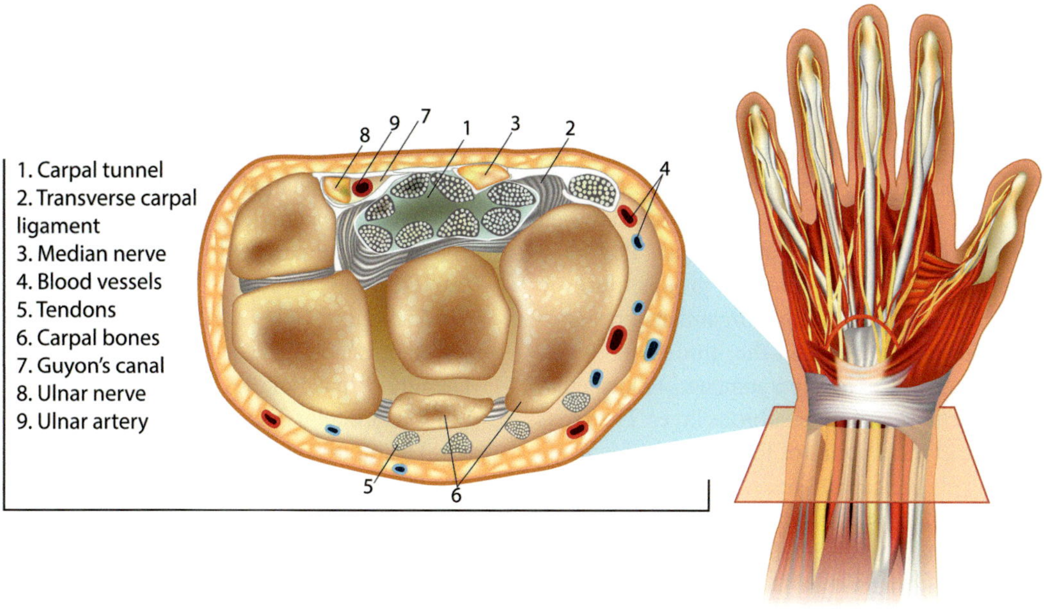

1. Carpal tunnel
2. Transverse carpal ligament
3. Median nerve
4. Blood vessels
5. Tendons
6. Carpal bones
7. Guyon's canal
8. Ulnar nerve
9. Ulnar artery

Fig. 11.4 Transverse section of the hand and anatomical structures in it (Sakurra/Shutterstock.com)

distal ends where they articulate with the finger bones are called *caput ossis metacarpalis*.

Attention!
The first metacarpal bone is the shortest and thickest. The epiphyseal line of the first metacarpal bone is close to the proximal, while the epiphyseal lines of all the phalanges and other metacarpal bones are close to the distal end. The longest metacarpal bone is the second metacarpal.

Clinical Information
Fractures that occur in the diaphysis (shaft) of the metacarpal bones are called boxer's fractures. Fractures of the first metacarpal bone are not included in this nomenclature.

The *phalanges* are 14 in total. There are two in the thumb and three in the other fingers. These bones can be named as the first, second, and third phalanges from proximal to distal, or they can be named as the proximal, middle, and distal phalanges. The surfaces of the phalanges that articulate with the metacarpal bones are called *basis phalangis* (base of phalanx), and their bodies (shaft) are called *corpus phalangis* (base of phalanx), and their distal ends are called *caput phalangis* (head of the phalanx). The epiphyseal lines of the phalanges are close to the proximal end. The distal ends of the distal phalanges do not have articular surfaces; here, there is a roughened, elevated area called the tuberosity of the distal phalanx. In living creatures, the nail (*unguis*) is located on the dorsal surface of this area.

11.2.2 Hand/Wrist Joint and Its Ligaments

The wrist joint (*the radiocarpal joint*) is located between the radius and the proximal carpal bones. The distal end of the ulna joins the joint via a discus. In the hand skeleton, the joints between the carpal bones are called the *intercarpal joints,* the joints between the carpal bones and the metacarpal bones are called the *carpometacarpal joints*, the joints between the metacarpal bones and the proximal phalanges are called the *metacarpopha-*

langeal joints, and the joints between the proximal and distal phalanges at the level of the fingers are called the *interphalangeal joints*.

The wrist ligaments maintain order between the carpal bones and provide the transfer of the forces loading on the bones to the forearm. Besides, they control the relationship between the carpal bones during movement. The wrist ligaments are divided into two groups, intrinsic and extrinsic. The intrinsic ligaments are intracapsular and lie between the fibrous and synovial layers. The extrinsic ligaments are located in the superficial part of the fibrous layer. The proximal attachment points of the extrinsic ligaments are outside the carpal bones; in the distal, on the other hand, they attach to the carpal bones. Both the proximal and distal attachment points of the intrinsic ligaments are located on the carpal bones. The wrist ligaments are named according to their starting and ending points, from the radius to the ulna. The joints located in the hand/wrist, the types of the joints, the movements occurring in the joints, and the ligaments are shown in Table 11.1.

The extrinsic ligaments:

1. The dorsal radiocarpal ligament
2. The radial collateral ligament
3. The palmar radiocarpal ligament
   (a) Radiocapital
   (b) Radioulnar
   (c) Radioscapholunate
4. The ulnocarpal complex
   (a) The articular disc
   (b) The ulnar collateral ligament
   (c) The palmar ulnocarpal ligament

The intrinsic ligaments:

1. Short ligaments of the distal row (palmar, dorsal, and interosseous)

Table 11.1 Joints in the hand/wrist, joint types, movements in the joints, and ligaments of the joints

Joint	Joint type	Occurring movements	Ligaments
Radiocarpal	Ellipsoid	• Flexion • Extension • Abduction • Adduction • Circumduction	• Dorsal radiocarpal • Palmar radiocarpal • Palmar ulnocarpal • Collateral ulnocarpal • Collateral radiocarpal
Intercarpal	Planar	• Limited gliding	• Palmar intercarpal • Dorsal intercarpal • Interosseous intercarpal
Mediocarpal	Medially ellipsoid Laterally planar	• Limited gliding	• Palmar intercarpal • Dorsal intercarpal
Carpometacarpal I	Sellar	• Flexion • Extension • Abduction • Adduction • Opposition • Circumduction	• Joint capsule
Carpometacarpals II–V	Planar	• Limited gliding	• Dorsal carpometacarpal• Palmar carpometacarpal
Intermetacarpal	Planar	• Limited gliding	• Dorsal metacarpal • Palmar metacarpal • Interosseous metacarpal
Metacarpophalangeal	Spheroid	• Flexion • Extension • Abduction • Adduction • Opposition • Circumduction	• Collaterals • Palmars • Deep transverse metacarpal
Interphalangeal	Ginglymus (trochlear)	• Flexion • Extension	• Collaterals • Palmars

2. The intermediate ligaments
   (a) Lunatriquetral
   (b) Scapholunate
   (c) Scaphotrapezial
3. The long ligament
   (a) Palmar intercarpal
   (b) Dorsal intercarpal

> **To Learn Easily**
> Radiocarpal and ulnocarpal ligaments limit the axial rotation of the hand with respect to the forearm and ensure the continuity of contact of the proximal row of carpal bones with the distal radius articular surface during wrist movements.

> **Clinical Information**
> The *Triangular Fibrocartilage Complex* (TFCC) is located between the proximal row of carpal bones and the distal articular surface of the ulna. It is the basic stabilizer of the distal radioulnar joint and the ulnar stabilizer of the radioulnocarpal joint. It transmits the axial load of the forearm to the hand by acting as a cushion for the ulnar side of the wrist. The TFCC is formed by the proximal and distal laminae, the volar and dorsal radioulnar ligaments, the ulnocarpal ligaments (ulnolunate and ulnotriquetral), the sheath of the extensor carpi ulnaris muscle, and the ulnomeniscal homolog.

> **Attention!**
> Radiocarpal and ulnocarpal ligament injuries cause instability in the radiocarpal joint. The triquetrum plays an important role in ulnar carpal instability patterns, as the ulnocarpal ligaments attach to the triquetrum.

11.2.3 Other Structures

11.2.3.1 Flexor and Extensor Retinacula

The *fascia antebrachii*, which is the deep fascia surrounding the forearm, is strengthened by the fibers extending in the transverse direction at the wrist, preventing the tendons from moving away from the joint axis during movements. This deep fascia, which attaches to the radius and ulna, is called the flexor retinaculum on the palmar side and the extensor retinaculum on the dorsal side. The extensor tendons on the dorsal aspect of the wrist are stabilized by the extensor retinaculum, preventing them from moving away from the bony tissues during hyperextension of the hand. These tendons are surrounded by a synovial sheath called *vaginae synoviales* in order to reduce their friction against the bone structures while passing through the dorsal part of the hand. This sheath forms the digital sheaths on the fingers as well.

> **Clinical Information**
> Painless swellings may appear on the hand, particularly on the dorsal part of the wrist, and may range in size from a grape to the size of an apricot. These swellings are thin-walled cystic structures with clear mucinous fluid and are called *ganglion cysts*. Although the cause is unknown, it is thought to occur as a result of mucoid degeneration. Repetitive and/or compulsive wrist flexion may cause enlargement of the cyst and pain. Ganglion cysts have connections with the synovial sheath (*vaginae synoviales*).

11.2.3.2 Palmar Fascia

The palmar fascia shows continuity with the fascia antebrachii and the dorsal surface fascia of the hand. While the palmar fascia is thin in the thenar and hypothenar regions, it thickens in the center to form the fibrous *palmaraponeurosis*.

The palmar aponeurosis has a triangular shape, and its proximal end (apex) continues with the retinaculum musculorum flexorum and the palmaris longus tendon. There is a medial fibrous septum that lies deep and stretches from the palmar aponeurosis to the fifth metacarpal bone. In the medial part of the medial fibrous septum, there is the *hypothenar compartment,* where the hypothenar muscles are located. Similarly, there is also a lateral fibrous septum that lies deep and stretches from the lateral edge of the palmar aponeurosis to the third metacarpal bone. At the lateral edge of this septum is the *thenar compartment,* in which the thenar muscles of the hand are located. Regarding the *central compartment*, it is located between the hypothenar and thenar compartments. The flexor muscle tendons and sheaths, lumbrical muscles, arcus palmaris superficialis, and digital vessels and nerves are located here. In the deepest part of the palmar surface of the hand is the *adductor compartment*, where the adductor pollicis is located. The thenar space and the midpalmar space cover the muscles located deep on the palmar surface of the hand and lie between the flexor tendons and the fascia. These spaces are bounded by fibrous spaces extending from the margins of the palmar aponeurosis to the metacarpal bones. Between them is the strong *lateral fibrous space* attached to the third metacarpal bone.

> **Clinical Information**
> Shortening, thickening, and fibrosis of the palmar fascia of the hand and the palmar aponeurosis are called *Dupuytren's contracture*.

11.2.3.3 Arteries of the Hand

The entire hand is supplied by the ulnar and radial arteries and their branches.

> **Clinical Information**
> On the anterior surface of the distal end of the radius, the region where the radial artery passes is one of the most commonly used areas for heart rate measurement. This region is located on the lateral side of the flexor carpi radialis tendon. The radial artery is covered only by fascia and skin in this region.

> **Attention!**
> While taking the pulse over the radial artery, the soft part of the palmar aspect of the thumb should not be used. Because this region has its own pulse, it can be confused with the pulse from the radial artery. If the pulse cannot be taken from one side of the patient, it should be checked from the same area on the other side. The reason is that the radial artery can sometimes have a variable course.

> **Clinical Information**
> Intermittent and bilateral ischemic attacks might occur in the fingers. The main symptoms are pallor of the skin, numbness, and pain in the hand. These findings characteristically occur with cold and emotional stimuli. If the cause of ischemia in the finger is idiopathic (unknown cause), it is called *Raynaud's phenomenon*, and the sympathetic nervous system is also affected.

11.2.3.4 Veins of the Hand

The veins of the hand are the cephalic vein on the lateral side and the basilic vein on the medial side.

11.2.3.5 Nerves of the Hand

The innervation of the hand is provided by the median, ulnar, and radial nerves. Branches from the lateral and posterior cutaneous nerves contribute to the innervation of the dorsal aspect of the hand.

The median nerve lesions most commonly occur by the nerve compression at the point where it passes through the carpal tunnel (Fig. 11.5). The flexor retinaculum is a strong fibrous band that continues with the palmar aponeurosis on the distal side. The carpal transverse ligament, which constitutes the main part of the flexor retinaculum, attaches to the pisiform and the hook of the hamate on the medial side. While extending towards the lateral, it is divided into two parts superficial and deep. The superficial part attaches to the tubercle of the scaphoid and the lateral border of the groove of the trapezium, and the deep part clings to the medial edge of this groove. The canal formed between these two parts and the carpal bones is called the *carpal tunnel*. The flexor muscle tendons and the median nerve pass through this structure. The borders of the carpal tunnel are formed by the flexor retinaculum on the palmar side, the pisiform and the hook of the hamate on the medial side, the scaphoid and trapezium on the lateral side, and the carpal bones on the dorsal side. The narrowest part of the carpal tunnel is at the level of the trapezium and hamate.

The canal between the pisiform and the hook of the hamate is called *Guyon's canal*. The ulnar artery and nerve pass through this canal (Fig. 11.4). The ulnar nerve may be compressed in Guyon's canal. In this case, loss of sensation in the area innervated by the ulnar nerve and weakness in the intrinsic muscles of the hand are observed. While the motor and sensory fibers of the ulnar nerve are together as a single branch in the proximal part of the canal, the motor and sensory branches proceed separately in the distal part.

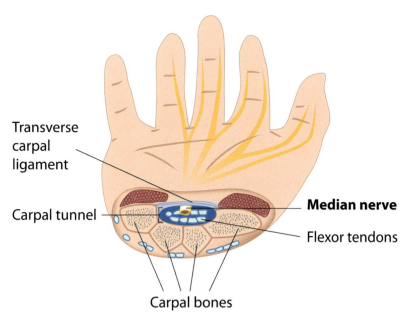

Fig. 11.5 Anatomical structures passing through the carpal tunnel (Alila Medical Media/Shutterstock.com)

The radial nerve does not innervate the hand muscles. It receives skin senses from the lateral 2/3 of the dorsal surface of the hand, the dorsal aspect of the thumb, and the proximal parts of the lateral 1.5 fingers.

To Learn Easily
Structures passing through the carpal tunnel (Fig. 11.5):

1. The flexor digitorum superficialis (four tendons)
2. The flexor digitorum profundus (four tendons)
3. The flexor pollicis longus
4. The median nerve

Attention!
It is often stated that the flexor carpi radialis tendon passes through the carpal tunnel. However, instead of through the tunnel, the tendon of the muscle passes through the fibers of the flexor retinaculum, which forms the roof of the carpal tunnel. This muscle has a fibro-osseous canal of its own.

Clinical Information
The median nerve is located on the radial side and is most superficial in the canal. The entrapment neuropathy caused by its compression in the carpal tunnel is called carpal tunnel syndrome. The median nerve gives the superficial palmar branch before entering the canal and divides into three terminal branches within the canal. Of these, two terminal sensory branches innervate the skin of the hand, while the terminal motor branch innervates three thenar muscles. Paresthesia, hypoesthesia, or anesthesia may be observed in the first three fingers and the lateral half of the fourth finger due to compression in the canal. In addition, the thumb coordination and strength may decrease, and the thumb may not be able to make the opposition movement. In this case, difficulties may be experienced during movements that are frequently used in daily life, such as buttoning up and hair brushing, and that require fine motor coordination of the thumb.

Clinical Information
Ape hand deformity is the inability of the thumb to move away from the other fingers of the hand, which occurs as a result of paralysis of the thenar muscles after median nerve damage. The thumb can only perform flexion and extension movements, whereas it performs the abduction movement within a limited angle and cannot do the opposition movement.

Clinical Information
As a result of ulnar nerve damage, significant motor and sensory loss occur in the hand. Atrophy is observed, especially in the interosseous muscles. This pathology is called *claw hand deformity*. The adductor muscles weaken as a result of the denervation arising in most of the intrinsic hand muscles. In case of an attempt to do flexion on the wrist, the hand is pulled laterally by the effect of the flexor carpi radialis innervated by the median nerve. As the fourth and fifth distal interphalangeal joints cannot be applied flexion, the patient has difficulty making a fist.

> **Attention!**
> While the motor and sensory fibers of the ulnar nerve are together as a single branch in the proximal of Guyon's canal, the motor and sensory branches progress separately in the distal. Therefore, the relationship between the clinical finding and the nerve compression site should not be ignored.

> **Clinical Information**
> Compression of the hook of the hamate due to the wrist staying in the extension position during long-term cycling causes entrapment of the ulnar nerve and is called *Cyclist's Palsy*. Loss of sensation in the medial half of the hand and weakness in the intrinsic hand muscles are observed.

> **Attention!**
> Loss of sensation is partial in radial nerve injuries. Even in the most severe radial nerve damage, the loss of sensation is limited to a small part of the lateral part of the dorsal aspect of the hand. However, when the radial nerve is damaged in the arm region, wrist extension cannot be performed due to paralysis of the forearm extensor muscles. In this condition, called the wrist-drop, the wrist and metacarpophalangeal joints remain in flexion. Thanks to the interosseous and lumbrical muscles (innervated by the ulnar and median nerves), a slight extension can be applied from the interphalangeal joints.

11.3 Contractile Structures Associated with the Hand/Wrist Joint

The hand and wrist muscles are divided into two groups: the extrinsic and intrinsic muscles. The proximal attachment points of the extrinsic muscles are located on the outside of the hand; the distal attachment points are located on the hand. Regarding the intrinsic muscles, both proximal and distal attachment sites of these muscles are located in the hand. The extrinsic muscles are divided into two: the extrinsic extensor and extrinsic flexor muscles. Although these muscles participate in the movements of the wrist and fingers, they are described in detail in Chap. 10 because they are located in the forearm region.

The intrinsic muscles of the hand are divided into three groups: thenar, hypothenar (Fig. 11.6), and metacarpal (Fig. 11.7) muscles (Table 11.2). The origins, insertion points, nerves, and functions of the intrinsic muscles of the hand are summarized in Table 11.3.

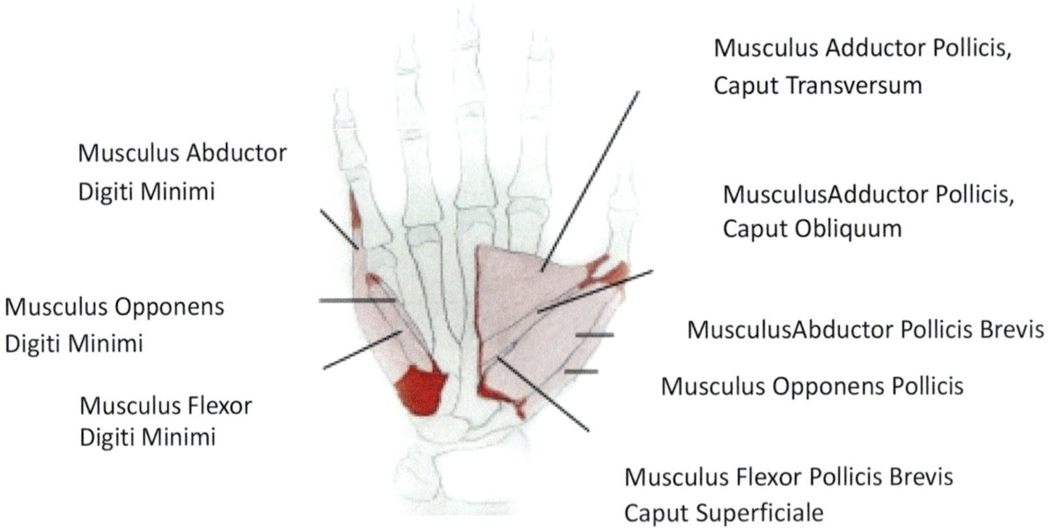

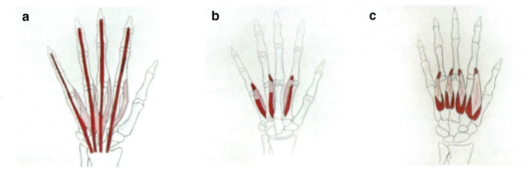

Fig. 11.6 Thenar and hypothenar muscles

Fig. 11.7 Metacarpal muscles. (**a**) Lumbrical muscles (I–IV) and flexor digitorum profundus muscle tendons, (**b**) Palmar interossei muscles (I–III), (**c**) Dorsal interossei muscles (I–IV)

Table 11.2 The intrinsic muscles of the hand

Thenar muscles	Hypothenar muscles	Metacarpal muscles
• Abductor pollicis brevis • Flexor pollicis brevis • Opponens pollicis • Adductor pollicis	• Abductor digiti minimi • Flexor digiti minimi brevis • Opponens digiti minimi • Palmaris brevis	• Lumbricals (I–IV) • Palmar interossei (I–III) • Dorsal interossei (I–IV)

Table 11.3 Origin, insertion, nerve, and functions of the intrinsic muscles of the hand

Muscle	Nerve	Origin	Insertion	Function
Abductor pollicis brevis	Median	Retinaculum musculorum flexorum, eminentia carpi radialis	The radial sesamoid bone of the first metacarpophalangeal joint, proximal phalanx of the thumb	Abduction and opposition of the first carpometacarpal joint, flexion of the first metacarpophalangeal joint
Flexor pollicis brevis	Superficial head: median nerve. Deep head: deep branch of the ulnar nerve	Superficial head: Retinaculum musculorum flexorum. Deep head: Capitatum, trapezium	The radial sesamoid bone of the first metacarpophalangeal joint, proximal phalanx of the thumb	Opposition and abduction of the first carpometacarpal joint, flexion of the first metacarpophalangeal joint
Opponens pollicis	Median and ulnar	Retinaculum musculorum flexorum, eminentia carpi radialis	The first metacarpal	Opposition of the first carpometacarpal joint
Adductor pollicis	Deep branch of the ulnar nerve	Oblique head: Hamatum, metacarpals II–IV. Transverse head: the third metacarpal	The ulnar sesamoid bone of the first metacarpophalangeal joint, proximal phalanx of the thumb	Abduction and opposition of the first carpometacarpal joint, flexion of the first metacarpophalangeal joint
Lumbricals I–IV	Median	Flexor digitorum profundus tendon	Dorsal aponeuroses of the second and fifth fingers (lateral band)	Flexion of the second and fourth metacarpophalangeal joints, extension of the second and fifth fingers
Palmar interossei I–III	Deep branch of the ulnar nerve	The ulnar aspect of the second metacarpal, the radial aspect of the metacarpals IV–V	Proximal phalanges and dorsal aponeuroses of the second, fourth, and fifth fingers (lateral band)	Flexion and adduction of the second, fourth, and fifth metacarpophalangeal joints, extension of second, fourth, and fifth fingers
Dorsal interossei I–IV	Deep branch of the ulnar nerve	Opposite aspects of the metacarpals I–V	Proximal phalanges and dorsal aponeuroses of the second and fourth fingers	Flexion and abduction of the second and fourth metacarpophalangeal joints, extension of second and fourth fingers
Palmaris brevis	Superficial branch of the ulnar nerve	The palmar aponeurosis	The skin of the hypothenar region	Stretches the skin of the hypothenar region
Abductor digiti minimi	Deep branch of the ulnar nerve	Pisiform, retinaculum musculorum flexorum	Proximal phalanx	Opposition of the fifth carpometacarpal joint, abduction of the fifth metacarpophalangeal joint
Flexor digiti minimi brevis	Deep branch of the ulnar nerve	Retinaculum musculorum flexorum, hook of hamate	Proximal phalanx of the fifth finger	Opposition of the fifth carpometacarpal joint, flexion of the fifth metacarpophalangeal joint
Opponens digiti minimi	Deep branch of the ulnar nerve	Retinaculum musculorum flexorum, hook of hamate	The fifth metacarpal	Opposition of the fifth carpometacarpal joint

11.4 Movements in the Hand/Wrist Joint

11.4.1 Movements in the Radiocarpal Joint

In the wrist joint, flexion-extension movements occur in the sagittal plane, and radial-ulnar deviation and the circumduction movements consisting of the sum of all these movements take place in the frontal plane (Fig. 11.8). On the wrist, the range of motion in extension is greater than in flexion. These movements take place with the participation of the mediocarpal joint, which is located between the proximal and distal rows of the carpal bones. The range of motion of the ulnar deviation of the hand is greater than the radial deviation. The ulnar deviation occurs mostly around the radiocarpal joint, while the radial deviation arises from the mediocarpal joint. The angular values of the movements around the wrist joint increase with the small-angle movements that occur in the intercarpal and mediocarpal joints.

11.4.2 Movements in the Intercarpal and Mediocarpal Joints

The joints between the carpal bones are called the intercarpal joints. A small amount of gliding movement occurs between these joints. By means of this limited gliding movement, the range of

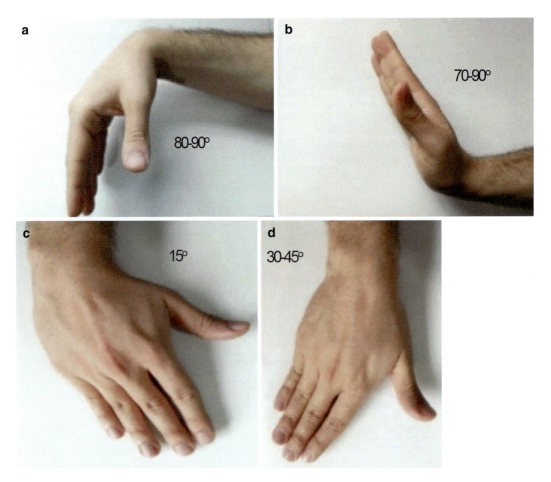

Fig. 11.8 Movements of the wrist. (**a**) Wrist flexion, (**b**) Wrist extension, (**c**) Radial deviation of the wrist, (**d**) Ulnar deviation of the wrist

motion of the wrist is increased. The mediocarpal joint is the articulation between the distal and proximal rows of the carpal bones, and it is very active during the flexion and extension movements of the hand.

> **To Learn Easily**
> The transverse axis of the radiocarpal joint passes through the lunate, and the transverse axis of the mediocarpal joint passes through the capitate. The dorsopalmar axis passes through the capitate. Flexion and extension movements occur at both the radiocarpal and mediocarpal joints, while radial and ulnar deviations occur only at the radiocarpal joint.

11.4.3 Movements in the Metacarpophalangeal and Interphalangeal Joints

In the metacarpophalangeal joints, the flexion-extension, abduction-adduction, and the circumduction (in the second and fifth fingers) movements occur; in all interphalangeal joints, the flexion-extension movements occur (Fig. 11.9).

> **Attention!**
> While the metacarpophalangeal, proximal interphalangeal, and distal interphalangeal joints are involved in finger extension, only the metacarpophalangeal joint is involved in abduction and adduction.

11.4.4 Movements in the Carpometacarpal and Intercarpal Joints

The flexion-extension, abduction-adduction, and circumduction movements take place in the first carpometacarpal joint (thumb joint) (Fig. 11.10). Although this joint can perform an angular movement in any plane, its axial rotation movement is limited. There is almost no movement at the second and third carpometacarpal joints. The fourth carpometacarpal joint has a limited ability of motion, while the fifth carpometacarpal joint is highly mobile. Especially when clenching fists, quite a lot of flexion and rotation movements occur.

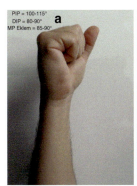
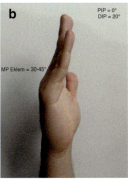
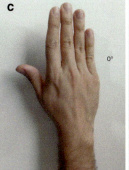
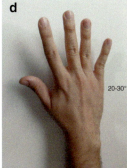

Fig. 11.9 Movements in the metacarpophalangeal and interphalangeal joints. (**a**) Finger flexion, (**b**) Finger extension, (**c**) Finger adduction, (**d**) Finger abduction. *MCP* Metacarpophalangeal joints, *PIP* Proximal interphalangeal joints, *DIP* Distal interphalangeal joints

Fig. 11.10 Carpometacarpal joint movements of the thumb. (**a**) Flexion, (**b**) Extension, (**c**) Adduction, (**d**) Abduction, (**e**) Opposition, (**f**) Reposition. *CMC* Carpometacarpal joint, *MCP* Metacarpophalangeal joint, *IP* Interphalangeal joint

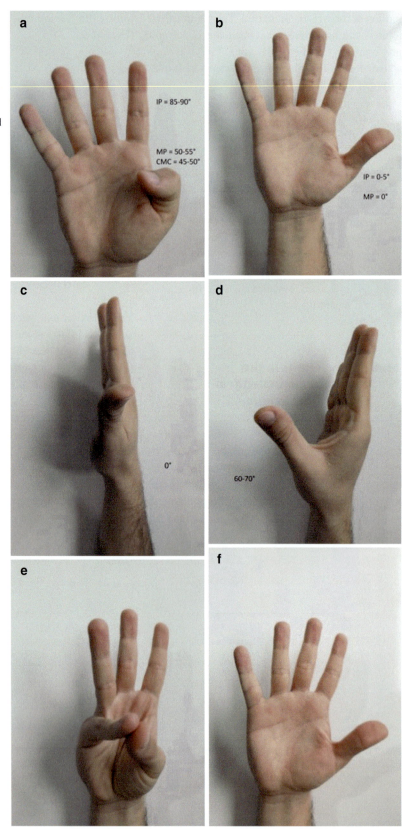

Attention!

Flexion and extension motions of the thumb occur in the carpometacarpal, metacarpophalangeal, and interphalangeal joints. Adduction, abduction, opposition, and reposition motions occur only in the carpometacarpal joint.

To Learn Easily

Abduction and adduction motions are defined according to the middle finger. Moving away from the middle finger is defined as abduction, and moving closer to it is defined as adduction.

Attention!

In post-surgery immobilization of the hand (such as plaster cast or splinting), the wrist and fingers should be positioned at correct angles. Otherwise, the hardness and adhesions that may occur in the soft tissues may adversely affect the functionality of the hand. The functional positioning of the hand is 10° flexion at the distal interphalangeal joints, 30° flexion at the proximal interphalangeal joints, 50–60° flexion at the metacarpophalangeal joints, and 30° extension at the radiocarpal joints (Fig. 11.11).

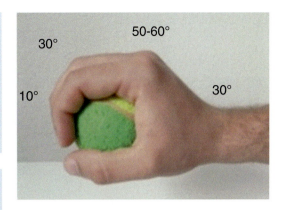

Fig. 11.11 Functional positioning of the hand

11.5 Palpation of the Structures Located in the Hand/Wrist Joint

Palpation of the hand usually starts from the dorsal side. Placing the hand and forearm on a flat surface while palpating the bony structures is important for the relaxation of the muscles. If relaxation is not achieved, the superficial tendons remain under tension, preventing palpation of the anatomical structures located in the deep. First of all, the bone structures listed in Table 11.3 are determined. After determining the dimensions and borders of the carpal bones, the soft tissues are palpated from the radial side to the ulnar side. The soft tissues to be palpated from the dorsal side are the radial fossa (*anatomical snuffbox*) (Fig. 11.3), extensor muscle tendons and their compartments, the radial nerve, the cephalic vein, and the radial artery (Table 11.3). The front and back views of the palpable bony structures in the hand are displayed in Fig. 11.12.

On the palmar surface, the radial styloid process, the ulnar styloid process, the pisiform, the hook of the hamate, the scaphoid, the trapezium, the lunate, and the capitate can be palpated (Fig. 11.13). After determining the dimensions and borders of the carpal bones, the soft tissues are palpated from the radial side to the ulnar side. The soft tissues that can be palpated from the palmar surface are the transverse carpal ligament, carpal tunnel, median nerve, flexor carpi radialis, radial artery, flexor pollicis longus, palmaris longus, flexor digitorum superficialis, flexor carpi ulnaris, ulnar artery, and ulnar nerve (Table 11.4).

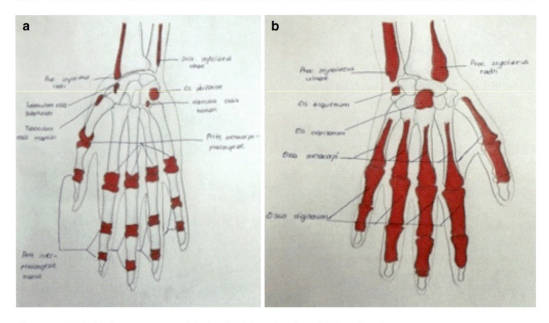

Fig. 11.12 Palpable bony structures of the hand. (**a**) Anterior view, (**b**) Posterior view

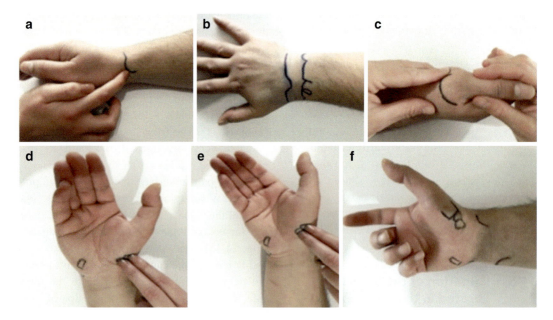

Fig. 11.13 Bone structures accessible from the palmar side. (**a**) Radial styloid process (protrusion), (**b**) Proximal and distal carpal bone borders, (**c**) First carpometacarpal joint space, (**d**) Palpation of the scaphoid via radial deviation of the hand, (**e**) Palpation of the trapezium via ulnar deviation of the hand, (**f**) Palmar view of palpable bony structures

Table 11.4 Palpable structures in the hand

Soft tissues that can be palpated from the dorsal aspect	Soft tissues that can be palpated from the palmar aspect
• The radial fossa (anatomical snuffbox) • Extensor tendons and Compartments • The radial nerve • The cephalic vein • The radial artery	• Transverse carpal ligament • Median nerve • Flexor carpi radialis • The radial artery • Flexor pollicis longus • Palmaris longus • Flexor digitorum superficialis • Flexor carpi ulnaris • The ulnar artery • The ulnar nerve
Bone structures that can be palpated from the dorsal aspect	**Bone structures that can be palpated from the palmar aspect**
• Triquetrum • Capitate • The radial styloid process[a] • The ulnar styloid process[a] • The carpometacarpal joints[a] • The metacarpophalangeal joints[a] • The interphalangeal joints[a] • Metacarpal bones[a] • Phalanges[a]	• The tubercle of the scaphoid bone • Protrusion of the trapezium bone • Pisiform • Hook of hamate • Lunate • The radial styloid process[a] • The ulnar styloid process[a] • The carpometacarpal joints[a] • The metacarpophalangeal joints[a] • The interphalangeal joints[a] • Metacarpal bones[a] • Phalanges[a]

[a] It can be palpated from both the dorsal and palmar aspects

> **To Learn Easily**
> When the patient is asked to flex their wrist and clench their fist, three tendons are observed in the middle of the wrist in the palmar direction. These tendons, from radial to ulnar, are flexor carpi radialis, palmaris longus, and flexor digitorum superficialis, respectively.

> **To Learn Easily**
> Finding the prominent points of the ulnar and radial bones by palpation of the carpal bones from the palmar aspect is crucial to determining the location of the carpal tunnel. First, the radial (scaphoid and trapezium) and ulnar (pisiform and the hook of the hamate) bone walls are detected. Next, the distal border of the forearm is palpated. The positions of the carpal bones (lunate and capitate) at the tunnel floor are determined by reference points. Finally, the carpal tunnel is determined by identifying the transverse carpal ligament (Fig. 11.9).

> **Clinical Information**
> The radial artery courses on the anterior surface of the distal end of the radius, and this area is frequently used for heart rate measurement. The radial artery lies lateral to the flexor carpi radialis tendon. If the fisted hand is tried to be flexed against the resistance, the flexor carpi radialis and palmaris longus tendons can be palpated. The flexor carpi radialis tendon is located in the anterior part of the wrist and slightly laterally. This tendon guides for finding the radial artery. Pulsation of the artery is taken from the lateral aspect of the tendon. Also, the abductor pollicis longus and extensor pollicis brevis tendons form the anterior edge of the ana-

tomical snuffbox. The extensor pollicis longus tendon forms the posterior wall of this box. The radial artery runs through this anatomical snuffbox, and its pulsation can also be taken from here. At the base of this box are the scaphoid and trapezium.

Clinical Information
The palmaris longus tendon can be palpated in the middle of the anterior aspect of the wrist. This tendon is a guide in locating the median nerve. The median nerve lies deep in the tendon. However, it should be noted that the palmaris longus muscle may not be found in everyone.

Clinical Information
The flexor carpi ulnaris tendon can be palpated as it crosses the anterior aspect of the wrist on the medial side, and this tendon attaches to the pisiform bone. The flexor carpi ulnaris tendon is used as a guide for palpation of the ulnar nerve and artery.

Attention!
Flexor digitorum superficialis tendons can be easily palpated during the flexion and extension motions of the fingers.

To Learn Easily
When the hand is at rest, the skin covering the dorsal side of the hand is thin and loose/lax. The laxity of the skin is due to the mobile subcutaneous tissue. When the wrist is extended against resistance and the fingers are abducted, the extensor digitorum tendons on the dorsal side of the hand are easily visible, especially in slim individuals. These tendons are not observed as they become thinner as they pass over the knuckles and form the dorsal aponeurosis. When one clenches a fist, joint lines are visible. On the dorsal surface of the hand, deep in the loose subcutaneous tissue and extensor tendons, the metacarpal bones can be easily palpated. Another structure that is prominently seen on the dorsal surface of the hand is the rete venosum dorsale manus, which is the vein network of the back of the hand.

Clinical Information
The skin of the palmar surface of the hand is thick because this surface is the area most likely to be exposed to trauma. While there are plenty of sweat glands in this region, sebaceous glands and hair are absent. The skin fold on the dorsal aspect of the wrist marks the location of the proximal edge of the retinaculum musculorum flexorum. The skin ridges on the fingertips are called fingerprints and are used for criminal identification since these prints belong only to that person. The main function of these epidermal ridges is to reduce slippage while holding objects.

11.6 Evidence-Based Exercises in Which Muscles Serving in the Hand/Wrist Joint Movements Work by Exercise Type

Evidence-based therapeutic exercises used for the hand and wrist are diverse, and what matters in the choice of exercise is our purpose, that is, what the patient needs. The purpose-oriented exercises are explained below.

Table 11.5 Exercise examples for the flexor and extensor muscles of the wrist

Muscle or muscle group	Type of exercise	How to do the exercise
Wrist and its flexors	Stretching	With the elbow extended, extension is applied to the wrist
Wrist extensors	Stretching	With the elbow extended, flexion is applied to the wrist
Wrist flexors	Concentric	The wrist is flexed with a free weight
Wrist flexors	Eccentric	In a controlled manner, the wrist moves with gravity from flexion to extension
Wrist extensors	Concentric	Wrist extension is done using a free weight
Wrist extensors	Eccentric	In a controlled manner, the wrist moves with gravity from extension to flexion

11.6.1 Musculotendinous Mobility Techniques

Through these exercises, which include active contraction of the hand muscles and unique movements of the fingers and the wrist, the mobility of the structures of the hand can be maintained or improved. These exercises are employed whenever possible in order to maintain or improve mobility, as adhesions between the anatomical structures of the hand can restrict joint movements. Tendon gliding exercises, tendon blocking exercises, and scar tissue mobilizations are examples. These include various gliding and isometric exercises in terms of exercise types.

11.6.2 Exercises to Improve Flexibility and Range of Motion

The purpose of the exercises that increase flexibility and range of motion is to stretch the muscles and connective tissue in the wrist and hand region and to maintain or restore the normal range of motion of the joints. They include general stretching techniques as well as stretching techniques for intrinsic and multi-joint muscles. They can be applied in the manner of passive, actively assisted, and active exercises.

11.6.3 Exercises to Improve Muscular Performance, Neuromuscular Control, and Coordinated Movement

In the subacute and chronic period of healing, tissues require only moderate or minimal protection; therefore, these exercises are used in the controlled movement phase of rehabilitation when returning to functional movements of the hand. In order for the patient to return to independent hand functions, they must have not only neuromuscular control and strength but also the muscular endurance, coordination, and fine motor skill (dexterity) necessary for the desired activity. Exercises to strengthen the hand and wrist muscles, exercises that increase grip strength and muscular endurance, develop fine finger dexterity, and functional skill activities can be included in this group. They can be performed as isometric, isotonic (concentric-eccentric), and isokinetic exercises. Various disc weights as well as auxiliary materials for resistance, such as putty, spring hand exercisers, and soft balls of various degrees and sizes, can be used during these exercises. In Table 11.5, examples of exercises for the flexor and extensor muscles of the wrist are given by the exercise types. These examples can be adapted for all the muscles involved in the wrist and hand movements.

> **Attention!**
> Regarding the hand, it is important to ensure the stability of all involved joints while stretching the muscles that span multiple joints.

> **Attention!**
> Before the muscle and connective tissue are stretched, normal gliding motion on the joint surfaces should be achieved first in order to prevent joint damage.

> **Attention!**
> In order to increase muscular performance and coordination and to provide neuromuscular control, it should be ensured that joint mobility and flexibility are provided before starting the exercises.

> **Attention!**
> In order to regain the functionality of the hand and wrist, the planned exercise programs should cover the entire upper extremity. As skills and functional activities, the patient can have exercises, such as picking up small objects of various sizes, turning and removing bolts, drawing, writing, tying a string or ribbon, opening and closing small bottles or cans, and typing with a keyboard.

> **Clinical Information**
> The movement pattern used by the patient must be observed, and it must be ensured that the patient does not use compensatory movements. Furthermore, due attention should be paid to joint stabilization during movements.

11.7 Conclusion

For hand rehabilitation, a good understanding of the anatomical structure, functions, palpation, and exercises of the hand is essential. Through this chapter, we present a clinical perspective, attempting to integrate the information about the hand.

Further Reading

Andayani NN, Wibawa A, Nugraha MHS. Effective ultrasound therapy and neural mobilization combinations in reducing hand disabilities in carpal Tunnel syndrome patients. Jurnal Keperawatan Indonesia. 2020;23(2):93–101.

Aparisi Gómez MP, Aparisi F, Battista G, Guglielmi G, Faldini C, Bazzocchi A. Functional and surgical anatomy of the upper limb: what the radiologist needs to know. Radiol Clin North Am. 2019;57(5):857–81.

Blanquero J, Cortés-Vega MD, Rodríguez-Sánchez-Laulhé P, Corrales-Serra BP, Gómez-Patricio E, Díaz-Matas N, et al. Feedback-guided exercises performed on a tablet touchscreen improve return to work, function, strength and healthcare usage more than an exercise program prescribed on paper for people with wrist, hand or finger injuries: a randomised trial. J Physiother. 2020;66(4):236–42.

Dahlin LB, Wiberg M. Nerve injuries of the upper extremity and hand. EFORT Open Rev. 2017;2(5):158–70.

Gitto S, Messina C, Mauri G, Aliprandi A, Sardanelli F, Sconfienza LM. Dynamic high-resolution ultrasound of intrinsic and extrinsic ligaments of the wrist: how to make it simple. Eur J Radiol. 2017;87:20–35.

Kisner C, Colby L. The wrist and hand. In: Kisner C, Colby L, editors. Therapeutic exercise: foundations and techniques. McGraw Hill, FA Davis Company; 2012. p. 651–708.

Kitridis D, Karamitsou P, Giannaros I, Papadakis N, Sinopidis C, Givissis P. Dupuytren's disease: limited fasciectomy, night splinting, and hand exercises—long-term results. Eur J Orthop Surg Traumatol. 2019;29(2):349–55.

Nguyen A, Vather M, Bal G, Meaney D, White M, Kwa M, et al. Does a hand strength-focused exercise program improve grip strength in older patients with wrist fractures managed nonoperatively?: a randomized controlled trial. Am J Phys Med Rehabil. 2020;99(4):285–90.

Orr CM. Locomotor hand postures, carpal kinematics during wrist extension, and associated morphology in anthropoid primates. Anat Record. 2017;300(2):382–401.

Phillips SG. An evidence-based review of overuse wrist injuries in athletes. Orthop Clin North Am. 2020;51(4):499–509.

Prasad G, Bhalli MJ. Assessing wrist pain: a simple guide. Brit J Hosp Med (Lond). 2020;81(5):1–7.

Roquelaure Y, Garlantézec R, Rousseau V, Descatha A, Evanoff B, Mattioli S, et al. Carpal tunnel syndrome and exposure to work-related biomechanical stressors and chemicals: findings from the Constances cohort. PLoS One. 2020;15(6):e0235051.

Sander A, Sommer K, Eichler K, Marzi I, Frank J. Mediocarpal instability of the wrist [Mediokarpale Instabilitäten der Handwurzel]. Unfallchirurg. 2018;121(5):365–72.

Takata SC, Wade ET, Roll SC. Hand therapy interventions, outcomes, and diagnoses evaluated over the last 10 years: a mapping review linking research to practice. J Hand Ther. 2019;32(1):1–9.

Xu Y, Zheng Y, Jiang D. The effect of finger exercises combined with local physiotherapy on recovery of hand function in postoperative with flexor tendon injury. Chinese J Pract Nurs. 2017;33(30):2327–30.

The Pelvis

Ayca Aklar

Abstract

The pelvis is a ring-shaped structure located between the trunk and lower extremities. The hip bone consists of three separate bones: the ilium, ischium, and pubis. These bones fuse in the acetabulum region, appearing as a single bone in adults. The sacrum consists of five fused vertebrae. The coccyx consists of four fused coccygeal vertebrae. The hip bones join with the sacrum posteriorly by the sacroiliac joint. Anteriorly, they unite by the symphysis pubis and take the form of a ring.

The term *"pelvis"* is used for the bones that make up the pelvic ring, which is composed of bony structures, and the stabilizing ligaments associated with them; the space enclosed by the bony structure located below the pelvic inlet and above the pelvic floor is called the *"pelvic cavity."* The pelvic floor muscles are located at the floor of the pelvic cavity and provide active support to the pelvic viscera. The ligament tissue and fascia surrounding these muscles form the pelvic diaphragm. In this chapter, the structures of the pelvis and their functions will be explained. Along with an explanation of palpation techniques and functional exercises, it would be helpful for pelvic floor dysfunctions specialists.

12.1 Noncontractile Structures in the Pelvis

The hip bone connects the lower extremity to the axial skeleton through its articulation with the sacrum. The right and left hip bones, together with the sacrum and coccyx, form the pelvis. The bony pelvis is composed of the right and left hip bones anteriorly and laterally, and the entire sacrococcygeal part of the vertebral column posteriorly. It refers to an irregular but fully bony ring. The pelvic *inlet*, which defines the upper border of the pelvic cavity, consists of the posterior sacral *promontory* (a protruding protuberance on the anterior aspect of the first sacral vertebra), the *linea arcuata* formed by the ilium and the superior ramus of the pubis on both sides, and anteriorly the crista pubica and the upper edge of the symphysis pubis.

In an upright person, the pelvis has a distinct anterior inclination so that the spina iliaca anterior superior and the upper edge of the symphysis pubis are in the same vertical plane. The tuber ischiadicums, the upper edge of the symphysis pubis, and the tip of the coccyx are in the same horizontal plane. The inner side of the bony pelvis contains a slightly wavy, compact bony ridge called the pelvic brim. In general, the plane of

A. Aklar (✉)
Physiotherapy and Rehabilitation, Health Sciences Faculty, Fenerbahce University, Istanbul, Turkey
e-mail: ayca.aklar@fbu.edu.tr

the pelvic inlet divides the bony pelvis into two parts: (1) the lesser pelvis (or true pelvis: the portion situated below the level of the pelvic brim), (2) the greater pelvis (or false pelvis: the portion above the pelvic inlet). The area enclosed by the lesser pelvis is the pelvic cavity, whereas the area enclosed by the greater pelvis is the lower part of the abdominal cavity and includes the right and left iliac fossae (Fig. 12.1). Due to the anterior tilt of the articulated pelvis described above, the plane of the pelvic brim makes an angle of 6° with the horizontal plane. The pelvis, which evolved with the onset of the bipedal period four to six million years ago, thus became suitable for locomotion. There are gender-specific differences in the pelvis in terms of anatomy (Table 12.1). The difference in the bone structure of the male and female pelvis also causes some changes in the muscles (Fig. 12.2).

12.1.1 Hip Bone (Coxa)

The adult hip bone consists of three regions: (1) Ilium: Large and fan-shaped upper part, (2) Ischium: posterior lower part, and (3) Pubis: Anteromedial part. The coxa, an irregular bone, is formed by the fusion of the ilium, pubis, and ischium. While these three bones fuse with the acetabular cartilage in the developmental stage, ossification occurs around the age of 18 (Fig. 12.3).

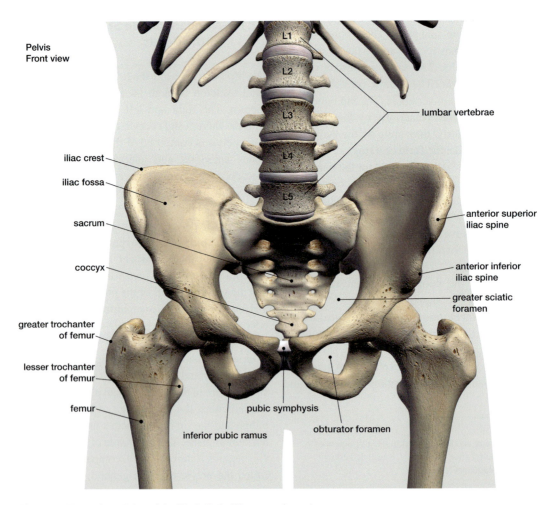

Fig. 12.1 Front view of the pelvis (Hank Grebe/Shutterstock.com)

12.1.2 Joints

The joints that make up the pelvis are the right and left sacroiliac joints, the symphysis pubis, and the sacrococcygeal joints. The pelvis articulates with the femoral head on both sides, forming the hip joint. The pelvis supports the vertebral column via the lumbosacral joint formed above by the fifth lumbar vertebra (L5) and the first sacral vertebra (S1). The two hip bones fuse anteriorly with the symphysis pubis. Posterolaterally, on both sides, the auricular articular surface at the medial edge of the ilium joins with the articular surface at the sacrum to form the sacroiliac joint. Finally, the lower end of the sacrum articulates with the upper surface of the coccyx to form the sacrococcygeal joint. The symphysis pubis and sacrococcygeal joints are examples of secondary cartilaginous joints (Fig. 12.2). The stability of the pelvic joints is ensured by strong ligaments. Important and strong ligaments of the pelvis are sacrotuberous, sacrospinous, iliolumbar, anterior sacroiliac, posterior sacroiliac, and interosseous sacroiliac ligaments.

Table 12.1 Differences between female and male pelvis

	Male	Female
Structure and weight of the bones	Thick and heavy	Thin and light
The shape of the pelvic inlet	Heart-shaped	Oval and rounded
The shape of the lesser pelvis	Deep and narrow	Shallow and wide
Subpubic angle (degree)	<70°	>80°
The shape of the pelvic outlet	Small	Wide and large

12.1.2.1 Lumbosacral Joint

L5 and S1 vertebrae join at the intervertebral joint through the largest fibrocartilaginous disc in the spine, located between the vertebral bodies. Posteriorly, they are articulated via the synovial zygapophyseal articular surfaces between the

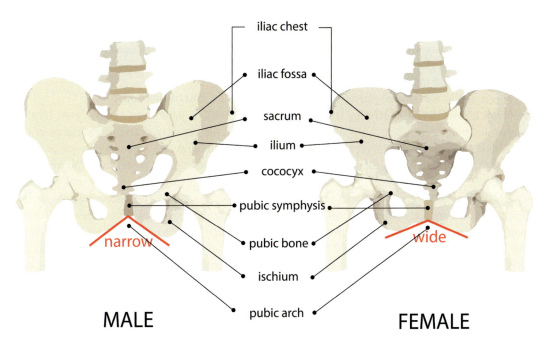

Fig. 12.2 Bone structures of female and male pelvis (narin phapnam/Shutterstock.com)

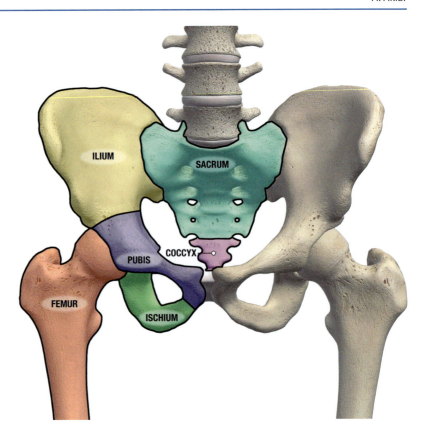

Fig. 12.3 Adult hip bone (Hank Grebe/Shutterstock.com)

articular protrusions. The intervertebral joint is fused on both sides by an amphiarthrodial symphysis, which consists of thin layers of hyaline cartilage. The anterior side of the intervertebral disc is longer. The synovial zygapophyseal articular surfaces are wider compared to the joints at the upper levels of the lumbar region and have facets oriented in the coronal plane. The sacrum sits below L5 with its base inclining forward and its apex inclining back.

Ligament support of the joint is provided by the vertebral ligaments including the intertransverse, interspinous, and supraspinous ligaments located at the higher levels of the spine, as well as the ligamentum flavum and the continuation of the zygapophyseal capsular elements located in the L5–S1 joint space. In addition, the iliolumbar ligaments support the joint laterally. Each one is attached to the pelvis via two bands, upper and lower, which begin at the tip of the transverse process of L5 (and often L4 too) and pass in front of the sacroiliac joint. The upper band attaches to the iliac crest, and from here, it continues with the thoracolumbar fascia. The lower band (also called the lumbosacral ligament) passes to the upper surface of the sacral area, and here, it blends with the anterior sacroiliac ligament.

12.1.2.2 Sacroiliac Joint

The sacroiliac joint is a synovial joint located between the ear-shaped articular surfaces of the sacrum and ilium and surrounded by the articular capsule anteriorly and posteriorly. The joint capsule is reinforced by the anterior and posterior sacroiliac ligaments. The interosseous ligament, consisting of many thick fibrous bands in adults (particularly in men), passes between the articular surfaces of the sacrum and ilium and fills the joint space. The dorsal longitudinal ligament, one of the important ligaments of the vertebral column, crosses the sacroiliac joint posteriorly and attaches to the sacrum and ilium (Fig. 12.4).

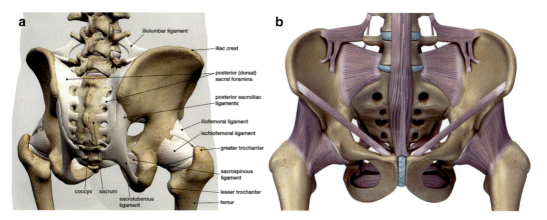

Fig. 12.4 Rear (**a**) (sciencepics/Shutterstock.com) and front (**b**) (Hank Grebe/Shutterstock.com) views of the joints and ligaments in the pelvis

Clinical Information

Since the dorsal longitudinal ligament is rich in nociceptors and proprioceptors, it is associated with posterior pelvic pain and absorbs the loads on the sacroiliac joint and hip. In cases where the tonus of the muscles surrounding the pelvis decreases, more load is placed on the ligaments surrounding the joint to maintain the stability of the sacroiliac joint. In the long term, this can result in pelvic pain. Evaluation of sensitive points on the ligament with good palpation and retraining the motor functions of the muscles surrounding the pelvis may be beneficial in reducing pain.

Sacroiliac joint stability is provided by the pitted and protruding articular surfaces (more specifically in males), passive stability (*form closure*), the tensile force generated by the inner and outer sacroiliac ligaments, and the contraction of the pelvic region, hip, and lumbar region muscles (*force closure*).

12.1.2.3 Symphysis Pubis

It is the secondary cartilaginous joint located between the bodies of the right and left ilium. Each of the opposing articular surfaces of the two pubic bones is covered with thin hyaline cartilage. A dense and strong fibrous disc connects the two articular surfaces. The symphysis pubis is supported superiorly and inferiorly by the superior pubic ligament and the arcuate pubic ligament (Fig. 12.4).

12.1.2.4 Sacrococcygeal Joint

It is a secondary cartilaginous type joint located between the sacrum and the upper surface (floor) of the coccyx (Fig. 12.4). The sacrococcygeal joint is supported anteriorly by the ventral sacrococcygeal ligament and posteriorly by the deep and superficial dorsal sacrococcygeal ligaments. On each side, a lateral sacrococcygeal ligament is located between the inferolateral angle of the sacrum and the transverse processes of the coccyx.

12.1.3 Ligaments

12.1.3.1 Sacroiliac Ligament

It consists of anterior, posterior, and interosseous sacroiliac ligaments. The anterior sacroiliac ligament forms the anterior part of the joint capsule and is thinner. The posterior sacroiliac ligament, on the other hand, supports the posterior part of the joint capsule. The interosseous sacroiliac ligaments lie deep between the sacrum and the ilium and, together with the fibers of the posterior sacroiliac ligament, run obliquely from the sacrum to the superior and lateral. Thanks to this placement of both ligaments, the sacrum is compressed between the two ilia.

12.1.3.2 Iliolumbar Ligament

It is not present in the newborn; develops with metaplasia of the muscle fibers of the quadratus lumborum in the 20s and undergoes degeneration from the 40s. It consists of two bands, the upper band extending from the medial of the transverse process of the fifth lumbar vertebra to the posterior end of the iliac crest, and the lower band blending into the anterior surface of the ventral sacroiliac ligament (Fig. 12.4). It is thought that the anterior and posterior bands of the iliolumbar ligament serve different functions, and this ligament develops due to the tensile stress occurring at the lumbosacral junction with upright posture. The posterior band is thinner than the anterior band and has a smaller attachment area at the iliac crest. The anatomical location of the iliolumbar ligament provides an anti-twist function in the pelvis. Since the grip area of the posterior band is smaller and thinner, it is more difficult to stabilize against bending. Therefore, it is often injured and causes pain, especially in athletes.

12.1.3.3 Sacrotuberous Ligament

It is a strong ligament that extends from the medial border of the ischial process to the lateral border of the sacrum and coccyx. The posterior surface of the ligament is partially attached to the gluteus maximus muscle (Fig. 12.4).

12.1.3.4 Sacrospinous Ligament

It is a triangular, fan-shaped ligament located on the inner side of the sacrotuberous ligament. Its apex is narrow and attaches to the end of the ischial spine. Its base is broad and adheres to the lateral side of the sacrococcygeal junction. The sacrospinous ligament, together with the spina ischiadicum, forms a boundary between the greater and lesser sciatic canals (Fig. 12.4). The sacrotuberous and sacrospinous ligaments protect the vertebral column by providing anterior movement of the lower end of the sacrum against excessive loads passing in front of the sacroiliac joint, such as in jumping from a height or lifting weights while standing.

12.1.4 A Transition Zone: Pelvis

The foramen ischiadicum majus and minus and the obturator foramen are openings that connect the pelvic cavity to the outside (Fig. 12.5). The foramen ischiadicum majus and minus is a transition site for

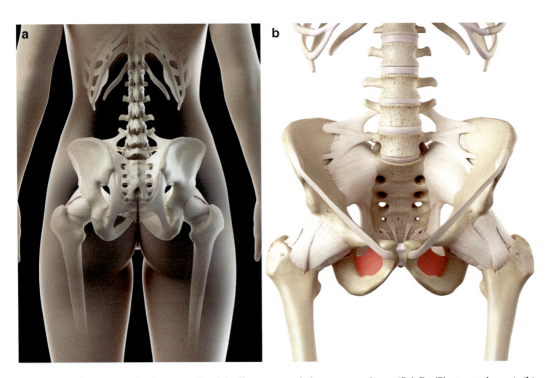

Fig. 12.5 (**a**) Lumbosacral region, sacroiliac joint ligaments, and obturator membrane (SciePro/Shutterstock.com), (**b**) foramen is chiadicum majus and minus (SciePro/Shutterstock.com)

anatomical structures located posterolaterally, transitioning from the pelvic cavity to the ipsilateral gluteal region. The obturator foramen is a large opening located in the anterior part of the hip bone and has a complete bony margin. This opening is a passageway for the anatomical structures leading to the adductor region (Fig. 12.1). It is almost completely enclosed by the obturator membrane with a dense and strong fibrous layer (Fig. 12.5b).

12.2 Contractile Structures Associated with the Pelvis

Pelvic muscles are divided into two groups: those attached to the pelvis and those located outside or inside the pelvic cavity. Muscles located outside the pelvic cavity: Lower extremity muscles (adductors, hamstrings, gluteals, rectus femoris, etc.); abdominal muscles (external oblique, internal oblique, and transverse abdominis). The inner part of the pelvic cavity: The iliacus muscle and the perineal muscle groups (many small and sensitive muscles attached to the inner surface of the ilium and the lower edge of the pelvic ring).

The piriformis, obturator internus, coccygeus, and levator ani are other muscles located on either side of the pelvic cavity. The piriformis is positioned in front of the sacrum, on the posterior wall of the pelvic cavity. The obturator internus is located on the inner surface of the foramen obturatum, which is covered by the obturator membrane, on the inside of the lateral wall of the pelvic cavity. The piriformis and obturator internus muscles are positioned inside the pelvic cavity. The tendons of both muscles leave the pelvis to attach to the greater trochanter of the femur (piriformis tendon from foramen ischiadicum majus; obturator internus tendon from foramen ischiadicum minus); they pass just behind the joint capsule to attach to the greater trochanter, and externally rotate the hip joint.

Pelvic floor musculature consists of three layers: superficial, middle, and deep, which extend in the shape of a funnel by attaching to the pubis and coccyx bones. The superficial layer of the pelvic floor includes the perineal muscles (superficial transverse perineal, ischiocavernosus, bulbocavernosus muscles, and external anal sphincter). The middle and deep layers contain the levator ani (LA) muscle. These pelvic floor layers play an important role in providing pelvic organ support and continence, in addition to the urethral and anal sphincter system (external and internal sphincter muscles and vascular elements in the submucosa). Laterally, the aponeurotic tissues of the pelvic floor muscles blend into the fascial layer above the obturator internus muscle. The main carrier of the pelvic floor is the levator ani muscle. This muscle, together with the fasciae covering the coccygeus muscle and itself from above and below, forms the pelvic diaphragm (Fig. 12.6). The right and left sides of the pelvic floor junction supply fibers to the perineal body, which lies superficially between the vagina and the rectum. The structure and effect of the muscles in each layer are summarized in Table 12.2. The combined action of these muscles creates a rising motion toward the heart with an upward force and a contracting motion around the sphincters.

> **Clinical Information**
> Depending on the increase in the level of sex hormones and relaxin hormone increases during pregnancy, the connective tissues in the pelvis relax. While this increases the amount of movement in the joints, it might also negatively affect the pelvic diaphragm, which provides urine control. With the increasing weight of the baby, the elongation/relaxation of the pelvic diaphragm may cause difficulty (incontinence) in urine control. Urinary incontinence might be seen during pregnancy (7–64%). The incidence of urinary incontinence within 2–3 months after birth is 3–38%.
>
> Besides, damage to structures such as ligaments, fascia, and peripheral nerves that make up the pelvic floor might occur during delivery. The high number of pregnancies and births is a significant risk factor in the occurrence of urinary incontinence complaints. It is thought that the mode of delivery affects stress urinary incontinence. Lower urinary system problems, seen 9 months after delivery, are more common in women who gave birth vaginally compared to women who gave birth by cesarean section. The pelvic floor exercises mentioned in this section are widely used in the treatment of urinary incontinence.

Anatomy

Fig. 12.6 Layers of the pelvic floor (molotoka/Shutterstock.com)

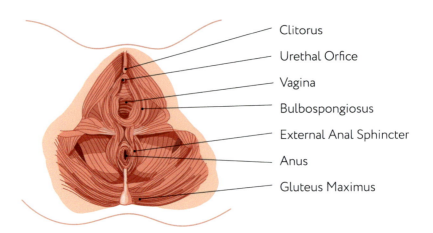

- Clitorus
- Urethal Orfice
- Vagina
- Bulbospongiosus
- External Anal Sphincter
- Anus
- Gluteus Maximus

Table 12.2 Pelvic floor anatomy

Muscle layer	Muscle	Function
The superficial muscles	Ischiocavernosus	Clitoris erection
	Bulbocavernosus	Narrowing of the introitus during sexual intercourse Clitoris erection
	Superficial transverse perineal	Fixation of the perineal body
	External anal sphincter	Closure of the anus
The urogenital diaphragm (The perineal membrane)	Deep transverse perineal	It creates pressure on the urethra and the anterior wall of the vagina
	Compressor urethrae	It supports the perineal body and introitus
	Urethrovaginal sphincter	It supports the perineal body and introitus
The pelvic diaphragm (Primary muscular support)	Levator ani • Pubococcygeus • Puborectalis • Iliococcygeus	It is primarily responsible for the movement of the pelvic floor The puborectalis helps to close the rectum
	Coccygeus	Flexion of the coccyx

12.3 Palpation of the Bones and Muscles of the Pelvis is Summarized in Table 12.3

Table 12.3 Muscle and bone palpation of the pelvis

Muscle	Palpation
Gluteus maximus	Crista iliaca, the major trochanter, and the ischial tuberosity are important bony points around the gluteal region The gluteal fold is an important determinant of the inferior border of the gluteus maximus muscle Besides, the muscle becomes apparent when the hip extension is performed in the prone and knee bent position
Gluteus medius	The anterior part of the crista iliaca and the upper border of the major trochanter are the defining bony points for this muscle The hand is placed as shown in the figure, and the patient is asked to do hip abduction against resistance A slight internal rotation can be added for the anterior fibers of the muscle

Table 12.3 (continued)

Piriformis	The piriformis muscle can be palpated in three stages: **Stage 1:** The person is placed on his/her side with the evaluated extremity up. The extremity is lifted toward the physiotherapist's chest and shoulder. In this position, the patient is asked to do abduction against resistance to detect the gluteus medius muscle **Stage 2:** The physiotherapist mobilizes the hip by placing his/her hand on the inside of the person's leg and tries to feel the major trochanter **Stage 3:** When the physiotherapist's hand is on the major trochanter and horizontal abduction of the hip joint is conducted against the resistance, the piriformis muscle is felt in the pit formed
Levator ani	In a lateral or supine position, flexion is applied to the hip joint After the thumb is placed on the medial of the tuber ischiadicum, the person is asked to cough It is the levator ani muscle felt under the hand
Bone—ligament	**Palpation**
Crista iliaca	In the lateral lying position, it is started by touching the spina iliaca posterior superior with the tips of the fingers and proceeded by touching the spina iliaca anterior superior The cristae or lateral and medial borders can be felt
Spina iliaca anterior superior	Palpation of this protrusion is quite easy It is the most apparent anterior point (protrusion) of the crista iliaca
Pubic tubercle	The major trochanter is felt on both sides using the hands, and the thumbs are moved medially in the horizontal plane. This protrusion-like structure is felt in the pubic region
Spina iliaca posterior superior	By following the crista iliaca, the most protruding surface is found posteriorly This protrusion that joins with the sacroiliac joint can also be found through the dimples it creates
Tuber ischiadicum	It is an oval structure with a broad posterosuperior ending When the hip is flexed, it becomes evident at the inferior border of the iliac bone, under the gluteus maximus muscle
Long dorsal ligament	The long dorsal ligament extends from the fifth lumbar vertebra (L5) to the coccyx. For its palpation, the person lies face down, and the therapist follows and feels with the fingertips, starting from L5 to the coccyx

12.4 Movements in the Pelvis

The pelvis has a stable structure. The transmission line of both the body weight force from above and the ground reaction force from below passes in front of the sacroiliac joints. The force due to body weight tends to tilt the sacrum forward; the ground reaction force, on the other hand, tends to rotate the hip bones backward. The pelvis is resistant to both forces due to its very strong ligaments that support the joints and the indented and protruding articular surfaces, especially in the sacroiliac joints. The two forces together provide a self-locking and screwed mechanism for maximum stability. It requires thousands of kilos of force to disrupt the pelvic stability obtained with this structural feature. It has been observed that when large forces are applied to the pelvis experimentally, the sacrum or ilium often breaks before the ligaments rupture or separate.

In general, three types of motion occur in the hip bones: (1) *Symmetrical motion:* It is the motion of both hip bones as a whole, associated with the sacrum. (2) *Asymmetrical motion:* It consists of the antagonistic motion of both hip bones, associated with the sacrum, and this movement also affects the symphysis pubis. (3) *Lumbopelvic motion:* It involves the rotation of both hip bones and the spine around the femoral head.

12.4.1 Symmetrical Motion

Symmetrical trunk and hip movements result in symmetrical movements in both sacroiliac joints. During trunk flexion or bilateral hip flexion, the sacral *nutation* occurs (from Latin, *nutatio*: nodding of the head) or the sacrum rotates toward the front. Thus, the apex moves dorsocranially, while the promontory moves ventrocaudally. The sacrum moves in the opposite direction (*contra-nutation*) during trunk extension or bilateral hip extension. During nutation and contra-nutation, a displacement (sliding) motion of a few millimeters occurs. During the nutation and contra-nutation movements of the sacrum, the hip bones (with the symphysis pubis fixed) also move symmetrically as a whole. Nutation, which is a combination of rotational and translational movements, causes the two tuber ischiadicum to move away from each other while bringing the iliac crests closer.

12.4.2 Asymmetrical Motion

Standing on one leg, especially mid-stance phase of gait, and asymmetric landings create asymmetrical force in the pelvis. Unilateral loading results in asymmetric and antagonistic movements in the sacroiliac joints, causing pelvic torsion.

> **Attention!**
>
> Although there is little motion in the symphysis pubis, it always accompanies asymmetric motions of the sacroiliac joint. However, relaxin, estrogen, and progesterone hormones released during pregnancy cause laxity in the joints, and this leads to an increase in the symphysis pubis motions. Therefore, movements that load the pelvis unilaterally in the later stages of pregnancy may result in pain in the symphysis pubis and inguinal region.

12.4.3 Lumbopelvic Rhythm

The sacroiliac joints have the important task of fixing the caudal end of the axial skeleton to the pelvis. As the pelvis flexes the hip on the femur, the lumbar vertebrae adapt as well. There are two types of lumbopelvic rhythms in the frontal and horizontal planes, in the same direction or the opposite direction. During the same directional lumbopelvic rhythm, the pelvis and lumbar spine rotate together in the same direction. During this time, the angular displacement of the body is maximum. However, during the opposite directional lumbopelvic rhythm, the lumbar spine and the pelvis rotate in the opposite direction; the thoracolumbar transition zone remains in an almost static position, as in walking (Fig. 12.7). Lumbopelvic rhythm workouts are among the exercises recommended for enhancing the motor control of the pelvic diaphragm and structures attached to the pelvis through the ilium and sacrum movements.

Elevation of the pelvis at one side (the other side is the depression of the pelvis) at the lumbosacral joint is analogous to the lateral flexion of the trunk at the lumbosacral joint. Therefore, erector spinae, transversospinalis group, quadratus lumborum, and latissimus dorsi muscles that perform lateral flexion of the trunk perform the elevation of the pelvis on one side (means the depression of the opposite pelvis) at the lumbosacral joint (Fig. 12.8a, c).

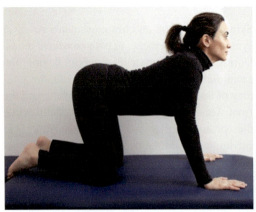 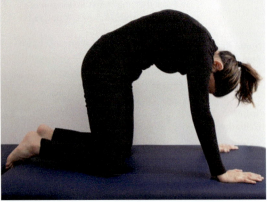

Fig. 12.7 Lumbopelvic rhythm exercises

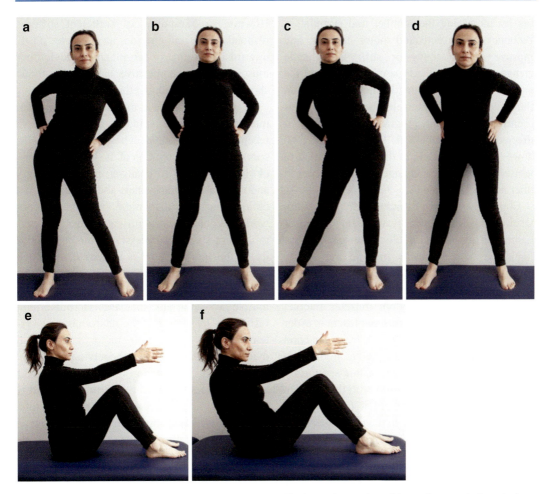

Fig. 12.8 Movements of the pelvis in the sagittal and frontal planes (**a**, **c**); Elevation of the pelvis to the right and the left, respectively, in the lumbosacral joint (**b**, **d**); Flexion and extension of the trunk respectively at the lumbosacral joint (**e**, **f**); Anterior and posterior tilt of the pelvis, respectively

The anterior tilt of the pelvis at the lumbosacral joint is similar to the extension of the trunk at the lumbosacral joint. Therefore, the erector spinae, transversospinalis group, quadratus lumborum, and latissimus dorsi muscles that carry out the extension of the trunk perform the anterior tilt of the pelvis at the lumbosacral joint as well (Fig. 12.8b, e).

The posterior tilt of the pelvis at the lumbosacral joint is similar to the flexion of the trunk at the lumbosacral joint. Therefore, the anterior abdominal wall muscles that flex the trunk, such as the rectus abdominis, external abdominal oblique, and internal abdominal oblique also perform the posterior tilt of the pelvis at the lumbosacral joint (Fig. 12.8d, f).

12.5 Evidence-Based Exercises by Which the Pelvic Muscles Work According to the Exercise Type

The pelvic floor muscles adapt to strength training like any skeletal muscle. The purpose of strength training is to increase strength and change muscle morphology by increasing the cross-sectional area, improve neurological factors by increasing the number and stimulation frequency of the activated motor neurons, and improve muscle tonus or stiffness. Specific changes depend on the type of exercise and the applied training program. It should be kept in mind that the targeted development at the end of a particular training program would also be affected by genetic and hereditary factors. However, if any muscle in the body is started to be used, physiological changes will also occur in other muscles activated.

Connective tissue (including epimysium, perimysium, and endomysium) is abundant inside and around all skeletal muscles. These connective tissue sheaths provide the tensile strength and viscoelastic properties (rigidity) of the muscles and the necessary support for muscle loading. The pelvic floor muscles interact with the supporting ligaments and fascia in order to protect the support for the pelvic organs and the connective tissue of the pelvic floor from excessive loads. The function of this supporting system is illustrated by Norton with the "boat in dry dock theory": Here, the pelvic floor muscles are compared to the water in the pool, the pelvic organs to the boat; and the amount of water in the pool determines the load on the anchors (ligaments and fasciae) holding the boat. If water is removed (loss of pelvic floor muscle tonus), the anchors (pelvic ligaments and fascia) are subjected to excessive tension.

In a blinded randomized controlled trial evaluating the effect of a six-month pelvic floor muscle training to prevent and treat pelvic organ prolapse (Brækken et al. 2010), when compared to the control group, the results indicated a 15.6% increase in pelvic floor muscle thickness, a 6.3% reduction in the levator hiatus area, a 6.3% reduction in muscle length, and an elevation of 4.3 and 6.7 mm respectively in the position of the bladder neck and rectal ampulla. It was also shown that during the Valsalva maneuver, the levator hiatus area and muscle length decreased, and pelvic floor muscle strength and autonomic function improved. The pelvic floor can be considered as a trampoline with its position in the pelvis. It will be difficult to jump if the trampoline is overstretched or sagging. However, a trampoline of sufficient stiffness responds faster and provides an effective "push" upwards. Therefore, when planning pelvic floor muscle training, connective and muscle tissue should be considered together.

As with other skeletal muscles, the levator ani muscle has muscle spindles and local nerve receptors in its tendons. These specialized sensors regulate the activation of the levator ani muscle by responding to changes in muscle length and tension. The transversus abdominis, internal oblique muscles, diaphragm, and pelvic floor work in coordination with each other to determine intra-abdominal pressure. Thus, the stability of the lumbar spine is increased. Although indirectly, the pelvic floor muscles support lumbopelvic stability. An increase in pelvic floor muscle activation also increases sacroiliac joint resistance. In summary, the neuromuscular system contributes to both motor control and dynamic stability of the lumbopelvic joints.

The order of excitation of the motor units is arranged according to the size principle and is relatively constant. According to this principle, motor neurons that innervate slow-twitch (type I) muscle fibers during light movements requiring low force (i.e., smaller motor units [with low threshold]) always work first. With increasing loads, the muscle needs more power, and gradually higher-threshold motor units (type II) are activated by stimulation. At higher shortening speeds, the submaximal forces may be maximum, or at least close to maximum. Some exceptions might be seen in the stimulation hierarchy of the motor units. For example, it is known that no activity occurs in type I fibers during an eccentric contraction, but activity occurs in type II fibers.

The two general loading strategies used to increase muscle strength can also be used in pelvic floor muscle training:

1. For strengthening, medium to high load is required to operate high threshold fast-twitch motor units, but the rate of contraction should be medium to slow.
2. Light to moderate loads performed at an explosive lifting speed should be included.

In muscle strengthening exercises for the pelvic floor muscles, the patient is first asked to contract the pelvic floor muscles close to the maximum, try to keep them at this contraction level, and finally, perform 3–4 rapid muscle contractions while maintaining the contraction.

An important part of adaptation in muscle training is to improve the ability of all motor units to participate in a given exercise. This is particularly important for the pelvic floor muscles because very few people are aware of these muscles or have voluntarily tried to contract them. Another important neural adaptation mechanism in training is the reduction of antagonist activation. It is difficult to say which muscles can be considered antagonists to the pelvic floor muscles. However, an abdominal contraction that occurs without a pelvic floor muscle contraction might be an antagonist contraction. This is because, under normal conditions, any increase in intra-abdominal pressure causes the pelvic floor muscles to contract automatically. This working principle of the muscles can be regarded as a goal during training.

It was shown that a coccyx motion occurred during a voluntary pelvic floor muscle contraction. Therefore, the contraction is concentric. However, the smallness of this motion suggests the presence of an isometric component. It was suggested that 6 s were required to achieve maximum contraction. However, holding times of 3–10 s are recommended for isometric contractions. Daily isometric training is superior to less frequent training, but performing it three times a week at maximum strength can produce significant increases in muscle strength. It was shown that isometric training performed alone without weights increases both protein synthesis (49%) and muscle hypertrophy of type I and type II muscle fibers. The pelvic floor muscle movement is eccentric during increases in abdominal pressure.

Although it is known that pelvic floor muscles work together with hip adductor, gluteal, and different abdominal muscle contractions, such contractions might not occur in people with pelvic floor dysfunction or might be inadequate compared to pelvic floor muscle training. For this reason, the person should first know how to use the pelvic floor muscles. Later, strength training can be advanced with the help of other muscles according to the needs of the person. For example, with a person who has urinary incontinence while lifting weights, pelvic floor muscle activation can be exercised during this movement to their needs. Figure 12.9 shows how the exercises can be progressed from easy to difficult.

> **Clinical Information**
>
> Although the ligaments and myofascial structures surrounding the pelvis are nociceptive structures, it is well known that neurophysiologically ongoing pain can be mediated both peripherally and centrally, and the forebrain largely regulates this process. Even in nociceptive pelvic girdle pain, the patient's cognitive status and psychosocial factors can affect the course and level of pain. Therefore, there is a need for the adoption of biopsychosocial approaches in evaluation and treatment.
>
> For example, decreased motor control of the muscles surrounding the pelvis (reduced *force closure*) may be associated with false beliefs, anxiety, and passive coping strategies. Interventions in such a situation must include motor learning methods such as supporting true beliefs, relaxation techniques, and active coping strategies. On the other hand, if the same situation (reduced *force closure*) includes true beliefs, active coping strategies, and a certain degree of functional disability, the main goal might be to treat physical disabilities for pain reduction. The exercises described in this section comprise strength and motor learning principles and can be used in situations where motor control is weakened.

Clinical Information
Normal pelvic floor function during urine filling and emptying

The pelvic floor is important for both storage and discharge of urine in the lower urinary tract. For normal storage without urinary incontinence, the urethra needs to be closed and supported. For effective support of the urethra, the anterior vaginal wall, the endopelvic fascia, and its connections with the arcus tendinous fascia pelvis (ATFP) must be intact. Besides, good tonus and strength of the middle part of the levator ani muscle support the anterior vaginal wall and associated fasciae. A healthy discharge of urine begins with the complete relaxation of the external urethral sphincter and levator ani muscles and becomes possible through coordinated events.

During voluntary contraction of the pelvic floor muscles, they move inward, closing the urethra and resisting the downward movement of the urethra. Thus, the movement of the urethra is restricted.

Clinical Information
Relationship between pelvic floor and bladder functions

Bladder filling depends on both structural and functional factors. While the levator ani muscle, endopelvic fascia, and ATFP comprise the structural components, the pudendal nerve, which stimulates the external urethral sphincter (EUS), and the levator ani nerve, which stimulates the pelvic floor muscles, constitute the functional components. These components are regulated by the coordinated operation of the central and peripheral nervous systems. Increased urethral pressure during urine storage causes an increase in the frequency of stimulation of the pudendal nerve, leading to an increase in the EUS activity. The normal storage of urine is dependent on the spinal reflex mechanism that activates the bladder outlet sympathetically and somatically and the tonic inhibitory system in the brain that suppresses the voiding reflex.

During bladder emptying, the urethra and pelvic floor muscles relax, reducing pressure at the bladder outlet. Relaxation creates a funnel-like effect at the bladder outlet and causes both the suppression of the spinal protection reflex on the EUS and the release of nitric oxide in the smooth muscles of the urethra as a result of increased parasympathetic stimulation. Simultaneously, the bladder muscles contract, and the bladder is emptied. Any condition that prevents the pelvic floor muscles from relaxing during bladder emptying causes problems during bladder emptying.

The structures in the pelvic floor are thought to vary in terms of nervous system connections. Direct roots from the pudendal nerve (three branches including dorsal, perineal, and rectal), levator ani nerve, and sacral roots provide the nervous system connections of the perineum. Providing nerve conduction in more than one way protects this area against injuries that might occur during birth.

Attention!

In pelvic floor muscle training, the correct contraction of the pelvic floor muscles should be taught first.

There are two phases to the correct contraction of the pelvic floor muscles:

These are (1) squeezing movements that close the openings in the pelvis and (2) upward movements toward the heart. 30% of women cannot perform the desired pelvic floor muscle contraction correctly. The main reasons for not correctly performing the voluntary pelvic floor muscle contraction are:

- The pelvic floor muscles are in the pelvis and cannot be seen from the outside.

- Neither men nor women are taught throughout their lives that these muscles can be contracted.
- Since these muscles are small, it is more difficult to control them voluntarily.
- The use of the pelvic and perineal regions has changed due to habits acquired during voiding and defecation (straining in the toilet).

When describing the correct contraction to men, they can be advised to lift the scrotum upwards. If necessary, a mirror can be used so that both men and women can see the inward lifting movement. However, some people may find it uncomfortable to observe their genitals, so the physiotherapist should show courtesy before recommending this method during training.

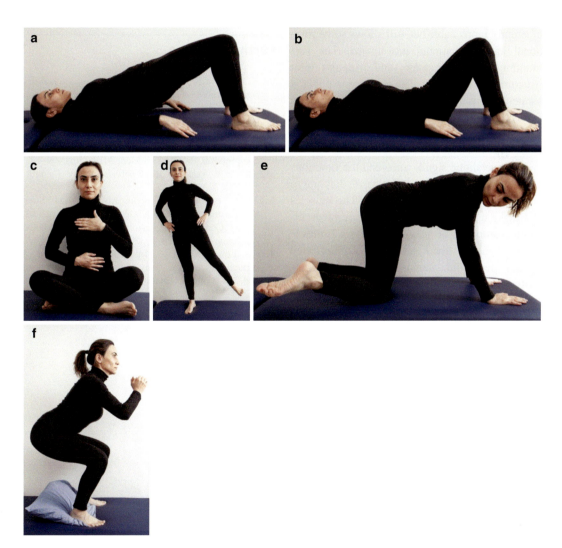

Fig. 12.9 Advancement of pelvic floor muscle training (**a**) when pelvic floor muscle training is given, especially in cases such as prolapse, positions against gravity are preferred, (**b**) the supine position, where pelvic floor muscle contraction can be followed with digital palpation, can be used in the initial phase, (**c**) then, pelvic floor muscle contractions can be conducted in coordination with the diaphragm and respiratory control, (**d–f**) the motor learning process is supported by different muscle groups, exercises that increase intra-abdominal pressure, and exercises against gravity

12.6 Conclusion

This section explains the anatomical and functional features of the pelvis, which has a very important role in the functional movements of the trunk and lower extremities. The pelvis has a bone and joint structure that is stable enough to support the body weight and also mobile enough to allow functional movement. The coronally situated articular surfaces of the fifth lumbar vertebra and the thick iliolumbar ligament supporting the joint support the lumbosacral joint against the anterior shearing force. The sacroiliac joint is inherently more stable but still allows some rotational and translational movements. The surrounding strong ligaments and irregular joint structure limit mobility. The symphysis pubis is located in the anterior part of the pelvis and is very slightly mobile.

The function of the pelvic diaphragm, which consists of three layers deep, middle and superficial, its metabolic significance and the functions of the muscles that make up the pelvic diaphragm are also mentioned in this section. The muscles that make up the pelvic diaphragm are predominantly composed of slow-twitch Type I muscle fibers. Type II fibers are more concentrated around the urethra, vagina, and anal openings. Furthermore, the section also refers to the functions of these muscles during micturition, defecation, sexual function, pelvic organ support, and delivery. While the palpation of the muscles, bones, and ligaments surrounding the pelvis is explained by visuals, evidence-based exercises are covered under a separate heading.

Symmetrical and asymmetrical motions that occur in the lumbosacral joint and the sacrum are emphasized. Finally, how these structures are controlled through the sympathetic and parasympathetic systems and the issues that we may encounter in the clinic are highlighted in the additional information sections.

Further Reading

Bø K, Mørkved S. Pelvic floor and exercise science. In: Bo K, Berghmans B, Morkved S, Van Kampen M, editors. Evidence-based physical therapy for the pelvic floor. Elsevier Health Sciences; 2015. p. 111–29.

Caetano AS, Suzuki FS, Lopes MH. Urinary incontinence and exercise: kinesiological description of an intervention proposal. Rev Bras de Med. 2019;25(5):409–12.

Mahadevan V. Anatomy of the pelvis. Surgery (Oxford). 2018;36(7):333–8.

Sayaca Ç, Eyüboğlu F, Tascilar LN, Çalık M, Kaya D. Kinesiology of the pelvis. In: Angın S, Şimşek İE, editors. Comparative kinesiology of the human body. Academic Press; 2020. p. 339–50.

Tixa S. Lower extremities. In: Tixa S, editor. Atlas of surface palpation: anatomy of the neck, trunk, upper, and lower limbs. Elsevier Health Sciences; 2016. p. 208–36.

The Hip

Muharrem Gokhan Beydagi

Abstract

The hip joint is a ball-and-socket joint surrounded by strong and well-balanced muscles. It is a stable joint with a wide range of motion in many planes. The hip joint, the structural link between the lower extremities and the axial skeleton, not only transmits forces from the ground but also absorbs forces from the trunk, head, neck, and upper extremities. Therefore, the hip joint is one of the most important joints in both daily life activities and sports activities. A good understanding of the hip anatomy and the forces acting on the joint can enhance current and future knowledge.

13.1 Hip Joint

The hip joint is a ball-and-socket synovial joint formed between the round head of the femur and the acetabulum of the pelvis and surrounded by strong and balanced muscles. The femoral head is stabilized by a deep socket surrounded and closed by a large connective tissue. It is a unique joint with both stability and a wide range of motion in three planes. It allows walking with weight-bearing by connecting the lower extremity to the pelvis. Any pathology or trauma to the hip adversely affects many daily life activities, such as walking, weight-bearing, climbing stairs, and so forth. In this chapter, detailed information is given about the structure of the hip joint and the bones, capsules, ligaments, and muscles associated with the joint. Muscles that produce force to create movement in the joint, important bony prominences to which the muscles attach, palpation of these protrusions and muscles, the function of the muscles and nerves, and evidence-based exercises for the muscles have also been explained.

13.2 Noncontractile Structures in the Hip Joint

13.2.1 Bone Structures

The hip joint is a spheroid-type (consisting of a ball and a socket where the ball is located) synovial joint (Fig. 13.1), located between the large, rounded head of the femur and the deep socket-type acetabulum of the pelvis. In the body, it is the joint that has the maximum range of motion after the shoulder joint. It is stable and has the ability to move in three planes.

M. G. Beydagi (✉)
Physiotherapy and Rehabilitation, Faculty of Health Sciences, Firat University, Elazig, Turkey
e-mail: mgbeydagi@firat.edu.tr

The Hip Joint

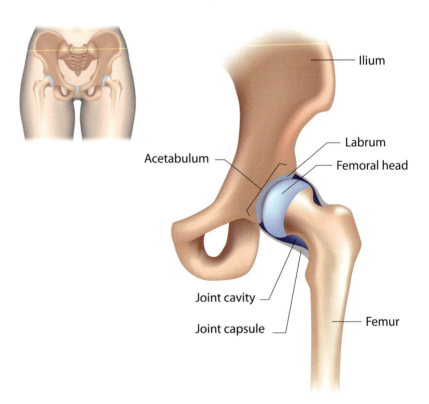

Fig. 13.1 Hip joint (Alila Medical Media/Shutterstock.com)

13.2.1.1 Proximal Femur

The femur is the longest and the strongest bone of the body (Fig. 13.2). The proximal femur consists of the femoral head (caput femoris), the femoral neck (collum femoris neck), and the greater and lesser trochanters. The region up to 5 cm distal to the greater and lesser trochanters is considered anatomically as the proximal femur.

The hip joint is located between the acetabulum and the femoral head. The femoral head, which looks like two-thirds of a sphere, is covered with hyaline cartilage. However, no cartilage is present at the attachment site of the ligamentum teres (ligamentum capitis femoris) (fovea capitis femoris). A branch of the obturator artery feeding the femoral head passes through the ligamentum teres and enters the bone.

The femoral head is connected to the femoral body (corpus femoris) by the femoral neck. At the junction of the femoral neck and body is the greater trochanter, which extends outward and backward and forms a raised mound. Prominent and easy to palpate, this bony prominence forms the distal insertion site of many muscles. On the medial surface of the greater trochanter is a small pit (trochanteric fossa), which is the distal insertion of the obturator muscle. Posteriorly, the femoral neck and femoral body meet at the intertrochanteric crista. The lesser trochanter projects from the lower end of this crista, which is a small conical projection extending posteriorly and inward. The lesser trochanter is the distal insertion site for the iliopsoas muscle and is the most important flexor of the hip. The line connecting the greater and lesser trochanters anteriorly is called the linea intertrochanterica, and the iliofemoral ligament attaches to it. Posteriorly, the intertrochanteric crista connects these two projections. Just below the trochanteric fossa is the quadrate tubercle, which rises slightly above the intertrochanteric crista and is the distal insertion of the quadratus femoris muscle.

The posterior part (middle one-third) of the femoral shaft is marked by a rough, line-shaped

Femur bone

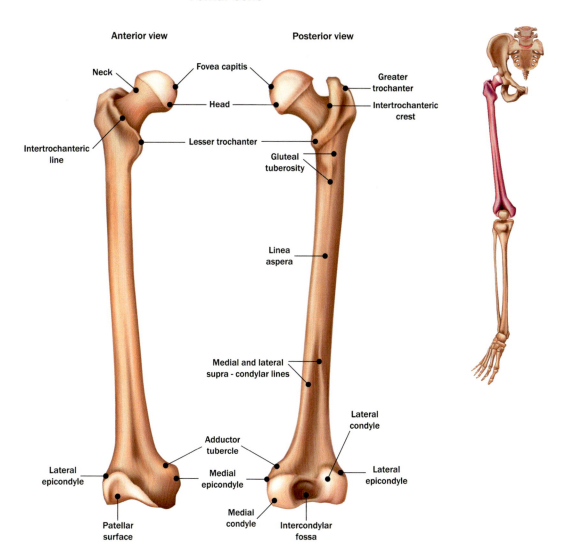

Fig. 13.2 Femur (studiovin/Shutterstock.com)

projection (linea aspera). This ascending line forms attachment sites for the vastus medialis, vastus lateralis, vastus intermedius, and most of the adductor muscles. This line divides proximally into the pectineal line (inner part) and gluteal ridge (outer part), forming a distal attachment point for some hip muscles.

Two important angles define the shape of the proximal part of the femur: inclination and torsional angles. *The inclination angle* is the angle formed between the femoral neck and body in the frontal plane, with the opening facing inward. Normally this angle is about 125° ± 5° in adults. If this angle is less than 120°, it is called *coxa vara*; if it is more than 130°, it is called *coxa valga*. *The torsional angle (anteversion angle)* is the angle used to describe the relative rotation that occurs between the femoral body and its neck. Normally, when viewed from above, the femoral neck is anterior to the plane passing through the femoral condyles. The normal value of this angle is considered to be 15°; if the angle is greater than 15°, it is called extreme anteversion, and if it is less than 15° (approaching 0°), it is called retroversion.

13.2.1.2 Acetabulum

The acetabulum is a cup-shaped structure that surrounds the femoral head in harmony with the hip joint. It is located anteriorly, laterally, and downwardly in the anatomical position and is formed by the three parts of the coxae. Of these three structures, the ilium and ischium are 80%, and the pubis is 20%. The acetabulum forms the socket part of the hip joint. This socket is an incomplete circle, with a downward opening. This opening is called the acetabular notch.

The femoral head contacts the lunate surface (facies lunata) of the acetabulum in the shape of a horseshoe (or half-moon), whose opening faces downward. The lunate surface is the thickest region of the acetabulum. It is lined with hyaline cartilage throughout its upper-anterior region. The highest joint strength during walking occurs in this thick cartilage area. The acetabular notch widens in the stance phase, where the joint force is the highest, thus increasing the contact area and reducing the force. With this natural mechanism, the load on the subchondral bone is reduced. A pit (acetabular fossa) is located deep in the base of the acetabulum and in the middle of the lunate surface. As this pit does not come into contact with the femoral head, it is not covered with cartilage. It contains adipose tissue, ligamentum teres, and blood vessels. The bone structures, important bony prominences, and the muscles attached to the hip joint are listed in Table 13.1.

Table 13.1 Muscle attachment points in the hip joint and the muscles attached to these points

Bone protrusions	Muscles
Originate from the outer surface of the ilium	• Gluteus medius • Gluteus minimus
Originate from the ischial prominence	• Adductor magnus • Gemellus inferior • Quadratus femoris • Semitendinosus • Semimembranosus • Biceps femoris (long head)
Attached to the lesser trochanter	• Iliacus • Psoas major
Attached to the greater trochanter	• Gluteus medius • Gluteus minimus • Piriformis • Gemellus superior • Gemellus inferior • Obturator externus • Obturator internus
Attached to linea aspera	• Adductor longus • Adductor brevis • Adductor magnus (the adductor magnus also attaches to the adductor tubercle of the femur)

surround the femoral neck. The fibers surrounding the femoral neck form a structure called the zona orbicularis. This condensed circular fiber group, together with the acetabular labrum, contributes to the stability of the joint. The inner surface of the capsule is covered by the synovial membrane. The synovial membrane also covers the acetabular fossa, the labrum, and the capsular portion of the femoral neck. The hip joint capsule is supported by four capsular ligaments.

13.2.2 Joint Capsule and Ligaments

13.2.2.1 Joint Capsule

In the hip joint, a strong fibrous capsule ensures the stability of the joint. Proximally, the capsule attaches to the bony rim of the acetabulum at a distance of about 6–8 mm from the labrum, encompassing the labrum and the transverse ligament. Distally, it has two endings, anterior and posterior. Anteriorly, it terminates at the intertrochanteric line and greater trochanter; and posteriorly, it terminates proximal to the intertrochanteric crista. Most of the capsular fibers run parallel to the femoral neck, while a smaller group of fibers

13.2.2.2 Joint Ligaments

The hip joint has four capsular (iliofemoral, pubofemoral, ischiofemoral, and zona orbicularis) and two intracapsular (transverse acetabular ligament and teres femoris ligament) ligaments (Fig. 13.3).

Iliofemoral Ligament (*Bigelow*'s Y Ligament, *Bertin*'s Ligament) (Anterior Ligament)

The iliofemoral ligament is the strongest and toughest of all capsular ligaments. It begins at the anterior inferior prominence of the spina iliaca of the ilium and ends at the intertrochanteric

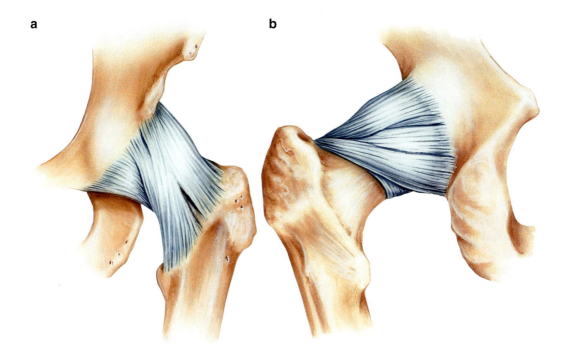

Fig. 13.3 Hip joint ligaments: (**a**) Anterior (Medical Art Inc/Shutterstock.com), (**b**) Posterior view (Medical Art Inc/Shutterstock.com)

line of the femur. Its base starts from above, and its two arms are connected above and below the intertrochanteric line in an inverted Y shape. It has two bands, the iliotrochanteric superior and inferior. The iliotrochanteric superior part is stronger and can withstand a force of 250 kg. The iliotrochanteric inferior part can withstand a force of 100 kg. Its most important task is to prevent hip hyperextension. When the hip is extended, it is taut, and together with the iliopsoas muscle, firmly fixes the anterior surface of the femoral head, helping us to stand. It stabilizes the hip joint by preventing excessive hip extension along with the ability to withstand a total force of approximately 350 kg.

Pubofemoral Ligament (Internal Lateral Ligament)

The pubofemoral ligament is a triangular ligament extending between the superior ramus of the pubis proximally and the intertrochanteric line distally, strengthening the anterior-lower part of the hip joint. It prevents excessive hip extension and abduction. In a low degree of external rotation, its fibers stretch to integrate with the inferior band of the iliofemoral ligament.

Ischiofemoral Ligament (Posterior Ligament)

The ischiofemoral ligament is thinner than the iliofemoral and pubofemoral ligaments. It starts from the ischial edge of the acetabulum and runs posteriorly and downward, ending at the femoral neck. It is spiral shaped and supports the capsule from behind. It stabilizes the hip joint in extension. The superficial fibers terminating near the apex of the greater trochanter spiral around the posterior aspect of the femoral neck. These superficial fibers are slightly stretched in full extension. However, they are most stretched at 10°–20° of abduction and internal rotation. Some of the deep fibers blend into the structure of the posterior and inferior capsule circular fibers (often referred to as the zona orbicularis) and are stretched at the final angles of hip flexion with the deeper portions of the capsule.

Zona Orbicularis

The Latin word orbicularis means a circular (orbis) or disk-shaped structure. This ligament wraps around the femoral neck and prevents it from protruding within the acetabulum. It is located deep into the iliofemoral, pubofemoral, and ischiofemoral ligaments, causing thickening of the joint capsule at the femoral neck. It is intertwined with the joint capsule. It is thought that the zona orbicularis also has an important role in the circulation of synovial fluid in the joint due to some fibers that travel close to the synovial membrane.

Capsular ligaments form most of the capsule and wrap around the head and neck of the femur. They stabilize the hip by limiting extension, abduction, and internal rotation of the femur. The connective tissues stretched at the final angles of movements in the hip joint are presented in Table 13.2.

Transverse Acetabular Ligament

The transverse acetabular ligament lies below the acetabulum and between the two edges of the acetabular notch. It is the part of the labrum in the fibrous cartilage structure in the acetabular notch. Together with the transverse acetabular ligament and the base of the acetabular notch, it forms a tunnel into the joint through which nerves and vessels enter.

Ligamentum Teres Femoris (Ligamentum Capitis Femoris)

The ligamentum teres femoris is a triangular, flat, and small intra-articular ligament. It extends from the edge of the transverse acetabular ligament and the acetabular notch to the pit in the femoral head. It runs inside the joint and is covered by the synovial membrane. Considering its size, it does not significantly contribute to joint stability. Within this ligament is the ramus acetabularis, a branch of the obturator artery responsible for the blood supply to the femoral head. When the hip is in the semi-flexion position, it is stretched during abduction or external rotation movements.

13.2.3 Other Structures

13.2.3.1 Acetabular Labrum

The acetabular labrum is a ring-shaped, flexible, and fibrous cartilage structure that surrounds the outer circular edge of the acetabulum. The transverse acetabular ligament completes this ring at the acetabular notch. This structure deepens the acetabulum cavity, restricts the translation of the femoral head, and creates negative pressure that prevents the hip joint from dislodging. It reduces the loads on the articular cartilage during walking and standing. It protects the synovial fluid on weight-bearing surfaces and increases the lubrication of the articular cartilage, thereby reducing the resistance of the cartilage to friction. It helps in mechanically distributing the stress that occurs due to the contact. The acetabular labrum provides significant mechanical stability to the hip joint by gripping the femoral head and deepening the acetabular cavity. It is responsible for proprioception, pain, and pressure sensations, thanks to the mechanoreceptors and nociceptors it contains.

13.3 Contractile Structures Associated with the Hip Joint

The hip joint has a large number of controlling muscles to provide a wide range of motion and good stability in all planes (Fig. 13.4). The muscles associated with the hip joint are responsible for dynamic stabilization and generate the necessary force for movement to occur. These muscles are grouped according to their location or function. The anterior muscles are defined as flexors, lateral muscles as abductors, posterior

Table 13.2 Connective tissues stretched during hip joint movements

Hip joint movement	Stretched tissue
Flexion (while knee is flexed)	Posterior and inferior capsule
Extension (while the knee is extended)	Some fibers of the iliofemoral ligament (primary), anterior capsule, and pubofemoral and ischiofemoral ligaments
Abduction	Pubofemoral ligament
Adduction	Superior part of the iliofemoral ligament
Internal rotation	Ischiofemoral ligament and posterior capsule
External rotation	Iliofemoral and pubofemoral ligaments

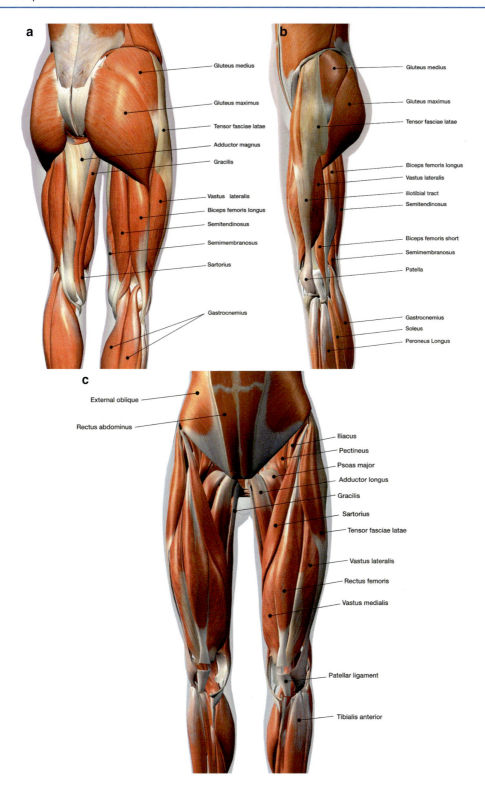

Fig. 13.4 Hip muscles responsible for joint movement: (**a**) Posterior (Hank Grebe/Shutterstock.com), (**b**) Lateral (Hank Grebe/Shutterstock.com), (**c**) Anterior view (Hank Grebe/Shutterstock.com)

muscles as extensors, and medial muscles as adductors. The actions and functions of the muscles associated with the hip joint movement are provided in Table 13.3, and the nerves responsible for the innervation of these muscles are listed in Table 13.4.

Table 13.3 Functions of the muscles involved in the movement of the hip joint

Muscle	Action	Function
Piriformis	• External rotation while extension • Abduction while flexion	When the sacrum is fixed, the piriformis muscle externally rotates, abducts, and flexes the femur. It assists in the posterior tilt of the pelvis when the femur is stationary and contracted bilaterally. It contributes to the internal rotation of the pelvis when contracted unilaterally ªExtending the leg when getting out of the car seat
Quadratus femoris	• External rotation	When the pelvis is fixed, the quadratus femoris muscle externally rotates the thigh. It assists in the posterior tilt of the pelvis when the femur is stationary and contracted bilaterally. It contributes to the internal rotation of the pelvis when contracted unilaterally
Obturator internus	• External rotation	When the pelvis is fixed, the obturator internus muscle externally rotates, flexes, and abducts the thigh. When the femur is fixed and contracts bilaterally, it tilts the pelvis anteriorly and makes an internal rotation
Obturator externus	• External rotation	When the pelvis is fixed, the obturator externus muscle externally rotates, flexes, and abducts the thigh. When the femur is stationary, it contracts anteriorly to the pelvis when it contracts bilaterally. When it contracts unilaterally, it tilts the pelvis posteriorly and makes an internal rotation
Psoas major	• Flexion	When the vertebral column is fixed, the psoas major muscle produces hip flexion. It also works as a weak adductor and external rotator. It flexes the trunk when the hip is fixed. ªStepping on the ladder.
Iliacus	• Flexion • External rotation	The iliacus muscle flexes the hip when the pelvis is fixed. When the femur is fixed, it tilts the pelvis when contracted bilaterally. It flexes the trunk when the hip is fixed ªStepping on the ladder
Gluteus maximus	• Extension • Internal rotation and flexion (anterior fibers) • External rotation and extension (posterior fibers)	Deep layer: When the femur is fixed, the gluteus maximus muscle tilts the pelvis posteriorly when it contracts bilaterally, and when it contracts unilaterally, it tilts the pelvis posteriorly and makes an internal rotation Superficial layer: It makes the femur in extension, external rotation, and abduction ªChanging from sitting position to standing position
Gluteus medius	• Abduction • Internal rotation and flexion (anterior fibers) • External rotation and extension (posterior fibers)	When the hip is fixed, the main task of the gluteus medius muscle is the abduction of the hip. When a person is on the ground on one foot, it makes the pelvis tilt laterally. It stabilizes the pelvis while walking or standing on one foot. Its anterior fibers assist in flexion and posterior fibers in extension. When the femur is fixed, it plays a role in both the anterior and the posterior tilt of the pelvis due to the contraction of its anterior or posterior fibers when it contracts bilaterally ªMovement of the hip in the direction of advancing when passing through a narrow space from side to side
Gluteus minimus	• Internal rotation • Abduction • Assist flexion	The most important task of the gluteus minimus muscle is to strengthen the anterior part of the gluteus medius. In addition to the abduction of the thigh, it also helps in flexion and internal rotation. When the femur is fixed, it assists in anterior tilt and external rotation of the pelvis when contracted bilaterally, and lateral tilt or external rotation of the pelvis when contracted unilaterally
Tensor fascia late	• Flexion • Abduction • Internal rotation	When the thigh and leg are fixed, the tensor fascia late muscle causes the pelvis to be anteriorly tilted when contracted bilaterally, and causes external rotation of the hip joint or lateral tilt of the pelvis when contracted unilaterally **It is active when balancing your body weight while standing on one leg. For example, kicking or falling off the block to ensure weight transfer from the hips to the feet when the goalkeeper is kicking

Table 13.3 (continued)

Muscle	Action	Function
Sartorius	• Flexion • Abduction • External rotation	When the thigh and leg are fixed, the sartorius muscle plays a role in the anterior tilt of the pelvis when contracted bilaterally, and in internal rotation or lateral tilt when contracted unilaterally [a]Crossing your legs
Adductor brevis	• Adduction • External rotation	When the thigh and leg are fixed, the adductor brevis muscle causes the pelvis to tilt anteriorly when contracted bilaterally, and laterally when contracted unilaterally [a]Hitting the ball with the inside of the foot
Adductor longus	• Adduction • External rotation	When the thigh and leg are fixed, the adductor longus muscle causes the pelvis to tilt anteriorly when contracted bilaterally, and laterally when contracted unilaterally [a]Kicking the ball with the inside of the foot
Adductor magnus	• Adduction • External rotation	When the thigh and leg are fixed, the adductor magnus muscle causes the pelvis to tilt anteriorly when contracted bilaterally, and laterally when contracted unilaterally [a]Kicking the ball with the inside of the foot
Pectineus	• Flexion • Adduction	The pectineus muscle helps stabilize the pelvis on the femur and allows for changes in the direction of movement
Gracilis	• Adduction • Flexion and internal rotation of knee	In adduction of the hip, the pectineus works together with the adductor brevis, adductor longus, and adductor magnus muscles. Gracilis is similar to sartorius in form and function [a]Putting the leg into car before sitting to the car seat
Gemellus superior	• External rotation	The obturator and gemellus muscles work together as a result, pulling the femur downward relative to the pelvis when the pelvis is stable, and pulling the pelvis upward relative to the femur when the femur is stationary. The obturator and gemellus muscles support the pelvis like a hammock
Gemellus inferior	• External rotation of the hip	

[a] Examples of muscle functions during activities of daily living

Table 13.4 Muscles responsible for hip joint movement and nerves that innervate them

Nerves	Muscles they innervate
Femoral	• Iliacus • Sartorius • Pectineus • Rectus femoris
Gluteus superior	• Gluteus medius • Gluteus minimus • Tensor fascia lata
Gluteus inferior	• Gluteus maximus
Sacral plexus (L_5–S_1)	• Quadratus femoris • Obturator internus • Gemellus superior • Gemellus inferior
Tibial branch of the sciatic nerve	• Semitendinosus • Semimembranosus • Biceps femoris (long head) • Adductor magnus (hamstring part)
Obturator	• Gracilis • Adductor magnus (anterior part) • Adductor longus • Adductor brevis • Obturator externus
Sacral plexus (L_5–S_{1-2})	• Piriformis
Anterior branches of the lumbar spinal nerves (L_{1-2-3})	• Psoas major
Lumbar spinal nerves (L_{1-2})	• Psoas minor
Peroneal branch of the sciatic nerve	• Biceps femoris (short head)

13.4 Palpation of Bones and Muscles in the Hip Joint

Palpation of the muscle and bony prominences of the hip joint helps in understanding the abnormal changes in these areas. Comparison of palpation by doing it bilaterally gives more meaningful results. Cold hands during palpation cause unwanted muscle contractions. In addition, clinical experience and knowledge of anatomy are necessary for the interpretation of palpation findings. How to palpate the muscle and bone in the hip joint is described in Table 13.5.

Table 13.5 Muscle and bone palpation of the hip joint

Muscle palpation	
Psoas	**Position:** The patient lies supine with hip and knee flexed **Palpation:** The iliac wing is found with the fingertips. The fingertips are slid upward, medially, and deeply toward the lateral vertebral bodies of the lumbar spine; then, the fingertips are moved back and forth to palpate the oblique fibers of the muscle. Meanwhile, resisted hip flexion is performed with the other hand and the psoas muscle is palpated
Iliacus	**Position:** The patient lies on his back **Palpation:** The iliac wing is found with the fingertips; the fingertips are slid inward, medially, and deeply along the anterior surface of the ilium, and the fan-shaped fibers of the iliacus are felt with the fingertips. At this time, resisted hip flexion is performed with the other hand and the iliacus muscle is palpated
Sartorius	**Position:** The patient lies supine with hip external rotation and knee flexion **Palpation:** Spina iliaca anterior superior (SIAS) is found with fingertips. The fingertips are slid down and medially along the lateral edge of the femoral triangle. The fingers are allowed to remain superficial to find the ribbon-like fibers of the sartorius. At this time, the muscle is palpated by performing resistant hip flexion and external rotation with the other hand
Tensor fascia lata	**Position:** The patient lies supine in the hip external rotation position **Palpation:** SIAS is found with fingertips. The fingertips are slid outward and downward on the femur. At this time, the muscle is palpated by performing resistant hip flexion and abduction with the other hand
Pectineus	**Position:** The patient lies on his back **Palpation:** The patient stands on the side facing the thigh. The upper ramus of the pubis is found with the fingertips. The fingertips are shifted outward and distally (toward the sartorius). Between the iliopsoas and medial adductors, the descending fibers of the pectineus are palpated by resisting hip flexion and adduction with the other hand
Adductor brevis	**Position:** The patient lies on his back with the hip externally rotated **Palpation:** The pubis is localized with the lateral edge of the palmar surface of the hand, and the palmar surface of the hand is displaced outward and downward toward the sartorius. The descending fibers of the adductor brevis are palpated by resisting hip flexion and adduction with the other hand, between the pectineus and the medial adductor
Adductor longus	**Position:** The patient lies supine with the hip externally rotated **Palpation:** The pubis is localized with the lateral edge of the palmar surface of the hand, and the thickest tendon is palpated by sliding the palmar surface of the hand outward and downward toward the sartorius. Resisted hip flexion and adduction are performed with the other hand **Caution:** The femoral triangle is adjacent to the adductor longus and contains the lymph nodes as well as the femoral nerve, artery, and vein. The distal inguinal fold should be palpated to avoid compressing these structures
Adductor magnus	**Position:** The patient lies face down **Palpation:** Fingertips and ischial protrusion are found. The fingertips are slid medially and distally toward the medial condyle. In the middle of the thigh, between the gracilis and the medial part of the hamstring, the descending fibers of the muscle are palpated by adduction of the resistant hip with the other hand
Piriformis	**Position:** The patient lies face down **Palpation:** The lateral edge of the sacrum is found with the fingertips. The fingertips are shifted laterally and distally toward the greater trochanter. With the other hand, resistive external rotation of the hip is performed, and the muscle fibers are palpated on the upper surface of the greater trochanter **Caution:** The sciatic nerve is located close to the muscle belly of the piriformis. It should be palpated, avoiding compression

Table 13.5 (continued)

Quadratus femoris	**Position:** The patient lies face down **Palpation:** The fingertips are localized proximal to the ischial process. The fingertips are shifted laterally and distally toward the greater trochanter. With the other hand, resisted external rotation of the hip is performed in knee flexion, and muscle fibers are palpated between the greater and lesser trochanters
Obturator internus	**Position:** The patient lies face down **Palpation:** The fingertips are localized on the lower surface of the obturator foramen, and the fingertips are slid lateral to the greater trochanter. With the other hand, resisted external rotation of the hip in knee flexion is made and the muscle fibers are palpated from the medial surface of the greater trochanter
Obturator externus	**Position:** The patient lies face down **Palpation:** The fingertips are localized proximal to the ischial process; the fingertips are shifted laterally and distally (toward the greater trochanter). The muscle fibers are palpated in the trochanteric fossa by performing the external rotation of the hip with resistance in knee flexion with the other hand
Gluteus maximus	**Position:** The patient lies face down **Palpation:** The lateral edge of the sacrum is found with the fingertips, and the fingertips are shifted laterally and distally (toward the greater trochanter). The superficial fibers of the muscle are palpated by performing a resistant hip extension with the other hand
Gluteus medius	**Position:** The patient lies face down **Palpation:** Iliac process is found with the fingertips, and the fingertips are slid toward the greater trochanter. With the other hand, resistive hip abduction is performed, and the muscle fibers are palpated lateral to the greater trochanter
Gluteus minimus	**Position:** The patient lies face down **Palpation:** The iliac process is found with the fingertips, and the fingertips are slid toward the greater trochanter. With the other hand, resistive hip abduction is performed, and the muscle fibers are palpated lateral to the greater trochanter
Gracilis	**Position:** The patient lies on his back with the hips externally rotated and the knees slightly flexed **Palpation:** The medial condyle of the femur is found with the palm of the hand; the most prominent tendon in this region is followed by sliding the palm toward the proximal pubis. With the other hand, resistive hip adduction and knee flexion are performed, and the proximal, long, thin fibers of the muscle are palpated proximally
Gemellus superior	**Position:** The patient lies face down **Palpation:** The fingertips are shifted laterally to the greater trochanter. The muscle fibers are palpated on the medial surface of the greater trochanter by performing the external rotation of the hip with resistance in knee flexion with the other hand
Gemellus inferior	**Position:** The patient lies face down **Palpation:** Fingertips are shifted laterally to the greater trochanter. The muscle fibers are palpated on the medial surface of the greater trochanter by performing the external rotation of the hip with resistance in knee flexion with the other hand
Bone palpation	
Spina iliaca anterior superior (SIAS)	**Position:** The patient lies on his back **Palpation:** Iliac wing is found with the fingertips. Fingertips are slid forward and downward. Under the hand, the large bony prominence SIAS is palpated
Spina iliaca anterior inferior (SIAI)	**Position:** The patient lies on his back **Palpation:** Iliac wing is found with the fingertips. The fingertips are slid forward and down, and the SIAS is found. Then, the fingertips are continuously slid forward and downward, and the SIAI is palpated, a small bony prominence deeper than the SIAS **Note:** It is a projection slightly below the SIAS
Spina iliaca posterior superior (SIPS)	**Position:** The patient lies face down **Palpation:** Lumbar spinous processes are found with the fingertips. Round and prominent SIPS are palpated by sliding the fingertips downward **Note:** Posteriorly, the line connecting the iliac crest passes through the L_{4-5} interspinous space. Posteriorly, the line connecting the SIPS passes through S_2; descending from S_2, the sacrum and coccyx can be palpated

(continued)

Table 13.5 (continued)	
Pubis ramus	**Position:** The patient lies on his back
	Palpation: The iliac wing is found with the fingertips. The fingertips are slid inward and slightly downward. A broad and flat protrusion, pubis ramus, is palpated
Ischial protrusion	**Position:** The patient lies face down
	Palpation: The greater trochanter is found with the fingertips. From the greater trochanter to the gluteal line, the large, rounded ischial prominence is palpated by deeply moving the fingertips downward and inward
	It is a rough, blunt projection of the lower part of the body that bears weight when sitting. It provides attachment to the hamstring and adductor magnus muscles
Greater trochanter	**Position:** The patient lies on his side with the palpable side up
	Palpation: The iliac wing is found by advancing laterally with the fingertips. Fingertips are slid downward so that the femur is parallel. A large, rounded protuberance is palpated a few centimeters below the iliac wing

13.5 Movements in the Hip Joint

The hip is the joint with the maximum range of motion in the body, after the shoulder joint. It has the ability to move in the directions of flexion–extension in the sagittal plane, abduction–adduction in the frontal plane, and internal–external rotation in the horizontal plane.

13.5.1 Joints Associated with Movements Occurring in the Hip Joint

The right and left hip joints are connected through the pelvis and lumbosacral joint. The movement of the hip joint is closely related to the movements of the pelvis and lumbar spine. The femur, pelvis, and spine move in concert to produce a greater range of motion than the joint range of motion produced by a single segment. Similar to the scapulohumeral movement, the combination of movements in several joints helps to increase the range of motion available for the distal segment. Table 13.6 shows the hip joint movements in the standing and upright positions and the associated movements between the pelvis and the lumbar spine.

Table 13.6 Associated movements between the hip joint, pelvis, and lumbar spine in the right extremity in standing and upright position

Hip joint movement (Right)	Pelvic movement (On the right)	Lumbar spine movement
Flexion	Anterior pelvic tilt	Lumbar extension
Extension	Posterior pelvic tilt	Lumbar flexion
Abduction	Lateral pelvic tilt (up)	Left lateral flexion
Adduction	Lateral pelvic tilt (down)	Right lateral flexion
Internal rotation	Forward rotation	Left rotation
External rotation	Backward rotation	Right rotation

13.6 Evidence-Based Exercises in Which the Muscles Involved in Hip Joint Movements Work According to the Exercise Type

The exercises based on evidence that the muscles involved in the movements occurring in the hip joint work according to the exercise type are shown in Table 13.7.

Table 13.7 Evidence-based exercises in which the muscles involved in hip joint movements work according to the exercise type

Muscle	Exercise type	Exercise name/position
Gluteus maximus	Concentric	• Squat • One-leg squat[a] • Deadlift, single-leg deadlift[a] • Clam exercise • Forward-back-to-side lunge • Step-up and step-down • Leg press • Bridging • Single-leg bridging
	Explosive	• Multiplanar hop
	Stretching	• Pulling knee to the abdomen in the supine position
Gluteus medius	Concentric	• Hip abduction in the side-lying position[a] • Hip abduction in the standing upright position • Clam exercise • Side walking with an elastic band • Hip hike • Side bridge
	Eccentric	• Hip drops
Gluteus minimus	Concentric	• Hip abduction and extension in the side-lying position[a] • Hip abduction in the side-lying position
Iliopsoas	Concentric	• Straight leg lift in the supine position
Adductor longus	Concentric	• Lunge • Step-up • Leg press
Adductor brevis	Concentric	• Lunge • Step-up • Leg press
Adductor magnus	Concentric	• Lunge • Step-up • Leg press
Tensor fascia lata	Concentric	• Hip abduction in the side-lying position • Hip abduction in the standing upright position • Clam exercise • Side walking with an elastic band
Gemellus superior, obturator externus	Concentric	• Clam exercise
Quadratus femoris	Concentric	• Step-down • One-leg squat
Sartorius	Concentric	• Lunge • Step-up • Leg press
Piriformis	Concentric	• Hip extension in the prone position with hip externally rotated (knee in full extension) • Clam exercise
	Stretching	• In the supine position, the ankle of the leg to be stretched is placed on the knee of the other leg and grasped under the knee and pulled to the chest
Gracilis	Concentric	• Step-up • Leg press

[a] The exercise with the highest muscle activation during workout

13.7 Conclusion

The hip joint is a ball-and-socket joint surrounded by strong and well-balanced muscles. It is a stable joint with a wide range of motion in many planes. The hip joint, the structural link between the lower extremities and the axial skeleton, not only transmits forces from the ground but also absorbs forces from the trunk, head, neck, and upper extremities. Therefore, the hip joint is one of the most important joints in both daily life activities and sports activities. A good understanding of hip anatomy and the forces acting on the joint can enhance current and future knowledge.

Further Reading

Bsat S, Frei H, Beaulé P. The acetabular labrum: a review of its function. Bone Joint J. 2016;98(6):730–5.

Castro MP, de Brito Fontana H, Fóes MC, Santos GM, Ruschel C, Roesler H. Activation of the gluteus maximus, gluteus medius and tensor fascia lata muscles during hip internal and external rotation exercises at three hip flexion postures. J Bodyw Mov Ther. 2021;27:487–92.

Field RE, Rajakulendran K. The labro-acetabular complex. J Bone Joint Surg Am. 2011;93(2):22–7.

Gulick DT, Fagnani JA, Gulick CN. Comparison of muscle activation of hip belt squat and barbell back squat techniques. Isonet Exerc Sci. 2015;23(2):101–8.

Hamstra-Wright KL, Bliven KH. Effective exercises for targeting the gluteus medius. J Sport Rehabil. 2012;21(3):296–300.

Jepson P, Beswick A, Smith T, Sands G, Drummond A, Sackley C. Assistive devices, hip precautions, environmental modifications and training to prevent dislocation and improve function after hip arthroplasty. Cochrane Database Syst Rev. 2013;11:CD01815.

Konrad A, Močnik R, Titze S, Nakamura M, Tilp M. The influence of stretching the hip flexor muscles on performance parameters. A systematic review with meta-analysis. Int J Environ Res Public Health. 2021;18(4):1936.

Lunn DE, Lampropoulos A, Stewart TD. Basic biomechanics of the hip. J Orthop Trauma. 2016;30(3):239–46.

Snell RS. The lower limb. In: Mehta V, Suri RK, editors. Snell's clinical anatomy. New Delhi: Wolters Kluwer India; 2018. p. 494–598.

Wyatt M, Freeman C, Beck M. Fractures of the hip. In: Castoldi F, Bonasia DE, editors. Anatomy of the hip joint. Springer; 2019. p. 1–18.

Ng KG, Jeffers JR, Beaulé PE. Hip joint capsular anatomy, mechanics, and surgical management. J Bone Joint Surg Am. 2019;101(23):2141.

Nelitz M. Femoral derotational osteotomies. Curr Rev Musculoskelet. 2018;11(2):272–9.

Zaghloul A, Mohamed EM. Hip joint: embryology, anatomy, and biomechanics. Biomed J Sci Tech Res. 2018;12(3):9304–18.

Malagelada F, Tayar R, Barke S, Stafford G, Field RE. Anatomy of the zona orbicularis of the hip: a magnetic resonance study. Surg Radiol Anat. 2015;37(1):11–8.

Lee KE, Baik SM, Yi CH, Kim SH. Electromyographic analysis of gluteus maximus, gluteus medius, hamstring and erector spinae muscles activity during the bridge exercise with hip external rotation in different knee flexion angles in healthy subjects. Phys Ther Korea. 2019;26(3):91–8.

Macadam P, Cronin J, Contreras B. An examination of the gluteal muscle activity associated with dynamic hip abduction and hip external rotation exercise: a systematic review. Int J Sports Phys Ther. 2015;10(5):573.

Moore D, Semciw AI, McClelland J, Wajswelner H, Pizzari T. Rehabilitation exercises for the gluteus minimus muscle segments: an electromyography study. J Sport Rehabil. 2019;28(6):544–51.

Morimoto Y, Oshikawa T, Imai A, Okubo Y, Kaneoka K. Piriformis electromyography activity during prone and side-lying hip joint movement. J Phys Ther Sci. 2018;30(1):154–8.

Ward SR, Winters TM, Blemker SS. The architectural design of the gluteal muscle group: implications for movement and rehabilitation. J Orthop Sports Phys Ther. 2010;40(2):95–102.

The Knee

14

Abdulhamit Tayfur and Beyza Tayfur

Abstract

The knee joint consists of tibiofemoral and patellofemoral compartments. The knee joint is vulnerable to traumatic injuries as it is located at the end of long lever arms of two long bones, the femur and tibia. The femoral condyles articulate with the nearly flat proximal articular surface of the tibia. Wide ligaments, joint capsule, menisci, and large muscles take part in the knee stabilization. Therefore, the stabilization is provided by ligaments and muscles surrounding the joint rather than the bone structures. Movements in the knee take place in two planes that allow flexion-extension and internal-external rotation. The soft tissues around the knee joint are usually exposed to large muscular or external forces during various activities. High functional loads on the knee often cause ligament, meniscus, and articular cartilage injuries. A better understanding of knee anatomy and kinesiology is important to understand most of the injury mechanisms and, as a result, to prescribe and implement appropriate rehabilitation programs. In this chapter, characteristics of the non-contractile and contractile anatomical structures of the knee joint, palpation of these structures, the movements occurring in the joint, and the evidence-based exercises for muscles involved in these movements will be explained.

14.1 Non-contractile Structures in the Knee Joint

14.1.1 Bone Structures

The bones that the muscles in the knee attached are the femur, patella, tibia, and fibula. The bony structures and important bony prominences in the knee and the muscles attached to these structures are shown in Table 14.1.

The femur is the longest bone in the human body (Fig. 14.1). At its proximal end is the spherical head of the femur. At the junction of the femoral neck and body, there is the greater trochanter on the projection extending upwards, and the lesser trochanter on the posterior, lower and inner side of it. Between the two trochanters, there are the intertrochanteric line anteriorly and the intertrochanteric crest posteriorly. The femoral body is slightly convex anteriorly. There is a rough surface called the linea aspera extending downwards in the posterior part of the femoral body and is

A. Tayfur
School of Physical Therapy and Rehabilitation,
Kırşehir Ahi Evran University, Kirsehir, Turkey
e-mail: abdulhamit.tayfur@ahievran.edu.tr

B. Tayfur (✉)
School of Kinesiology, University of Michigan,
Ann Arbor, MI, USA
e-mail: beyzat@umich.edu

Table 14.1 Bone protrusions in the knee joint and the muscles attached to these protrusions

Bone protrusions	Muscles
Attaches to the base of the patella (via the quadriceps tendon) and the tibial tuberosity (via the patellar tendon)	Rectus femoris
Starting from the linea aspera (medial lip) and intertrochanteric line of the femur, it attaches to the medial edge of the patella and the tibial tuberosity (via the patellar tendon)	Long head of vastus medialis
Starting from the linea aspera (distal part) and the supracondylar line of the femur, it attaches to the knee joint capsule, medial surface of the patella, medial to the quadriceps tendon and to the tibial tuberosity (via the patellar tendon)	Vastus medialis oblique
Starting from the linea aspera, the greater trochanter (lower part) and the intertrochanteric line of the femur, attaches to the base and lateral edge of the patella (via the quadriceps tendon), the tibial tuberosity (via the patellar tendon) and the knee joint capsule	Vastus lateralis
Starting from the upper, lateral, and anterior surface of the two-third of the femoral body, it attaches to the lateral base of the patella, the lateral tibial condyle, and the tibial tuberosity (via the patellar tendon)	Vastus intermedius
Attaches to the lateral to the head of the fibula and the fibular collateral ligament	Long head of biceps femoris
Starting from the linea aspera and the lateral condyle of the femur, it attaches to the lateral tibial condyle	Short head of biceps femoris
Attaches to the proximal body of the tibia, the medial tibial condyle (lower part), the tibial tuberosity, and the pes anserine	Semitendinosus
Attaches to medial tibial condyle (lower part) and the oblique popliteal ligament	Semimembranosus
Starting from the medial condyle of the femur, the popliteal surface of the femur, and the knee joint capsule	Medial head of gastrocnemius
Starting from the lateral condyle of the femur, the lateral surface of the femur, the supracondylar line of the femur, and the knee joint capsule	Lateral head of gastrocnemius
Starting from the lateral condyle of the femur and the popliteal ligament, it attaches to the adjacent posterior margin of the lateral meniscus, the head of the fibula (via the popliteofibular ligament), and the linea musculi solei on the posterior surface of the tibia	Popliteus
Starting from the lateral supracondylar line of the femur	Plantaris
Attaches to the medial body of the tibia, the medial part of the tibial tuberosity, and the pes anserine	Gracilis
Attaches to the proximal medial surface of the tibial body, the medial part of the tibial tuberosity, and the knee joint capsule	Sartorius
Attaches to the lower one-third of the femur via the iliotibial band	Tensor fascia lata (TFL)
Attaches to the middle part of the linea aspera (via the aponeurosis) of the femur	Adductor longus
Attaches to the upper part of the linea aspera (via the aponeurosis) of the femur	Adductor brevis
Attaches to the linea aspera (via the aponeurosis), the adductor tubercle on the medial supracondylar line, and the medial condyle of the femur	Adductor magnus

divided into two parts, medial lip and lateral lip towards the middle part of the body. On the outer side of the upper lateral lip, there is the gluteal tuberosity, and on the outer side of the medial lip, there is the pectineal line. These two parts are separated from each other and borders the popliteal surface externally and internally in the posterior distal part of the femoral body. The distal end of the femur consists of the medial and lateral condyles and the intercondylar fossa between the condyles and is thicker than the proximal femur. The articular surfaces on the condyles unite to form the patellar surface. The most protruding parts of the distal end are called the medial and lateral epicondyles. Above the medial epicondyle is the adductor tubercle.

The tibia is a long bone located medial to the leg (Fig. 14.1). On the anterior side of its proximal

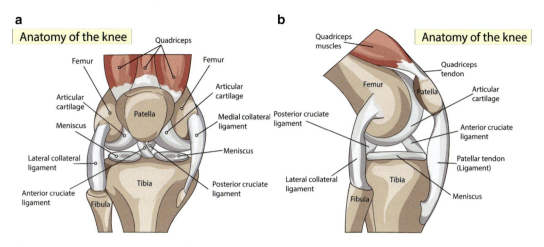

Fig. 14.1 (**a**, **b**) Knee anatomy (Viktoriia_P/Shutterstock.com)

end, there is a large and wide protuberance called the tibial tuberosity, and on the upper side, there are medial and lateral condyles that articulate with the femur condyles. While the articular surface on the lateral tibial condyle is round, the articular surface on the medial tibial condyle is oval and deeper than the lateral one. Between these two articular surfaces is the intercondylar eminence. The posterior and inferior part of the lateral tibial condyle is the articular surface that articulates with the head of the fibula. The body of the tibia has three aspects (medial, lateral, and posterior) and three edges (anterior, medial, and interosseus (or lateral)). On the posterior aspect is the soleal line.

The patella is the largest sesamoid bone in the human body, containing the thickest cartilage layer and located within the junction of the patellar and quadriceps tendons (Fig. 14.1). It resembles an inverted triangle as its base is above and its apex is below. It has five surfaces: superior, inferior, lateral, medial, and odd. The anterior surface of the patella is raised and rough, while the posterior surface is slightly concave. The main function of the patella is to increase the force released by the quadriceps femoris muscle by acting as a lever. Since the patella keeps the quadriceps tendon away from the movement axis, it increases the efficiency of the extension during the last 30° of extension movement. Patella also acts as a guide for the quadriceps and patellar tendon, reduces the friction of the quadriceps mechanism (extension mechanism consisting of

> **Clinical Information**
> In chondromalacia patella (early degeneration of the patellar cartilage) or patellofemoral pain syndrome, the odd facet is the most common and first affected part of the patella.

the quadriceps tendon, patella, and patellar tendon), controls the capsular tension in the knee, and acts as a bone shield for the cartilage tissue on the femoral condylar surface.

The fibula is a long bone located lateral to the leg (Fig. 14.1). At its proximal end are the head of the fibula and the articular surface. The upper two-third of the body of the fibula has four edges (anterior, posterior (or lateral), medial, and interosseus) and four aspects (anterior, posterior, medial, and lateral).

14.1.2 Joint Capsule and Ligaments

14.1.2.1 Joint Capsule

The joint capsule is a fibrous tissue that surrounds the knee joint. It is supported by fascia, muscles, and ligaments. The anterior part of the joint capsule contains the patella, the quadriceps tendon, and the patellar tendon. It is also surrounded by the quadriceps muscle and medial and lateral patellar retinacular fibers. The lateral part of the joint capsule contains the lateral collateral ligament, the lateral patellar retinacular fibers, and the iliotibial band. The biceps femoris muscle, the popliteus muscle tendon, and the lateral head of the gastrocnemius muscle are important structures that support the lateral joint capsule. The posterior part of the capsule is surrounded by oblique and arcuate popliteal ligaments. The popliteus, gastrocnemius, and hamstring muscles, especially the fibrous extensions of the semimembranosus tendon, are important muscles that support the posterior part of the joint capsule. The postero-lateral portion of the joint capsule is supported by the arcuate popliteal ligament, the lateral collateral ligament, the popliteus tendon, and the popliteofibular ligament. The tendons and ligaments associated with the postero-lateral portion of the joint capsule are collectively referred to as the "posterolateral corner." The posterolateral corner is a vulnerable area and is frequently injured along with other ligaments in the knee (such as the medial collateral ligament or the anterior cruciate ligament). Medial part of the joint capsule starts from the patellar tendon and extends to the medial of the posterior capsule. The anterior of the medial capsule is reinforced by the medial patellar retinacular fibers, while the medial of the capsule is additionally supported by the superficial and deep fibers of the medial collateral ligament. Posterior of the medial capsule starts from the adductor tubercle and continues by merging with the extensions of the semimembranosus tendon. Since the tissue is quite prominent, it is also supported by the pes anserine tendon, which is also called the "posterior oblique ligament" and formed by the union of the sartorius, gracilis, and semitendinosus muscles. This structure is very important in providing knee joint stability.

14.1.2.2 Cruciate Ligaments

Cruciate ligaments are one of the most important intra-articular structures in stabilizing the knee joint. The cruciate ligaments covered by the synovial membrane are supplied by the medial genicular artery. Blood flow is mostly provided by small veinlets in the synovial membrane. The cruciate ligaments are called anterior and posterior cruciate ligaments according to their attachment points on the tibia bone. Both ligaments are quite thick and strong. Due to their structure and anatomical location, they prevent excessive movements that may occur in the knee joint and contribute greatly to stabilization. Their most important task is to limit the anterior and posterior gliding and shearing movements that occur between the tibia and femur bones. Due to their diagonal and oblique positions, they contribute to stabilization by limiting the excessive movement of the joint, especially during pivoting and cutting movements. Cruciate ligaments are also rich in mechanoreceptors. In this way, besides mechanical knee stabilization, they provide important proprioceptive feedback to the central nervous system about the joint position.

Anterior Cruciate Ligament

The anterior cruciate ligament starts from the medial side of the lateral femoral condyle and attaches to the anterior of the tibial plateau between the two condyles (Fig. 14.1). The collagen fibers of the ligament rotate around each other, forming a spiral structure. This spiral structure divides the ligament into two main bundles, anteromedial and posterolateral. The tension and spiral structure of these bundles change during knee flexion and extension movements. In particular, the posterolateral bundle is stretched during full extension of the knee, while it relaxes with increasing flexion of the knee. The posterior joint capsule together with the posterolateral bundle, the posterior parts of the collateral ligaments, and the knee flexor muscles remain tense during knee extension, thereby stabilizing the knee joint. These structures can be damaged as a result of forcing the joint into excessive extension.

> **To Learn Easily**
>
> The ACL is located in the direction of inserting the hand into the pocket. It attaches to the eminence of the tibia, starting from proximal lateral to anterior, medial, and distal. In this position, the same directional forces that move your middle finger can stretch the ligament and cause it to break.

During the last 60° of knee extension, the quadriceps femoris muscle begins to pull the tibia forward, causing the tibia to slide forward under the femur. The anterior cruciate ligament restricts the forward sliding movement of the tibia on the femur to keep this movement within safe limits. The force of the quadriceps muscle that is pulling the tibia forward, hence the tension force on the anterior cruciate ligament, increases as the knee is extended and reaches its maximum in the full extension position. This is because the angle of attachment of the patellar tendon to the tibia changes during knee extension. Therefore, the quadriceps femoris muscle is seen as an antagonist of the anterior cruciate ligament. When the muscle contracts, the fibers of the ligament are stretched, stabilizing the joint.

> **Clinical Information**
> The anterior cruciate ligament is one of the most important structures in the control of pivoting movement. It controls the rotational movement of the tibia under the femur due to its diagonal position. When the ligament cannot fulfill its function, the tibia rotates in the anterolateral direction.

The anterior cruciate ligament is the most vulnerable ligament to injury in the knee due to its anatomical location and function. It prevents most movements in the knee joint from occurring excessively. For this reason, forcing the physiological limits of knee movements also forces the anterior cruciate ligament. The anterior cruciate ligament is most commonly injured during landing, sudden deceleration, cutting, or excessive trunk rotation while on one leg. In general, the ligament may be overstretched and ruptured with a strong contraction of the quadriceps femoris during full extension or slight flexion of the knee, excessive valgus of the knee when landing after the jump, and excessive internal rotation of the femur on the fixed tibia. In general, the ligament may be overstretched and ruptured with a strong contraction of the quadriceps femoris during full extension or slight flexion of the knee, excessive valgus of the knee when landing after the jump, and excessive internal rotation of the femur on the fixed tibia. In addition to the anterior cruciate ligament, injuries to the posterior part of the joint capsule and medial collateral ligament may also occur in excessive knee extension injuries.

Posterior Cruciate Ligament
The posterior cruciate ligament attaches between the condyles on the posterior surface of the tibia, starting from the lateral of the medial femoral condyle (facing the articular surface). It is thicker than the anterior cruciate ligament. It consists of two bundles, anterolateral and posteromedial which are smaller in size. The fibers of the posterior cruciate ligament also change their spiral structure and tension during the knee movement similar to the anterior cruciate ligament. The tension on the posterior cruciate ligament increases with knee flexion angle, especially between 90 and 120°. For this reason, posterior cruciate ligament injuries are often seen in the knee flexion position. The hamstring muscles pull the tibia by sliding it backwards under the femur during knee flexion. The posterior cruciate ligament begins to stretch with knee flexion to keep this sliding movement within normal limits. Because of this relationship, the hamstring muscles are considered the antagonist of the posterior cruciate ligament. The antagonist relationship increases in parallel with the knee flexion degree and ligament resistance with muscle pulling force. In addition to flexion, the posterior cruciate ligament also limits excessive varus-valgus stresses and excessive rotations of the knee.

The posterior cruciate ligament is stretched when the squat is performed suddenly, as it also prevents the femur from sliding forward on the tibial plateau. The joint capsule and surrounding muscles also help the posterior cruciate ligament to prevent the femur from sliding forward on the tibia. Especially the tendon of the popliteus muscle supports the posterior lateral part of the knee diagonally, hence restricts the forward sliding of the femur and helps the posterior cruciate ligament. Posterior cruciate ligament injuries are rare. If the ligament is injured, the anterior displacement of the femur on the tibia cannot be controlled. The posterior cruciate ligament is usually injured in accidents that cause multiple injuries to the knee joint, such as traffic accidents, or in situations that force the ligament, such as falling on the knee when the knee is fully flexed.

> **Clinical Information**
> One of the most common injury mechanisms of the posterior cruciate ligament is the excessive forward sliding of the femur on the tibia due to sudden stop of a vehicle while sitting in it with the knee in the flexion position. In posterior cruciate ligament injuries, there is difficulty in joint stabilization in activities such as going downstairs or running downhill.

14.1.2.3 Collateral Ligaments

The collateral ligaments take part in the stabilization of the medial (medial collateral ligament) and lateral (lateral collateral ligament) knee joint. Especially during full extension of the knee, collateral ligaments are stretched together with the posteromedial joint capsule, the flexor muscles of the knee, and the anterior cruciate ligament.

Medial Collateral Ligament

The medial collateral ligament is flat and wide and is located medial to the knee joint (Fig. 14.1). It consists of two main parts which are called superficial and deep parts due to their locations. The superficial part is outside the joint capsule and starts from the medial condyle of the femur, blends with the medial retinacular fibers of the patella, and attaches to the medial and proximal part of the tibia. The deep part is inside the joint capsule and starts from the medial condyle of the femur, joins the posteromedial of the joint capsule, the medial meniscus, and the tendon of the semimembranosus muscle. The main task of the medial collateral ligament is to prevent excessive medial movement (e.g., valgus) of the knee joint. The medial collateral ligament is stretched during full extension of the knee joint and might be injured due to valgus loads occurring in this position. During this loading, the anterior cruciate ligament and joint capsule may also be affected.

Lateral Collateral Ligament

The lateral collateral ligament is a narrow strip structure and is a strong ligament (Fig. 14.1). Starting from the lateral epicondyle of the femur, it mixes distally with the biceps femoris muscle tendon and attaches to the head of the fibula. In contrast to the medial collateral ligament, the lateral collateral ligament does not unite with its neighbor, the lateral meniscus, because the tendon of the popliteus muscle passes between these two structures. The main task of the lateral collateral ligament is to prevent excessive lateral movement (e.g., varus) of the knee.

14.1.2.4 Medial Patellofemoral Ligament

The medial patellar retinacular fibers are a wide ligament that starts from the medial corner of the patella and attaches to the femur, tibia, medial meniscus, and distal part of the vastus medialis muscle. It is responsible for the medial stabilization of the patella. It is stretched more during the last 30° extension of the knee joint. At this angle, the tension of the ligament is further increased by the contraction of the vastus medialis muscle. This ligament is important for medial stabilization of the patella, as the patella moves away from the groove in the distal femur during knee extension. It can be injured during lateral dislocations of the patella.

14.1.2.5 Oblique Popliteal Ligament

The oblique popliteal ligament starts from the posteromedial of the joint capsule and the tendon of the semimembranosus muscle, runs laterally and superiorly, and ends by mixing with the joint capsule fibers close to the lateral femoral condyle. It is stretched during the tibial external rotation, which occurs during the full extension of the knee.

14.1.2.6 Arcuate Popliteal Ligament

It is divided into two parts, starting from the head of the fibula. The larger of these parts takes a curved shape and forms an *"arch"* and attaches to

Fig. 14.2 Meniscus anatomy (Alila Medical Media/Shutterstock.com)

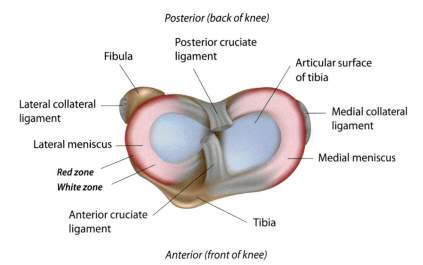

the side of the popliteus tendon, between the condyles at the posterior part of the tibia. Together with the posterior capsule, it helps to stabilize the posterior of the knee. The smaller part attaches posterior to the lateral femoral condyle and often to the sesamoid bone, which is embedded in the lateral head of the gastrocnemius muscle.

14.1.2.7 Popliteofibular Ligament

It lies between the popliteus tendon and the head of the fibula. It supports the knee joint capsule postero-laterally.

14.1.3 Other Structures

14.1.3.1 Meniscus

Menisci are crescent-shaped fibrocartilage structures. There are two, medial and lateral, which attach to the joint capsule on the outside and the intercondylar region of the tibia on the inside (Fig. 14.2). The parts that attach to the intercondylar region are called anterior and posterior horns. The menisci are attached to the joint capsule and tibia by coronary (menisco-tibial) ligaments. Since these ligaments are loose, they allow the menisci to move during knee joint movements. In addition, in the anterior part, the two menisci are connected to each other by a weak transverse ligament. Owing to their shape, they form light pads on the superior surface of the tibia where the femoral condyles can be placed and play an important role during stabilization.

The medial and lateral meniscuses have different shapes and attachments. The medial meniscus is oval in shape and its outer part is mixed with the fibers of the medial collateral ligament and joint capsule. On the other hand, the lateral meniscus is more rounded in shape and is attached to the outer fibers of the joint capsule without any ligaments. The popliteus tendon passes between the lateral meniscus and the joint capsule. There are also muscles that are connected to the menisci. The quadriceps and semimembranosus muscles are connected to both the medial and lateral meniscus, while the popliteus muscle is connected only with the lateral meniscus. These connections contribute to the stability and movement adaptability of the menisci during muscle contraction.

The main task of the menisci is to ensure the proper distribution of loads passing through the knee joint and to reduce the compression forces passing through the joint by acting as a buffer between the bones. The menisci prevent the joint surfaces from being damaged by contributing to the softer and smoother movement of the bone surfaces. At the same time, owing to their shape, they play an important role in stabilizing the joint and ensuring harmony between the tibia and the femur during movement. Menisci also make an important contribution to the sense of proprioception.

The blood supply to the menisci is provided by the genicular branches of the popliteal artery in the outer one-third part, and the outer part is called the "red zone" (Fig. 14.2). There is no blood supply in the inner parts of the menisci, this area is nourished by the synovial fluid. Thus, this area is called the "white zone." The thin part between the red and white zone is called the "red-white zone" due to its low blood supply. Healing capacity of the menisci after injury is directly related to the level of blood supply. While the healing capacity of the outer parts is high due to blood supply, the healing capacity of the inner parts is low due to no blood supply. The menisci are one of the most commonly injured structures in the knee. Strong rotational forces affecting the knee in flexion or weight-bearing positions constitute the most common injury mechanism of the menisci.

> **Clinical Information**
> It is very important to protect the menisci, especially due to its role in load distribution. Injury or surgical removal (meniscectomy) of the meniscus causes an increase in the load on the cartilage and, consequently, its wear. In this case, the risk of developing knee osteoarthritis increases.

> **Clinical Information**
> The medial meniscus is injured more often than the lateral meniscus. The most common injury mechanism in the medial meniscus is the position where forces are applied in the direction of knee valgus and internal rotation. In addition, it is injured along with structures such as the medial collateral ligament and the medial joint capsule.

14.1.3.2 Iliotibial Band

The iliotibial band is the continuation of the tensor fascia lata muscle and attaches to the lateral tubercle of the tibia by blending with the lateral patellar retinacular fibers. It assists in the lateral stability of the knee joint when the knee is in the extension position.

14.1.3.3 Plicas

The plicas are structures formed as a result of the folding of the synovial membrane in the inner layer of the knee joint capsule. Although their size is variable, they are most commonly located close to the patella (suprapatellar), inferior and medial to the knee. The plicas prevent excessive stretching of the synovial surface during joint movements, but they do not have any functional contributions. Plicas may not exist in every person. In cases where they are too large, they may cause knee pain. Especially the medial plica is the most common one and if it is large, it may cause medial knee pain due to trauma or irritation.

14.1.3.4 Bursae

Bursae are sacs filled with synovial fluid. It is usually found in areas where stress and friction are intense. They prevent tissue trauma that may occur as a result of repeated friction and increased stress between tissues. Due to the complex connections between tendons, ligaments, bones, joint capsule, and muscles in the knee joint, there are many bursae around the knee joint. The largest of these is the suprapatellar bursa, located on the patella, between the femur and the quadriceps femoris muscle. There are deep and superficial bursae below the patella (infrapatellar). The deep bursae are between the tibia and the patellar tendon, and the superficial bursae are between the lower border of the patella and the skin.

14.1.3.5 Medial and Lateral Patellar Retinacula

Medial and lateral patellar retinacular fibers are connective tissue extensions that surround the vastus lateralis, vastus medialis, and iliotibial band. These fibers form a web connection between the femur, tibia, patella, quadriceps and patellar tendon, collateral ligaments, and menisci. They are called medial or lateral according to their position.

14.1.3.6 Hoffa Fat Pad

Fat pads are structures that have similar functions to bursae, are located in areas where repetitive movements are frequent, and reduce stress and friction. In the knee joint, the suprapatellar and the deep infrapatellar bursae are associated with fat pads. Irritation of the infrapatellar fat pad (Hoffa fat pad) can be seen between the patella and the femoral condyle due to compression as a result of direct impact. In particular, repetitive and uncontrolled knee extension may cause irritation. Fat pads are among the most sensitive structures in the knee and their irritation is very painful.

14.1.4 Knee Joint and Associated Joints

The knee joint consists of two joints, the tibiofemoral and patellofemoral joints. Although the proximal tibiofibular joint is located in the knee region, it has no role in knee joint movements.

The tibiofemoral joint is the largest joint in the body. It is a hinge-type joint and connects the articular surfaces of the two long bones, the femur and tibia. Femoral condyles are convex, while tibial condyles are smaller and flatter. The tibiofemoral joint is closely related to the collateral and cruciate ligaments and the menisci. There are two menisci attached to the tibia to partially fill the joint space between the tibia and the femur and increase the harmony between the articular surfaces. Since the harmony between the bone surfaces forming the joint is insufficient, joint stability is mostly provided by muscles, ligaments, joint capsules, and menisci. Since the condyles of the femur provide a wide articular surface in the sagittal axis, the flexion-extension range of motion is high. The synovium around the joint is very large and is directly related to many structures around the knee joint.

> **Clinical Information**
> Since the wide range of motion and joint stabilization are mostly provided by the soft tissues, the knee joint is open to injuries.

The patellofemoral joint is a modified planar joint located in the anterior part of the knee between the patella and the trochlear groove of the femur. The patellofemoral joint capsule continues with the tibiofemoral joint capsule. The patellofemoral joint is directly related to the medial-lateral retinaculum, patellofemoral ligaments, quadriceps, and patellar tendon. Stabilization of the patellofemoral joint is provided by the alignment of the articular surfaces, the quadriceps muscle, and other soft tissues around it.

The proximal tibiofibular joint is a planar type synovial joint located between the tibia and the head of the fibula. It is supported by anterior and posterior ligaments of the same name as the joint. The movement also occurs in this joint during any activity associated with the ankle. The fibula can bear up to one-sixth of the body weight. Hypomobility, limitation, or loss of function in this joint can cause knee pain during activity. In approximately 10% of the population, the proximal tibiofibular joint capsule is fused with the tibiofemoral joint capsule.

14.2 Contractile Structures Associated with the Knee Joint

The muscles associated with the knee joint are mainly grouped as the muscles that flex, extend and rotate the knee (Fig. 14.3). The muscles involved in the knee joint, their movement and functions are given in Table 14.2, and the nerves responsible for innervation of these muscles are given in Table 14.3.

The primary muscle responsible for knee extension is the quadriceps femoris. It consists of

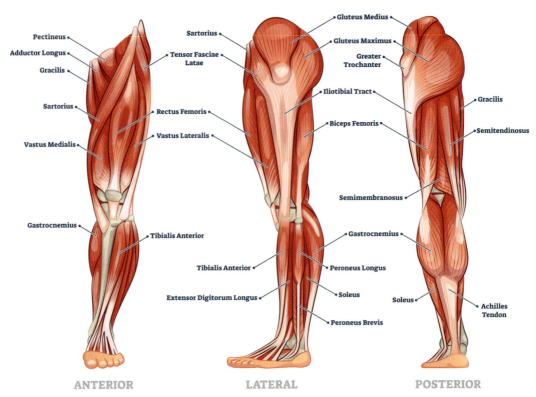

Fig. 14.3 Muscles around the knee (VectorMine/Shutterstock.com)

four parts: the rectus femoris, vastus medialis, vastus lateralis, and vastus intermedius. The rectus femoris starts in the pelvis from the anterior inferior iliac spine, while all other parts originate from the femoral body. The four parts of the quadriceps muscle fuse distally to form the quadriceps tendon and attach to the patella. The quadriceps femoris continues with the patellar tendon in the lower part of the patella and attaches to the tibial tuberosity. The patella and patellar tendon alignment is called the "knee extensor mechanism." While the vastus medialis, vastus lateralis, and vastus intermedius are responsible for knee extension, the rectus femoris muscle anatomically assists hip flexion in addition to knee extension, as it also crosses the hip joint.

The vastus lateralis is located lateral to the femur, the vastus medialis is located medial, the rectus femoris is located in the midline, and the vastus intermedius is located deep to the rectus femoris. While some of the vastus medialis muscle fibers are oblique, some are longitudinal. The oblique muscle fibers (vastus medialis obliquus) attach more distally to the patella at an angle of approximately 50°. The longitudinal fibers (vastus medialis longus) attach to the patella more flat and at an angle of about 15°. In particular, oblique fibers are important for medial movement and stabilization of the patella. Deeper to the vastus intermedius muscle is the articularis genu muscle, which is not very prominent. Starting from the distal anterior part of the femur and attaching to the anterior part of the joint capsule, the articularis genu muscle pulls the joint capsule and synovial membrane proximally during knee extension.

Except for the gastrocnemius muscle, the muscle group consisting of hamstrings, sartorius,

Table 14.2 Movements and functions of muscles involved in knee joint movement

Muscles	Movement	Function
Rectus femoris	• Knee extension • Hip flexion	Lock the knee joint in extension. They are active at the beginning of the stance phase of the gait (heel strike and loading), in the middle of the stance phase (extension begins after maximum flexion in the mid-stance phase), in the middle and end of the swing phase (lock the knee at the end of the deceleration). They work actively during many activities such as running, jumping, lunge, and kicking the ball
Vastus medialis, Vastus lateralis, Vastus intermedius	• Knee extension	
Long head of biceps femoris	• Knee flexion and external rotation • Hip extension and external rotation	They are active at the beginning of the stance phase of the gait (loading), in the middle of the stance phase (maximum flexion in the mid-stance phase), at the end of the stance phase (heel off and push), at the beginning and middle of the swing phase (acceleration). They work actively during many activities such as running, jumping, lunge and kicking the ball
Short head of biceps femoris	• Knee flexion and external rotation	
Semitendinosus	• Knee flexion and internal rotation • Hip extension and internal rotation	
Semimembranosus	• Knee flexion and internal rotation • Hip extension and internal rotation	
Gastrocnemius	• Knee flexion • Ankle plantarflexion and eversion	Helps knee flexion during walking. It is more active in ankle movements
Popliteus	• Knee flexion and internal rotation (when the proximal joint is fixed)	It initiates knee flexion by unlocking the knee joint. Therefore, it works in the first phase of all activities that require flexion when the knee is in full extension
Plantaris	• Knee flexion • Ankle plantarflexion	Helps knee flexion during walking. It is more active in ankle movements
Gracilis	• Knee flexion and internal rotation • Hip flexion and adduction	It positions the thigh and leg during crossed legs. It helps the medial collateral ligament and joint capsule during knee flexion and medial stabilization of the knee
Sartorius	• Knee flexion and internal rotation • Hip flexion, abduction, and external rotation	It positions the thigh and leg during crossed legs. It helps the medial collateral ligament and joint capsule during knee flexion and medial stabilization of the knee

Table 14.3 Nerves that innervate the muscles responsible for knee joint movement and the muscles they innervate

Nerves	The muscles they innervate
Femoral nerve	• Quadriceps femoris • Sartorius
Tibial nerve	• Long head of biceps femoris • Semitendinosus • Semimembranosus • Gastrocnemius • Popliteus • Plantaris
Common peroneal nerve	• Short head of biceps femoris
Obturator nerve	• Gracilis • Adductor longus

gracilis, and popliteus is called the knee flexor rotators, since all of the muscles that flex the knee joint also perform internal or external rotation of the knee.

Of the hamstring muscles, the semimembranosus, semitendinosus, and long head of the biceps femoris originate from the ischial tuberosity, and the short head of the biceps femoris originates from the lateral linea aspera of the femur. Distally, they cross the knee joint and attach to the tibia and fibula. The semimembranosus muscle attaches distally to the posterior part of the medial condyle of the tibia. It is also connected to the medial collateral ligament, the menisci, and the oblique popliteal ligament. The semitendinosus tendon runs deep into the semimembranosus muscle along the femur and comes out just proximal to the knee joint and attaches to the anteromedial of the tibia. The biceps femoris muscle is attached to the head of the fibula and has connections with the lateral collateral ligament, the tibiofibular joint capsule, and the lateral tubercle of the tibia. The long and short heads of the biceps femoris muscle are collectively called the lateral hamstring, and they perform external rotation in addition to knee flexion. The semimembranosus and semitendinosus muscles are expressed as medial hamstring, and they perform internal rotation in addition to knee flexion. For these rotational movements to take place, the knee must be in the flexion position. This mechanism will be explained in detail in the section for movements in the knee joint. Additionally, all hamstring muscles cross both the hip and knee joints, except the short head of the biceps femoris muscle. Therefore, they also take part in hip extension.

The tendon of the sartorius muscle, which is the longest muscle in the body, starting from the anterior superior iliac spine of the pelvis, and the tendon of the gracilis muscle, starting from the anterior pubis of the pelvis, fuse with the tendon of the semitendinosus muscle medial to the knee joint and attach to the anteromedial of the tibia. The structure formed by these three tendons is called the pes anserinus. The three muscles together generate the knee flexion and internal rotation movements. At the same time, they take part in the medial stabilization of the knee by helping the medial collateral ligament and joint capsule.

The popliteus is a triangular muscle located in the popliteal fossa. It passes proximally between the lateral collateral ligament and the lateral meniscus and attaches to the lateral condyle of the femur. The popliteus tendon attaches to the head of the fibula just below the knee joint line via the popliteofibular ligament, and more distally, to a large area posterior to the tibia. It provides flexion and internal rotation of the knee joint.

The gastrocnemius muscle has two heads starting from the medial and lateral condyles of the femur and passes behind the knee joint and joins the Achilles tendon at the ankle. It provides flexion of the knee joint and plantarflexion and eversion of the ankle joint.

The plantaris muscle originates from the supracondylar line on the lateral condyle of the femur, behind the knee joint, and attaches medially to the Achilles tendon. It provides flexion of the knee joint and plantarflexion of the ankle joint.

14.3 Palpation of the Bones and Muscles of the Knee Joint

Palpation of the bones and muscles associated with the knee joint is shown in Table 14.4.

Table 14.4 Palpation of bones and muscles associated with the knee joint

Bone	Palpation
Femur greater trochanter	Palpation of the thigh is usually started by positioning the greater trochanter. In the supine position, it lies approximately at the same level as the pubic tubercle on the proximal lateral thigh. It is quite large (about 4 × 4 cm) and superficial, so it is quite easy to palpate
Femur lesser trochanter	It is located in the proximal medial thigh. In the supine position, the distal aspect of the psoas major muscle is found and followed as distally as possible. Then, the psoas major muscle is relaxed with hip flexion and external rotation and pressed against the femur in this position
Patella	It is a prominent bone located in front of the distal femur. For palpation, the patient is positioned in supine with the lower extremity relaxed
Femur trochlear groove	In sitting position, the knee joint is flexed to approximately 90°. The quadriceps femoris muscle is relaxed. In this position, the trochlear groove becomes prominent. It is palpated proximal to the patella in the anterior midline of the femur.
Knee joint	In sitting position, when the knee joint is flexed approximately 90°, the inferior of the patella descends and the knee joint line can be palpated both medially and laterally. It is palpated medially and laterally from anterior to posterior in the articular cavity between the femur and tibia
Femoral condyles	While the knee joint is flexed at approximately 90° in sitting position, the lower edges of the medial and lateral condyles are palpated by pressing the proximal femur, above the knee joint line on both sides of the patella
Tibial condyles	While the knee joint is flexed at approximately 90° in the sitting position, the upper edges of the medial and lateral condyles are palpated by pressing the distal tibia, down the knee joint line on both sides of the patella
Head of fibula	It is located posterolateral to the knee and is the most prominent point proximal to the fibula. In a sitting position, with the knee joint flexed to approximately 90°, continue to palpate along the upper edge of the lateral condyle of the tibia to reach the head of the fibula and palpate anteriorly, posteriorly, and laterally. Caution: The common peroneal nerve is superficial near the head of the fibula. Therefore, palpation should be done carefully
Tibial tuberosity	In a sitting position, with the knee joint flexed approximately 90°, it is a prominent point located in the center of the anterior upper part of the tibia body, approximately 2.5–5 cm from the inferior edge of the patella and is easily palpated
Muscle	Palpation
Quadriceps femoris Rectus femoris Vastus medialis Vastus lateralis Vastus intermedius	In supine position, the thighs are on the bed and the legs are hanging off. The palpating hand is placed proximally on the anterior aspect of the thigh. In proximal, the rectus femoris lies between the sartorius and tensor fascia lata (TFL) muscles. Continuing laterally and distally from the proximal tendon of the sartorius (or medially and distally from the proximal tendon of the TFL) the rectus femoris is detected. The rectus femoris contraction is felt by extending the knee. With the other hand, resistance can be applied just proximal to the ankle joint, and its localization can be determined by the eye. The rectus femoris is palpated by placing the hand distally towards the tibial tuberosity, perpendicular to the muscle fibers For vastus medialis, the knee is extended. It is palpated and felt immediately proximal and anteromedial to the patella. The vastus medialis lies superficially and is easy to palpate from distal thigh. However, because it is deeper proximally, it may be difficult to distinguish from neighboring muscles and palpate For vastus lateralis, the knee is extended. It is palpated and felt immediately proximal and anterolateral to the patella. The vastus lateralis is palpated following perpendicular to the fibers along the anterolateral, lateral (below the iliotibial band), and posterolateral (just behind the iliotibial band) of the thigh. Although vastus lateralis is superficial in the anterolateral and posterolateral aspects of the thigh and deeper towards to the lateral of the iliotibial band, it is very easy to palpate. However, it can be difficult to palpate as its connection to the linea aspera is very deep The vastus intermedius muscle is very difficult to distinguish and palpate because it is located deep in the rectus femoris and vastus lateralis muscles and performs the same function as the other quadriceps femoris muscles

(continued)

Table 14.4 (continued)

Hamstring **Long head of biceps femoris** **Semitendinosus** **Semimembranosus**	In prone position, with the knee joint partially flexed, the hand is placed just distal to the ischial tuberosity. The leg is supported over the ankle joint with the other hand. Resistance is given to the knee flexion, and it is palpated just distal to the ischial tuberosity to feel the contraction of the hamstring muscles. If the fibers are continued perpendicular to the fibula head laterally, the long head of the biceps femoris is palpated. Likewise, semitendinosus is palpable if you proceed from the ischial tuberosity to the medial side of the knee. After each of the hamstring muscles has been identified, the patient can be asked to relax, and the resting tone can be palpated **Alternative Palpation Position (Sitting):** When sitting with the feet flat on the floor, the leg can be rotated at the knee joint and the distal tendons of the biceps femoris, semitendinosus, and gracilis muscles can be found. For the biceps femoris, it can be easily palpated with external rotation on the lateral side. The semitendinosus and gracilis tendons can be felt with internal rotation on the medial side. The semitendinosus tendon is greater, more lateral, and closer to the midline of the thigh than the gracilis tendon Distally, the tendon of the medial and lateral hamstring is easy to distinguish, as they are quite far apart. However, proximally they are difficult to distinguish because of their very close position. Tendons can be easily distinguished by rotation at the knee joint. Internal rotation is performed for the medial hamstring and external rotation is for the lateral hamstring. Among the medial hamstring, the semitendinosus tendon is very prominent distally. Semimembranosus can be palpated especially on the medial side of the semitendinosus tendon The vastus lateralis is just in front of the biceps femoris muscle body. Borders can be easily distinguished by flexing and extending the knee joint. Proximally, the adductor magnus is located just in front of the medial hamstring and their borders can be determined by flexing the knee (the adductor magnus is loose during flexion)
Sartorius	In a supine position, thighs are on the bed and the legs are hanging off. Knowing the palpation methods of the Sartorius and TFL muscles is important to distinguish the two muscles. Both muscles start from the ASIS and flex the hip joint. However, the TFL internally rotates the hip, while the sartorius externally rotates it. Therefore, the sartorius is felt just distal and slightly medial to the ASIS by external rotation and flexion of the hip against gravity. Additionally, the sartorius can be felt better with hip abduction and knee flexion. If necessary, resistance is given at the distal with the other hand from the anteromedial of the thigh. The sartorius is palpated by following the fibers perpendicular to the distal attachment point. After the sartorius is detected, the patient is asked to relax, and the resting tone is also palpated **Alternative Palpation Position (Supine, entire lower extremity on bed):** Contraction of the sartorius is felt just distal and slightly medial to the ASIS by external rotation and flexion of the hip against gravity. The proximal medial edge of the sartorius forms the lateral border of the femoral triangle. There are the iliopsoas and pectineus muscles, and the femoral nerve, artery, and vein within the femoral triangle Although the sartorius is superficial, the distal 1/2 of the sartorius is often difficult to palpate and distinguish from neighboring muscles. One way of locating it is by extending the knee first to locate the vastus medialis at the distal (usually quite prominent). After identifying the vastus medialis, continue posteromedially towards the sartorius. Next, the knee is flexed to feel the sartorius contraction

Table 14.4 (continued)

Gracilis	In the supine position, the legs are hanging off the bed from the knee joint. The palpating hand is placed medially, proximal to the thigh. The gracilis is adjacent to the adductor longus anteriorly and the adductor magnus posteriorly on the proximal thigh. First, the proximal tendon of the adductor longus should be found as it is the most prominent tendon in the region. Then, gracilis is detected by continuing posteromedially. By asking the patient to flex the knee to push the bed (the adductor longus and adductor magnus remain relaxed on both sides), the gracilis can be easily distinguished proximally. Proceeding distally, the gracilis muscle is palpated perpendicular to the fibers **Alternative Palpation Position (Sitting):** The gracilis distal tendon can be easily identified. When sitting with the feet flat on the floor, the knee is internally rotated and two stretched tendons are felt significantly in the distal posteromedial thigh. The gracilis tendon is smaller and located more medially (the structure that is larger, more lateral, and closer to the midline of the thigh is the semitendinosus tendon). Once identified, the gracilis is palpated, following perpendicular to the fibers proximal and towards the pubic bone. At distal, hip abduction (the sartorius contracts) and adduction (the gracilis contracts) movements can be used to separate gracilis from sartorius **Alternative Palpation Position (Prone):** When palpating the gracilis in the prone position, it should be noted that the gracilis is located in front of the adductor magnus **Alternative Palpation Position (Side Lying):** In this position, the gracilis in the lower extremity that is closer to the bed is palpated. To access the gracilis, the lower extremity that is away from the bed is lifted crossing over the other lower extremity by hip and knee flexion. By flexing the knee that is on the bed against resistance, the contraction of the gracilis can be felt
Gastrocnemius	In the prone position and with the knee joint fully extended, the palpating hand is placed on the posterior proximal leg and the other hand on the plantar surface of the foot. The patient is asked to do plantarflexion against resistance and the contraction of the gastrocnemius is felt. On the posterior proximal leg, the medial and lateral body of the gastrocnemius can be palpated separately at their insertion on the posterior surfaces of the femoral condyles. Perpendicular to the fibers, the gastrocnemius muscle body is followed proximally. The lateral head is medial to the biceps femoris distal tendon, and the medial head is lateral to the semitendinosus and semimembranosus tendons. After entering the popliteal region, the femoral condyle connections of both heads of the gastrocnemius are palpated by flexing the knee joint passively to approximately 90° to loosen the hamstring. However, palpation should be done carefully because of the artery, vein, tibial and common peroneal nerves in the popliteal region **Alternative Palpation Position (Standing):** The gastrocnemius can easily be palpated while standing. The patient is asked to rise on their toes and the contraction of the gastrocnemius is felt
Plantaris	Since the plantaris is a small muscle, it is very difficult to distinguish it from gastrocnemius. Plantaris is side by side with the lateral head of the gastrocnemius and produces the same joint movement. The plantaris muscle is located medial to the lateral head of the gastrocnemius at proximal. In the prone position, palpation can begin gently in the center of the popliteal fossa with the knee joint fully extended. Then, it is palpated by continuing slowly in the lateral direction until the presence of muscle tissue contraction is felt by ankle plantarflexion

(continued)

Table 14.4 (continued)

Popliteus	In prone position, with 90° of knee flexion, the palpating hand is placed proximally, posterior to the medial edge of the tibia. The contraction of popliteus is felt by internal rotation of the knee joint. If resistance is required, it is given with the other hand just proximal to the ankle joint in the opposite direction. After the tibial insertion of the popliteus is felt, the person is asked to internally rotate the knee joint and then relax. Simultaneously, palpation is continued over the gastrocnemius towards the proximal insertion of the popliteus on the lateral femoral condyle. Since most of the body of popliteus is located under gastrocnemius, gentle pressure while palpating over gastrocnemius may be helpful to feel the slight contractions during movement. At a certain point, the proximal connection of the popliteus enters the knee joint space and cannot be palpated. After detecting the popliteus, the person can be asked to relax, and the resting tone can be palpated The proximal insertion of popliteus on the lateral femoral condyle can also be directly palpated. The lateral surface of the lateral femoral condyle (just behind the lateral collateral ligament) is detected, and tension of the popliteus distal tendon is felt with internal rotation of the knee against resistance **Alternative Palpation Position (Sitting):** In sitting position with the feet flat on the floor, it may be easier to internally rotate the knee as the person can see their knees. The popliteus is palpated by following the steps applied while in prone position

14.4 Movements in the Knee Joint

The main movements of the knee joint are flexion and extension. In addition, internal and external rotation movements occur when the knee is in a flexed position. An average of 130–150° of flexion movement and 5–10° of hyperextension (0° is considered as full extension of the knee) is seen in the knee joint. The knee joint is mechanically locked in full extension and most ligaments are stretched in this position. Therefore, no rotational movement occurs in full knee extension. In addition, the force applied by the hamstring muscles, which rotate the knee when the knee is in full extension, decreases because the force arm is short. As the knee progresses from extension to flexion, the capacity of the rotation increases and rotation can be reached up to a total of 45° (internal and external in total) in approximately 90° flexion. The external rotation range of motion is greater than the internal rotation range, approximately twice as high. Internal and external rotation of the knee joint is defined by the position of the tibial tuberosity against the anterior aspect of the femur. If the tibial tuberosity moves laterally with respect to the anterior surface of the femur, it is called external rotation, and if it moves medially, it is called internal rotation.

Flexion-extension movement in the knee joint can be defined in two different ways. One of them is the movement of the tibia relative to the femur. For example, when the knee moves from flexion to extension in a sitting position, the tibia moves while the femur is fixed. The other movement is the flexion-extension movement of the femur on the fixed tibia. An example of this is the movement that occurs during standing up from a squat position. The femur moves on the fixed tibia. As the tibia moves over the femur (e.g., knee extension in a sitting position), the articular surface of the tibia rolls under the condyles of the femur and slides forward. As the femur moves on the tibia (e.g., rise from a squat), the femoral condyles roll over the tibia and slide backward.

The knee locking mechanism (Screw-home mechanism) is important for understanding knee mechanics and movements. In order for the knee joint to fully extend, it must perform an external rotation of approximately 10°. In the last 30° of extension, the knee joint is externally rotated due to the mechanical structure of the articular surfaces. This involuntary rotation occurs depending on the flexion-extension movement. The most important factor in the formation of the mechanism is the shape of the medial femoral condyle. The medial femoral condyle is positioned approximately 30° laterally as it extends into the trochlear groove. Since the articular surface of the medial condyle is longer than the lateral condyle and extends anteriorly, the tibia moves with this lateral orientation during extension. As a result, external rotation occurs along with knee extension. In addition to the structure of the femoral condyles, the tension force emerging in the anterior cruciate ligament during knee extension and the lateral pulling force of the quadriceps muscle are also effective in the knee locking mechanism.

In order for the knee joint to flex, it must be unlocked in the full extension position. First, the internal rotation movement must occur in the joint. Popliteus is the main muscle in unlocking the joint with internal rotation movement. Popliteus unlocks the knee joint and initiates knee flexion by initiating internal rotation of the tibia.

In order for internal and external rotation to occur in the knee joint, the knee joint must be in a flexed position. During rotational movements, the menisci change shape and adapt as they are exposed to compression and rotational forces between the femur and tibia. Meanwhile, the stability of the menisci is provided by popliteus and semimembranosus muscles.

Patellofemoral joint is another joint in which movement occurs in the knee. During knee flexion and extension movements, the patella glides in the trochlear groove between the condyles of the femur. As the tibia moves relative to the femur (e.g., the knee flexion in a sitting position), the patella glides in the trochlear groove. The patella is pulled towards the tibia during knee flexion as it is strongly attached to the tibial tuberosity via the patellar tendon. As the femur moves relative to the tibia (e.g., squat), the femur glides under the patella. The harmony between the patella and femoral trochlear groove and the ratio of the surface contacting to each other varies according to the knee position. Only the superior border of the patella is in contact with the femur when the knee is flexed to approximately 135°. As the knee extends, the contact surface between the patella and femur continues to increase. About 90°–60° of flexion position, the fit between the patella and the trochlear groove of the femur reaches its highest level, and approximately one-third of the lower surface of the patella is in contact with the femur. As the knee joint extends, the contact area shifts towards the inferior border of the patella. The fit and contact surface between the patella and trochlear groove is reduced. In full knee extension, the patella remains completely above the trochlear groove, on the suprapatellar fat pad. If the quadriceps is relaxed, patella can be moved freely in the desired direction passively. Chronic lateral dislocations of the patella occur most frequently in positions close to knee extension, due to this patella-femur alignment that decreases gradually towards knee extension.

14.5 Evidence-Based Exercises for the Muscles Involved in Knee Joint Movements Based on Exercise Type

In order to provide stability and function in the knee joint, it is important to maintain different types of contractions and flexibility of the muscles around the joint. It is necessary to know the most appropriate exercises according to the type of contraction in order to restore the function of the muscles around the knee joint both in the prevention of injuries and in the rehabilitation process after injury. Physiotherapists should tailor the type and intensity of exercises to the needs of patients. The patient's cause of injury, current clinical picture, and, if applied, the form of the surgical method and the characteristic features of the tissue to which the intervention was performed are important factors while selecting exercises. For example, if the patient has undergone anterior cruciate ligament reconstruction surgery, the load on the ligament should be taken into account while working the quadriceps femoris muscle and the exercises should be chosen accordingly. Another important criterion in the choice of exercise is the needs of the patient. For example, the exercises to be given to an individual over the age of 50 who are not interested in sports versus an active athlete at the age of 25 should be different. Table 14.5 lists the evidence-based exercises for the muscles around the knee.

Table 14.5 Evidence-based exercises for the muscles involved in knee joint movements based on the exercise type

Muscle	Exercise type	Exercise/position
Quadriceps	Isometric	Standing in a squat position (solar22/Shutterstock.com)
	Concentric	Knee extension in open kinetic chain (weight can be added around the ankle) (APword/Shutterstock.com)
		Knee extension in closed kinetic chain with leg press machine (weight adjustable) (Lio putra/Shutterstock.com)
		Rise up from squat (can be made more difficult by putting weight on hands) (solar22/Shutterstock.com)
		Getting up from lunge (can be made more difficult by putting weight on hand) (solar22/Shutterstock.com)

Table 14.5 (continued)

	Eccentric	Controlled return to flexion position after knee extension in open kinetic chain (weight can be added around the ankle) (APword/Shutterstock.com)
		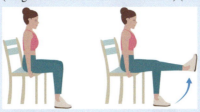
		Controlled return to knee flexion position from full knee extension with leg press machine (weight adjustable) (Lio putra/Shutterstock.com)
		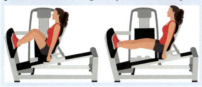
		Squat (can be made more difficult by putting weight on hand) (solar22/Shutterstock.com)
		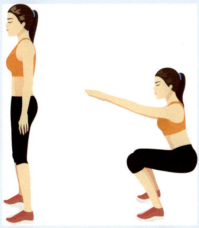
		Lunge (can be made more difficult by putting weight on hand) (solar22/Shutterstock.com)
		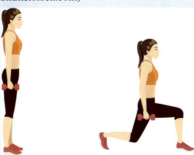

(continued)

Table 14.5 (continued)

	Stretching	While standing or in prone position, the knee is bent by holding the ankle and the quadriceps is stretched without allowing hip flexion (solar22/Shutterstock.com)	
	Explosive	Squat jumps (solar22/Shutterstock.com)	
		Lunge jumps (solar22/Shutterstock.com)	
Hamstring	Isometric	In bridge, the person lies in supine and raises their hips while keeping their feet and shoulders on the ground. With the hips in a fixed position above, the hamstring works isometrically (solar22/Shutterstock.com)	

Table 14.5 (continued)

	Eccentric	In the Nordic hamstring exercise, the person stands on the ground on their knees, slowly leaning forward with the ankles fixed and without hip flexion (michelangeloop/Shutterstock.com) 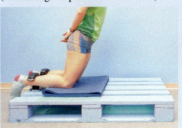
		With the torso upright, knee extended, controlled leaning forward from the hip (with hip flexion) with weight in hand (solar22/Shutterstock.com) 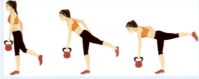
	Concentric	In the leg curl movement, knee flexion with weight or resistance at the ankle while in prone position (solar22/Shutterstock.com) 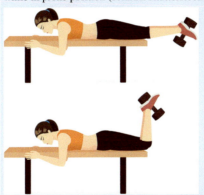
		The kettlebell swing exercise is started with a weight in the hand, feet shoulder-width apart, hips and knees flexed. Then the hips and knees are extended while the arms are flexed at the same time. Return to the initial position by squatting after full standing stance (solar22/Shutterstock.com) 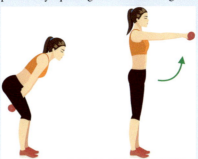

(continued)

Table 14.5 (continued)

	Stretching	In supine position, the hip and opposite leg are fixed on the floor, while the entire leg is raised without impairing full extension of the knee. Support can be given in the form of a towel or band wrapped around the ankle to be pulled with hands. In addition, starting from the hips and knees flexion at 90° in the supine position, the knees can be extended while keeping the hips fixed (solar22/Shutterstock.com)

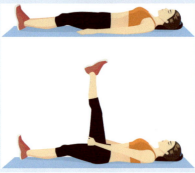

In the long sitting position, the hamstrings are stretched by leaning forward without bending the knees (solar22/Shutterstock.com)

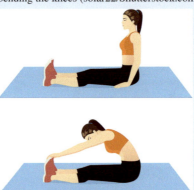

While standing, the hamstrings are stretched by leaning forward with hip flexion without impairing knee extension (solar22/Shutterstock.com)

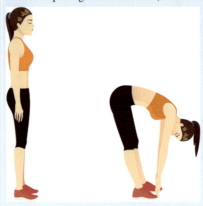

Table 14.5 (continued)

	Explosive	Jumping on one or both legs with deep knee flexion (robuart/Shutterstock.com) Jump from the ground onto the box (solar22/Shutterstock.com)

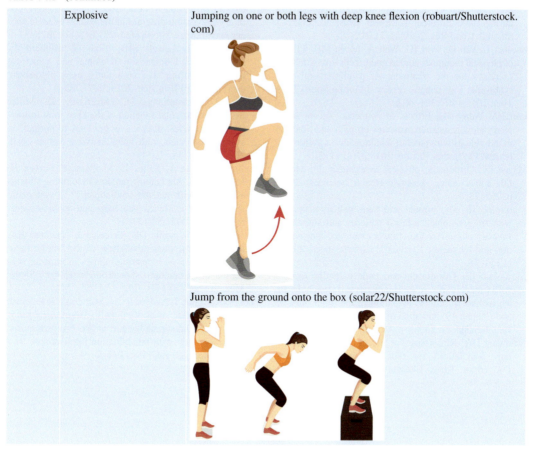

14.6 Conclusion

Due to its anatomical structure, the knee is a complex and important joint that needs to be evaluated. Knowledge of knee anatomy and kinesiology is an important factor in understanding most injury mechanisms and deciding on effective rehabilitation interventions. In the clinic, it will be easier to evaluate and plan the treatment process in light of the information given in this chapter for the knee joint.

Further Reading

Avers D, Brown M. Daniels and Worthingham's muscle testing: techniques of manual examination and performance testing. In: Avers D, Brown M, editors. Testing the muscles of the lower extremity. Elsevier Health Sciences; 2018. p. 423–38.

Bourne MN, Timmins RG, Opar DA, Pizzari T, Ruddy JD, Sims C, et al. An evidence-based framework for strengthening exercises to prevent hamstring injury. Sports Med. 2018;48(2):251–67.

Brukner P, Khan K. Clinical sports medicine. In: Brukner P, Khan K, editors. Chapter 30: Anterior thigh pain, Chapter 31: Posterior thigh pain, Chapter 32: Acute knee injuries, Chapter 33: Anterior knee pain and Chapter 34: Lateral, medial and posterior knee pain. McGraw-Hill; 2016. p. 579–734.

Buckthorpe M, Villa FD. Optimising the 'Mid-Stage' training and testing process after ACL reconstruction. Sports Med. 2020;50(4):657–78.

Buckthorpe M, La Rosa G, Villa FD. Restoring knee extensor strength after anterior cruciate ligament reconstruction: a clinical commentary. Int J Sports Phys Ther. 2019;14(1):159–72.

Davies G, Riemann BL, Manske R. Current concepts of plyometric exercise. Int J Sports Phys Ther. 2015;10(6):760–86.

Del Monte MJ, Opar DA, Timmins RG, Ross JA, Keogh JW, Lorenzen C. Hamstring myoelectrical activity during three different kettlebell swing exercises. J Strength Cond Res. 2020;34(7):1953–8.

Kooiker L, Van De Port IG, Weir A, Moen MH. Effects of physical therapist–guided quadriceps-strengthening exercises for the treatment of patellofemoral pain syndrome: a systematic review. J Orthop Sports Phys Ther. 2014;44(6):391–402.

Lim HY, Wong SH. Effects of isometric, eccentric, or heavy slow resistance exercises on pain and function in individuals with patellar tendinopathy: a systematic review. Physiother Res Int. 2018;23(4):e1721.

Magee DJ. Orthopedic physical assessment. In: Magee DJ, editor. Knee. Elsevier Health Sciences; 2014. p. 765–78.

Muscolino JE. The muscle and bone palpation manual with trigger points, referral patterns and stretching. In: Muscolino JE, editor. Lower extremity bone palpation and ligaments. Elsevier Health Sciences; 2008a. p. 113–36.

Muscolino JE. The muscle and bone palpation manual with trigger points, referral patterns and stretching. In: Muscolino JE, editor. Palpation of the thigh muscles and Chapter 19: Palpation of the leg muscles. Elsevier Health Sciences; 2008b. p. 413–86.

Neumann DA. Kinesiology of the musculoskeletal system: foundations for rehabilitation. In: Neumann DA, editor. Knee. Elsevier Health Sciences; 2013. p. 538–88.

Silvers-Granelli H, Mandelbaum B, Adeniji O, Insler S, Bizzini M, Pohlig R, et al. Efficacy of the FIFA 11+ injury prevention program in the collegiate male soccer player. Am J Sports Med. 2015;43(11):2628–37.

Struminger AH, Lewek MD, Goto S, Hibberd E, Blackburn JT. Comparison of gluteal and hamstring activation during five commonly used plyometric exercises. Clin Biomech. 2013;28(7):783–9.

Tayfur B, Charuphongsa C, Morrissey D, Miller SC. Neuromuscular function of the knee joint following knee injuries: does it ever get back to normal? A systematic review with meta-analyses. Sports Med. 2021;51:321–38.

Tayfur A, Haque A, Salles JI, Malliaras P, Screen H, Morrissey D. Are landing patterns in jumping athletes associated with patellar tendinopathy? A systematic review with evidence gap map and meta-analysis. Sports Med. 2022;52:123–37.

van der Horst N, Smits DW, Petersen J, Goedhart EA, Backx FJ. The preventive effect of the Nordic hamstring exercise on hamstring injuries in amateur soccer players: a randomized controlled trial. Am J Sports Med. 2015;43(6):1316–23.

Zebis MK, Skotte J, Andersen CH, Mortensen P, Petersen HH, Viskær TC, et al. Kettlebell swing targets semitendinosus and supine leg curl targets biceps femoris: an EMG study with rehabilitation implications. Br J Sports Med. 2013;47(18):1192–8.

The Foot and Ankle

15

Serdar Demirci and Gurkan Gunaydin

Abstract

The foot and ankle are complex structures with serious tasks in activities such as standing still, walking, and running in daily life. Contractile and noncontractile structures that make up the foot skeleton are frequently exposed to traumas due to various reasons, especially sports injuries. Good knowledge of functional anatomy is among the most important concepts to understand the injuries occurring in the foot skeleton better, develop preventive strategies for the prevention of injuries, and plan the post-injury conservative or postsurgical treatment modalities. In this chapter, the contractile and noncontractile structures of the foot and ankle joints and their palpation, the joints that generate the ankle complex and these joint motions, and evidence-based exercises for the muscles responsible for foot/ankle function are explained.

15.1 Foot and Ankle Joints

When the foot and ankle are considered a functional unit, they form a complex structure with serious tasks in activities such as standing still, walking, and running and are often exposed to traumas. Good knowledge of functional anatomy is among the important concepts to understand injuries of this nature and plan an appropriate treatment program following injuries. Considering the foot skeleton functionally, it is made up of three anatomic regions, the rearfoot, midfoot, and forefoot (Fig. 15.1). The rearfoot forms the talus and calcaneus. The rearfoot is the first part of the foot to contact the ground in the gait cycle influencing the function and movement of the other two parts. The navicular, medial cuneiform, middle cuneiform, lateral cuneiform, and cuboid bone form the midfoot. The mechanics of this part of the foot provide stability and mobility when transmitting motion from the rear-

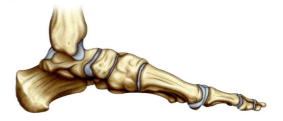

Fig. 15.1 Rearfoot, midfoot, and forefoot (ilusmedical/Shutterstock.com)

S. Demirci (✉)
Physiotherapy and Rehabilitation, Faculty of Health Sciences, Balikesir University, Balikesir, Turkey
e-mail: serdar.demirci@balikesir.edu.tr

G. Gunaydin
Physiotherapy and Rehabilitation, Faculty of Health Sciences, Aydin Adnan Menderes University, Aydin, Turkey

© The Author(s), under exclusive license to Springer Nature Switzerland AG 2023
D. Kaya Utlu (ed.), *Functional Exercise Anatomy and Physiology for Physiotherapists*,
https://doi.org/10.1007/978-3-031-27184-7_15

foot to the forefoot. The forefoot is made up of metatarsals and phalanges and provides the adaptation of the foot to the ground, forming the last part of the foot touching the ground in the stance phase.

With all these structures and the contractile and noncontractile tissues that make up these structures, the ankle joint and the foot perform three main functions: (1) to act as a shock absorber during the heel contact, which is the starting of the stance phase, (2) adapt to the ground surface, and (3) create necessary stable support to push the body forward. To perform these functions, the foot must become rigid or flexible at the right time. The functional anatomy of the foot skeleton must be well known to understand all these functions. The contractile and noncontractile structures of the foot/ankle joint and their palpation, the joints that make up the foot/ankle complex, and evidence-based exercises for the muscles responsible for foot/ankle function will be discussed in this section.

15.2 Noncontractile Structures in the Foot and Ankle

15.2.1 Bone Structures

There are 26 bones in the foot skeleton, which carry the weight of the body (Fig. 15.2). These bones form three groups from proximal to distal: tarsal bones, metatarsals, and phalanges. The tarsal bones consist of seven bones; talus, calcaneus, navicular, medial cuneiform, middle cuneiform, lateral cuneiform, and cuboideum. The largest bone in the foot is the calcaneus, and the largest metatarsal bone is the most medial, with two phalanges forming the big toe in front of it. The other metatarsals of the foot have three phalanges. These bones in the foot skeleton and their prominences form attachment points for the muscles in the foot/ankle. The muscles that are attached to the bones and special bone prominences in the foot skeleton are given in Table 15.1 according to the origo and insertio points. Muscles that origi-

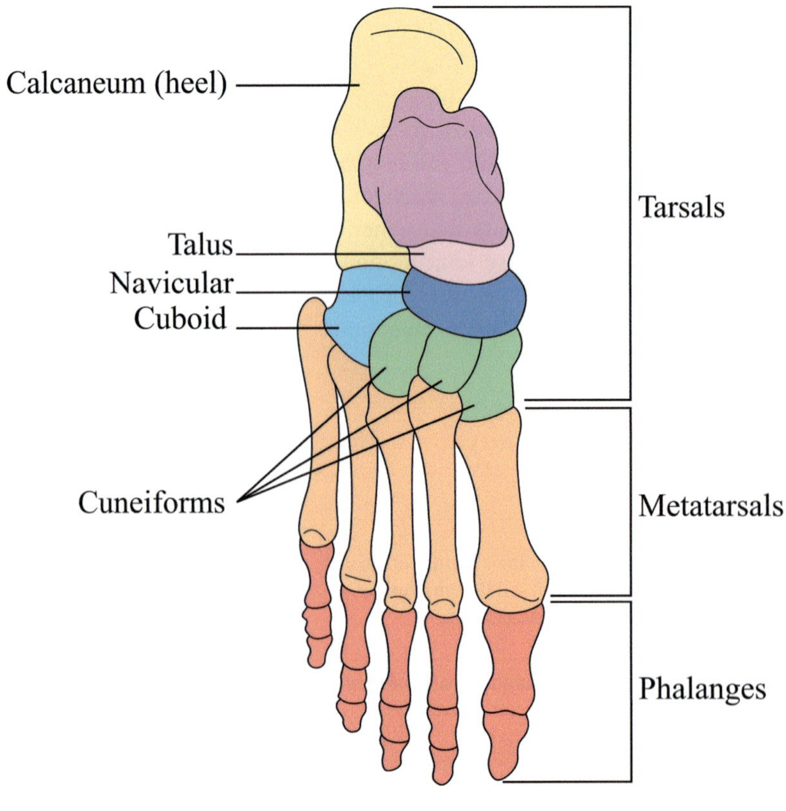

Fig. 15.2 The bones of the foot (Excellent Dream/Shutterstock.com)

Table 15.1 Muscles located on bony prominences according to origo and insertio points

Extrinsic muscles	
Starting from the bone/bony prominences/ anatomic structure	Muscles
Femur	• Gastrocnemius • Plantaris
Tibia	• Soleus • Tibialis anterior • Tibialis posterior • Extensor digitorum longus • Flexor digitorum longus
Fibula	• Soleus • Tibialis posterior • Extensor hallucis longus • Extensor digitorum longus • Peroneus longus • Peroneus brevis • Peroneus tertius • Flexor hallucis longus (FHL)
Interosseous membrane	• Tibialis anterior • Tibialis posterior • Extensor hallucis longus • Extensor digitorum longus • Peroneus longus • Peroneus tertius • Flexor hallucis longus

Intrinsic muscles	
Starting from the bone/bony prominences/ anatomic structure	Muscles
The dorsal side of the calcaneus	• Extensor digitorum brevis (EDB) • Extensor hallucis brevis (EHB)
The lateral side of the calcaneus	• Extensor digitorum brevis
The medial protrusion of the calcaneal tubercle	• Abductor hallucis • Flexor digitorum brevis • Abductor digiti minimi pedis • Quadratus plantae
The lateral protrusion of the calcaneal tubercle	• Abductor digiti minimi pedis • Quadratus plantae
Cuboideum	• Flexor hallucis brevis
Lateral cuneiform	• Flexor hallucis brevis
Metatarsal bones	• Dorsal interossei
The basis of 2–4th metatarsals	• Adductor hallucis • Plantar interosseous
The 5th metatarsal basis	• Flexor digiti minimi brevis
The basis of 3–5th metatarsal bones	• Plantar interossei

Table 15.1 (continued)

Flexor digitorum longus tendons[a]	• Lumbricales
Long plantar ligament[a]	• Quadratus plantae • Flexor digiti minimi brevis
Plantar aponeurosis[a]	• Abductor hallucis • Flexor digitorum brevis • Abductor digiti minimi

Ending on bone/bony prominences/ anatomic structure	Muscles
Calcaneal tubercle	• Gastrocnemius • Soleus, plantaris
Medial cuneiform	• Tibialis anterior • Peroneus longus • Tibialis posterior
2–3th cuneiform	• Tibialis posterior
Navicular tubercle	• Tibialis posterior
Basis of the 1st metatarsal bone	• Tibialis anterior • Peroneus longus
Basis of 2–4th metatarsal bones	• Tibialis posterior
Basis of the 5th metatarsal bone	• Peroneus tertius • Peroneus brevis
Base of the proximal phalanx of the thumb	• Extensor hallucis brevis (i.e., attaches to the dorsal surface) • Abductor hallucis (i.e., attaches to the plantar surface) • Flexor hallucis brevis (i.e., attaches to the plantar surface) • Adductor hallucis (i.e., attaches to the plantar surface)
Base of the distal phalanx of the thumb	• Extensor hallucis longus (i.e., attaches to the dorsal surface) • Flexor hallucis longus (i.e., attaches to the plantar surface)
Basis of the proximal phalanx of 2–5th fingers	• Lumbricales
Dorsal aspect of the medial and distal phalanges of the 2–5th fingers	• Extensor digitorum longus
Base of the distal phalanges of the 2–5th fingers	• Flexor digitorum longus
Medial phalanx of 2–5th fingers	• Flexor digitorum brevis
Proximal phalanx of 2–4th fingers	• Dorsal interossei (attaching to the dorsal surface)

(continued)

Table 15.1 (continued)

Basis of the proximal phalanges of 3–5th fingers	• Plantar interossei
Basis of the proximal phalanx of the 5th finger	• Abductor digiti minimi pedis • Flexor digiti minimi brevis
Flexor digitorum longus tendon [a]	• Quadratus plantae
Extensor digitorum longus tendons [a]	• Extensor digitorum brevis (in the form of 3 tendons to 2-4th fingers)

Additional information: The talus is the only tarsal bone to which no muscle is attached

[a] In the foot-ankle complex, some muscles start and end from tendons or ligaments

nate from the leg are given under the heading of extrinsic muscles. The muscles that originate from the tarsal bones are given under the heading of intrinsic muscles.

15.2.2 Foot and Ankle Joints

The ankle joint is the only one between the foot and leg controlling the foot in the sagittal plane. It is responsible for adjusting the line of gravity during standing and providing the necessary push and restraint during walking. The second joint in the foot skeleton is the subtalar joint between the talus and the calcaneus playing an important role in transmitting body weight to the foot in both static and dynamic conditions. The third joint is the transverse tarsal joint, which is a functional joint in the middle of the tarsus. This last joint plays an important role in the push-off phase of gait, allowing the forefoot to adjust itself relative to the rearfoot. In this way, the sole of the forefoot can maintain full contact with the surface independently of the rearfoot. These three joints provide a high degree of stability while allowing the foot to adapt to any surface while walking. The joint structures that make up the foot skeleton, the movements occurring in these joints, and the ligaments associated with the joints are summarized in Table 15.2.

15.2.2.1 Ankle Joint (i.e., Talocrural Joint)

The ankle joint is a synovial hinge (i.e., ginglymus)-type joint between the articular surface at the distal ends of the tibia and fibula and the trochlea tali of the talus and is made up of three joints: tibiofibular, tibiotalar, and fibulotalar (Fig. 15.3). The joint between the tibia and talus bears most of the weight. The joint axis passing through the malleolus is oblique and makes an angle of approximately 20–25° with the frontal plane because the medial malleolus is located more proximally and anteriorly than the lateral malleolus. The joint axis passes through the middle of the lateral malleolus and below the medial malleolus. Two movements occur in the joint, namely, dorsiflexion and plantar flexion in the sagittal plane. Talar rotation, fibular slip, and rotation movements are also present because of the oblique axis. The forward or backward movement of the center of gravity, which falls in front of the ankle joint during a normal stance, is regulated in the ankle so that it remains within the restrictions of the support surface.

15.2.2.2 Foot Joint

The foot joint is divided into the following four groups:

1. Intertarsal
2. Tarsometatarsal and intermetatarsal
3. Metatarsophalangeal (i.e., MTF)
4. Interphalangeal (i.e., IF)

Intertarsal Joints

These are the subtalar, talocalcaneonavicular, calcaneocuboid, transverse tarsal, cuneonavicular, intercuneiform, and cuneocuboid joints. The transverse tarsal joint is a functional joint and includes the talocalcaneonavicular joint medially and the calcaneocuboid joint laterally and is also known as the "Chopart" joint. All joints are characterized by interosseous, dorsal, and plantar ligaments, with the plantar ligaments much stronger than the dorsal.

Table 15.2 Foot and ankle joints and related structures

Ankle joint	Type	Synovial hinge type
	Articular surfaces	The distal end of the tibia, the inner surface of the medial and lateral malleolus, and the trochlea and lateral surfaces of the talus
	Capsule	The thin and loose capsule attaches anteriorly to the articular margins except for the talus neck
	Ligaments	Deltoid ligament (i.e., medial collateral ligament) Lateral collateral ligament: • Anterior and posterior talofibular ligaments • Calcaneofibular ligament • Anterior and posterior capsular ligaments
	Stabilization	Provided by joint surfaces, ligaments, and muscles
	Movement	Dorsiflexion, plantar flexion
Subtalar joint	Type	Synovial planar type
	Joint surfaces	Concave facet on the lower surface of the talus and convex facet on the upper surface of the calcaneus
	Capsule	The thin and loose capsule attaches to the joint margins
	Ligaments	Interosseous talocalcaneal ligament Cervical talocalcaneal ligament Medial talocalcaneal ligament Lateral talocalcaneal ligament Posterior talocalcaneal ligament
	Stabilization	Provided by ligaments (especially interosseous ligaments)
	Movement	Inversion and eversion of the foot
Talocalcaneonavicular joint	Type	Synovial planar type
	Joint surfaces	Posterior concave surface of the navicular, anterior calcaneus, lower surface and head of the neck of the talus with the plantar calcaneonavicular ligament
	Capsule	Attaches to joint edges
	Ligaments	Plantar calcaneonavicular (i.e., spring) ligament Calcaneonavicular part of the bifurcated ligament Dorsal talonavicular ligament
	Stabilization	Provided by the spring, bifurcated ligament, and tibialis posterior muscle
	Movement	Inversion and eversion of the foot
Calcaneocuboid joint	Type	Synovial planar type
	Joint surfaces	Anterior surface of calcaneus and posterior surface of cuboid
	Capsule	Attaches around the joint (thick inferior and superior)
	Ligaments	Dorsal calcaneocuboid ligament Plantar calcaneocuboid ligament The calcaneocuboid part of the bifurcated ligament Long plantar ligament
	Stabilization	Provided by the plantar ligaments and the peroneus longus muscle
	Movement	Forefoot pronation, supination
Cuneonavicular joint	Type	Synovial planar type
	Joint surfaces	The posterior concave surface of the cuneiform bones and the facet on the anterior surface of the navicular
	Capsule	Joint circumference
	Ligaments	Dorsal cuneonavicular ligament Plantar cuneonavicular ligament
	Movement	Limited sliding
Intercuneiform joint	Type	Synovial planar type

(continued)

Table 15.2 (continued)

Cuneocuboid joint	Type	Synovial planar type
	Joint surfaces	The posterior surface of the cuboid bone and the posterolateral surface of lateral cuneiform
	Ligaments	Dorsal cuneocuboid ligament Plantar cuneocuboid ligament Interosseous cuneocuboid ligament
	Stabilization	Stabilization is provided by the associated ligaments
	Movement	Limited sliding
Tarsometatarsal joint	Type	Synovial planar type
	Joint surfaces	Anterior surface of cuboid and cuneiform bone and base of metatarsal
	Capsule	Attaches to joint edges
	Ligaments	Dorsal tarsometatarsal ligament Plantar tarsometatarsal ligament Interosseous tarsometatarsal ligament
	Stabilization	Provided by ligaments and muscles that cross and/or attach to bones
	Movement	Dorsiflexion, plantar flexion
Intermetatarsal joint	Type	Synovial planar type
Metatarsophalangeal joint	Type	Synovial ellipsoid type
	Joint surfaces	Rounded metatarsal head and base of proximal phalanx
	Capsule	Loose, replaces the plantar ligament at the plantar surface
	Ligaments	Collateral ligament Plantar ligament Deep transverse metatarsal ligament
	Movement	Dorsiflexion and plantar flexion of the fingers
Interphalangeal joint	Type	Synovial hinge type
	Joint surfaces	Head of the proximal phalanx and base of the next distal phalanx
	Capsule	Completely covers the joint and is strengthened by collateral ligaments replacing the plantar
	Ligaments	Collateral ligament Plantar ligament
	Stabilization	Provided by ligaments and tendons passing through the joint
	Movement	Dorsiflexion and plantar flexion of the fingers

Subtalar joint (i.e., the talocalcaneal joint): It is a synovial planar-type joint between the concave facet on the lower surface of the talus body and the convex posterior facet on the upper surface of the calcaneus. The axis of motion of the subtalar joint is oblique, and pronation (i.e., dorsiflexion, abduction, and calcaneal eversion) and supination (i.e., plantar flexion, adduction, and calcaneal inversion) movements occur. While the calcaneus is displaced medially and the talus laterally during the inversion movement, the calcaneus moves laterally and the talus moves medially during eversion.

Talocalcaneonavicular joint: It is a planar-type joint between the talus, calcaneus, and navicular bones and is also referred to as an irregular and synovial ball-socket-type joint in some sources with no definite axis. It has an oblique axis running from inside to outside, front to back, and top to bottom with sliding movements, which creates less inversion and eversion movements in the foot than in the subtalar joint.

Calcaneocuboid joint: It is a planar-type joint between the facet on the anterior surface of the calcaneus and the facet on the posterior surface of the cuboideum with a limited sliding motion.

Cuneonavicular joint: It is the planar-type joint between the navicular and the three cuneiform bones with limited sliding movements.

Cuboidonavicular joint: It is a syndesmosis-type joint with strong ligaments between the articular surfaces. Although it is also known as a fibrous or immovable joint in the literature, it has little or no movement.

Intercuneiform joint: It is a synovial planar-type joint between the three cuneiform bones with a limited sliding motion.

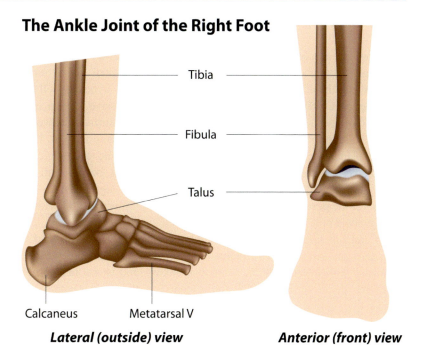

Fig. 15.3 The ankle joint (Alila Medical Media/Shutterstock.com)

Cuneocuboid joint: It is a planar-type joint between the cuboideum and the lateral cuneiform with a limited sliding motion.

Tarsometatarsal (i.e., Lisfranc) and Intermetatarsal Joint

Tarsometatarsal joint: It is a planar-type joint between the cuboideum and the bases of the fourth and fifth metatarsals and between the three cuneiforms and the bases of the first, second, and third metatarsal bones. It is also known as the "*Lisfranc*" joint with minimal occurrence of flexion-extension and supination-pronation movements.

Intermetatarsal joint: It is a small synovial plane-type joint between the bases of the lateral four metatarsal bones and the facets on their adjacent sides with no connection between the bases of the first and second metatarsals because they are connected only by interosseous fibers with a limited sliding motion.

Metatarsophalangeal Joint

It is a synovial ellipsoid-type joint between the head of the metatarsal bones and the proximal phalanx. Dorsiflexion, plantar flexion, abduction, adduction, and circumduction movements occur in the metatarsophalangeal joints.

Interphalangeal Joint

It is a hinge (i.e., ginglymus)-type joint between the head of the proximal phalanx and the base of the distal phalanx. Only flexion and extension movements occur in the interphalangeal joints because of the shape of the articular surfaces.

> **Clinical Information**
> Full dorsiflexion of the ankle is the position in which the talus is most stable. Subtalar joint dislocations are extremely rare because of the joint structure and the strong ligaments in the surrounding area. The "subtalar neutral" position is used as a reference to determine the level of much the pathologies in the ankle. "Subtalar neutral" position is the position where the head of the talus can be palpated equally from both medial and lateral sides, the foot is not in pronation or supination, and the subtalar joint is at a neutral angle during which the fourth and fifth metatarsal heads are on the same plane as the other metatarsal heads.

15.2.3 Joint Capsule and Ligaments

The fibrous capsule completely surrounds the ankle joint. It attaches above to the joint edges of the tibia and fibula, below just outside the corresponding joint surface edges of the talus, and to the neck of the talus. The capsule is thin and weak (i.e., anteriorly and posteriorly) to accommodate plantar flexion and dorsiflexion of the joint and is supported by collateral ligaments laterally and medially. The capsule posteriorly attaches to the posterior tibiofibular ligament.

Ligaments play important roles in the stabilization and function of the foot and ankle complex. The anatomic locations and functions of the ligaments associated with the foot and ankle joints are given in Table 15.3 and shown in Fig. 15.4.

> **Clinical Information**
> Approximately 80–90% of ankle ligament injuries are lateral collateral ligament injuries and 10–15% are medial malleolus fractures associated with deltoid ligament injuries.

15.2.4 Other Structures

15.2.4.1 Synovial Bursae

Synovial bursae are flat, fluid-filled sacs lined with synovial cells and located in areas with excessive friction and pressure and act as a sliding surface between areas of high pressure, reducing friction. Under chronic pressure, it can become pathological and its walls can thicken, swell, become inflamed, or even rupture. There are significant differences between bursae in terms of both location and size.

15.2.4.2 Subcutaneous Bursae

Subcutaneous bursae are located on the medial and lateral malleoli of the ankle joint. Although there are anatomic and structural differences, subcutaneous retro-Achilles tendon bursae (i.e., between the posterior surface of the Achilles tendon and the skin) and subcalcaneal bursae were defined. There are subcutaneous bursae on the dorsomedial surface of the first metatarsal head and the dorsolateral surface of the fifth metatarsal head. The plantar subcutaneous bursae are located on the first and fifth metatarsal heads. The subcutaneous bursae may also be seen over the proximal interphalangeal joints.

Table 15.3 The anatomic placement and functions of ligaments in foot and ankle joints

Posterior ankle ligaments		
Ligament	Anatomic localization	Functions
Posterior talocalcaneal ligament	The posterior of the talus and superior of the calcaneus	Restricts the posterior movement of the talus over the calcaneus
Posterior tibiofibular ligament	The posterior distal of the tibia and the posterior distal of the fibula	Provides the stability of the distal tibiofibular joint
Posterior talofibular ligament	The posterolateral of the talus and the posterior distal end of the lateral malleolus	Prevents the separation of the fibula from the talus
Interosseous membrane	Between the tibia and the fibula	Strengthens the connection between the tibia and the fibula
Lateral ankle ligaments		
Ligament	Anatomic localization	Functions
Anterior tibiofibular ligament	The anterior surface of the lateral malleolus and the medial inferior edge of the tibia	Provides the stability of the anterior tibiofibular joint
Lateral collateral ligament		Restricts excessive inversion of the ankle
• Posterior talofibular ligament	The lateral malleolus and the posterolateral of the talus	Prevents the separation of the fibula from the talus It prevents the ankle joint from sliding backward

Table 15.3 (continued)

• Calcaneofibular ligament	The apex of the lateral malleolus and the lateral tubercle of the calcaneus	Restricts the talar tilt in the direction of adduction
• Anterior talofibular ligament	Anterior of the lateral malleolus and anterior of the talus	• Restricts the internal rotation movement and the anterior gliding movement in the socket within the ankle joint of the talus • It also plays restrictive roles in the ankle plantar flexion movement
Interosseous talocalcaneal ligament	The inferior surface of the talus and the superior of the calcaneus	Restricts the separation of the talus from the calcaneus
Dorsal talonavicular ligament	The dorsal surface of the talus and the dorsal surface of the navicular	Restricts the separation of the navicular from the talus
Bifurcate ligament		Restricts the separation of the navicular and cuboid from the calcaneus
• Calcaneonavicular	Distal of the calcaneus and proximal of the navicular	
• Calcaneocuboid	Distal of the calcaneus and proximal of the cuboid	
Dorsal cuboidonavicular ligament	The lateral surface of the cuboid and the dorsal surface of the navicular	Restricts the separation of the navicular from the cuboid
Dorsal cuneonavicular ligament	The navicular and the three cuneiforms	Restricts the separation of the cuneiform from the navicular
Dorsal intercuneiform ligament	Between the cuneiform bones	Restricts the separation of the cuneiforms
Dorsal tarsometatarsal ligament	Between dorsal of tarsal bones and the corresponding metatarsal bones	Strengthens the tarsometatarsal joint
Medial ankle ligaments		
Ligament	**Anatomic localization**	**Functions**
Deltoid ligament (i.e., medial collateral ligament)		Restricts the medial and inferior valgus movement of the talus and its anterior translation Strengthens the calcaneonavicular ligament Restricts excessive dorsal and plantar flexion Supports the medial longitudinal arch
• Posterior tibiotalar ligament	Between the posteromedial of the medial malleolus and the medial of the talus	Restricts the eversion of the ankle
• Tibiocalcaneal ligament	Anterior distal of the medial malleolus to the sustentaculum tali	Restricts the ankle eversion
• Tibionavicular ligament	Proximal of the navicula and medial malleolus	Restricts the ankle eversion
• Anterior tibiotalar ligament	Between the anterior of the medial malleol and talus	Restricts the ankle eversion
Medial talocalcaneal ligament	The posterior of the sustentaculum tali and talus medial tubercle	Restricts the posterior movement of the talus over the calcaneus
Plantar calcaneonavicular (spring) ligament	Posteroinferior of navicula and sustentaculum tali	Supports the longitudinal arch of the foot
Plantar foot ligaments		
Ligament	**Anatomic localization**	**Functions**
Long plantar ligament	Between the plantar surface of the calcaneus and the cuboid	Supports the arch of the foot
Plantar calcaneocuboid ligament (i.e., short plantar ligament)	The anteroinferior surface of the calcaneus and the inferior surface of the cuboid	Supports the arch of the foot
Plantar calcaneonavicular ligament (i.e., spring)	Posterioinferior of the talus and the sustentaculum tali	Supports the longitudinal arch of the foot

(continued)

Table 15.3 (continued)

Plantar cuboidonavicular ligament	Inferior of the navicula and inferomedial of the cuboid	Restricts the separation of the cuboid from the navicular and supports the arch
Plantar tarsometatarsal ligament	Between the tarsal bones that correspond to the 1–5th metatarsal on the plantar side	Restricts the separation of the metatarsal bones from the corresponding tarsal bones
Collateral ligament	Between the distal of the proximal phalanx and the proximal of the distal phalanx	Strengthens the capsule of the interphalangeal joint
Plantar ligament (i.e., *plate*)	The plantar surface of the joint capsule	Strengthens the plantar surface of the interphalangeal and metatarsophalangeal joints
Deep transverse metatarsal ligament	Between the metatarsophalangeal joints on the plantar side	Restricts the separation of the metatarsophalangeal joint

ANKLE JOINT

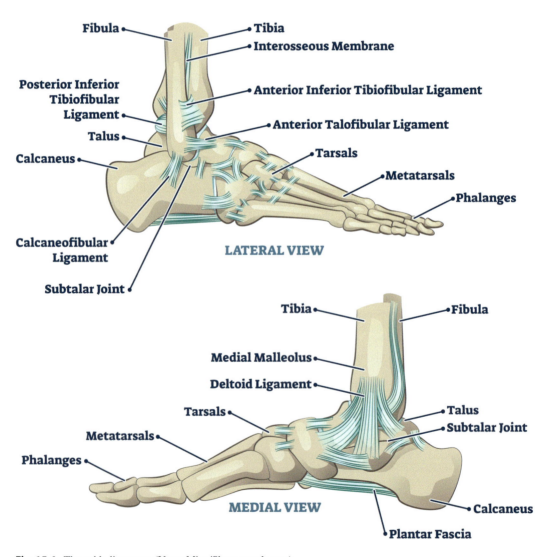

Fig. 15.4 The ankle ligaments (VectorMine/Shutterstock.com)

15.2.4.3 Subfascial Bursae

Subfascial synovial bursae can be examined in two groups.

Group I: This group includes bursae localized between the place where a tendon begins or attaches and the bone. It is the most well-known retrocalcaneal bursa in this group. However, some bursae correspond to the insertion of the Achilles tendon bursa, tibialis anterior and tibialis posterior tendons, interosseous tendons and bursae localized between the metatarsophalangeal joint, the flexor hallucis brevis, and the common origin of the first cuneiform, short flexor tendons, and the base of the fifth metatarsal and the fifth finger.

Retrocalcaneal bursae: The retrocalcaneal bursae are located between the deep surface of the Achilles tendon and the superior prominence of the calcaneus. The anterior wall of this bursae consist of a fibrocartilaginous structure overlapping the calcaneus, and their posterior wall are indistinguishable from the epitendons of the Achilles tendon. The bursae contain a small amount of fluid and reduce the friction of the anterior tendon surface against the calcaneus under normal conditions. Dorsiflexion of the ankle increases pressure on the bursae, and plantar flexion of the foot reduces pressure on the bursae.

Group II: This group includes bursae under the tendon or muscle passing through the bony prominence, between tendons and ligaments, and between tendons and muscles sliding over or close to each other.

15.2.4.4 Plantar Fascia

It is the thickest connective tissue supporting the arches on the plantar surface of the foot. After starting from the anterior of the calcaneal tubercle, the plantar fascia runs along the plantar surface of the foot, extends to the metatarsophalangeal joint, and attaches to the proximal phalanges in the form of five bands. The plantar fascia is made up of medial, central, and lateral bands, starting from the medial. The medial and lateral bands are thin, while the central band is thick. The medial band attaches to the calcaneus and continues toward the front of the foot, covering the plantar surface of the abductor hallucis longus muscle. The central band attaches to the medial tubercle of the calcaneus and forms the thickest part of the plantar fascia. The central band is also called the plantar aponeurosis and has a triangular shape. It wraps around the flexor digitorum longus tendon at the midfoot level and the lateral band attaches to the calcaneus and covers the abductor digiti minimi muscle at the midfoot level and runs toward the front of the foot. The plantar fascia has an important role in weight-bearing because of its anatomic localization and helps to transfer the body weight forward in the push-off phase of the gait. Especially the "Windlass Mechanism" facilitates the push-off phase. With the extension of the first metatarsophalangeal joint, the plantar aponeurosis is stretched and the medial longitudinal arch rises at the end of the stance phase. The foot becomes a rigid lever with the supination of the subtalar joint. This is called the windlass mechanism.

> **Clinical Information**
>
> Five-degree dorsiflexion is needed to ensure full sole contact while transitioning from the mid-stance phase of the gait cycle to the heel lift phase. Dorsiflexion movement is restricted and anterior translation of the tibia is prevented in the short gastrosoleus, which is compensated by pronation of the subtalar joint. Excessive pronation of the foot causes increased stress on the plantar fascia during the push-off phase of gait. In such a case, it can cause plantar fasciitis. Also, the absence of the windlass mechanism affects the supination of the subtalar joint and may cause plantar fasciitis.

15.2.4.5 Arches of the Foot

The foot undertakes important tasks such as shock absorption during stance and walking, proper distribution of body weight, adapting to changes in the ground, and pushing the body forward because it is the point of contact with the ground. To perform these tasks, the foot is

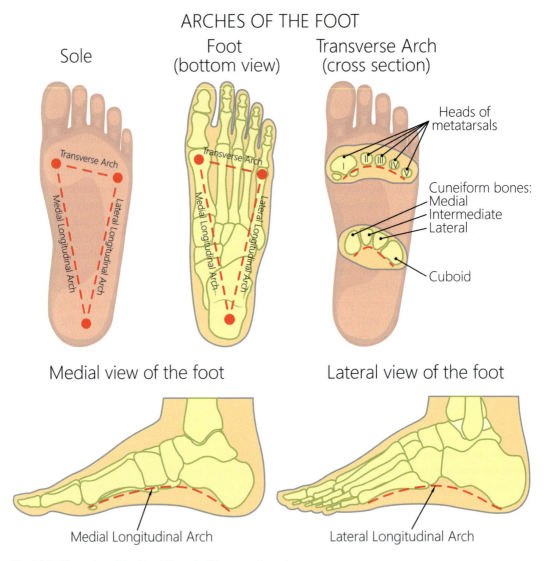

Fig. 15.5 The arches of the foot (Aksanaku/Shutterstock.com)

supported by the foot bones and the strong ligaments that support these bones, the muscles, and the foot arches formed by the fascia on the plantar surface of the foot. There are three arches in the foot, two longitudinal and one transverse, medial, and lateral (Fig. 15.5).

Medial Longitudinal Arch

It is the widest arch of the foot and starts from the posteromedial of the calcaneus and forms anteriorly by the talus, navicular, three cuneiforms, and first three metatarsal bones. The talus is at the top of the arch and is often called the "keystone" because it bears body weight. The arc drops slightly during weight-bearing and then returns to its original state when the weight is lifted. Normally, the medial longitudinal arch does not touch the ground or flatten and is supported by the flexor hallucis longus, tibialis anterior, tibialis posterior, long plantar ligament, short plantar ligament, and spring ligament.

Lateral Longitudinal Arch

It is the arch of the foot that comes into contact with the ground following the heel contact during walking, starting from the posterolateral of the calcaneus and formed by the cuboideum and 3–4th metatarsal bones anteriorly. The cuboideum forms the apex of the arc. The peroneus longus and the long and short plantar ligaments have the most important support for this part.

Transverse Arch

It is an arch that is formed by the wedge-shaped union of the tarsal bones and metatarsals. This arc provides transverse stability of the midfoot and collapses slightly during weight-bearing and allows the body weight to be shared between the five metatarsal heads. It is supported dynamically by intrinsic and extrinsic muscles such as the tibialis posterior, peroneus longus, and connective tissue. The middle cuneiform forms the keystone of the arch.

15.3 Contractile Structures Associated with the Ankle Joint

The muscles of the foot and ankle are divided into two groups, the extrinsic and intrinsic muscles. Extrinsic muscles originate from the tibia, fibula, and femur, while intrinsic muscles originate from the tarsal bones. Appropriate joint kinematics is formed with the coordinated movements of these muscles and the functions of the foot-ankle complex are maintained. The muscles are separated by regions (Fig. 15.6). The functions of these muscles are given in Table 15.4, and the nerves responsible for the innervation of these muscles are given in Table 15.5.

> **Clinical Information**
>
> The role of the muscles in supporting the arches of the feet is small during a static normal stance. However, the muscles become active with activities such as walking, running, and jumping. Standing for a long time, carrying heavy loads, and using unsuitable shoes can cause arcs to collapse, which is especially seen in occupational groups that work for a long time. EMG studies suggest that especially tibialis posterior function loss is associated with pes planus. For this reason, it is very important to do exercises for the development of the muscles that support the arches in the foot and to choose the appropriate shoes for the foot that support the arches. However, the situation in children and infants is somewhat different. Babies are usually born with a flexible low sole. A prevalence of 50% lower arch was reported in children who are aged 2–6 years, but this rate decreases toward primary school age, and the arches of the foot are structurally mature in children aged 12–13 years.

> **Clinical Information**
>
> The overactivity of the tibialis anterior explains the wear-tear patterns on the posterolateral side of the heel because of frictional forces between the shoe and the ground.

> **Clinical Information**
>
> The tibialis posterior controls pronation eccentrically during the mid-stance phase and foot flate phase of the gait cycle. Any weakness of this muscle can cause excessive pronation of the subtalar joint and result in plantar fasciitis.

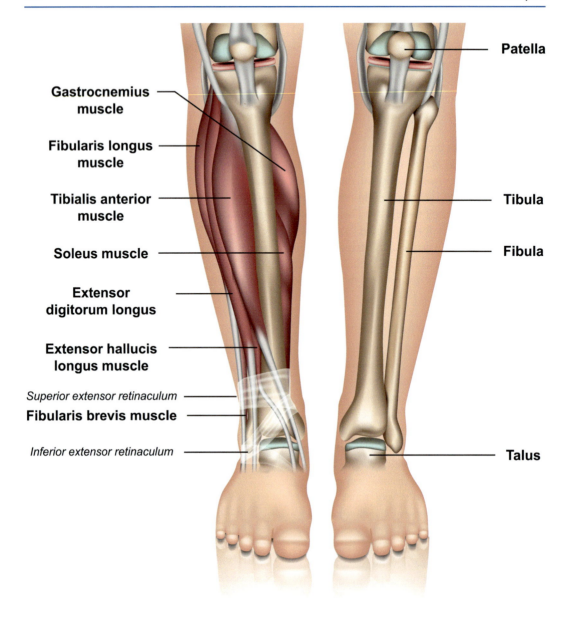

Fig. 15.6 The leg muscles (medicalstocks/Shutterstock.com)

Table 15.4 Muscles associated with the foot and ankle joints and their functions

Superficial posterior muscles of the leg		
Muscle	Action	Function
Gastrocnemius	Ankle plantar flexion and the knee flexion	It provides significant propulsion during walking, running, and jumping activities
Soleus	Ankle plantar flexion	Ensures that the leg is fixed on the foot while standing and is constantly active
Plantaris	Assists plantar flexion of the ankle and knee flexion	–

Table 15.4 (continued)

Muscle	Action	Function
Deep posterior muscles of the leg		
Tibialis posterior	Inverts foot and assists in ankle plantar flexion	Helps to maintain the balance of the tibia on the foot, especially during the lateral displacement of body weight. Being a strong invertor muscle, it controls the forefoot during activities such as walking and running, preventing the medial arch of the foot from fully straightening
Flexor hallucis longus	Flexes big toe and assists with ankle plantar flexion	Producing most of the final push in the foot while walking It also plays an important role in maintaining the medial longitudinal arch
Flexor digitorum longus	Flexes 2–5th digits, assists with plantar flexion of the ankle, and supports the longitudinal arch of the foot	It presses the fingertips firmly against the ground to achieve maximum grip and thrust during the toe lift in the push phase of running, jumping, or walking The toes tend to grasp the ground for balance when standing
Lateral muscles of the leg		
Peroneus (i.e., fibularis) longus	Everts foot and assists in plantar flexion	Helps maintain an upright position while standing, along with other surrounding muscles Prevents the body from falling to the opposite side while standing on one leg Controls the mediolateral sway by pressing the medial side of the foot to the ground However, its main functional activity occurs during vigorous movements of the foot (e.g., running on uneven ground). Here, the control over the tibialis anterior and the medial side of the foot and the first metatarsal is very important
Peroneus (i.e., fibularis) brevis	Everts foot and assists in plantar flexion	Helps prevent mediolateral oscillation while standing Prevents the body from falling to the opposite side while standing on one leg Plays an important role in controlling the position of the foot when walking or running, especially on uneven ground, and prevents the foot from over-inversion
Peroneus (i.e., fibularis) tertius	Dorsiflexes ankle and everts foot	Helps prevent excessive inversion during sports activities
Anterior muscles of the leg		
Tibialis anterior	Dorsiflexes ankle and inverts foot	It provides the balance of the body on the foot, as in the other muscles in the leg Works with the surrounding muscles to maintain balance during activities that change the weight distribution of the upper body
Extensor digitorum longus	Extends the 2–5th digits and assists with ankle dorsiflexion	Raises the toes while walking and running
Extensor hallucis longus	Extends the big toe and assists with ankle dorsiflexion and inversion	Brings the big toe into the extension position before heel contact during walking. In this way, the heel becomes ready for the weight transfer phase The extension of the interphalangeal joint is entirely dependent on the extensor hallucis longus because the thumb has no associated lumbrical or interosseous muscle
Muscles of the dorsum of the foot		
Extensor digitorum brevis	Extends the 2–4th digits at the metatarsophalangeal joint	Helps the extensor digitorum longus and extensor hallucis longus to lift the toes off the ground while running and walking

(continued)

Table 15.4 (continued)

Extensor hallucis brevis	Assists with the extension of the big toe at the metatarsophalangeal joint	Raises the big toe during walking
Dorsal interossei	Flexes the metatarsophalangeal joint and abducts 2–4th digits	Positions the foot and big toe for balance

First layer of muscles: the sole of foot

Muscle	Action	Function
Abductor hallucis	Abducts the big toe and assists with big toe flexion	Acts as a beam for the arch when the foot is used to propel the body forward because of its location on the medial side of the foot It helps control the central position of this toe when flexed because it attaches to the medial side of the big toe It must not be forgotten that the big toe moves medially when the muscle contracts hard, but more importantly, the foot is positioned laterally, improving the relationship between the big toe and the medial side of the foot
Flexor digitorum brevis	Flexes the 2–5th digits	Takes part in the generation of push from the toes when the need increases like the flexor digitorum longus This muscle also supports the longitudinal arch and stabilizes the foot during walking or running
Abductor digiti minimi	Abducts and assists the flexion of the fifth digit at the metatarsophalangeal joint	Acts as a beam for this arch, similar to the function of the abductor hallucis muscle located on the medial side of the foot because it extends from the posterior to the anterior of the lateral longitudinal arch It also protects the arc during activities such as running and jumping

Second layer of muscles: the sole of foot

Muscle	Action	Function
Lumbricales	Flexes the proximal phalanges of the 2–5th digits and extends the middle and distal phalanges of the 2–5th digits	Its activation prevents the toes from clawing during the pushing phase of gait. Paralysis of these muscles results in the extensor muscles pulling the toes from the metatarsophalangeal joints into hyperextension
Quadratus plantae	Assists in flexion of the 2–5th digits	Plays an important role in gait when the ankle joint is in plantar flexion It exerts a force on the long flexor tendons and the toes can bend to grip the ground, providing support and thrust during the pushing phase, which may suggest that the flexor digitorum longus is strongly acting on two joints at the same time

Third layer of muscles: the sole of foot

Muscle	Action	Function
Flexor digiti minimi brevis	Flexes the proximal phalanx of the fifth digit	Supports the lateral longitudinal arch of the foot
Adductor hallucis (transverse head)	Adducts big toe	Adductor hallucis helps to control the position of the big toe by working with abductor hallucis. In this way, active flexion can be produced, providing the final push needed in walking, running, or jumping It also helps protect the anterior metatarsal arch of the foot because of its diagonal position along the forefoot The pull of the adductor hallucis is almost at a right angle to the phalanx and for this reason, it has a better mechanical advantage than abductor hallucis
Adductor hallucis (oblique head)	Adducts big toe	Positions the big toe for balance and push
Flexor hallucis brevis	Flexes proximal phalanx of the big toe	Helps the flexor hallucis longus in the final push-off phase, when the foot is off the ground during the activity

Table 15.4 (continued)

The deep interosseal muscles		
Muscle	**Action**	**Function**
Plantar interossei	Flexion of the metatarsophalangeal joint and adduction of the 2–4th digits	Helps control the position of the third, fourth, and fifth toes during the pushing phase of walking and running with the help of the dorsal interossei and abductor digiti minimi It helps prevent the toes from spreading when weight is applied suddenly to the forefoot
Dorsal interossei	Flexion of the metatarsophalangeal joint and abduction of 2–4th digits	They are strong muscles. Their activity along with the plantar interossei controls the orientation of the toes during vigorous activity. In this way, it enables the long and short flexors to perform their appropriate actions These muscles can flex these joints because of their relationship with the metatarsophalangeal joint. In this way, they can help protect the anterior metatarsal arch by raising the heads of the second, third, and fourth metatarsals They also help to a restricted extent to protect the medial and lateral longitudinal arches of the foot

Table 15.5 The nerves and nerve roots providing innervation of the muscles associated with the foot and ankle joints

Nerves	Nerve roots	Muscles
Tibial nerve	L4, L5, S1, S2, S3	• Semitendinosus • Semimembranosus • Biceps femoris • Adductor magnus • Gastrocnemius • Soleus • Plantaris • Flexor hallucis longus • Flexor digitorum longus • Tibialis posterior
Medial plantar nerve	S2, S3	• Flexor hallucis brevis • Abductor hallucis • Flexor digitorum brevis • Lumbricales
Lateral plantar nerve	S2, S3	• Adductor hallucis • Abductor digiti minimi • Quadratus plantae • Lumbricales • Flexor digiti minimi brevis • Interossei
Deep fibular nerve	L4, L5, S1	• Tibialis anterior • Extensor digitorum longus • Extensor hallucis longus • Fibularis tertius • Extensor digitorum brevis • Extensor hallucis brevis
Superficial fibular nerve	L5, S1, S2	• Peroneus longus • Peroneus brevis

15.4 Palpation of Bone Structures and Muscles in the Ankle Joint

The explanations of the bone structures in the foot/ankle complex and their palpation are given in Table 15.6, and the visuals of these palpation points are given in Fig. 15.7. The explanations of the muscles associated with the foot/ankle complex and their palpation are given in Table 15.7, and images of these palpation points are given in Fig. 15.8.

> **Attention!**
> Palpation positions of I patient and the therapist in the images are given as examples. In the palpation of the muscle and bony prominences, the most comfortable position for tissue evaluation must be chosen, considering the functional status of the patient and the ergonomics of the therapist.

Table 15.6 The palpation of the bone structures in the foot and ankle

Bone structures	Palpation
Distal fibular shaft	The fibula is palpated from the lateral malleolus and can be palpated from the muscles in the proximal part of the leg to the area where the bone structure cannot be felt while ascending (Fig. 15.7a)
Medial malleoli	The medial malleolus is the most prominent bony prominence at the distal end of the tibia medial to the ankle joint. The fingers can be palpated by placing them on a large projection felt below the anteromedial shaft of the tibia (Fig. 15.7b)
Lateral malleoli	The lateral malleolus can be palpated by placing the fingers on the most prominent bony prominence at the distal end of the fibula, lateral to the ankle joint. It is larger than the medial malleolus and extends more distally and posteriorly (Fig. 15.7c)
Ankle joint	The ankle joint lies in a horizontal line 1 cm above the end of the medial malleolus and 2 cm above the end of the lateral malleolus and can be easily palpated on the dorsal surface. Starting from the medial, the joint can be identified by applying firm pressure along the inner border of the medial malleolus. If the extensor tendons are pulled aside, the lower end of the tibia and the medial edge of the lateral malleolus can be palpated
Talus head	The talus head is located behind the navicular. The talonavicular joint between the talus and the navicular is very prominent and easily palpable during the inversion and eversion of the foot
Anterior surface of the talus	If the foot is passively inversion and plantar flexed, most of the anterior surface of the talus can be palpated. The anterior surface of the trochlea of the talus can be palpated by placing the fingers on the lateral malleolus and sliding them distally and medially (Fig. 15.7d)
Sustentaculum tali	When the medial malleolus is localized with the thumb and descended approximately 1–1.5 cm distal from the medial malleoli end, the sustentaculum tali can be palpated (Fig. 15.7e) *Alternative method: It can also be palpated when moving approximately 2.5 cm posterior from the navicular tubercle and when the head of the talus is descended slightly posteriorly in the plantar direction. The sustentaculum tali forms a shelf-like structure on which the talus sits. The joint line between the tali of the sustentaculum and the talus located proximal can be easily palpated*
Medial tubercle of the talus	If the thumb is placed medial to the calcaneus and moved slowly proximally and anteriorly, the medial tubercle of the talus can be palpated slightly posteriorly and proximal to the sustentaculum tali (i.e., posterior and plantar face of the medial malleolus)
Sinus tarsi	Depression is felt when the thumb is placed in the lateral malleolus and shifted distally and anteromedially. This depression is the upper part of the tarsal sinus, which is an opening between the talus and the calcaneus into the subtalar joint space. Pressure is directed medially and inward for the best palpation of the tarsal sinus (Fig. 15.7f)
Calcaneus	The calcaneus can be palpated by placing the thumb and fingertips behind the heel (Fig. 15.7g)
Calcaneal tubercle	The calcaneal tubercle can be easily palpated on the plantar aspect of the foot. The thumb is placed on the plantar surface of the calcaneus. The plantar face can be palpated by applying firm pressure to both sides of the midline of the calcaneus. The medial surface of the calcaneal tuberosity is usually more prominent compared to the lateral surface (Fig. 15.7h)
Peroneal (i.e., fibular) tubercle	It can be palpated by placing the thumb on the lateral malleolus and sliding it distally to the lateral surface of the calcaneus. *Alternative method: The lateral surface of the calcaneus is felt under the subcutaneous tissue when the cuboid is palpated and moved proximally along the lateral surface of the foot. The peroneal tubercle over the calcaneus can be palpated approximately 2 cm below and anterior to the lateral malleolus tip*
Navicular tubercle	It can be palpated when the thumb is placed on the medial malleolus and slide distally and anteriorly (i.e., medial longitudinal posteriorly) (Fig. 15.7i) *Alternative method: It can also be palpated by moving the thumb proximal to the first cuneiform*
Medial cuneiform	The flat surface of the cuneiform can be palpated when the thumb is placed on the navicular and the foot is moved from dorsal to distal (Fig. 15.7j) *Alternative method: It can also be palpated over the joint line between the first metatarsal and the first cuneiform just near the base of the first metatarsal located medial and dorsal*

Table 15.6 (continued)

Bone structures	Palpation
2nd and 3rd cuneiforms	The second and third cuneiforms can be palpated from the dorsum of the foot Second cuneiform is proximal to the second metatarsal and the third cuneiform is proximal to the third metatarsal. The tarsometatarsal joint line between the metatarsal and the cuneiform is felt when palpating proximal to the base of the second and third metatarsals The cuneiform can be easily held with the hand proximal to the joint line
Cuboideum	The dorsal surface of the cuboid can be palpated by placing the thumb lateral to the calcaneus and sliding it distally and anteriorly (Fig. 15.7k) *Alternative method: There is a depression extending to the cuboid on the lateral side of the foot, just proximal to the fifth metatarsal, which is formed by the expansion of the base of the fifth metatarsal and the concave shape of the lateral edge of the cuboid. The cuboid can be palpated with firm pressure medial to this depression*
Metatarsals	The metatarsals are easily palpable subcutaneously proximal to the MTF joint line of each finger (Fig. 15.7l)
1–5th metatarsal head	Metatarsal bone heads can be palpated from the plantar surface of the foot. Although all five metatarsals can be palpated by hand, the first and fifth metatarsal heads are most prominent because of the concavity of the transverse arch of the foot (Fig. 15.7m). After palpating the fifth metatarsal head the other four metatarsal heads can also be palpated by moving towards the medial. Above the plantar surface of the first metatarsal head are two small sesamoid bones. When the first metatarsal head is palpated on the plantar surface, what is felt are the two sesamoid bones
Sesamoids	The big toe is extended and the distal end of the first metatarsal is palpated. Two sesamoid bones located side by side proximal to the first MTF joint are palpable (Fig. 15.7n)
1st metatarsophalangeal joint	The joint line of the first metatarsophalangeal joint is felt if palpation is continued proximally from the medial surface of the proximal phalanx of the big toe
2–4th metatarsophalangeal joint	The MTF joint line can be felt if palpation is continued from the proximal phalanges of the 2–4th toes proximally on the dorsal aspect of the foot (Fig. 15.7o)
5th metatarsophalangeal joint	The fifth MTF joint line is felt if palpation is continued proximally from the lateral surface of the proximal phalanx of the fifth toe *N.B.: The proximal phalanx of the fifth toe is slightly more proximal than the other proximal phalanges of the foot. For this reason, the fifth MTF joint is located more proximal than the other MTF joints*
Big toe phalanges and interphalangeal joint	The distal and proximal phalanges of the big toe and the interphalangeal joint between them can be palpated from the distal medial of the foot
2–4th phalanges and interphalangeal joints	2–4th phalanges are easily palpable from the dorsum of the foot. Starting from the distal, the distal phalanx, middle phalanx, and proximal phalanx of each finger and the joint lines between these phalanges, and also proximal interphalangeal joint and distal interphalangeal joint can be palpated.
Phalanx and interphalangeal joints of the little finger	The phalanx and interphalangeal joints of the little finger can be palpated from the lateral distal of the foot to the proximal, middle, and distal phalanx. The proximal and distal interphalangeal joints can also be palpated between the phalanges

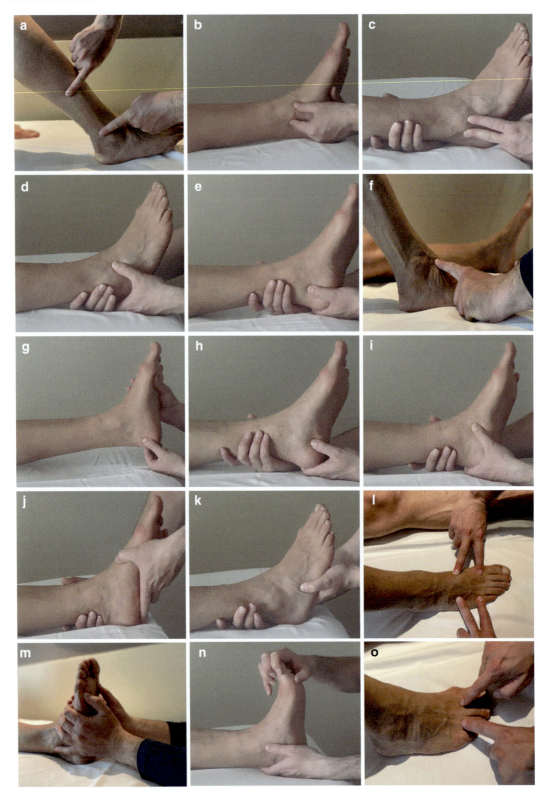

Fig. 15.7 The palpation of the bone structures in the foot skeleton (**a**) Distal fibular shaft, (**b**) Medial malleoli, (**c**) Lateral malleoli, (**d**) Anterior surface of the talus, (**e**) Sustentaculum tali, (**f**) Sinus tarsi, (**g**) Calcaneus, (**h**) Calcaneal tubercle, (**i**) Navicular tubercle, (**j**) Medial cuneiform, (**k**) Cuboideum, (**l**) Metatarsals, (**m**) 1–5th metatarsal head, (**n**) Sesamoids, (**o**) 2–4th metatarsophalangeal joint

Table 15.7 The palpation of the muscles associated with the foot and ankle joints

Muscles	Palpation
Gastrocnemius	When descending behind the knee joint, the two major muscle bodies of the gastrocnemius can be felt on either side of the upper leg. The medial head of the muscle is slightly more bulky and lower than the lateral head. Both are felt to be joined by a flat broad tendon just below the half of the leg *For easy palpation: The lateral and medial muscle body of the muscle can be seen and palpated when resisting plantar flexion of the ankle, proximal to the posterior of the leg (Fig. 15.8a). It can be palpated as the gastrocnemius tendon (i.e., Achilles tendon) in the lower half of the leg up to the insertion site in the calcaneus*
Soleus	The soleus is not easy to palpate because it is located below the gastrocnemius. Its lateral border is felt like a flat elevation below and lateral to the gastrocnemius when resistance is applied to the plantar flexion of the ankle with the knee flexed to 90° (Fig. 15.8b). The calcaneal tendon narrowing and rounding at the ankle joint can be felt when the palpated hand is lowered down the leg
Plantaris	The body of the plantaris muscle is located medial to the proximal insertion of the lateral head of the gastrocnemius. It can be palpated by placing the thumb posterior to the head of the fibula and sliding it medially and distally between the two heads of the gastrocnemius. Palpation must be started from the distal border of the popliteal fossa because of the vascular nerve bundle in the popliteal fossa (Fig. 15.8c). *For easy palpation: Begin with gentle palpation in the center of the popliteal fossa and resist plantar flexion of the ankle and slowly move down until you feel the contraction. Plantaris is difficult to distinguish from the lateral head of the gastrocnemius because both muscles have the same functions*
Tibialis posterior	It is not possible to palpate the body of the muscle because of other overlying muscles. The fingers are placed on the medial edge of the tibia in the prone position, with the knee flexion. The superficial fibers can be palpated partially if the fingers are slid posteriorly and pressed deeply in a hook shape (Fig. 15.8d). However, it is easy to feel the tendon as it passes behind the medial malleolus and jointly as it attaches to the tubercle of the navicular *For easy palpation: When plantar flexion and inversion against resistance is performed while lying on the supine, the tendon can be felt behind the medial malleolus and the contraction of the body of the muscle can be felt when the posterior midline of the leg is pressed lightly and the foot is inverted*
Flexor digitorum longus	Flexor digitorum longus (i.e., FDL) is very difficult to distinguish. However, the tendon can only be identified when passing by the sustentaculum tali A portion of the body of the flexor digitorum longus is superficial between the soleus and the tibial shaft distal and medially of the leg. When the 2–5th fingers are flexed, contraction can be felt *For easy palpation: More comfortable contraction is felt if resistance is given to the flexion of the 2–5th fingers. The distal tendon of the FDL is usually palpable at the level of the medial malleolus and can sometimes be seen posterior and distal to the medial malleolus (Fig. 15.8e). The medial malleoli are located a little further away from the distal tendon of the tibialis posterior. The distal tendons of the FDL are quite superficial on the plantar surface of the foot. FDL can be palpated by flexing and relaxing the fingers at two to five metatarsophalangeal and interphalangeal joints. However, it is sometimes difficult to distinguish the location and boundaries of these tendons precisely because of adjacent muscle and soft tissue. The body of the muscle can be felt by gently pressing the posteromedial part of the leg and flexing the 2–5th fingers during contraction*
Flexor hallucis longus	The flexor hallucis longus is almost impossible to palpate since it is deep within the leg muscles, flexor retinaculum, plantar aponeurosis, and foot muscles, and its tendon is deeply located on both the calf and the plantar side of the foot. A small distal portion of the flexor hallucis longus (i.e., FHL) body is superficial on the distal medial surface of the leg between the FDL and the calcaneal tendon. The contraction of the FHL is felt if resistance is also applied when the big toe is bent (Fig. 15.8f). The distal tendon is deep at the level of the medial malleolus and is difficult to palpate. If alternately flexed and relaxed from the MTF and interphalangeal joints of the big toe, the distal tendon of the FHL on the sole can be palpated. However, it is quite difficult to precisely distinguish the location and boundaries of its tendon from adjacent muscle and soft tissue. A contraction can be felt when the posterolateral aspect of the leg is pressed lightly and the big toe is flexed to palpate the body of the FHL

(continued)

Table 15.7 (continued)

Muscles	Palpation
Peroneus (i.e., fibularis) longus	The fingers are placed lateral to the knee joint in the side-lying position. The head of the fibula is palpated just below the joint level. The fingers are slid down from the head of the fibula to the lateral side of the fibula. The long and vertical body of the muscle is felt when the toes are held in this position and the outside of the foot is lifted. The tendons of the peroneus longus and brevis are palpated if the same maneuver is performed by placing the fingers under and behind the lateral malleolus. The peroneus longus passes below and the peroneus brevis passes above when the peroneal tubercle is observed *For easy palpation: The peroneus longus continues as a tendon down about half of the leg. The distal of the tendon can usually be palpated fairly easily just behind the lateral malleolus by perpendicular friction to the tendon. Contraction of the muscle can be felt from the lateral leg if the eversion of the foot is resisted by the tarsal joints* (Fig. 15.8g)
Peroneus (i.e., fibularis) brevis	Peroneus brevis is difficult to palpate because it is located deep to the peroneus longus. When the fingers placed on the body of the peroneus longus are moved down from the lower half of the fibula (but in the same vertical line) and the foot is everted and plantar flexed, the muscle body of the peroneus brevis can be palpated (Fig. 15.8h) *For easy palpation: Resistance is given to ankle eversion and plantar flexion to better feel the muscle. The distal tendon can be palpated distal to the lateral malleolus and its tendon can be easily traced to the groove just above the fibular tubercle and then its insertion to the fifth metatarsal tubercle can be followed*
Peroneus (i.e., fibularis) tertius	Peroneus tertius is very difficult to palpate. However, the muscle can be partially felt inside the small pit when the fingers are slid down the anterior part of the lateral malleolus. Its tendon can be felt in the groove on the medial side of the base of the fifth metatarsal bone *For easy palpation: A tendon going to the fifth metatarsal is felt when the distal tendon of the extensor digitorum longus that goes to the little toe on the back of the foot is found and palpated laterally. Friction can be applied to feel the tendon. It can be felt by resisting dorsiflexion and eversion of the foot If the tendon is still not felt. The muscle body can be palpated from the inside of the leg by going proximal From this position* (Fig. 15.8i)
Tibialis anterior	When the thumb is placed on the tibial shaft and shifted laterally, the muscle body can be palpated. *For easy palpation: When the foot is resisted by dorsiflexion and inversion of the ankle, the distal tendon of the tibialis anterior can be seen medial to the ankle joint. When the fingers are placed vertically on the distal tendon and moved back and forth, the tendon can be felt. Continuing to palpate proximally toward the lateral tibial condyle, the muscle body can be palpated on the anterior of the leg just next to the shaft of the tibia* (Fig. 15.8j)
Extensor hallucis longus	The tendon of the muscle can be traced to its insertion at the base of the distal phalanx as it crosses the first metatarsophalangeal joint If the big toe is extended. It can be felt and seen as it passes from the lateral of the tibialis anterior tendon to the anterior of the ankle joint If traced along the tendon with the fingers. From here, it can be felt that the tendon moves upward and laterally before it enters deep into the surrounding muscles. The muscle can be felt to contract under the toes as the toes are move about 12 cm higher and a little laterally and the big toe is rhythmically extended and flexed *For easy palpation: If resistance is applied to the extension of the thumb from the metatarsophalangeal and interphalangeal joints, the tendon can be seen and palpated by perpendicular friction. The muscle may not be palpable when the friction is continued proximally because it is located deep in the tibialis anterior and extensor digitorum longus. A deep contraction of other muscles can be felt with the extension of the big toe* (Fig. 15.8k)
Extensor digitorum longus	The extensor digitorum longus muscle can be easily palpated from the anterolateral aspect of the leg. The fingers are placed on the lateral side of the leg, about 2 cm downward and medially from the head of the fibula. The muscle may be felt to contract when lifting the toes off the ground. The tendon can be easily distinguished lateral to the tibialis anterior and extensor hallucis longus when the fingers are placed in front of the ankle joint *For easy palpation: The extensor digitorum longus (i.e., EDL) tendons become visible on the dorsum of the foot if resistance is applied to the extension of the metatarsophalangeal and interphalangeal joints of the 2–5th toes. The fingers can be palpated by moving them back and forth by placing them distally perpendicular to the tendon. If the palpation is continued proximally, much of the body of the muscle is found to be located between the tibialis anterior and peroneus longus* (Fig. 15.8l)

Table 15.7 (continued)

Muscles	Palpation
Extensor digitorum brevis, extensor hallucis brevis	The fingers are placed on the tendon, where the extensor digitorum longus is divided into four parts. The extensor digitorum brevis (i.e., EDB) tendon can be felt immediately laterally and deeply when the toes are extended. It is difficult to follow the tendon distally The body of the EDB is 2.5 cm distal to the lateral malleolus on the proximal dorsolateral surface of the foot; extensor hallucis brevis (i.e., EHB) can be palpated on its dorsomedial surface. The body of the muscle can be seen and palpated if 2–4th fingers are extended with resistance from the metatarsophalangeal joint (Fig. 15.8m). The same procedure is followed for EDB to palpate EHB. However, the supporting hand is placed on the proximal phalanx of the big toe to provide resistance to the extension of the big toe. The tendons of these muscles can be palpated distally by contracting and relaxing the distal against resistance and perpendicular friction to the tendon. The distal tendons of these muscles are difficult to palpate and separate from each other. The distal of EDB and EHB can be palpable and difficult to distinguish. The tendons will (also) be stretched by extension of the proximal phalanges of the toes because they are located deep within the distal tendons of the extensor digitorum longus
Lumbricales	These muscles are covered with many small muscles and long flexor tendons on the sole and it is not possible to palpate them because they are located deep on the soles of the feet
Quadratus plantae	Quadratus plantae is not palpable because the muscle is located deep on the sole. The quadratus plantae muscle is located deep to the flexor digitorum brevis and flexes the 2–5th fingers. For this reason, it is difficult to distinguish these two muscles from each other
Flexor digitorum brevis	The flexor digitorum brevis is very difficult to palpate as it is covered by the thickest fascia of the body and its tendons are deep in the foot. The fingers are placed on the proximal plantar midline of the foot. Place the fingers of the supporting hand on the plantar surface of the proximal or middle phalanges of the 2nd to 5th toes if resistance is needed. Contraction is felt when flexion of the 2–5th fingers from the metatarsophalangeal joint is requested and resistance is given
Flexor hallucis brevis	This muscle is located too deep on the plantar surface of the foot and is not palpable. Only the sesamoid bones in their tendons can be palpated *For easy palpation: Fingers are placed on the plantar surface of the first metatarsal bone. Muscle contraction is felt when flexion of the big toe is requested from the metatarsophalangeal joint. The muscle can be felt better by resisting the flexion of the big toe* (Fig. 15.8n)
Flexor digiti minimi pedis	Flexor digiti minimi pedis can be felt when deep pressure is applied to the midsection of the lateral plantar surface of the foot during flexion of the little finger *For easy palpation: Fingers are placed on the plantar surface of the foot on the fifth metatarsal bone. Contraction is felt if resistance is applied to the flexion of the little finger at the metatarsophalangeal joint* (Fig. 15.8o)
Abductor hallucis	The fingers are placed on the medial plantar surface of the foot below the medial longitudinal arch. The body of the muscle can be easily palpated toward the heel when bending the toes and the tendon of the muscle can be felt by tracking forward from the heel *For easy palpation: The toes are placed on the medial side of the foot close to the plantar surface. The contraction of the muscle is felt if abduction of the big toe is desired from the metatarsophalangeal joint. The muscle can be felt better by applying resistance from the medial side of the proximal phalanx of the big toe*
Abductor digiti minimi	This muscle is difficult to palpate. The fingers are placed on the distal and the lateral aspect of the foot close to the plantar surface. Resistance can be applied and contraction of the muscle can be felt while abducting the proximal phalanx of the little finger from the metatarsophalangeal joint
Dorsal interossei	Muscle contraction can be felt when the fingers are placed on the dorsum of the foot between the proximal parts of the metatarsals and the toes are abducted
Adductor hallucis	*This muscle is too deep to be palpable*
Plantar interossei	*This muscle is too deep to be palpable*

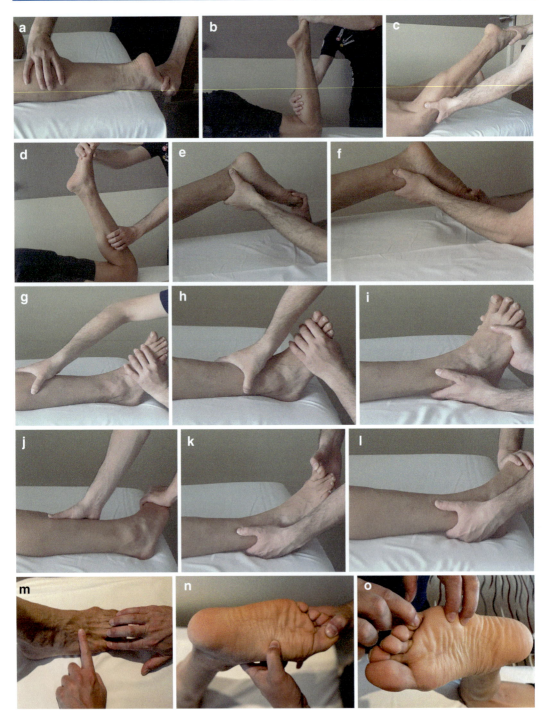

Fig. 15.8 The palpation of the foot skeletal muscles (**a**) Gastrocnemius, (**b**) Soleus, (**c**) Plantaris, (**d**) Tibialis posterior, (**e**) Flexor digitorum longus, (**f**) Flexor hallucis longus, (**g**) Peroneus (i.e., fibularis) longus, (**h**) Peroneus (i.e., fibularis) brevis, (**i**) Peroneus (i.e., fibularis) tertius, (**j**) Tibialis anterior, (**k**) Extensor hallucis longus, (**l**) Extensor digitorum longus, (**m**) Extensor digitorum brevis, extensor hallucis brevis, (**n**) Flexor hallucis brevis, (**o**) Flexor digiti minimi pedis

15.5 Movements in the Ankle Joint

The ankle joint complex is made up of the leg and foot, forming the kinetic link allowing the lower extremity to interact with the ground. As it is already known, this is an important requirement for walking and other activities of daily living. Although the bone and ligament structure of the ankle is exposed to high compression and shear forces during walking, it provides the joint to work with high stability and is also more resistant to degenerative processes (e.g., osteoarthritis) when compared to similarly load-bearing hip and knee joints, if not associated with previous traumas.

15.5.1 Ankle Movements

The key movements of the ankle joint complex are plantar and dorsiflexion in the sagittal plane, abduction and adduction in the transverse plane, and inversion and eversion in the frontal plane. The combination of these movements in both subtalar and tibiotalar joints creates 3D movements (i.e., supination and pronation), which are defined by the position of the plantar surface of the foot. While the combination of plantar flexion, inversion, and adduction during supination causes medial movement of the sole, dorsiflexion, eversion, and abduction movements during pronation cause lateral movement of the sole. The basic muscles and assistive muscles responsible for the movements in the foot skeleton are summarized in Table 15.8.

15.5.2 Rotation Axis of the Ankle

Although it is accepted by most researchers that the tibiotalar joint is a simple hinge-type joint, it is also argued that it is multiaxial because of internal rotation during dorsiflexion and external rotation during plantar flexion. The axis of rotation of the ankle joint complex in the sagittal plane is around the line passing through the medial and lateral malleoli; the axis of rotation in the coronal plane occurs at the intersection between the malleolus and the long axis of the tibia; the axis of rotation in the transverse plane occurs around the long axis of the tibia and intersects the midline of the foot. The axis of the subtalar joint is an oblique axis running from posterior to anterior and forming an angle of approximately 40° with the anterior-posterior axis in the sagittal plane and 23° with the midline of the foot in the transverse plane. Similar to the tibiotalar joint, the subtalar joint creates multiple motions during plantar and dorsiflexion, resulting in pronation and supination.

15.5.3 Joint Range of Motion

Ankle movements occur mainly at the tibiotalar joint between 10 and 20° dorsiflexion and 40–55° plantar flexion in the sagittal plane, and the ankle has a total range of motion between 65° and 75°. There are also 23° inversion and 12° eversion in the frontal plane. However, the range of motion that is needed in daily life is less. For example, a joint range of motion of 30° is sufficient for walking, 37° for climbing stairs, and approximately 56° for descending stairs.

> **Attention!**
> In addition to the method used in the evaluation of ankle range of motion, it must be kept in mind that joint range of motion varies considerably among individuals because of geographical and cultural differences based on activities of daily living.

Table 15.8 The muscles that are involved in movements in the foot skeleton

Movements in the foot and ankle joints and the muscles responsible for movement	
Movement	**Muscles involved in the movement**
Dorsiflexion	• Tibialis anterior • Peroneus tertius • *Extensor digitorum longus* • *Extensor hallucis longus*
Plantar flexion	• Gastrocnemius • Soleus • Plantaris • Peroneus longus • Peroneus brevis • Tibialis posterior • *Flexor digitorum longus* • *Flexor hallucis longus*
Inversion	• Tibialis anterior • Tibialis posterior
Eversion	• Peroneus longus • Peroneus brevis • Peroneus tertius
Movements in the toes and the muscles responsible for movement	
Movement	**Muscles**
Extension to the fingers	• Extensor hallucis longus (i.e., MTF, IF) • Extensor digitorum longus (i.e., MTF, PIF, DIF) • Extensor digitorum brevis (i.e., MTF, PIF, DIF) • Lumbricales (i.e., PIF, DIF)
Flexion to the fingers	• Flexor digitorum longus (i.e., MTF, PIF, DIF) • Flexor digitorum brevis (i.e., MTF, PIF) • Flexor hallucis longus (i.e., MTF, IF) • Flexor hallucis brevis (i.e., MTF) • Plantaris quantae (i.e., MTF, PIF, DIF) • Flexor digiti minimi brevis (i.e., MTF) • Interossei (i.e., MTF) • Lumbricales (i.e., MTF)
Abduction to the fingers	• Abductor hallucis (i.e., MTF) • Abductor digiti minimi (i.e., MTF) • Dorsal interossei (i.e., MTF)
Adduction to the fingers	• Adductor hallucis (i.e., MTF) • Plantar interossei (i.e., MTF)

Attention!
1. Muscles whose main function is to flex and extend the toes and play assistive roles during foot and ankle movements are given in italics
2. Two joints in the big toe, metatarsophalangeal (i.e., *MTF*) and interphalangeal (i.e., *IF*). There are three joints in each of the other four toes: Metatarsophalangeal metatarsophalangeal (i.e., *MTF*), proximal interphalangeal (i.e., *PIF*), and distal interphalangeal (i.e., *DIF*). Joints in which the muscles play roles are given in parentheses in their abbreviated forms

15.5.4 Kinematics of Walking

There are two phases of gait: stance and swing. The stance phase is divided into three subphases during a normal gait cycle as the heel, ankle, and forefoot activation, depending on the sagittal motion of the ankle. The heel activation phase continues from the heel strike with slight plantar flexion until the foot is flat on the ground. The dorsi flexors contract eccentrically to lower the foot to the ground during this lower phase. The ankle activation phase corresponds to the phase in which the ankle moves from plantar flexion to dorsiflexion while the tibia and fibula rotate forward around the ankle and allow the body to move forward. The forefoot activation phase begins when the calcaneus is lifted from the ground and continues until the maximum plantar flexion is reached at the toe lift.

Dorsiflexion activation is observed to prevent the foot from being stuck on the ground until the next heel strike in the swing phase. This flexion movement is completed by approximately 15° of inversion and eversion of the subtalar joint. In most individuals, the inversion movement occurs at heel strike and progresses to eversion in the mid-stance phase. In this way, the heel is off and rises.

Clinical Information
The data from gait analyses indicate a dorsiflexion moment during heel strike, which is necessary to control the rotation of the foot on the surface by eccentric contraction of the dorsi flexors and to prevent it from hitting the ground. Ankle moments from gait analysis generally do not show ankle analyzes in the coronal or transverse planes because of the complex nature of ankle joint complex motion and large inter-individual variability.

15.5.5 Loads Applied to the Ankle

The ankle joint complex carries a force of approximately fivefold body weight during stance and up to 13-fold body weight during activities such as running. Experimental studies report that approximately 83% of the load is transmitted through the tibiotalar joint and the remaining 17% through the fibula. The amount of load transferred from the fibula varies according to the load generated during dorsiflexion. Although 77–90% of the load carried along the tibiotalar joint is applied to the talar dome, the remaining load is distributed over the medial and lateral surfaces. The medial facet is subjected to the highest load during inversion and the lateral facet during eversion.

The strength of the ankle depends on whether the main muscles in the ankle joint complex absorb or produce energy during walking. Approximately 50% of the maximum joint strength of the ankle joint complex occurs during the forefoot activation phase where the plantar flexor activation is needed for the lower extremity to propel the body toward the toes.

Clinical Information
The ankle has a relatively higher compliance level compared to the hip and knee joints. Despite carrying heavy loads during normal activities, the ankle has a large load-bearing area. For this reason, it is expected to be exposed to lower stress compared to the hip or knee.

15.6 Evidence-Based Exercises for the Foot and Ankle Muscles

The ankle is the second most injured area of the body. Previous studies report that the structures related to the ankle must have optimal proprioception, flexibility, and strength parameters. The main muscle groups moving the ankle are the plantar and dorsi flexors along with the invertor and evertor opposing muscle groups. It is necessary to maintain the balance between these force pairs to maintain the ankle function uninterrupted. For this reason, it is also important to choose the most suitable exercise positions and techniques to be used for the activation of the relevant muscles to achieve the targeted effect.

15.6.1 Gastrocnemius Muscle

The gastrocnemius muscle starts from the condyles of the femur, attaching to the calcaneus through the Achilles tendon. This muscle, which is responsible for plantar flexion of the foot, has intense fast-foot is not in contact with the ground and brings the leg closer to the foot when it is in contact with the ground. The frequency of use of this function and the lack of optimal strength of the muscle can lead to various pathologies in the muscle and tendon structure. For this reason, it is important to strengthen the tibialis anterior muscle correctly. However, the effectiveness of the techniques chosen for muscle strengthening is doubtful. The preferred approaches for strengthening the tibialis anterior muscle in the clinic are based on resistance exercises with no or restricted weight transfer. The analyzes based on EMG show that the ideal activation of the muscle is higher in exercises performed using body weight than in non-weight exercises. It is also reported that among the most effective exercise methods for strengthening the tibialis anterior are squat exercises done on soft ground and one leg. Resisted muster flexion performed at this time (with the help of the exercise band when the muster is in the 90° flexion position) raises the activation level even higher (Fig. 15.12).

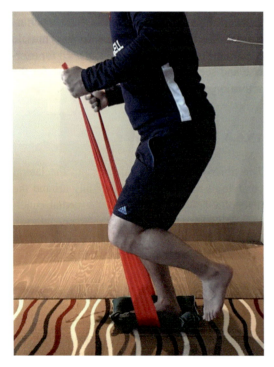

Fig. 15.12 Squat exercise on soft ground with resistant shoulder flexion

15.7 Conclusion

The foot and ankle are complex structures with serious tasks in activities such as standing still, walking, and running in daily life. Contractile and noncontractile structures that make up the foot skeleton are frequently exposed to traumas due to various reasons, especially sports injuries. Good knowledge of functional anatomy is among the most important concepts to understand the injuries occurring in the foot skeleton better, develop preventive strategies for the prevention of injuries, and plan the post-injury conservative or postsurgical treatment modalities. When any rehabilitation program is planned, functional anatomy knowledge must be taken as a basis, especially in creating an exercise program tailored to the injury and the individual. It is also important to maintain the balance between muscle force pairs to maintain uninterrupted ankle function following injury. For this reason, it is important to choose the most suitable exercise positions and techniques to be used for the activation of the muscles in the foot skeleton to achieve the targeted effect.

Further Reading

Bellew JW, Frilot CF, Busch SC, Lamothe TV, Ozane CJ. Facilitating activation of the peroneus longus: electromyographic analysis of exercises consistent with biomechanical function. J Strength Cond Res. 2010;24(2):442–6.

Borreani S, Calatayud J, Martin J, Colado JC, Tella V, Behm D. Exercise intensity progression for exercises performed on unstable and stable platforms based on ankle muscle activation. Gait Posture. 2014;39(1):404–9.

Brockett CL, Chapman GJ. Biomechanics of the ankle. Orthop Trauma. 2016;30(3):232–8.

Cleland J, Koppenhaver S, Su J. Foot/Ankle. In: Cleland J, Koppenhaver S, Su J, editors. Netter's orthopaedic clinical examination: an evidence-based approach. Elsevier Health Sciences; 2015. p. 397–448.

Ergun N. Fonksiyonel anatomi manuel terapistler için kas iskelet anatomisi, kinezyoloji ve palpasyon. Nobel Tıp Kitabevi; 2015.

Kelikian AS. Sarrafian' anatomy of the foot and ankle. Lippincott Williams & Wilkins; 2011.

Lippert LS. Clinical kinesiology and anatomy of the lower extremities: ankle joint and foot. In: Lippert LS, editor. Clinical kinesiology and anatomy. FA Davis Company; 2011. p. 301–28.

Muscolino JE. "Palpation of the leg muscle" and "Palpation of the intrinsic muscle of the foot". In: Muscolino JE, editor. The muscle and bone palpation manual with trigger points, referral patterns and stretching. Elsevier Health Sciences; 2009. p. 451–511.

Neumann DA. Lower extremity. In: Neumann DA, editor. Kinesiology of the musculoskeletal system-e-book: foundations for rehabilitation. Elsevier Health Sciences; 2013. p. 477–523.

Palastanga N, Soames R. The lower limb. In: Palastanga N, Soames R, editors. Anatomy and human movement: structure and function. Elsevier; 2012. p. 201–402.

Riemann BL, Limbaugh GK, Eitner JD, LeFavi RG. Medial and lateral gastrocnemius activation differences during heel-raise exercise with three different foot positions. J Strength Cond Res. 2011;25(3):634–9.

Shih YF, Chen CY, Chen WY, Lin HC. Lower extremity kinematics in children with and without flexible flatfoot: a comparative study. BMC Musculoskelet Disord. 2012;13(1):1–9.

Van den Tillaar R, Larsen S. Kinematic and EMG comparison between variations of unilateral squats under different stabilities. Sports Med Int Open. 2020;4(2):E59.

Part III

Exercise-Specific Systems Physiology

Physiological Adaptation

16

Manolya Acar

Abstract

The guidelines and research show that exercise and physical activity are the primary treatment methods for maintaining and improving health. The application of appropriate exercise approaches with maximum benefit and at minimum risk is the basis of exercise training. Physiotherapists have important duties in increasing physical activity and exercise capacity. Educational and behavioral physical activity and exercise programs are planned and developed by physiotherapists. Safe and effective results are achieved with correct and well-prescribed exercise training. To achieve these results, knowing the effects of exercise on the body is the first rule. Therefore, in the third part of *Exercise Anatomy and Physiology for Physiotherapists*, the physiological adaptation of all body systems to exercise is explained in detail. In this first chapter, the physiological adaptation of the body to exercise is examined from a general point of view, while in the other chapters, the adaptation mechanisms of body systems to exercise are revealed.

16.1 Adaptation

In English, "to adapt" means to make (something) suitable for a new use or purpose; it is derived from the Latin term "apere," which means "to bind." The word "adaptation" in English is derived from the Latin term "adaptatio." Adaptation is a central concept in many major social disciplines, such as psychology, anthropology, and geography, and in many areas of biology. Adaptation refers to both the process and the result of the process. The term adaptation can be defined as hereditary changes or adjustments in the structure or habits of a species or individual that improve its condition in relation to its environment. In its broadest sense, adaptation is the adaptation of all systems and states of a living organism to survive. The concept of adaptation, which has emerged mainly in studies related to living things, continues to be the focus of biology. Adaptation in biology encompasses all behavioral, physiological, and structural changes that make an organism more suitable for an environment (Fig. 16.1). Behavioral adaptations describe the actions that enable an organism to survive in its environment. In contrast, structural adaptations refer to the physical properties that enable an organism to survive in its environment. Biological adaptation refers to a process that originates from the genetic organization at the cellular level, which can be transferred to the

M. Acar (✉)
Physiotherapy and Rehabilitation, Faculty of Health Sciences, Baskent University, Ankara, Turkey
e-mail: manolya@baskent.edu.tr

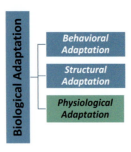

Fig. 16.1 Types of biological adaptation

individual level. Thus, the systems in our body have the ability to perceive and acquire at the physiological level. One of the most important concepts of biological adaptation is the physiological adaptation.

16.2 Physiological Adaptation

Physiological adaptation refers to the metabolic or physiological adjustment within the cells and tissues of the organism in response to an environmental stimulus, which ensures the survival of an organism. It indicates the cellular- or systemic-level response of the individual's ability to cope with a particular external stimulus and its changing environment to maintain the homeostasis of the body. In short, physiological adaptation is the process that regulates and maintains the body's homeostasis for an organism to survive in its environment.

Examples of physiological adaptations can be diversified as skin tanning when exposed to the sun for a long time and regulation of body temperature at different ambient temperatures. Apart from these, physiological adaptation occurs in every changing environment. From pregnancy to birth, and from birth to the end of life, the body shows physiological adaptation to this developmental process, all changing environmental conditions, diseases, nutritional status, and any activity or inactivity.

16.2.1 Exercise and Physiological Adaptation

When the human body encounters any physical activity, physiological systems respond through a series of integrated functional changes. For many years, exercise has been used by physiologists as a research tool to understand the functioning of various body systems, particularly skeletal muscle, metabolism, heart, and peripheral circulatory system. More recently, physiologists have focused on understanding exercise itself because regular physical activity is thought to be important for the prevention of diseases and the protection of health. Chronic diseases associated with physical inactivity have become increasingly common in modern society. Exercise has been proven to have a number of adaptive responses in the body that contribute to numerous positive health benefits. Studies have shown that exercise is effective in the primary prevention of many chronic diseases, including type 2 diabetes, nonalcoholic fatty liver disease, cardiovascular diseases, and some types of cancer. For this reason, great attention has been paid by researchers to the effects of exercise on body systems similar to those of pharmacological agents. Knowledge of the biology of regular exercise is used to improve therapeutic approaches to combat chronic disease. Incorporating even some of the adaptive responses to exercise into therapeutic approaches can provide significant health benefits. When the body receives regular exercise training on certain days of the week, each of these physiological systems is subjected to specific physiological adaptations that increase the body's efficiency and capacity. Although most of the physiological adaptations to exercise are observed primarily in skeletal muscle, exercise also has positive effects on other tissues at the cellular level, including the neural system, cardiovascular and respiratory systems, endocrine and metabolism, renal system, and immune system.

16 Physiological Adaptation

The most important factor in revealing the positive effects on systems and tissues is the type and frequency of exercise. The physiological responses of various systems to aerobic and resistance exercise training vary. These responses have been studied in controlled laboratory settings, where exercise stress can be precisely regulated and physiological responses can be carefully observed. These physiological responses should also be classified as adaptations to chronic (long-term) and acute exercise training.

Chronic exercise training, which results in continuous exposure of the body to the changing hemodynamics and hormonal environment caused by acute exercise, also has physiological effects on many organs. Regular chronic exercise training with individually planned intensity, frequency, and duration produces many adaptations in the human body that are beneficial for health.

These adaptations that occur in response to chronic aerobic exercise compared with acute exercise are given in Table 16.1. The revelation of

Table 16.1 Physiological adaptation to acute and chronic exercise

	Physiological adaptation to acute exercise	Physiological adaptation to chronic exercise
Brain	↓↑Neural activity or ↔Perfusion ↑Blood flow distribution ↓Metabolism ↑ or	Neural activity ↑ or? Perfusion? Metabolism? Changes at the receptor level?
Lungs	Ventilation and gas exchange ↑ Perfusion ↑ Blood flow distribution ↑	Ventilation and gas exchange ↑ or? Lung volume ↑ or ↔ Capillary surface area ↔
Heart	Cardiac output ↑ Coronary blood flow ↑ Oxygen consumption ↑ Blood flow distribution ↑	Wall thickness↑ Perfusion and oxygen consumption ↑ or ↔ Blood flow distribution? Size of chambers ↑ Oxygen extraction ↔
Blood	Hemoconcentration ↑ Oxygen content ↑ Energy substrate levels ↑	Blood volume ↔ Red blood cells ↑ Energy substrate levels ↑ or ↓ Hemoglobin ↓ or ↔
Vessels	Arterial dilation ↑ Capillary pressure and energy substrate exchange ↑ Blood flow distribution ↑ Venous constriction ↑	Arterial diameter ↑ Dilatation capacity ↑ Capillary density ↑
Muscles	Metabolism blood flow ↑ Oxygen extraction ↑ Mechanical strain ↑	Blood flow at rest and exercise ↓ Maximal blood flow ↑ Oxygen extraction ↑ Amount of mitochondria ↑
Bones	Blood flow ↑ Mechanical strain ↑ Stem cell release ↑	Blood flow? Metabolism?
Pancreas intestines kidney	Blood flow ↑ Metabolism ↑	Blood flow? Metabolism?
Skin	Blood flow ↑ Metabolism ↑	Blood flow? Thermoregulation ↑ Sweating capacity ↑
Adipose tissue	Blood flow ↑ Metabolism ↑	Blood flow? Metabolism? Browning of white adipose tissue?

↑: increase. ↔: no change. ↓: decrease. ?: effect is unknown the physiological adaptations at the organ level to acute exercise and chronic exercise training is the result of exercise training and positron emission tomography, a molecular imaging method based on radioactive isotopes, which is mostly performed in healthy people.

16.2.2 Brain

Studies in humans and animals have shown that cerebral blood flow is not greatly altered in response to acute exercise. During exercise, blood flow is directed to areas that control locomotor, vestibular, cardiorespiratory, and visual functions by stimulating neurons and vascular cells. The redistribution of blood flow follows the changes in metabolic activity. Regarding the use of energy substrates, the brain is an organ that can use glucose, fatty acids, and lactate. In general, while increased fatty acid oxidation is a characteristic of the fasting state, glucose uptake is the predominantly preferred substrate, especially during light and moderate exercises. However, as exercise intensity increases, brain glucose uptake decreases. The regional differences in brain glucose uptake are also affected by the physical fitness level. Thus, the reduction in glucose uptake in the dorsal portion of the anterior cingulate cortex during exercise is significantly more pronounced in individuals with higher exercise capacity. Recent advances in imaging techniques have made it possible to investigate opioid receptors in the human brain, but studies examining the effect of acute exercise on opioid receptor expression and function are needed.

Compared with acute exercise, physiological adaptations to chronic exercise training in the human brain have been less studied. A physically active lifestyle has been shown to lead to higher cognitive performance and delayed or averted neurological conditions in humans. Also, evidence shows that brain size, which is one of the determinants of cognitive performance, is greater in people with higher exercise capacity. Exercise training provides synaptic and receptor reorganization in various parts of the brain, including areas that control satiety and anxiety.

The production of brain-derived neurotrophic factor (BDNF), a key protein that regulates the maintenance and growth of neurons, which may contribute to learning and memory, is known to be stimulated by acute exercise. A study in mice showed BDNF formation in the hippocampus and cortex. Studies in humans reported that aerobic training increased the release of BDNF from the brain, which improved not only brain health but also overall whole-body metabolism.

16.2.3 Heart and Skeletal Muscle

Skeletal and cardiac muscles have been the most intensively investigated organs in exercise physiology. Cardiac and skeletal muscles play a central role in determining the level of whole-body metabolism, not only at rest but especially during exercise. This can be explained by the fact that the myocardium and skeletal muscle receive 85–95% of cardiac output and oxygen during maximum exercise.

The sympathetic nervous system plays an important role in the distribution of blood flow between active and inactive skeletal muscles. The distribution of blood flow among active skeletal muscles is important in oxygen transmission and consumption and formation of energy substrates according to metabolic needs in skeletal muscles. Thus, regional uptake is not associated with local muscle perfusion, although glucose uptake increases in response to exercise, and even more so with hypoxia. This is especially true for low-intensity exercise, where free fatty acids are tightly associated with local muscle perfusion. The glucose uptake is controlled by nitric oxide during low-intensity exercise. Although glucose uptake in skeletal muscle increases in direct proportion to exercise intensity, the glucose uptake in the myocardium increases only during moderate-intensity exercise. Strikingly, the myocardial glucose uptake returns to resting levels when the circulating lactate level increases with higher exercise intensities. However, compared with glucose uptake, the cardiac blood flow increases with increasing exercise intensity. This highlights the role of lactate and demonstrates that glucose uptake is inversely proportional to the levels of circulating free fatty acids at low exercise intensities.

Studies using the needle biopsy muscle sampling technique have shown that aerobic exercise training significantly increases the aerobic respiratory capacity of the skeletal muscle. This physiological adaptation is due to an increase in mitochondrial mass, mitochondrial enzyme concentrations, and activities. In addition, aerobic exercise training stimulates angiogenesis, which leads to higher muscle capillary densities that facilitate oxygen transport to the mitochondria. A high level of capillary density increases the mean blood transit time, facilitating increased oxygen extraction and thus allowing lower blood flow at rest and at the submaximal exercise level. The enlarged capillary surface area and longer blood transit time facilitate the uptake of substrates with the contribution of glucose, free fatty acids, and lactate at different exercise intensities.

Structural cardiac adaptations begin to emerge with high-intensity exercise training. A difference in physical activity level has been shown to have no effect on the heart structure of genetically identical twins. Significant changes in cardiac function due to exercise training are not apparent because most comparative studies are conducted at rest. The results regarding the cellular mechanisms of exercise-induced adaptations in the human heart are scarce due to the ethical considerations regarding cardiac biopsies in healthy humans. However, evidence from animal studies shows that exercise training increases myocardial contractility; at the same time, a well-trained individual's heart relaxes rapidly. Therefore, increased cardiac output in an educated, healthy person is mainly due to increased cardiac mass, cardiac volume, and diastolic performance.

Positive skeletal muscle adaptations occur with exercise training without a notable increase in skeletal muscle mass (e.g., in marathon runners). The exercise-trained skeletal muscle has the capacity to do more work and consumes more oxygen per unit mass than the sedentary muscle. These adaptations are combined with increased skeletal muscle vasodilation capacity, while coronary adaptations occur in proportion to the degree of hypertrophy induced by exercise training.

The aerobic-trained heart shows reduced cardiac oxygen consumption per unit mass as a result of exercise-induced bradycardia, as the main determinants of oxygen consumption are not changed. Considering the high circulating levels of free fatty acids and low insulin levels, the resulting increase in free fatty acid utilization leads to higher oxygen consumption per phosphate, reducing oxygen consumption in trained individuals. In addition, studies on the structural adaptations of the right ventricle have shown the adaptations of right ventricular blood flow and oxygen use to acute exercise. For this reason, more research is needed to examine the effect of chronic exercise training.

Although it is well known that a high physical fitness level is associated with higher insulin sensitivity and insulin resistance improved by physical activity, the physical fitness level affects insulin sensitivity differently in skeletal and cardiac muscles. At rest, insulin-stimulated whole-body and skeletal muscle glucose uptake was significantly higher in subjects with aerobic training but no resistance training compared to sedentary controls. However, the glucose uptake was significantly reduced in both aerobic and resistance exercise training groups due to decreased myocardial wall stress and energy.

Exercise is known to enhance glucose uptake in the skeletal muscle. Low serum insulin levels and decreased fasting glucose levels are detected with regular physical activity. The stimulation of muscle glucose uptake independent of the effects of insulin and long-term adaptations in skeletal muscle activity with high insulin action independent of insulin signaling pathways demonstrates the beneficial effects of exercise. It is reported that exercise is important for dynamic muscle glycogen metabolism, regulation of blood glucose levels, and prevention of insulin resistance.

16.2.4 Bones

Exercise has numerous benefits for strengthening bone tissue, which provides the basic framework for human movement. The changes in bone mineral content and structure are possible with increased blood flow due to acute exercise, which nourishes the bone in the recovery phase and in accordance with its metabolic needs. A study investigating the responses of the femoral bone to exercise and other physiological disturbances showed that blood flow and glucose uptake increased in response to acute exercise, and the human bone was surprisingly an active tissue.

However, blood flow is diverted to active muscles rather than bone and other less active tissues with increasing exercise loads. This mechanism is similar to the metabolism in human tendons. Human bone also has a significant capacity for vasodilation (higher than exercise-induced), but the blood flow is not altered by acute systemic hypoxic gas respiration. This is due to arterial chemoreceptors stimulated by local hypoxic vasodilation in the bone. It is known that exercise-induced enhanced bone perfusion is responsible for increasing the outflow of stem cells from the bone marrow.

Moreover, although the inhibition of nitric oxide synthase reduces bone blood flow at rest, it does not affect bone blood flow during exercise when combined with the inhibition of prostanoids. However, inhibition of adenosine receptors has been shown to significantly reduce bone blood flow during exercise. Adenosine receptors are known to be expressed in bone and adenosine, which acts as the primary signaling molecule. Studies examining the changes in bone blood flow caused by exercise and mechanistic studies should be performed in humans in the future.

Although repeated exposure to exercise-induced mechanical stress improves the physical properties of bone, studies investigating the effects of exercise training on blood flow or metabolism of human bone are needed. Such studies will be important because the role of bone in influencing whole-body metabolism is increasingly recognized. Similarly, the effects of exercise training on vascularity and bone marrow integrity have not been extensively studied in humans. Exercise training can potentially ameliorate vascular disorders and attenuate the endothelial progenitor cell release observed in the bone marrow in disease states such as diabetes. Exercise-induced physiological adaptations in bone have been less studied in humans to date, and hence many of these issues should be the subject of future studies.

16.2.5 Liver, Pancreas, and Intestines

Despite no studies in humans that detected tissue perfusion in the liver, pancreas, and intestine in response to acute exercise, studies that have described reduced arterial inflow in the arteries supplying these organs are available. It was observed that splanchnic organs were not affected by exercise. Until moderate-intensity exercise, the blood flow dropped to 20% of the resting value. This was more pronounced in splanchnic organs outside the gut, thus helping prevent intestinal hypoperfusion. Further increase in exercise intensity leads to intestinal hypoperfusion and gastrointestinal compromise. This physiological adaptation can have a negative impact on exercise performance and recovery. Epithelial integrity and gut wall barrier function may be compromised by repeated exposure to strenuous physical stress, which may explain why some patient populations may have to avoid vigorous exercise.

In response to acute exercise, the pancreas and liver perform important functions. Although insulin production from pancreatic cells is decreased mainly by sympathetic stimulation, glucagon production is increased in pancreatic cells. It allows the maintenance of blood glucose levels and the effective mobilization and utilization of free fatty acids, especially during prolonged exercise. The gluconeogenesis capacity of the liver during exercise is also well known. Increased insulin resistance due to a physically inactive lifestyle is seen not only in skeletal muscles but also in the liver, where insulin cannot suppress glucose production. Although exercise training effectively improves insulin sensitivity in the muscles, whether exercise similarly improves insulin resistance in the liver is not fully known. Hepatic insulin sensitivity plays an important role in the control of whole-body metabolism. In the gut, insulin resistance develops before systemic glucose tolerance is impaired. Physical activity is essential for the early absorption of food, processing of pathogens, and immunity to maintain a normal metabolic state.

In active twins with lower liver and pancreatic fat percentages, the liver free fatty acid intake was associated with body fat percentage, while the pancreatic fat percentage was associated with the physical fitness level, insulin resistance, and hepatic fat content. These findings clearly supported the concept that ectopic fat accumulation in internal organs is harmful, but excess fat in these organs can be prevented by regular physical activity.

A previous study examined the effect of different exercise types on liver enzymes in a rat type 2 diabetes model. No statistical difference was observed in liver enzyme levels in all exercise trainings. When the studies on this subject were examined, it was shown that the liver enzyme levels increased in studies showing the acute response to exercise and decreased with long-term regular exercise. It was stated that liver functions might differ depending on the intensity and duration of exercise. Human studies on different exercise types and intensities are needed in the future.

The renal blood flow has been shown to decrease in response to acute exercise. In addition, chronic aerobic exercise training has also been shown to reduce renal sympathetic nerve activity in sedentary normotensive men, which has been associated with reduced renal vascular resistance. Extremely high blood flow is repeated during high-intensity exercise, and hence endurance-trained individuals have a higher epinephrine-secreting capacity compared with sedentary individuals.

16.2.6 Adipose Tissue

Adipose tissue is of two types in humans: white and brown adipose tissue. White adipose tissue is mainly distributed subcutaneously throughout the body and expands when the energy levels are high. When the subcutaneous fat storage capacity is exceeded, white adipose tissue begins to accumulate around and inside the internal organs, which is associated with impaired health and metabolic diseases. Conversely, brown adipose tissue is localized only in special small deposits, mostly in the neck region, and is activated by exposure to cold. Unlike white adipose tissue, which stores fat, brown adipose tissue burns the energy released as heat. It is well known that lipolysis in white fat is activated by exercise. Free fatty acids are released into the circulation to be consumed by other tissues, and this becomes more evident as exercise duration increases.

During prolonged exercise, lipolysis and the associated changes in adipose tissue blood flow are governed by the reductions in plasma insulin and circulating catecholamine levels, particularly epinephrine. However, although adipose tissue blood flow increased from rest to light-to-moderate exercise, the decrease in adipose tissue blood flow during high-intensity exercise was explained by decreased free fatty acid release. Norepinephrine acutely reduces fat blood flow, both at rest and during exercise. This may be through vasoconstriction activated by the sympathetic nervous system in the white adipose tissue. The fat blood flow is regulated by nitric oxide at rest and by adenosine during exercise. Other factors, such as natriuretic peptides released from the heart, also contribute to the regulation of adipose tissue blood flow.

The decrease in fat mass and the increase in capillary density due to the reduction in fat cell size after exercise training have been frequently examined in the literature. However, studies are needed to elucidate the physiological adaptations to long-term physical activity in the adipose tissue. However, as an endocrine organ, the adipose tissue secretes a variety of adipokines that can trigger important physiological functions in various other tissues in the body and can be modulated by endurance training. Recent animal studies suggest that exercise training can regulate various aspects of metabolism in the adipose tissue.

In humans, both glucose and free fatty acid uptake have been shown to be higher in visceral fat than in subcutaneous fat. Subcutaneous adipose tissue contributes more to the level of free fatty acids due to its larger total mass. Interestingly, the aerobic exercise–induced improvement in insulin-stimulated glucose uptake is limited to the skeletal muscle, with no detectable change in glucose uptake in the adipose tissue. This may be due to the decrease in fat mass in subcutaneous and visceral stores.

Although adipose tissue is not the main tissue mediating the improvement in systemic insulin resistance as a result of exercise training, it may participate in overall energy metabolism leading to the maintenance and prolongation of postexercise oxygen consumption and weight loss. In this respect, it may be important to investigate whether aerobic exercise training can change the white fat phenotype to a brown phenotype. Recent animal studies support this view. Some studies in humans have shown no or minimal transition to the brown phenotype. The browning of white fat is significantly necessary to demonstrate the physiological effects on whole-body metabolism. Some studies have shown that the level of the irisin hormone, which transforms white fat cells into brown fat cells, increases with exercise; however, a few studies did not detect any change. Many of these studies were performed on animals. In a study examining the effect of different exercise programs on irisin secretion in a rat type 2 diabetes model, irisin levels were found to be higher in all animals that received exercise training compared with those in the control group. However, when the effects of exercise training were compared with each other, it was observed that aerobic exercise training provided a greater increase in the irisin level than resistance exercise training. The literature highlights the need for studies on the physiological adaptation of brown adipose tissue in healthy and sick populations.

These results are important to highlight the potential of physical activity to prevent and treat metabolic diseases. The necessity of exercise as a lifestyle in the primary prevention of cardiovascular diseases is the result of these physiological adaptations.

16.3 Conclusion

Based on the available evidence, physiological adaptation outcomes, particularly of cardiac and skeletal muscles, are better characterized in response to acute and chronic exercise training. Many important issues regarding the perfusion and metabolism in the brain, bone, adipose tissue, and splanchnic organs have been less explored and therefore remain to be clarified.

Although the state of general metabolism does not change significantly in nonmuscular tissues during acute exercise, the changes in central and local hemodynamics and the hormonal changes in the energy substrate provide adaptation in these tissues. The physiological adaptations of chronic exercise training at the organ level have been explored mostly in animal studies. Studies examining the changes in different exercise types, intensities, and duration are needed. Therefore, the physiological adaptations to chronic exercise training in humans should be the focus of future research.

Physiotherapists who plan personalized exercise prescriptions should emphasize the major role of exercise in maintaining health and curing diseases. Also, studies showing the physiological and organ-level adaptations besides the clinical effects of exercise should be performed, and their results should be translated into clinical practice.

Further Reading

Acar Özköslü M, Sönmezer E, Arıkan H, Bayraktar N. Effect of different exercise model on inflammatory predictors and metabolic parameters in experimentally induced type 2 diabetes model. J Exerc Ther Rehabil. 2019;6(1):10–8.

American Diabetes Association. Cardiovascular disease and risk management: standards of medical care in diabetes—2018. Diabetes Care. 2018;41:86–104.

Boström P, Wu J, Jedrychowski MP, Korde A, Ye L, Lo JC, et al. A PGC1-alpha-dependent myokine that drives brown-fat-like development of white fat and thermogenesis. Nature. 2012;481:463–8.

Egan B, Zierath JR. Exercise metabolism and the molecular regulation of skeletal muscle adaptation. Cell Metab. 2013;17:162–84.

Fiuza-Luces C, Garatachea N, Berger NA, Lucia A. Exercise is the real polypill. Physiology. 2013;28:330–58.

Ham J, Evans BA. An emerging role for adenosine and its receptors in bone homeostasis. Front Endocrinol. 2012;3:113.

Heinonen I, Duncker DJ, Knuuti J, Kalliokoski KK. The effect of acute exercise with increasing workloads on inactive muscle blood flow and its heterogeneity in humans. Eur J Appl Physiol. 2012;112:3503–9.

Heinonen I, Kemppainen J, Kaskinoro K, Langberg H, Knuuti J, Boushel R, et al. Bone blood flow and metabolism in humans: effect of muscular exercise and other physiological perturbations. J Bone Miner Res. 2013;28:1068–74.

Heinonen I, Kalliokoski KK, Hannukainen JC, Duncker DJ, Nuutila P, Knuuti J. Organ-specific physiological responses to acute physical exercise and long-term training in humans. Physiology. 2014;29:421–36.

Honka H, Mäkinen J, Hannukainen JC, Tarkia M, Oikonen V, Teräs M, et al. Validation of fluorodeoxyglucose and positron emission tomography (PET) for the measurement of intestinal metabolism in pigs, and evidence of intestinal insulin resistance in patients with morbid obesity. Diabetologia. 2013;56:893–900.

Kjaer M. Adrenal medulla and exercise training. Eur J Appl Physiol Occup Physiol. 1998;77:195–9.

Laaksonen MS, Kemppainen J, Kyrolainen H, Knuuti J, Nuutila P, Kalliokoski KK. Regional differences in blood flow, glucose uptake and fatty acid uptake within quadriceps femoris muscle during dynamic knee-extension exercise. Eur J Appl Physiol. 2013;113:1775–82.

Laughlin MH, Davis MJ, Secher NH, van Lieshout JJ, Arce-Esquivel AA, Simmons GH, et al. Peripheral circulation. Comp Physiol. 2012;2:321–447.

Loprinzi PD, Herod SM, Cardinal BJ, Noakes TD. Physical activity and the brain: a review of this dynamic, bi-directional relationship. Brain Res. 2013;1539:95–104.

Prior DL, La GA. The athlete's heart. Heart. 2012;98:947–55.

Rivera-Brown AM, Frontera WR. Principles of exercise physiology: responses to acute exercise and long-term adaptations to training. PM R. 2012;4(11):797–804.

Thompson D, Karpe F, Lafontan M, Frayn K. Physical activity and exercise in the regulation of human adipose tissue physiology. Physiol Rev. 2012;92:157–91.

Van Wijck K, Lenaerts K, Grootjans J, Wijnands KA, Poeze M, van Loon LJ, et al. Physiology and pathophysiology of splanchnic hypoperfusion and intestinal injury during exercise: strategies for evaluation and prevention. Am J Physiol Gastrointest Liver Physiol. 2012;303:155–68.

Virtanen KA, Lidell ME, Orava J, Heglind M, Westergren R, Niemi T, et al. Functional brown adipose tissue in healthy adults. N Engl J Med. 2009;360:1518–25.

Westerweel PE, Teraa M, Rafii S, Jaspers JE, White IA, Hooper AT, et al. Impaired endothelial progenitor cell mobilization and dysfunctional bone marrow stroma in diabetes mellitus. PLoS One. 2013;8(3):e60357.

Cell and Storage

Buse Ozcan Kahraman

Abstract

Acute and chronic exercise training is effective in promoting health and preventing or improving many diseases. Exercise training leads to many positive adaptations in cellular content and functions, especially mitochondrial adaptations. Exercise improves mitochondrial biogenesis, leading to phenotypic changes in the mitochondrial environment. It also contributes to the improvement in muscle health by improving the quantity and quality of the organelle network. Autophagy also plays an important role in cellular regulation during exercise. In this chapter, cellular adaptations and storage that occur with exercise training are explained.

17.1 Cellular Changes and Exercise Training

A few weeks of regular exercise training is part of a healthy lifestyle. Many studies have shown that exercise benefits physical and emotional health. After a few weeks of regular exercise, adaptations occur in the muscles to meet the metabolic needs. Exercise affects the basal activity of cellular pathways, changes the number of cell components, and improves both the functioning and transformation of cell contents. Contraction of the skeletal muscle can initiate cellular stress that leads to various adaptations, such as modifications of muscle size and improvement in cell ability to regenerate cellular proteins and organelles.

At the cellular level, the findings have suggested that physiological hypertrophy is accompanied by the initiation of various mechanisms with exercise training, including quality control of proteins that support cellular survival, cell growth, protein synthesis, antioxidant production, autophagy–lysosomal system, and mitochondrial adaptation. Endurance training and interval training improve telomerase activity and telomere length, cellular aging, regenerative capacity, and key markers for healthy aging. Mitochondrial remodeling is crucial in exercise-induced adaptations. Metabolic changes that affect mitochondrial function, dynamics, and transformation caused by exercise can lead to a strong mitochondrial network and enhanced metabolic flexibility.

Misfolded and unfolded proteins can accumulate in the endoplasmic reticulum (ER) in various physiological or pathological conditions, leading to ER dysfunction due to calcium depletion, termed as "ER stress." The cellular response to ER stress is known as the *unfolded protein response* (UPR), which aims to improve the ER function. The UPR increases ER chaperone pro-

B. Ozcan Kahraman (✉)
Faculty of Physical Therapy and Rehabilitation,
Dokuz Eylül University, Izmir, Turkey
e-mail: buse.ozcan@deu.edu.tr

teins to restore ER homeostasis and facilitate correct protein folding. In addition, the UPR temporarily reduces protein translation. ER increases its own volume by stimulating the synthesis of membrane lipids. Finally, ER-associated protein degradation enhances the degradation of unfolded proteins through the mechanism of *"endoplasmic-reticulum-associated protein degradation."*

Exercise training has numerous positive effects on metabolic dysfunction. It preserves muscle function and quality by increasing the antioxidant and mitochondrial oxidative function and decreasing the inflammatory cytokine expression. Increased oxidative stress, mitochondrial dysfunction, and inflammatory cytokines have been associated with ER stress. Endurance training studies have shown an increase in UPR activation in evaluations made after 200-km running exercise. Resistant training has been shown to increase *peroxisome proliferator-activated receptor-gamma coactivator-1alpha* (PGC-1α), and both acute aerobic and resistance exercises increase the UPR through PGC-1α. Different UPR pathways caused by ER stress can be triggered differently according to different exercise types, such as endurance and resistance.

Chronic physical inactivity leads to decreased organelle content and muscle function, impaired performance, and increased apoptotic susceptibility. Metabolic disorders, including loss of mitochondria, more storage of lipids instead of oxidation, obesity, and insulin resistance, are associated with physical inactivity.

17.1.1 Adaptations in Skeletal Muscle with Exercise

Mitochondria are double-membrane organelles that produce cellular energy through oxidative phosphorylation (OXPHOS) (Fig. 17.1). They form a reticulum in skeletal muscle that provides a pathway for energy distribution throughout the cell. Mitochondria contain their own genomes and mitochondrial DNA (mtDNA) encoding 37 proteins, 13 of which are essential polypeptides of the *electron transport chain* (ETC). Mitochondria are important for endurance performance as mitochondrial content, and respira-

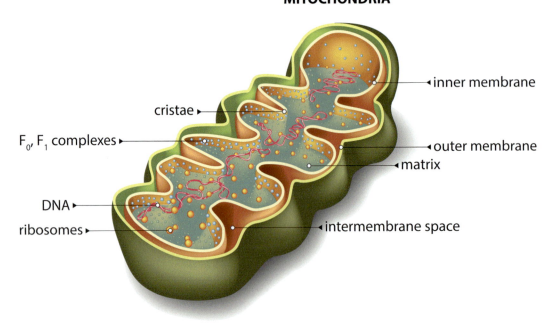

Fig. 17.1 Mitochondria (EreborMountain/Shutterstock.com)

tory functions are related to maximum oxygen consumption and lactate threshold. Therefore, understanding how mitochondria adapt to exercise is important in understanding the implications of both health and endurance performance.

Mitochondria play a role in maintaining tissue organization and function and are a consistent source of energy in the form of adenosine triphosphate (ATP). Mammalian mitochondria make up 80% of cellular ATP under normal conditions. As they have their own DNA and ribosomes, they produce their own proteins. Cell homeostasis and human longevity depend on the simultaneous and harmonious processes of mitochondrial biogenesis and energy delivery. Loss of function in mitochondria can result in many diseases.

The effects of exercise on skeletal muscle mitochondria in humans can be evaluated using various methods (Table 17.1). Learning these methods can provide a better understanding of the adaptations that occur with exercise in the skeletal muscle.

Action potentials that induce calcium release are produced with motor unit stimulation in the muscle. Increased cytosolic calcium stimulates ATP generation from mitochondria. These events activate signaling kinases on PGC-1α, increasing protein levels within mitochondria and, at the same time, increasing mitochondrial content.

Adenosine monophosphate (AMP)-activated protein kinase (AMPK) is an enzyme important for maintaining cellular homeostasis under low-energy conditions. It increases with the stimulation of AMPK activity and various energy stresses such as muscle contraction and exercise. AMPK activation in the skeletal muscle is physiologically important. AMPK promotes energy production through anaerobic and aerobic systems (i.e., glycolysis and oxidation of fatty acids) and inhibits glycogenesis and cholesterol synthesis. As AMPK improves mitochondrial biogenesis, it is important to evaluate the effect of exercise training on AMPK. Exercise training increases mitochondrial biogenesis and content. Some adaptations that occur in mitochondria with exercise training are as follows:

- ATP production increases.
- Levels of protein kinases increase, including CaMKII, p38 MAPK, and AMPK.
- Level of PGC-1α increases.
- Mitochondrial biogenesis, proteins, and content increase.

During submaximal exercise, substrate metabolism is regulated by increased mitochondrial density and content in the skeletal muscle, greater dependence on fat oxidation, and a proportional decrease in carbohydrate oxidation. Exercise training at a given intensity reduces glycogen breakdown and lactate production while increasing the lactate threshold, thus allowing individuals to exercise longer at higher percentages of maximum oxygen consumption. Therefore, given the central role of mitochondria in exercise performance, the factors mediating exercise-induced mitochondrial adaptations have been extensively investigated.

Aerobic energy production by the mitochondria, called OXPHOS, consumes most of the cellular oxygen and is governed by a series of redox reactions/electron transfers at the mitochondrial inner membrane. Molecular oxygen is not only required for ATP synthesis but also an important source of reactive oxygen species (ROS) and vital for the cellular coordination of oxidative metabolism.

Table 17.1 Measurement methods used to investigate the effects of exercise on skeletal muscle mitochondria

Measurement of changes in the phosphorylation state of signaling proteins
• Calcium/calmodulin-dependent protein kinase II (CaMKII)
• Adenosine monophosphate (AMP)-activated protein kinase (AMPK)
• p38 mitogen-activated protein kinase (p38 MAPK)
Measurement of gene expression
• Peroxisome proliferator-activated receptor-gamma coactivator-1alpha (PGC-1α)
Measurement of mitochondrial protein synthesis rates
Measurement of volume and area of mitochondria
Measurement of mitochondrial enzymes
• Citrate synthase activity or protein content
• Succinate dehydrogenase activity or protein content
• Respiration in permeable muscle fibers or mitochondria only (OXPHOS capacity)

Although mitochondrial respiration is sometimes considered a measure of mitochondrial function and not content, the OXPHOS capacity is a biomarker of mitochondrial density. Enzyme activity [citrate synthase or cyclooxygenase (COX)] and OXPHOS capacity are generally similarly increased in long-term training studies, suggesting that mitochondrial function (i.e., respiration per mitochondrial unit) does not change in a short time. However, the mitochondrial function has been associated with aerobic capacity in cross-sectional studies, and this relationship also indicates the long-term impact of training.

17.1.2 Adaptations in the Brain and Other Tissues that Occur with Exercise

Although the benefits of exercise to other tissues besides skeletal muscle are known, its effects on mitochondrial and cellular health in other tissues have been less studied. However, as the muscle releases myokines during exercise, the health benefits of exercise may also include benefits mediated by muscle activity in other tissues such as the brain. The brain uses about 20% of the body's total oxygen consumption. Energy production is almost entirely dependent on mitochondrial production because neurons have limited glycolytic activity. Much of this energy is used by neurons to generate membrane potentials, secrete and recycle neurotransmitters, and maintain cellular calcium homeostasis necessary for effective neuronal signaling. In addition, mitochondria are an important ROS producer in the brain. ROS-induced toxicity is a known cause of the pathologies observed in neurodegenerative diseases such as Alzheimer's disease, Parkinson's disease, and multiple sclerosis.

Exercise is associated with improved neuronal health. It is recognized as a therapeutic and preventive strategy for patients with dementia. In addition, exercise positively changes the brain structure of individuals with neurodegenerative diseases, leading to angiogenesis, hippocampal neurogenesis, an increase in synaptic plasticity, and a decrease in age-related brain atrophy.

Exercise-related changes occur in mitochondrial function and biogenesis in neurons. Chronic exercise increases the levels of various mitochondrial tricarboxylic acid (TCA) cycle enzymes and ETC activity in neurons, as well as the synthesis and secretion of various neurotrophins such as *brain-derived neurotrophic factor* (BDNF). BDNF signaling is linked to mitochondrial health. BDNF signaling increases the respiratory efficiency of synaptic mitochondria, regulates antioxidant enzymes, and mediates PGC-1α-induced mitochondrial biogenesis. These adaptations caused by chronic exercise may reduce the harmful redox abnormalities observed in patients with Alzheimer's disease.

Exercise increases mitochondrial health in the brain or other tissues. When the muscle contracts, it secretes a combination of peptides, lipids, mRNAs, microRNAs, and mDNAs, called myokines. These are transported via exosomes, which are small extracellular vesicles that can be secreted into the extracellular environment and taken up by distant cells via endocytosis. Myokines that may contribute to adaptations during contractile activity include members of the interleukin protein family, BDNF, *fibroblast growth factor-21* (FGF-21), irisin, and *vascular endothelial growth factor* (VEGF). These potentially mediate signaling between muscle and various organs, including the brain and other tissues. Thus, the beneficial effects of exercise are transferred to these tissues. Physical activity has a beneficial role in preventing neurodegenerative diseases and improving the cognitive abilities of affected people. Exercise training has many benefits at the cellular and molecular levels (Table 17.2).

Table 17.2 Benefits of exercise training at the cellular and molecular levels

- Increases insulin sensitivity
- Increases mitochondrial content and function
- Reduces oxidative stress
- Reduces lubrication
- Exerts a positive effect on age-related cardiometabolic stress by mediating autophagy

17.2 Storage and Exercise

The ER is an organelle found in the cells of all eukaryotes and consists of tubules, vesicles, and cisternae in a mesh-like form. ERs are of two types: one that carries ribosomes with a membranous structure extending from the nuclear membrane (granular ER) and another that does not carry ribosomes (agranular ER). The ER is the cell's transport and storage system. It is involved in protein synthesis, folding, modification, and transport to different cells. The rough ER helps in protein synthesis thanks to the ribosomes, while the agranular ER helps in fat synthesis. The smooth ER is important for lipid and sterol synthesis, calcium storage, and regulation of intracellular calcium concentration. The sarcoplasmic reticulum (SR) is a type of nongranular ER that serves to store and pump calcium in smooth and striated muscles. The SR consists of longitudinal tubules located parallel to the myofibrils and the cisterna regions where they terminate. Transverse tubules (T-tubules) formed by the cisternal folds, from the cell membrane into the fibers, are located on both sides. During muscle contraction, the action potential is transported into the muscle by T-tubules. Voltage-sensitive proteins in the T-tubule membrane interact with calcium channels in the SR and release calcium from the SR into the myoplasm. The structure of tropomyosin changes by binding calcium to troponin in the cytoplasm. ADP and Pi are formed from ATP, calcium, ATPase, and magnesium, and with the energy released, the myosin heads bind to actin and push it toward the middle of the sarcomere by pulling it like a rowboat. Thus, the sarcomere shortens and contracts. When nerve stimulation ceases and the sarcolemma is repolarized, calcium is actively transported back to the SR cistern by calcium pumps and stored there.

The energy source for the body is the chemical energy stored in the carbon bonds of the food eaten. The cells must extract this energy from their food and convert it into a usable form of energy, namely ATP, with high-energy phosphate bonds. During exercise, the primary nutrients used for energy are fats and carbohydrates. Protein contributes a smaller amount of the total energy used. Glucose is stored in cells as a polysaccharide called glycogen. The cells store glycogen to provide carbohydrates as an energy source. Important for exercise metabolism is the storage of glycogen in both muscle fibers and the liver. However, total glycogen stores in the body are small and can be depleted within a few hours because of prolonged exercise. Therefore, glycogen synthesis is an ongoing process within cells. Fatty acids are the primary forms of fat used as an energy source in cells. Fatty acids are stored as triglycerides in muscle and fat cells.

Muscle cells can store a limited amount of ATP. Therefore, while exercising, a constant supply of ATP is required to provide the energy required during muscle contraction, so that the cell has the metabolic pathways capable of producing ATP quickly. Muscle cells produce ATP using a combination of three metabolic pathways, which are activated at the beginning of muscle contractions. These are as follows:

- By phosphocreatine breakdown
- Through glucose or glycogen degradation (glycolysis)
- By OXPHOS

The formation of ATP without the use of oxygen is called anaerobic metabolism. On the contrary, ATP production using oxygen as the final electron acceptor is called aerobic metabolism. The ATP–phosphocreatine system and glycolysis are two anaerobic metabolic pathways that can produce ATP without oxygen, while ATP formation by OXPHOS is the aerobic pathway (Fig. 17.2).

The aforementioned three metabolic pathways are described as follows:

- In the first metabolic pathway, ATP is broken down into ADP + Pi at the beginning of the exercise. This sudden increase in ADP concentration stimulates creatine kinase to trigger the breakdown of phosphocreatine, which is required to resynthesize ATP. As muscle cells store only small amounts of phosphocreatine, the total amount of ATP that can be formed through this reaction is limited. The combina-

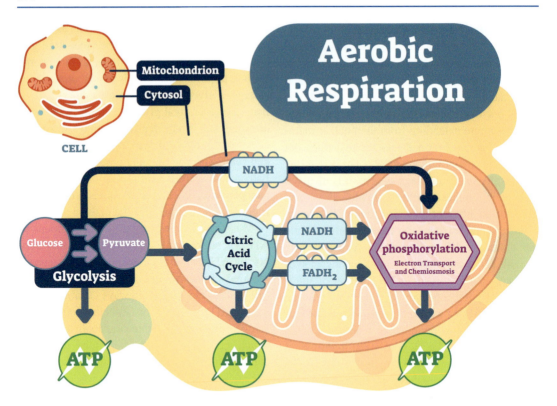

Fig. 17.2 Aerobic respiration (VectorMine/Shutterstock.com)

tion of stored ATP and phosphocreatine is called the "ATP–phosphocreatine system" or "phosphagen system." This system is the first energy store to provide energy for muscle contraction at the start of exercise and during short-term, high-intensity exercise. This energy is stored in the cytosol of the cell, and not in the mitochondria.
- The second metabolic pathway, glycolysis, involves the breakdown of glucose or glycogen to form two pyruvate or lactate molecules. It is the anaerobic pathway used to transfer bond energy from glucose to Pi and back to ADP. Glycolysis occurs in the sarcoplasm of the muscle cells, with two molecules of ATP and two molecules of pyruvate or lactate gained per molecule of glucose.
- In the third metabolic pathway, aerobic ATP production occurs with the citric acid cycle and electron transport chain (ETC) working together in the mitochondria. Although energy production is slower with OXPHOS, more ATP is produced. The primary function of the citric acid cycle (also called Krebs cycle or TCA) is to complete the oxidation of carbohydrates, fats, or proteins using nicotinamide adenine dinucleotide and flavin adenine dinucleotide as hydrogen carriers. The energy released by the electrons of their hydrogen can be used to combine ADP + Pi to reform ATP in ETC.

During high-intensity, short-term exercises (2–20 s), the ATP production of the muscle is dominated by the ATP– phosphocreatine system. Intense exercise lasting more than 20 s uses more anaerobic glycolysis to produce most of the ATP needed. A combination of the ATP–phosphocreatine system, glycolysis, and aerobic system is used to produce the required ATP in high-intensity events lasting longer than 45 s, while half the anaerobic and aerobic systems are used to produce the ATP needed for exercise lasting between 2 and 3 min. The main energy source during prolonged low and moderate exercises is OXPHOS.

Acute exercise causes a rapid depletion of glycogen in the skeletal muscle. After acute exercise, glycogen is resynthesized, and the glycogen content is stored back within 24 h. This suggests that exercise increases glucose uptake and storage. In response to acute exercise, the glycogen storage capacity of the skeletal muscle increases. That is, exercise increases the resynthesis of glycogen. It also contributes to the changes in muscle biochemistry and cells. Many of the acute effects of exercise are related to improved glucose metabolism and improved skeletal muscle insulin sensitivity.

Evidence shows that exercise acutely increases the conversion and oxidation of free fatty acids in both healthy and trained individuals. Therefore, adipose tissue is an important fuel source with increased movement of free fatty acids from adipocytes, which acts as an important substrate in prolonged exercises. On the contrary, in response to long-term vigorous exercise training programs, significant changes are seen in the level of oxidative metabolism, with increased mitochondrial oxygen uptake and respiratory enzyme activity in the skeletal muscle. This leads to an increase in the aerobic working capacity.

17.3 Adaptations Formed by Different Exercise Types

In accordance with the specificity principle of exercise, endurance training is associated with improved aerobic energy metabolism and endurance to fatigue for increased capacity, while resistance training is associated with muscle hypertrophy and increased force-generating capacity.

Different types of exercises can provide a powerful stimulus for mitochondrial biogenesis. In this section, acute and chronic adaptations that occur with high-intensity exercise, moderate-intensity continuous training (MICT), sprint interval training (SIT), high-intensity training (HIT), and high-intensity interval training (HIIT) are discussed.

For exercise training to cause adaptations at the cellular level, it must be done for a certain period, frequency, and intensity. Along with a strong increase in mitochondrial content, exercise provides an improvement in OXPHOS and mitochondrial respiratory capacity. Also, prolonged training reduces ROS production, which is indicative of an enhanced capacity for electron flow through the ETC.

Mitochondrial volume and maximum oxygen consumption are interrelated. Endurance training, which is considered the primary way to achieve mitochondrial adaptations, leads to an increase in total mitochondrial proteins, including β-oxidation, TCA cycle, and ETC, thus improving the energy supply capacity of the muscle that is active during exercise training. Long-term endurance training causes the mitochondrial volume to increase by approximately 40–50%, and this increase in content is parallel to the improvement in the respiratory and oxidative capacities of the mitochondria. In addition, mitochondrial adaptations due to exercise vary between different fiber types, depending on the initial organelle content and motor unit grade during the training session.

In the human body, slow-twitch (Type I) fibers contain the highest percentage of mitochondria, followed by fast-twitch red (Type IIa) fibers and white Type IIx fibers. Exercise training can increase the mitochondrial content in any of these fiber types. This suggests that mitochondrial adaptations are not dependent on the myosin-based fiber type, but rather on the stimulus and the fiber involved. The relationship between training intensity and duration is important in determining mitochondrial adaptation for each fiber type. Type I fibers work at 40% of maximum oxygen consumption and lower exercise intensity. As the workload increases (more than 40% of maximum oxygen consumption), Type IIa fibers come into play. Only when exercise intensity exceeds by approximately 75% of maximum oxygen consumption, Type IIx fibers come into play. According to this principle, different mitochondrial adaptations can occur in the muscle according to training approaches.

Resistance exercise training is mainly associated with muscle hypertrophy and improvement in power generation capacity, along with increasing resistance to fatigue and improving aerobic energy metabolism. Examining the effect of resistive exercise shows that it has the potential to produce significant improvements in maximal combined respiration measured in permeable myofibers, although no parallel increase occurs in mitochondrial gene expression or mitochondrial mass. These adaptations may be more pronounced in older individuals or in diseased muscles such as sporadic inclusion body myositis, as mitochondrial gene expression and basal-state content are reduced.

The abundance of ribosomal RNA (rRNA) and ribosomal biogenesis after resistance exercise training appear to be the key factors for muscle hypertrophy. After resistance exercise training, high responders to muscle hypertrophy have a greater increase in rRNA abundance than low responders. In addition, blunted ribosome biogenesis after acute resistance exercise during aging may contribute to the attenuation of exercise-induced hypertrophy. Protein synthesis and modulation of ribosome biogenesis markers occur in human skeletal muscle during both acute and chronic resistance exercises. One study compared exercises performed at two different exercise volumes (low, one set; medium, three sets) for 12 weeks of full-body resistance training.

Immunohistochemistry and mRNA genetype profiling analyses showed that multiset resistance training was more important. The level of total RNA was higher in the 2nd and 12th weeks for multiset training compared with single-set training. According to these data, both protocols led to an increase in ribosomal biogenesis, and multiset training produced higher effects. These results supported the idea that chronic resistance exercise could increase protein translation and ribosomal biogenesis in a volume-dependent manner.

17.3.1 Exercise Intensity and Cellular Adaptations

The use of interval training modalities, such as HIIT and SIT, has increased in recent years. With interval training protocols, an adaptation level similar to traditional endurance training can be gained in a shorter time with less exercise volume. As with endurance exercise, periods of HIT promote the activation of several signaling kinases that converge on PGC-1α to promote organelle synthesis. However, exercise at higher intensities leads to faster ATP hydrolysis and more calcium release to build strength, which, in turn, leads to increased activation of signaling kinases such as p38 MAPK, AMPK, and CaMKII (Fig. 17.3). Both HIIT and SIT provide increases in mitochondrial content by 25–35% after repeated six to seven sessions. ATP conversion is greater for high-intensity exercise based on carbohydrate oxidation and use of more glycogen than that for low-intensity exercise. In studies where total work done was matched, high-intensity exercise was associated with greater activation of certain kinases and greater expression of mtRNA for PGC-1α, a key regulator of mitochondrial biogenesis, compared with low-intensity exercise. In addition, mitochondrial protein synthesis was found to be higher in high-intensity exercise performed in continuous training than in lower-intensity exercise. According to this result, a higher rate of mitochondrial biogenesis occurs when a given exercise volume is performed at a higher intensity.

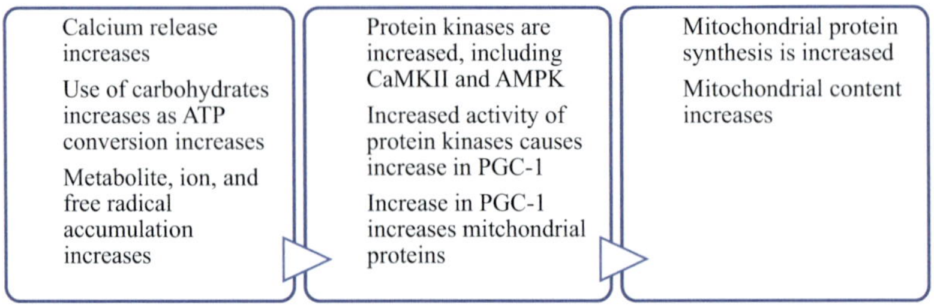

Fig. 17.3 Adaptations caused by high-intensity exercises

Calcium release increases	Protein kinases are increased, including CaMKII and AMPK	Mitochondrial protein synthesis is increased
Use of carbohydrates increases as ATP conversion increases	Increased activity of protein kinases causes increase in PGC-1	Mitochondrial content increases
Metabolite, ion, and free radical accumulation increases	Increase in PGC-1 increases mitchondrial proteins	

The activation of mitochondrial biogenesis in response to exercise in low-volume SIT is thought to be partially linked to ROS production. SIT induces ROS-dependent degradation of the ryanodine receptor, which is involved in the post-exercise increase in intracellular calcium concentration, a signal for mitochondrial biogenesis. In addition, SIT inhibits aconitase activity through the increase in ROS.

Improvements in interval training can be explained by the response of the skeletal muscle to rest–work cycles. When a moderate-intensity exercise session is divided into 1-min intervals (i.e., given rest intervals), AMPK phosphorylation is more elicited than when the session is continuously administered for 30 min. However, the chronic implications of these acute differences in signaling patterns are not yet clear. The intermittent nature of interval training plays a role in the size of the adaptations. The maximum activity of citrate synthase increased with interval training at the same workload but did not change with continuous training. Moreover, HIIT provided a greater increase in mitochondrial content, as assessed by the maximum activity of citrate synthase and OXPHOS capacity in permeable muscle fibers, compared with MICT. On the contrary, an increase in mitochondrial content was found to be similar after HIIT and MICT protocols were applied by matching workloads. Studies examining the effect of severity on the lactate threshold generally report similar increases between protocols. Some studies reported that a small volume of exercise performed at very high intensity could elicit similar skeletal muscle adaptations compared with large volumes of moderate-intensity exercise.

Comparing a low-volume SIT with a high-volume HIIT showed that the increase in mitochondrial respiration was only significant after SIT. Low-volume SIT increased the lactate threshold to a similar extent, a variable strongly associated with skeletal muscle mitochondrial content than larger MICT and HIIT volumes. It caused greater increases in the maximal activity of citrate synthase for MICT than for SIT in work-matched SIT and MICT comparisons. Similar decreases in blood lactate concentrations were achieved during submaximal exercise, and the maximum activity of citrate synthase was higher in the post-training SIT group. AMP and ADP concentrations were the highest after the first exercise session, and glycogenolysis and lactate accumulation was strongly suppressed during the third exercise compared with the first exercise. In other words, the metabolic signal did not increase with the increase in the number of sessions. Moreover, the expression of genes involved in mitochondrial biogenesis was similar for SIT and MICT with or without the same workload.

17.3.2 Acute Exercise and Cellular Adaptations

Mitochondria respond quickly to short-term training (Table 17.3). In fact, a single endurance exercise is sufficient to increase the function of the organelle network necessary to initiate structural changes in the mitochondrial network. Similar to MICT, a single session of HIIT or SIT activates signaling pathways associated with mitochondrial biogenesis, such as phosphorylation of AMPK and p38 MAPK and expression of PGC-1α mRNA. Regular and repeated activation of these pathways leads to increases in mitochondrial density. Examining the adaptation process to short-term HIIT, mRNA expression (e.g., PGC-1α) has been shown to increase acutely and transiently after each HIIT session. Studies reported that the maximum activity of citrate synthase increased after the third session compared with the baseline level, and the protein content and enzyme activity of citrate synthase increased regularly over seven sessions. Other studies reported significant increases in citrate synthase activity 24 h after a single SIT or MICT session. After six to seven sessions of HIIT or SIT, the mitochondrial content, as measured by citrate synthase or cyclooxygenase (COX) activity,

Table 17.3 Some adaptations of acute exercise training

p38 MAPK and AMPK ↑
Expression of PGC-1α and mRNA ↑
Protein content and enzyme activity of citrate synthase ↑
Mitochondrial biogenesis and content ↑

increases by 25–35%. The mitochondrial content has been shown to stabilize after 5 days of training when the intensity and duration of exercise are held constant. However, when the severity increases progressively, the mitochondrial content continues to increase for at least a few weeks.

17.3.3 Training Duration, Frequency, and Cellular Adaptations

The effects of duration at the cellular level depend on the intensity of the exercise. The effects of 10-day cycling for 30 or 60 min per day at a low, moderate, or high intensity (60%, 70%, and 86% of maximum oxygen consumption, respectively) were examined. After moderate and vigorous training, AMP and ADP accumulation and phosphocreatine and glycogen depletion decreased from more than 60 min of exercise to 30 min of exercise. These results indicated an increase in mitochondrial content. Comparing two 11-week training programs consisting of different exercise modes and intensities, similar increases in mitochondrial content and markers were observed in the groups that underwent HIT of approximately 3800 kcal/week and a moderate-intensity training of approximately 2000 kcal/week.

In one study, 4 weeks of normal-volume training (3 sessions/week), followed by 20 days of high-volume training (2 sessions/day), followed by 2 weeks of reduced-volume training (5 sessions) was performed. After high-volume training, the mitochondrial respiration and citrate synthase activity, protein content of ETS subunits, and PGC-1α, NRF1, mitochondrial transcription factor A, PHF20, and p53 levels increased compared with the baseline levels. Studies reported that after reduced-volume training, all measured mitochondrial parameters, except citrate synthase activity, increased compared with the baseline values. These results supported that increasing HIIT volume by increasing the duration and frequency, while keeping the intensity constant, increases the mitochondrial content and provided evidence that increases in high-intensity exercise volume could also increase the mitochondrial content.

17.4 Autophagy, Mitophagy, and Exercise

Autophagy is defined as recycling aged or damaged cellular organelles and proteins for the resynthesis of new organelles and ATP, often under stress conditions such as starvation and increased physical activity (Fig. 17.4). In the first step, proteins or other cellular components (e.g., mitochondria, ribosomes, peroxisomes, ER, lipids, and polysaccharides) are enclosed in a double-membrane vesicle called an autophagosome. Next, the contents of the autophagosome are removed by another vesicle called the lysosome, which contains acid hydrolases. Specific recognition and degradation of damaged or redundant organelles can also be achieved by selective autophagy as a specific form of autophagy. Mitophagy (selective autophagy of mitochondria) has an important role in situations where energy stress, such as hunger, obesity, and physical activity, occurs. In the final stage of mitophagy, the autophagosome needs to fuse with lysosomes to be degraded by proteolytic enzymes in the lysosome lumen. Therefore, lysosomal health is extremely important for the maintenance of mitochondrial quality in muscles. Although timely removal of aged or damaged cell mitochondria in the heart is essential for cardiac homeostasis, excessive or pathological mitophagy is considered harmful to the organism. Studies have shown that exercise not only temporarily triggers cardioprotective mitophagy but also helps maintain an appropriate level of mitophagy. Therefore, mitophagy helps better understand how exercise affects the overall health of the organism.

Although the activation of the organelle biogenesis pathway leads to an increase in mitochondrial content because of exercise training, it is also vital to eliminate mitochondrial segments that outlive their usefulness through mitophagy so as to maintain or improve the quality of the mitochondrial pool. The main mitophagy pathway investigated in the context of exercise includes PTEN-mediated putative kinase protein 1 (PINK1) and Parkin proteins. Normally, PINK1 is degraded by resident proteases upon arrival at

Autophagy

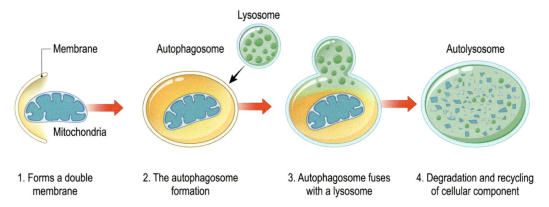

Fig. 17.4 Autophagy (Designua/Shutterstock.com)

the mitochondria. An increase in autophagy and mitophagy markers occurs in the muscle in response to repetitive exercises performed as endurance training. After training, Parkin localization to mitochondria and Parkin production in muscles increase. However, the exercise-induced increase in mitophagy flow decreases after training. Some studies showed that the mitophagy flow in the basal state decreased after endurance training as a chronic contractile activity. According to these studies, the improvement in mitochondrial function that occurred with such exercises reduced the need for mitophagy signaling. In addition, an increase in TFEB protein, as well as lysosomal markers, in lysosome-associated membrane proteins occurred with chronic exercise. These results supported the idea that chronic exercise induced the expression of lysosomes and autophagy-related genes, allowing the muscle to be ready to clear dysfunctional organelles, including mitochondria. Given the similar increases in mitochondrial content and function observed in HIIT and SIT compared with traditional endurance training, mitochondrial transformation may be induced to a similar degree in these alternative training modalities. Therefore, exercise can be an effective therapeutic modality to balance disease with defects in organelle replacement.

Mitophagy is regulated by numerous cellular stresses, including the energy imbalance caused by acute exercise. During exercise, the AMP/ATP ratio increases, thereby activating AMPK and autophagy-activating kinase 1 (ULK1). It also inhibits mTORC1, a known suppressor of the process. These initial steps are known to occur 6 h after exercise and activate mitophagy. Acute exercise has been shown to have a faster effect by promoting Parkin localization to mitochondria. With LC3-II, p62, and ubiquitin, an increase in mitophagy flux occurs immediately after exercise. In addition, exercise acts as a stimulus for PGC-1α induction to regulate both organelle biogenesis and mitophagy. Therefore, these proteins play a critical role in maintaining the health of the mitochondrial pool within the skeletal muscle.

The ER stress is linked to autophagy, a tool for the control of protein quality. It also protects against diseases such as autophagy, inflammatory diseases, aging, insulin resistance, and cancer. As autophagy is directly linked to mitochondria and mitochondrial dysfunction can lead to ER stress, exercise can reduce ER stress by affecting mitochondrial protein homeostasis. Endurance exercise stimulates autophagy in the skeletal muscle and heart. Autophagy is required for skeletal muscle adaptation and improvement in physical performance induced by exercise training. Autophagy and ER stress appear to respond differently during/after exercise based on the stage of the exercise. During exercise, the mTOR pathway decreases, resulting in increased autophagy. In particular, mTOR, which increases after exercise, reduces autophagy. In trained individuals, repetitive exercise training appears to stimulate the adaptive arm of the UPR and protect the skeletal muscle against the increased stress caused by exercise in subsequent exercises.

An increase in the expression of autophagy genes and proteins has been noted in humans following ultra-endurance exercise (running on a treadmill for 24–28 h). In addition, lifelong exercise with calorie restriction is known to ameliorate the reduction in autophagy observed with aging and reduce the age-related increase in oxidative damage and apoptosis. This suggests that exercise may be a potential treatment modality for myopathies characterized by impaired autophagy, with disease-specific evaluation.

17.5 Conclusion

- Exercise leads to changes in the skeletal muscle, particularly increasing mitochondrial content and improving the health of the mitochondrial pool, which are key to increased metabolic capacity.
- Endurance training leads to improved muscle health by improving mitochondrial biogenesis, function, and the content and quality of organelles. As alternative exercise training modalities, shorter training at the same workload has shown similar developments in mitochondria.
- Short-term, high-intensity activities produce higher amounts of anaerobic ATP, while longer activities cause higher aerobic metabolism.
- Exercise increases the release of autophagy-related genes and proteins, making the muscle ready to clear dysfunctional organelles, including mitochondria.

Further Reading

Bækkerud FH, Solberg F, Leinan IM, Wisløff U, Karlsen T, Rognmo Ø. Comparison of three popular exercise modalities on V˙O2max in overweight and obese. Med Sci Sports Exerc. 2016;48:491–8.

Bernardo BC, Ooi JYY, Weeks KL, Patterson NL, McMullen JR. Understanding key mechanisms of exercise-induced cardiac protection to mitigate disease: current knowledge and emerging concepts. Physiol Rev. 2018;98:419–75.

Carter HN, Kim Y, Erlich AT, Zarrin-Khat D, Hood DA. Autophagy and mitophagy flux in young and aged skeletal muscle following chronic contractile activity. J Physiol. 2018;596:3567–84.

Chen CCW, Erlich AT, Hood DA. Role of Parkin and endurance training on mitochondrial turnover in skeletal muscle. Skelet Muscle. 2018;8:10.

Granata C, Oliveira RS, Little JP, Renner K, Bishop DJ. Mitochondrial adaptations to high-volume exercise training are rapidly reversed after a reduction in training volume in human skeletal muscle. FASEB J. 2016;30:3413–23.

Groennebaek T, Vissing K. Impact of resistance training on skeletal muscle mitochondrial biogenesis, content, and function. Front Physiol. 2017;8:713.

Hammarström D, Øfsteng S, Koll L, Hanestadhaugen M, Hollan I, Apró W, et al. Benefits of higher resistance-training volume are related to ribosome biogenesis. J Physiol. 2020;598:543–65.

Hood DA, Tryon LD, Vainshtein A, Memme J, Chen C, Pauly M, et al. Exercise and the regulation of mitochondrial turnover. Prog Mol Biol Transl Sci. 2015;135:99–127.

Hood DA, Memme JM, Oliveira AN, Triolo M. Maintenance of skeletal muscle mitochondria in health, exercise, and aging. Annu Rev Physiol. 2019;81:19–41.

Ju JS, Jeon SI, Park JY, Lee JY, Lee SC, Cho KJ, et al. Autophagy plays a role in skeletal muscle mitochondrial biogenesis in an endurance exercise-trained condition. J Physiol Sci. 2016;66:417–30.

Kim HJ, Jamart C, Deldicque L, An GL, Lee YH, Kim CK, et al. Endoplasmic reticulum stress markers and ubiquitin–proteasome pathway activity in response to a 200-km run. Med Sci Sports Exerc. 2011;43:18–25.

Kim Y, Triolo M, Erlich AT, Hood DA. Regulation of autophagic and mitophagic flux during chronic contractile activity-induced muscle adaptations. Pflugers Arch. 2019;471:431–40.

Kristensen DE, Albers PH, Prats C, Baba O, Birk JB, Wojtaszewski JF. Human muscle fibre type-specific regulation of AMPK and downstream targets by exercise. J Physiol. 2015;593:2053–69.

Larsen FJ, Schiffer TA, Ørtenblad N, Zinner C, Morales-Alamo D, Willis SJ, et al. High-intensity sprint training inhibits mitochondrial respiration through aconitase inactivation. FASEB J. 2016;30:417–27.

Luan X, Tian X, Zhang H, Huang R, Li N, Chen P, et al. Exercise as a prescription for patients with various diseases. J Sport Health Sci. 2019;8:422–41.

MacInnis MJ, Gibala MJ. Physiological adaptations to interval training and the role of exercise intensity. J Physiol. 2017;595:2915–30.

MacInnis MJ, Zacharewicz E, Martin BJ, Haikalis ME, Skelly LE, Tarnopolsky MA, et al. Superior mitochondrial adaptations in human skeletal muscle after interval compared to continuous single-leg cycling matched for total work. J Physiol. 2017;595:2955–68.

Mancini A, Vitucci D, Randers MB, Schmidt JF, Hagman M, Andersen TR, et al. Lifelong football training: effects on autophagy and healthy longevity promotion. Front Physiol. 2019;10:132.

Marques-Aleixo I, Santos-Alves E, Balça MM, Rizo-Roca D, Moreira PI, Oliveira PJ, et al. Physical exercise improves brain cortex and cerebellum mitochondrial bioenergetics and alters apoptotic, dynamic and auto(mito)phagy markers. Neuroscience. 2015;301:480–95.

Memme JM, Erlich AT, Phukan G, Hood DA. Exercise and mitochondrial health. J Physiol. 2021;599:803–17.

Park JS, Davis RL, Sue CM. Mitochondrial dysfunction in Parkinson's disease: new mechanistic insights and therapeutic perspectives. Curr Neurol Neurosci Rep. 2018;18:21.

Rosenkilde M, Reichkendler MH, Auerbach P, Bonne TC, Sjödin A, Ploug T, et al. Changes in peak fat oxidation in response to different doses of endurance training. Scand J Med Sci Sports. 2015;25:41–52.

Sanchez AM, Candau R, Bernardi H. Recent data on cellular component turnover: focus on adaptations to physical exercise. Cells. 2019;8:542.

Silvennoinen M, Ahtiainen JP, Hulmi JJ, Pekkala S, Taipale RS, Nindl BC, et al. PGC-1 isoforms and their target genes are expressed differently in human skeletal muscle following resistance and endurance exercise. Physiol Rep. 2015;3:e12563.

Trovato E, Di Felice V, Barone R. Extracellular vesicles: delivery vehicles of myokines. Front Physiol. 2019;10:522.

Adaptation of the Musculoskeletal System to Exercise

18

Aslihan Cakmak

18.1 Introduction

Regular exercise training plays an important role in improving musculoskeletal fitness. Skeletal muscles could be remodeled with a variety of physiological stimuli. Exercise elicits several molecular, metabolic, and morphological responses in skeletal muscles. These reactions may include increased muscle strength and endurance, as well as the prevention of injury. It is necessary to understand the structure and function of the muscle to understand the musculoskeletal response to exercise. In this section, the musculoskeletal system, and acute and chronic responses of the musculoskeletal system to aerobic exercise will be explained.

18.2 Musculoskeletal Anatomy: An Overview of the Musculoskeletal System

The musculoskeletal system connects and supports tissues and organs and is constituted by muscles, bones, cartilage, tendons, ligaments, joints, and connective tissues.

A. Cakmak (✉)
Faculty of Physical Therapy and Rehabilitation, Hacettepe University, Ankara, Turkey
e-mail: aslihancakmak@hacettepe.edu.tr

The skeletal system supports soft tissue, protects internal organs, and provides movement. It acts as an important source of nutrients and blood components. In a long bone, the main part is called the shaft or diaphysis of the bone, and the ends are called the epiphysis. The epiphyses are covered with articular cartilage. Cartilage is a connective tissue form that reduces friction in the synovial joints and spreads the load on the joint over a wide area, reducing the stress in contact with the joint surface. Joints are connections between bones. They form the joints system together with the bones and ligaments. Ligaments are fibrous connective tissues that connect bones to other bones. The joints are classified as fibrous, cartilaginous, and synovial. Fibrous joints are where the bones are joined by dense fibrous connective tissue. Cartilaginous joints are where the bones connected with cartilage. Synovial joints are the type of joints that consist of a joint capsule and synovial membrane surrounding a joint cavity filled with synovial fluid. The most common joints of the human body are synovial joints. Perfusion of the joints is provided by numerous arterial branches, and innervation is provided by branches of nerves that supply the adjacent muscle and overlying skin. Proprioceptive feedback and pain, which are important in regulating movement and preventing injury, occur as a result of high sensory fiber density in the joint capsule.

Muscle tissue is evaluated within three separate muscle groups: Skeletal, cardiac, and smooth

© The Author(s), under exclusive license to Springer Nature Switzerland AG 2023
D. Kaya Utlu (ed.), *Functional Exercise Anatomy and Physiology for Physiotherapists*,
https://doi.org/10.1007/978-3-031-27184-7_18

muscle. The human body contains over 600 skeletal muscles that make up 40–50% of the entire body weight. Force generation for movement, respiration, and postural support, and heat generation at cold stress are important functions of skeletal muscles. In addition, skeletal muscles are known to be endocrine organs and take a key part in regulating various organ systems of the body.

Dense connective tissue, called tendons, connects skeletal muscles to bones. During the contraction of muscles, one end of the muscle is attached to a still bone (origin) and the other end to a moving bone (insertion). Movements depend on the type of joints and the muscles involved. The joint angle decreasing muscles are called flexors, while the joint angle increasing muscles are called extensors.

18.3 Musculoskeletal Physiology: Structure of Skeletal Muscle, Types of Muscle Fiber, and Contraction, Sliding, and Rotating Filaments by Muscle Contraction

18.3.1 Structure of Skeletal Muscle

Skeletal muscles are a complex structure that includes long, multinucleated cells called muscle fibers (myofiber/muscle cells) as well as various elements, including nervous tissue, blood, and various connective tissues. The elements comprising the muscle tissue are primarily water (75%), protein (20%), and others (5%) such as inorganic salts, minerals, fat, and carbohydrates. Muscle mass is relevant to the balance of protein synthesis and degradation. Both protein synthesis and protein degradation are responsive to factors such as physical activity, exercise, hormonal balance, nutritional status, and injury.

Skeletal muscle architecture is defined as a very specific and fine organization of muscle fibers and associated connective tissue. Tendons are the structures that connect the muscle to the bone. Tendons connect the muscle to the periosteum of the bone. Wide and flat tendon structures are called **aponeurosis**. Although it is not separated from the tendon with a clear line, the outer connective tissue surrounding the entire muscle, different from the tendon, is called the **epimysium (deep fascia)**. Composed of collagen, reticular, and elastic fibers, the epimysium provides the muscle its shape and includes blood vessels and nerves. In the inner part of the muscle, the **perimysium** surrounds the muscle fiber bundles. The bundle of muscle fibers surrounded by the perimysium is called the **muscle fascicle**. The connective tissue of the perimysium contains vessels, nerves, and proprioceptors (muscle spindles, Vater-Pacini corpuscles, Ruffini corpuscles). The **endomysium** surrounds each muscle fiber. The endomysium contains many capillaries and nerve fibers, except for lymph capillaries. These connective tissues occupy 10–15% of the muscle volume and create a sort of skeleton regulating and controlling muscle activity (Fig. 18.1).

The **sarcolemma** is the encompassing membrane of the muscle fiber. A group of precursor cells in muscle, **satellite cells**, are found between the sarcolemma and the basal lamina. Satellite cells are described as adult stem cells of the skeletal muscles. These cells are involved in the muscle growth, repair, and regeneration. The **sarcoplasm**, the cytoplasm containing cell proteins, organelles, and myofibrils, lies underneath the sarcolemma. The **sarcoplasmic reticulum** is a special network of membranous channels surrounding each myofibril that stores, releases, and reuptakes calcium ions (Ca^{++}) in the muscle sarcoplasm. The **transverse tubules (T tubules)** are membranous channels passing through the sarcolemma to the muscle fiber and extending along the fiber. The enlarged areas of the sarcoplasmic reticulum surrounding the transverse tubules are called **terminal cisternae**.

Muscle fibers are innervated by somatic efferent (motor) neurons. Each one of the skeletal muscle fibers is linked with a branch of nerve fiber from a nerve cell. These nerve cells are called as motor neurons. Motor neurons, axon terminals, and the skeletal muscle fibers they innervate form the motor unit. Each muscle consists of tens or hundreds of motor units. The contraction process commences with the excita-

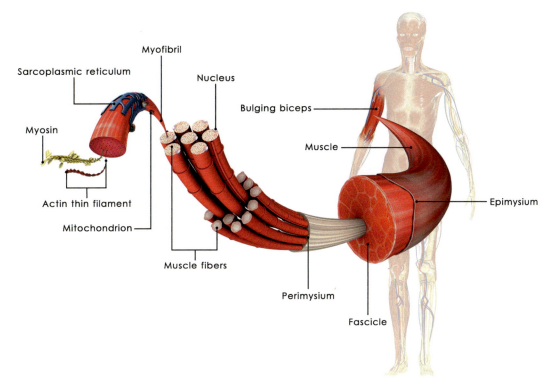

Fig. 18.1 Structure of Skeletal Muscle (sciencepics/Shutterstock.com)

tion of motor neurons. The **neuromuscular junction** is the area where the motor neurons and the muscle cells cross. The sarcolemma forms a pocket called the **synaptic cleft** at this junction. The synaptic cleft separates the end of the motor neuron and the muscle fiber. When an impulse reaches the end of the motor nerve, the neurotransmitter acetylcholine (ACh) is released and propagates across the synaptic cleft in order to bind with ACh receptor areas. Consequently, this increases the sarcolemma permeability to sodium, which results in a depolarization called the endplate potential. The endplate potential is a signal that is at or strong enough to exceed the threshold to initiate the contraction process. At the neuromuscular junction, a synaptic connection occurs, which allows communication with the motor neuron and the muscle fiber it innervates.

One of the most deterministic features of skeletal muscles is their striated microscopic appearance. This appearance is due to the thin and thick extensions called **myofilaments** that form the muscle fibers. According to the estimates, each muscle fiber consists of several hundred or several thousand myofibrils and includes billions of myofilaments. **Actin (thin filament)** and **myosin (thick filament)** myofilaments, **troponin and tropomyosin** proteins in actin, and other support proteins form sarcomeres, the essential contractile units for skeletal muscles. Troponin and tropomyosin regulate muscle contraction by controlling the interactivity between actin and myosin. Z disc separates the sarcomeres from each other. Additionally, the Z line of the sarcomere serves as a connection point of the actin myofilament. The H zone is the middle part of the A band and consists of myosin only when the muscle is at rest. The I band contains actin only, while the A band consists of both actin and myosin. The M line is located in the middle of the Z discs (Fig. 18.2).

Other proteins contributing to the muscles in terms of both mechanical and physiological proper-

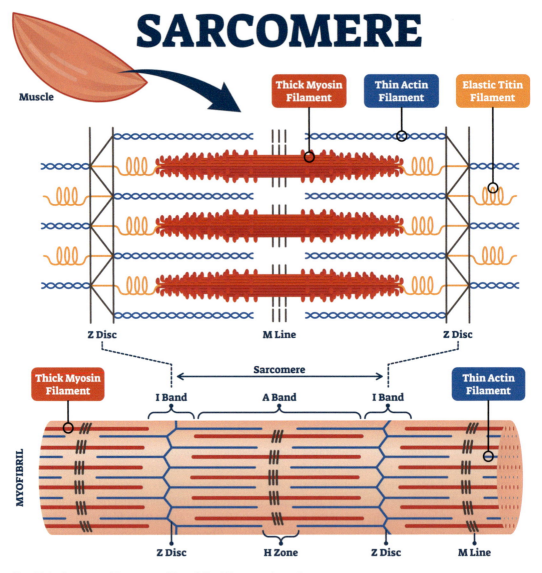

Fig. 18.2 Structure of Sarcomere (VectorMine/Shutterstock.com)

ties are called **titin** and **nebulin**. A large-elastic protein called titin binds to the Z disc and myosin of the sarcomere and helps stabilize and align. Nebulin, on the other hand, integrates with other proteins in actin-containing thin filaments. These proteins partake in the integrity of the sarcomere, influencing the passive tension and stiffness properties of cells. Titin is thought to be involved in the formation of strength in due course of muscle movements. Furthermore, **desmin** protein binds the Z disc to the sarcolemma and extracellular matrix.

18.3.2 Muscle Fiber and Contraction Types

Muscle has three biochemical properties important to function: oxidative capacity, the myosin isoform type, and the contractile protein level of the fiber. The number of mitochondria, the number of capillaries around the fiber, and the amount of myoglobin within the fiber determine the oxidative capacity of a muscle fiber. The increase in the number of mitochondria increases the capacity for adenosine triphosphate (ATP) production aerobically. Numerous capillaries surrounding a muscle fiber ensure that the fiber receives sufficient oxygen during the contraction process. An oxygen-binding protein called myoglobin is found in skeletal muscle fibers and cardiac muscle. Myoglobin carries oxygen from the muscle cell membrane to the mitochondria. The high myoglobin concentration facilitates the transport of oxygen from the capillaries to the mitochondria.

In humans, there are three main isoforms of myosin, and these isoforms differ in their activity, the rate of ATP breakdown. The muscle fibers containing ATPase isoforms with high ATPase activity cause high-speed muscle shortening.

The main factor regulating the maximum shortening rate of fibers is myosin ATPase activity. Accordingly, fibers having high myosin ATPase activities are called fast fibers, and fibers having low myosin ATPase activities are called slow fibers.

Skeletal muscle fiber types are classified in humans as types I, IIa, and IIx. Type I fibers have slow strength generation characteristics with a dominant oxidative metabolism, high myoglobin content, high energy efficiency, and high resistance to fatigue, while type IIa fibers (fast-twitch) provide fast strength generation using both oxidative and glycolytic metabolisms. Type IIx muscle fibers have a glycolytic profile with a fast contraction rate, low myoglobin content, low energy efficiency, and low resistance to fatigue.

The process of creating force by skeletal muscle is called muscle contraction. Muscle movement can be classified as dynamic (isotonic, isokinetic, and plyometric) or static (isometric). Static action (isometric contraction) is common in postural muscles such as standing and sitting to maintain a static body position. Muscle movements resulting in the body parts' movements are called dynamic (isotonic exercise). During dynamic action, concentric (positive phase) or eccentric (negative phase) contraction occurs.

18.3.2.1 Static Contraction

Isometric contraction is a contraction that does not cause any change in muscle length, although there is a change in tension and energy. The force produced during an isometric contraction depends entirely on the length of the muscle during the contraction. Isometric contraction is performed in static positions whereby the joint angle and length of the muscle remain the same. Isometric contraction is performed against an object that cannot be moved (e.g., push-up stance/position "plank hold/pose," side push-up position "side plank pose," sitting against a wall "wall-sit").

18.3.2.2 Dynamic Contraction

Isotonic contraction involves muscle contractions in which the muscle length changes against resistance. In this contraction type, the change in muscle length produces force. Isotonic contractions can be concentric or eccentric. In both contractions, a dynamic contraction occurs, which is produced during dynamic exercise with movement. Dynamic exercise is a type of exercise contributing joint movement.

Concentric contraction occurs when the length of the muscle is shortened, with no change in tension. The muscle commences to shorten when activated and has to withstand a load.

Eccentric contraction, in contrast to concentric contraction, is a condition in which muscles are lengthened in response to a greater opposing force. As the load on the muscle continues to increase, the external force on the muscle reaches a point that is greater than the force the muscle can generate. Therefore, despite the muscle becoming fully active, it is forced to lengthen due to the excess external load. The absolute tensions obtained with eccentric contraction are fairly high regarding the capacity of the muscle in order to produce maximum tetanic tension. Furthermore, absolute stress is relatively independent of the elongation rate. This indicates that skeletal muscles are very resistant to elongation.

Isokinetic contraction occurs during the shortening of the muscle at a constant rate and endeavors maximum tension throughout its entire range of motion. This is achieved with specially designed equipment adjusting the resistance automatically throughout the motion range.

A plyometric contraction refers to a concentric contraction that occurs immediately after an eccentric contraction.

18.3.3 Muscle Contraction, Sliding and Winding Filaments

Muscle contraction process involves numerous cell proteins and energy systems. The contraction mechanism of the muscle is described by the theory of sliding filaments. According to this theory, the muscle contracts by shortening myofibrils due to the sliding of actin on myosin. During muscle contraction, the Z lines move closer together, and the sarcomere shortens. The interaction between actin and myosin filaments is responsible for muscle contraction as multiple cross-bridges extending from myosin attach to actin and cause the filaments to slide over each other. The binding of myosin cross-bridges to actin pulls actin towards the center of the sarcomere and results in the shortening of the muscle. Muscle contraction requires energy, which is provided by the myosin ATPase enzyme located at the top of the myosin cross-bridge. The enzyme breaks down ATP, converting it into adenosine diphosphate (ADP) and inorganic phosphate (Pi), which releases energy and pulls actin onto myosin, causing muscle shortening. The process of myosin cross-bridge attracting the actin molecule is known as the contraction cycle, power stroke. A single power stroke of all cross-bridges in a muscle shortens the muscle by only 1% of its resting length, and therefore, the cycle needs to be repeated many times to achieve significant shortening. Some muscles can shorten by more than half their resting length. This demonstrates that the contraction cycle needs to be reiterated many times.

18.3.3.1 Excitation-Contraction Coupling

Excitation-contraction coupling is a series of events in which a nerve stimulus (action potential) reaches the muscle membrane, then causes shortening of the muscle with cross-bridge activity, and subsequently, muscle depolarization (excitation) and force production (contraction) occur. Muscle contraction processes are excitation, contraction, and relaxation.

Excitation: Excitation commences with the impulse reaching the neuromuscular junction. The action potential of the motor neuron creates the ACh release into the synaptic cleft. ACh binds to receptors on the motor endplate, creating an endplate potential that leads to muscle cell depolarization. This depolarization descends through the transverse tubules and deeper into the muscle fiber. Muscle depolarizes and Ca^{++} is released from the sarcoplasmic reticulum through the sarcoplasm.

Contraction: Depolarization of the transverse tubules causes the Ca^{++} releasing to be occurred at the sarcoplasmic reticulum through the sarcoplasm of the muscle fiber. Ca^{++} binds to troponin on actin. With the connection of Ca^{++} to troponin, tropomyosin, which is directly bound to troponin, is shifted. This exposes the myosin connecting areas on actin. Myosin cross-bridges bind to the active area on actin. The linking of the cross-bridges commences the energy release that is kept inside the myosin. That allows the movement of the cross-bridge, resulting in the muscle shortening. This happens over and over as long as the neuromuscular stimulation continues.

Relaxation: The first step of muscle relaxation happens when the motor neuron stops firing. When neurostimulation of the muscle ceases, ACh releasing stops and the muscle fiber repolarizes. When motor neuron firing and muscle stimulation cease, Ca^{++} is pumped from the sarcoplasm to the sarcoplasmic reticulum for storage. In the absence of free Ca^{++} in the cytosol, troponin closes the myosin connection areas on actin with tropomyosin. The presence of tropomyosin at the active areas on actin inhibits myosin-actin cross-bridge creation and relaxes the muscle.

The theory of sliding filaments aligns with the observed properties of muscles, including the force-velocity relationship and the force-length relationship of the concentric portion. Although this mechanism is widely acknowledged for isometric and concentric contraction, there remain uncertainties concerning the underlying mechanism of eccentric contraction. After an eccentric contraction, there is an increase in isometric force surpassing the force generated by a complete isometric contraction at the same muscle length and activation level. This phenomenon is known as residual force enhancement after stretch (RFE). Furthermore, residual force depression occurs when muscles are actively shortened, resulting in a smaller isometric force than the force obtained during purely isometric contractions at the same muscle length and activation level. This phenomenon cannot be accounted for by the cross-bridge theory, leading to alternative explanations such as the sarcomere length non-uniformity and titin mechanism. The non-uniformity of sarcomere length is on the basis of the concept that sarcomere lengths and strengths are unstable in the decreasing portion of the force-length relationship. However, RFE is also observed in the ascending part of the force-length relationship, a single mechanically isolated sarcomere can also produce large amounts of RFE, and RFE also occurs in the absence of sarcomere length uniformities. These findings show that RFE cannot be fully explained by the non-uniformity of sarcomere length.

Based on the titin mechanism, since titin binds to the thick filaments in the A band and the thin filaments in the Z disc, the movement of the thin filaments by the cross-bridges causes titin's movement. This initiates a process that can keep elastic potential energy when isometric strength increases and during active stretching. The winding filament pattern is a mechanism whereby titin contributes to muscle strength enhancement and active shortening.

The winding filament hypothesis is based on the proline, glutamate, valine, and lysine (PEVK) segment of titin wrapping on actin during strength enhancement, and cross-bridges rotate the PEVK segment on actin in active muscles. The N2A region of titin separates the tandem immunoglobulin (Ig) domains from the hard PEVK region. Hence, modulation of titin stiffness is achieved by Ca^{++}-dependent binding to actin. In passive tension, the proximal tandem Ig segments unfold to nearly their length when the sarcomere is stretched further its relaxed length. Once the proximal tandem Ig segments reach their length, the PEVK segment is extended by further stretching. In active stretching of muscle sarcomeres, the N2A domain of titin binds to actin, following Ca^{++} influx. Cross-bridges rotate the PEVK segment over actin in active muscles. Consequently, when Ca^{++}-activated sarcomeres are stretched, only the rigid PEVK segment elongates, resulting in higher force generation.

There is evidence to suggest that in the absence of actin-myosin interactions, RFE results from titin stiffening via Ca^{++} binding to the PEVK segment and specific immunoglobulin domains. In this case, it is thought that there are unknown components associated with the activation of Ca^{++} and the binding of titin to actin, which causes RFE.

18.4 The Acute Response of the Musculoskeletal System to Aerobic Exercise

Skeletal muscles could be remodeled with a variety of physiological stimuli. Exercise elicits molecular, metabolic, and morphological responses in skeletal muscles. Acute responses to exercise are sudden changes that occur with a single exercise session. Chronic responses, on the other hand, are changes and adaptations that occur regularly for a certain period of time, at rest and during exercise. Exercises are can be classified as aerobic/endurance and resistance/strength exercises. Endurance exercises are performed against a low load for a long period of time, while strength exercises are performed against a higher load for a short period of time.

The adaptation mechanism that takes place in skeletal muscle in response to exercise depends on the stimulus. Resistance exercise is designed to withstand the stress of lifting heavy loads. Resistance exercise leads to the increase in muscle mass and muscle fiber cross-sectional area, neural adaptations, and maximum force production. On the other hand, endurance exercise induces metabolic adaptations to increase maximal oxygen consumption and mitochondrial biogenesis, improve energy source selection, and provide resistance to fatigue.

Responses to exercise in muscle fibers are the result of an increase in the number of certain proteins. Exercise-induced synthesis of cellular proteins occurs when exercise stress stimulates cell signaling pathways that activate transcriptional activators in contracting muscle fibers. These transcriptional activators activate certain genes to synthesize new proteins. This gene activation results in the transcription of messenger RNA (mRNA), which contains the genetic information for the amino acid sequence of a particular protein. After being synthesized, the mRNA moves to the ribosome, where it translated into a specific protein. The distinct types of the proteins present in a muscle fiber determines its properties and capacity to perform specific types of exercise. A single session of exercise causes a temporary increase in the number of certain mRNAs. This increase peaks between the first 4–8 h after exercise, returning to basal levels within 24 h. This exercise-induced increase in mRNA increases the synthesis of specific muscle proteins. Further studies are needed to investigate the responses of the musculoskeletal system to acute aerobic exercise.

18.5 The Chronic Response of the Musculoskeletal System to Aerobic Exercise

Aerobic exercise training causes various adaptations in skeletal muscle, tendons, and bone tissue.

18.5.1 Skeletal Muscle Adaptations

Endurance exercise enhances the ability of muscle fibers to maintain homeostasis during the exercise. Additionally, endurance exercise creates a shift in muscle fiber type from fast to slow, increasing the number of capillaries surrounding muscle fibers, mitochondria size in exercising muscles, fat oxidation, and muscle antioxidant capacity. In addition, the acid-base balance is maintained due to the fact that the muscles produce less lactate and H^+ with exercise training.

18.5.1.1 Muscle Fiber Type Shifting
The muscle fiber type shifts from fast to slow resulting from endurance training due to a decrease in the amount of fast myosin in the muscle and an increase in the slow myosin isoforms. Despite slow myosin isoforms having lower myosin ATPase activity, they can do more with less ATP usage. This fast-to-slow shifting in myosin isoforms improves mechanical efficiency. The fiber type shifting induced by exercise depends on the duration, intensity, and frequency of endurance training. Although there is a fiber type shifting from fast to slow with endurance training, this change does not result in a complete transition from fast fibers to slow fibers.

18.5.1.2 Increase in the Mitochondrial Content of the Muscle
Endurance training increases the mitochondrial content of the skeletal muscle fibers. In skeletal muscle, there are two subgroups of mitochondria: below the sarcolemma (subsarcolemmal mitochondria) and around the contractile proteins (intermyofibrillary mitochondria—80% of the total mitochondria). Endurance training increases the volume of both mitochondrial subsets in active skeletal muscle fibers. The muscle mitochondrial volume may increase up to 50–100% in the first 6 weeks of endurance training. The amount of exercise-induced increase in mitochondria depends on the exercise intensity and duration.

The increase in mitochondrial volume with exercise is caused by an increase in mitochondrial size rather than an increase in their number. This increase results in a boost in oxidative capacity and a greater ability to utilize fat as a source of energy. As a consequence, the body can prevent the depletion of limited carbohydrate stores in the liver and muscles during exercise.

18.5.1.3 Increase in Muscle Capillarization

The moderate-intensity aerobic exercise training (45 min, 3 times/week, walking training for 24 weeks, at 70% of heart rate reserve) increases myofibrillar protein synthesis, capillarization, peak oxygen consumption, and quadriceps muscle strength. The enhanced capillarization is believed to improve exercise capacity by facilitating oxygen distribution, as well as promote adaptations in myofibrillar protein synthesis. The increase in skeletal muscle capillarization facilitates nutrient delivery and removal of waste products, increasing the ability to transport nutrients across the sarcolemma.

18.5.1.4 Changes in Energy Source Use

Plasma glucose is the main fuel for the nervous system. Therefore, maintaining its level is critical. Endurance training causes biochemical changes in skeletal muscles that help maintain blood glucose level during the prolonged submaximal exercise. Endurance training causes a decrease in glucose (carbohydrate) use as an energy source and an increase in fat metabolism during the prolonged submaximal exercise. Consequently, these changes preserve plasma glucose and increase the use of fat as an energy source in skeletal muscle during exercise.

The presence of a glucose transport protein (GLUT4) in the sarcolemma is required for the glucose uptake into skeletal muscles during contraction. Endurance exercise training increases the number of GLUT4 glucose transporters and the ability of insulin to transport glucose into the muscle, increasing the capacity to transport glucose to skeletal muscle. Thus, the dependence on carbohydrates as an energy source decreases during prolonged submaximal exercise. In trained individuals, glucose uptake and oxidation from the blood are reduced during submaximal exercise. As a result, trained individuals can better maintain their blood glucose levels during prolonged exercise.

The ability of the muscles to metabolize fat increases with exercise training. This increase occurs as a result of increased capillary density, which increases the delivery of free fatty acids to the muscles, and the increased ability of free fatty acids to be transported from the cytoplasm to the mitochondria and across the sarcolemma. The conversion of free fatty acids to acetyl coenzyme A by beta-oxidation in the Krebs cycle takes place in the mitochondria. The increase in the volume of mitochondria in the muscle fiber with exercise training also increases the ability of the muscle to metabolize fat. The increase in lipid oxidation and less need for carbohydrate metabolism during exercise ensure the preservation of muscle and liver glycogen stores.

18.5.1.5 Increase in Muscle Antioxidant Capacity

Free radicals are molecules that have an unpaired electron in their outer orbital. These molecules are highly reactive due to this unpaired electron. They can damage proteins, membranes, and DNA. Cells have a network of antioxidants that neutralize the radicals and protect against the radical-induced damage. Antioxidants can be divided into two groups produced in body cells (endogenous) and derived from the diet (exogenous). Free radicals are produced during muscle contraction, and radical production can disrupt cellular homeostasis. Free radicals can increase oxidative damage to muscle contraction proteins and cause muscle fatigue in situations requiring long-term endurance. Endurance training can increase the endogenous antioxidant levels in the muscles and protect the muscle fibers from radical-induced damage. The improvement in muscle antioxidant capacity neutralizes free radicals produced during exercise and preserves muscle fiber.

18.5.1.6 Maintenance of Acid-Base Balance

High-intensity interval training can increase the buffering capacity of the exercising muscles. Regular endurance training causes less change in blood pH level in submaximal exercise. This is because the muscles produce less lactate and H$^+$ with submaximal endurance training. Lactate is formed when there is an accumulation of NADH and pyruvate in the cytoplasm of cells with lactate dehydrogenase. Increasing the capacity of using fat as fuel reduces the need for carbohydrate oxidation. If less carbohydrates are used, less pyruvate is formed. Moreover, an increase in the number of mitochondria increases the uptake of pyruvate into the mitochondria for oxidation in the Krebs cycle, rather than being converted to lactate in the cytoplasm. NADH formed in glycolysis is transported more rapidly to the mitochondria as a result of endurance training, thus producing less lactate and H^+.

Muscle hypertrophy is another adaptation seen with endurance exercise training. In a study, 12 weeks of endurance training was shown to increase the muscle mass by 7–11%. These increases in muscle mass, which occur with endurance training, have been mostly observed in the quadriceps muscle. In the aforementioned study, exercise training was performed on a cycle ergometer by the individuals who do not exercise regularly or who are sedentary. It has been noted that the hypertrophy of the quadriceps muscle occurring with endurance training depends on the frequency and the intensity of exercise training. Studies comparing aerobic exercise modalities are needed to clarify the muscle hypertrophy associated with endurance training.

Research is ongoing to evaluate how aerobic exercises affect the function of muscle protein synthesis and satellite cells. The increase in mRNA and specific muscle protein synthesis with one exercise session has a cumulative effect on regularly repeated exercise. Accordingly, a gradual increase in specific muscle proteins occurs that improves muscle function with exercise training. Skeletal muscle stem cells, known as satellite cells as well, are thought to play a key role in the adaptive process to exercise. Resistive exercise training is associated with an increase in satellite cell content. However, the effects of aerobic exercise on the function of satellite cells are still unclear. It has been stated that the ability to modulate the function of satellite cells by increasing skeletal muscle capillarization and mitochondrial biogenesis with aerobic exercise training may be beneficial in improving skeletal muscle health in various muscle-wasting conditions such as aging. The effects of aerobic exercise on satellite cells need to be clarified.

Slow-twitch muscle fibers, which have a high capacity to produce ATP aerobically, contain high myoglobin content. Studies in animals show that the myoglobin content of the muscle is related to the level of physical activity. However, the effect of regular physical activity on myoglobin levels in humans remains unclear.

18.5.2 Aerobic Exercise and Tendon

Although many studies have been conducted on the effects of resistance exercise training on tendons, studies investigating the effects of endurance training on tendons are limited. It has been stated that increased muscle extracellular matrix-tendon unit stiffness with endurance training improves exercise performance. This results in an enhanced capacity to store and utilize elastic energy more efficiently. For instance, runners with a musculotendinous system that is longer and stiffer tend to have a lower oxygen uptake during submaximal running speeds.

Endurance athletes have been shown to have tendon stiffness similar to or higher than untrained individuals. It has been stated that although running training for 9 months in sedentary individuals provides cardiovascular improvements, it does not change the mechanical properties of the Achilles tendon. Evidence suggests that runners have a larger Achilles tendon cross-sectional area, more prominently near the insertion, compared with non-runners. The greater cross-sectional area distal to the tendon may result from site-specific hypertrophy in response to the habitual load of running. Considering that tendon hypertrophy in response to loading represents tension-bearing components, namely collagen fibrils, the larger cross-section means that stress is reduced across the tendon and may play an important role in injury prevention. These results are based on a large number of conflicting data. These conflicting results may be due to the differences in populations of the studies, tendon types and regions, and exercise protocols. More studies are needed to

18.5.3 Aerobic Exercise and Bone Tissue

As one of the most common forms of aerobic exercise, the effects of walking on bone mineral density have been broadly researched, despite that they are not always consistent across various studies. There is no evidence of a close relationship between increased bone mineral density and walking exercises. Walking as a stand-alone exercise did not have a significant effect on the mineral density of the bone in perimenopausal and postmenopausal women. However, walking exercise interventions lasting longer than 6 months have been reported to have positive effects on femoral neck bone mineral density in this population.

This type of exercise has proven less effective in preventing osteoporosis, as walking provides only a slight increase in the loads on the skeleton against gravity. Resistance exercise training, on the other hand, is seen as a strong stimulant to increase and maintain bone mass during the aging process. However, while combined resistance exercise protocols were effective in maintaining the bone mineral density of the femoral neck and lumbar spine in postmenopausal women, resistance protocols alone did not create a significant change. Multi-component exercise programs including resistance, aerobic, weight-bearing, and whole-body vibration training can increase bone mass or prevent its age-related decline.

18.6 Adaptation Mechanisms in Different Exercise Types

The muscle fiber type shifting with aerobic training is considered as a result of muscle plasticity. The increase in fat oxidation with aerobic training occurs with the increase in blood flow to the muscle, increase in the enzymes that metabolize fat, and increase in the mitochondrial capacity of the muscle. Increased fat catabolism in submaximal activity preserves glycogen reserves, which are important during prolonged intense exertion. Factors such as decreased muscle glycogen utilization, reduced glucose production (decreased hepatic glycogenolysis and gluconeogenesis), and plasma-derived glucose utilization contribute to reduced use of carbohydrate as a substrate and increased fat oxidation. Hepatic gluconeogenic capacity improved by exercise training provides greater resistance to hypoglycemia during prolonged activity.

There is no clarity about the mechanisms for the responses of skeletal muscle to different types of exercise. It is known that primary signals play a role in exercise-induced adaptation in skeletal muscle. These primary signals are mechanical stimuli, an increase in cellular calcium, an increase in free radicals, and a decrease in muscle phosphate/energy levels.

18.6.1 Primary Signals

Mechanical stimuli trigger signaling processes to promote adaptation in resistance exercise training. Passive stretching of a muscle fiber results in activation of a mechanoreceptor that stimulates biochemical signaling in the sarcolemma and induces an increase in contractile protein synthesis. Mechanical load-induced signaling events with resistive exercise play an important role in exercise induced-muscle fiber adaptation. This indicates that muscle fibers can detect differences in the intensity and duration of mechanical stimuli (i.e., resistance versus endurance exercise). In particular, mechanical stretching along the sarcolemma with resistance exercise training is the primary signal that promotes contractile protein synthesis and causes muscle hypertrophy.

Calcium has an important role in cell signaling mechanism. Free calcium in the cytoplasm has the ability to activate many enzymes and other signaling molecules that support protein synthesis. The increase in cytosolic calcium activates an important kinase called calmodulin-dependent protein kinase (CaMK). The calmodulin-dependent kinase is an enzyme that promotes the phosphorylation of various protein substrates. The level of free calcium in the sarcoplasm is determined by the type and intensity of exercise. Long-term endurance exercises cause high calcium levels in the sarcoplasm for a long time, while resistance exercise causes high cytosolic calcium levels for a short time. These differences in cytosolic calcium levels according to exercise types determine calcium-mediated signaling events that lead to the synthesis of specific muscle proteins.

Exercise causes the free radicals and oxidants production in active skeletal muscles. During exercise, signals are activated that promote the expression of various muscle proteins, including antioxidant enzymes, which protect the muscle against exercise-induced oxidative stress by the generation of free radicals.

Primary signals (calcium release, increased adenosine monophosphate (AMP)/ATP ratio, and free radical production) are responsible for the activation of secondary signaling events.

18.6.2 Secondary Signals

Secondary signals are 5′ AMP activating protein kinase (AMPK), mitogen activated protein kinase p38 (p38), peroxisome proliferator activated receptor-gamma coactivator 1α (PGC-1α), CaMK, calcineurin, and nuclear factor kappa B (NFκB). These secondary signals give rise to mitochondrial biogenesis, fiber type shifting, and increased expression of antioxidant enzymes.

Exercise accelerates ATP consumption in exercising muscles and increases the AMP/ATP ratio in muscle fibers. This change causes the activation of AMPK, which plays an important role in adaptation. AMPK is a signaling molecule activated by high-intensity interval and prolonged endurance exercise. During exercise, it regulates multiple energy production pathways by the stimulation of glucose uptake and the fatty acid oxidation.

During endurance exercise, a signal molecule called mitogen-activated protein kinase p38 (p38) in muscle fibers is activated. p38 activates receptor-gamma coactivator 1α (PGC-1α), which is responsible for regulating mitochondrial biogenesis. Both high-intensity interval training and submaximal endurance exercise activate PGC-1α. PGC-1α regulates several changes induced by endurance exercise in skeletal muscle, such as new capillary formation (angiogenesis), fast to slow muscle fiber type shift, and synthesis of antioxidant enzymes. Activation of AMPK, CaMK, and p38 supports mitochondrial biogenesis through activation of PGC-1α. Additionally, increases in cytosolic calcium activate calcineurin, leading to a shift from fast to slow muscle fiber type.

The increase in free radicals activates p38 and NFκB. Activated NFκB induces the expression of several antioxidant enzymes protecting against damage.

Until this part, adaptation mechanisms to endurance training have been mentioned. There are differences in adaptation mechanisms to resistance exercise training. Factors such as motor unit firing, stimulus frequency, muscle tension, and type II motor units creating more tension than type I motor units play a role in increasing strength with resistant exercise training. That is, resistance exercise training increases muscle strength with changes in the nervous system and increases muscle mass. Resistance exercise training increases the synthesis of contractile proteins in the muscle. This causes an increase in the cross-sectional area of the fiber. The increase in protein synthesis with resistance exercise training is controlled by the mammalian target of the rapamycin (mTOR) signal pathway. mTOR is a protein kinase described as the master regulator of protein synthesis and muscle size. A secondary signaling molecule mTOR is involved in adaptation of muscle to resistance exercise training, activated by the stimulation of mechanoreceptor on the sarcolemma.

Satellite cells are a source of myonuclei (muscle fiber nuclei) in muscle fibers. In a muscle fiber, the number of myonuclei could be increased as a result of the fusion of the satellite cell with the muscle fiber. Resistance exercise training results in increases in muscle fiber cross-sectional area and the number of myonuclei. Hypertrophy occurs as a result of increase in the myonuclei number in fibers in response to resistance exercise training.

The health benefits of exercise in the prevention and treatment of many system related-pathologies are widely recognized. However, the complexity of molecular networks and biological mechanisms for exercise adaptation and the resulting health benefits are not fully understood. The implementation of "-omics" technologies to exercise may facilitate understanding the complexity of biological networks underlying the systemic health benefits of exercise. Omics-based themes (genome/epigenome, transcriptome, proteome, secretome, phosphoproteome, acetylome, metabolome, and lipidome) have been identified to map various aspects of exercise biological networks and explore responses and adaptations to exercise in health and disease. Future research using these omic-based technologies may help to better understand exercise-related mechanisms.

18.7 Factors Affecting Adaptation to Exercise

The adaptation to exercise is influenced by various factors, including the individual's initial level of physical fitness, as well as the type, intensity, duration, and frequency of the exercise. Physiological changes and increases in performance capacity that occur with exercise are higher in individuals with lower initial fitness level than in individuals with higher fitness level. Studies indicate that with an identical exercise regimen, sedentary middle-aged men with heart disease experience a 50% increase in maximal oxygen consumption, whereas active healthy adults only experience a 10–15% increase. Nevertheless, even a small improvement in aerobic capacity, such as 1–2%, can be significant for an athlete. Typically, endurance training can result in a 5–25% improvement in aerobic capacity, with some of the gains occurring within the first week of training.

Exercise intensity is the most important factor affecting adaptation to exercise. As a practical approach to determine the appropriate intensity of aerobic exercise, percentages of maximum heart rate are used. Training at levels between 60 and 90% of maximum heart rate can lead to substantial improvements in aerobic capacity.

The adaptation to exercise is affected by the duration and intensity of the activity, which interact with one another. While there is no definitive time threshold for achieving the optimal increase in aerobic capacity, any potential threshold is contingent on various factors such as the total workload, intensity, frequency of exercise, and initial fitness level. Evidence suggests that increasing exercise duration may not always lead to greater improvements, especially among physically active individuals.

The impact of altering exercise frequency while maintaining constant duration and intensity remains uncertain. Some research suggests that changes in exercise frequency can influence cardiovascular improvements, while others propose that the effects of frequency are not as significant as those of intensity or duration. Research has indicated that the changes in maximal oxygen consumption were similar when high-intensity interval exercise training was performed twice a week versus five times a week.

Responses to exercise training due to the principle of specialization vary significantly depending on the type of exercise training and testing. Besides, specialization refers to the types of adaptations that occur in the muscle as a result of training. Endurance exercise training gives rise to the primary adaptations such as capillaries and mitochondria volume increase, while the primary adaptation to resistance training is an increase in the number of contractile proteins.

Genetics is an important determinant of individuals' adaptive responses to exercise. There is great variation among people in increasing oxygen consumption in response to training. An average of 15–20% increase in oxygen consumption with exercise training is classified as low responders, and those with 50% are classified as high responders. These differences in response to exercise training indicate that genetics plays a large role in training adaptation. It has been noted that this large variation in adaptive responses to exercise is due to genes that are major players in adaptation to exercise training.

18.8 Possible Complications During/After Exercise in Musculoskeletal Pathologies and Their Management

Musculoskeletal diseases constitute a remarkable reason for a worldwide disability and morbidity, with significant costs to health and social care. Common musculoskeletal diseases include back pain, fibromyalgia, gout, osteoarthritis, tendinitis, and rheumatoid arthritis. These diseases result in pain and functional inability that affect quality of life and productivity. The management of musculoskeletal disorders should begin with appropriate and comprehensive pain management.

It is known that exercise reduces pain and improves function in musculoskeletal diseases. However, poorly planned exercise programs can cause acute or chronic muscle, tendon, and ligament injuries, traumatic fractures, and other injuries. Eccentric contractions, non-specific exercises, and multiple strenuous exercise sessions cause temporary muscle damage and lead to delayed onset muscle soreness (DOMS). Symptoms usually appear within 24–72 h. These are often in the form of pain, restriction of movement, stiffness, swelling, and intramuscular edema. Therapeutic modalities such as thermal therapies, compression during/after exercise, intermittent compression, active recovery, low-intensity exercise, flexibility exercises, whole-body vibration, and massage can be used to prevent or reduce DOMS symptoms.

Performing excessive and non-specific exercises and a poorly planned exercise program can lead to overtraining/overtraining syndrome. This situation, which could be seen frequently in athletes, is generally defined as the deterioration of the balance between training and rest. This causes chronic fatigue during exercise and recovery. Related symptoms cover poor exercise performance, frequent infections, fatigue, acute and chronic changes in systemic inflammatory responses, mood disorders, and general malaise.

It is crucial to design personalized exercise programs to avoid potential complications that may arise during and after exercise in individuals with musculoskeletal pathologies. Therefore, the increases of the workload should be done in a planned, systematic, and gradual manner, with adequate rest intervals.

18.9 Comparison of the Adaptation Mechanism of the Musculoskeletal System to Exercise: A Healthy Individual and a Patient with Fibromyalgia

Clinical Inference from the Cases: Suggestions and Don'ts When Planning Exercise Training

The comparison of the adaptation mechanism of the musculoskeletal system to exercise in patient with fibromyalgia and healthy individual is given in Table 18.1.

In fibromyalgia, symptoms of pain and fatigue may fluctuate daily, and there may be variability in the patient's participation in exercise. This can directly affect progress and the intensity and type of exercise that can be tolerated. Exercise testing and training should be personalized to minimize or prevent pain and fatigue and improve their physical performance. In addition, protocols should be progressed in slow increments in order not to cause an increase in pain, eccentric exercises should be limited, and strength training should be planned with one-day intervals and rest between repetitions.

Table 18.1 Comparison of responses to exercise in healthy individuals and patients with fibromyalgia

Case 1. Healthy individual	Case 2. Patient with fibromyalgia
35 years old K.C. (Male) is 1.80 m tall and weighs 88 kg. He works in a bank K.C. consults a physiotherapist to improve her physical fitness. He states that he does not perform exercise regularly for the last 3 years. He does not have any diagnosed disease and does not smoke	48 years old S.N. (Female), 1.58 m and 72 kg, is a teacher. She was recently diagnosed with fibromyalgia. She does not smoke. and had been walking regularly every day until the last year, has been living a sedentary life for the last 1 year due to chronic, widespread pain in his trunk and extremities. She gained 5 kg in the last year due to inactivity and overeating.
Evaluation of cases	
Case 1	**Case 2**
Medical history Family history Evaluation of body composition Joint range of motion assessment Assessment of muscle strength and endurance Assessment of cardiorespiratory fitness Pain assessment Fatigue, sleep quality, and anxiety assessment	Medical history Family history Evaluation of body composition Joint range of motion assessment Evaluation of muscle strength and endurance Evaluation of cardiorespiratory fitness Pain and trigger point assessment Fatigue, sleep quality, and anxiety assessment
Treatment program	
Case 1	**Case 2**
Aerobic exercise training ≥5 days/week—moderate-intensity exercise or ≥3 days/week—vigorous exercise or ≥3–5 days/week—a combination of moderate and vigorous exercise If moderate: ≥30 min/day, 150 min/week If vigorous exercise: ≥ 20 min/day, 75 min/week **Strength training** Moderate to vigorous, 2–4 sets, 8–12 reps, 2–3 days (non-consecutive)/week **Flexibility exercises** Static stretching 10–30 s, 2–4 reps, 2–3 days/week	**Aerobic exercise training** Light to moderate exercise 20–30 min, 3 days/week Aerobic, weight-bearing exercises (e.g., aqua therapy, cycling, walking, swimming) are recommended to reduce pain **Strength training** 40–80% of one max rep 1–3 sets, 5–20 reps, 2–3 days/week A personalized approach to rest between sets and exercises is recommended based on tolerance **Flexibility exercises** In a painless range, 10–30 s, 2–4 reps, 2–3 days/week
Musculoskeletal system adaptation to exercise	
Case 1. Healthy individual	**Case 2. Patient with fibromyalgia**
Acute response to aerobic exercise	
↑ In temporary amounts of certain mRNAs for the synthesis of specific muscle proteins	There are different results in studies comparing the pain response to acute aerobic exercise between individuals with fibromyalgia with healthy individuals
Chronic response to aerobic exercise	
↓ Fast amount of myosin ↑ Slow myosin isoforms ↑ Capillary density ↑ Mitochondrial density ↑ Mitochondria volume ↑ Lipid oxidation as an energy source ↓ Need for carbohydrate metabolism ↑ Antioxidant capacity of muscle ↑ Buffering capacity of the muscle Acute response to strength exercise training	↑ Health-related quality of life ↓ Pain intensity ↑ Physical function ↓ Fatigue ↓ Stiffness

(continued)

Table 18.1 (continued)

A single-session resistance exercise increases muscle protein synthesis by 50–150% within 1–4 h after exercise in both trained and non-trained individuals. This increase in protein synthesis, which occurs with exercise, remains high for 30–48 h, depending on the training status of the individuals. Post-exercise protein synthesis remains elevated for longer in non-trained subjects than in trained subjects. This explains why exercise-induced muscle hypertrophy occurs more rapidly in non-trained subjects than in trained subjects	Studies investigating the acute responses to a single-session resistance exercise in fibromyalgia are needed
Chronic response to strength exercise training	
↑ Muscle strength ↑ Muscle mass ↑ Increase in muscle fiber size (More in type II muscle fiber size than type I ↑) ↑ Muscle cross-sectional area (mostly in type II fibers) ↑ Sarcoplasmic reticulum and T-tubule volume ↑ Pennation angle and fascicle length ↓↔ Capillary density ↓↔ Mitochondrial density ↑ Number of mitochondria ↑ ATP, creation phosphate and glycogen stores ↓ Myoglobin ↑ Buffering capacity ↑ Bone mineral density ↑ Tendon and ligament cross-sectional area ↑ Collagen synthesis ↑ Tendon stiffness	↓ Pain ↓ Fatigue ↓ Number of trigger points ↓ Depression and anxiety ↑ Functional capacity ↑ Quality of life

18.10 Conclusion

To conclude, resistance exercise training increases the muscle mass and muscle fiber cross-sectional area, neural adaptations, and maximum force production, while endurance exercise training improves muscle mitochondrial biogenesis, energy source selection, and resistance to fatigue. Primary signals such as mechanical stimuli, increase in cellular calcium and free radicals, and decrease in muscle phosphate/energy levels and secondary signals activated by primary signals play a role in exercise-induced adaptations in skeletal muscle. The adaptation to exercise is influenced by various factors, including the individual's initial level of fitness as well as the type, intensity, duration, and frequency of the exercise. It is critical to design personalized exercise programs to minimize the risk of complications that may arise during and after exercise in individuals with musculoskeletal pathologies. The increases in the workload should be done gradually and adequate rest intervals should be ensured.

Further Reading

American College of Sports Medicine. Preliminary section: background materials functional anatomy. In: Swain DP, Brawner CA, Chambliss HO, Nagelkirk PR, Paternostro-Bayles M, Swank AM, editors. ACSM's resource manual for guidelines for exercise testing and prescription, 7th ed. Philadelphia: Wolters Kluwer Health/Lippincott Williams & Wilkins; 2014a. p. 2–31. isbn:978-1609139568.

American College of Sports Medicine. Adaptations to resistance training. In: Swain DP, Brawner CA, Chambliss HO, Nagelkirk PR, Paternostro-Bayles M, Swank AM, editors. ACSM's resource manual for guidelines for exercise testing and prescription, 7th ed. Philadelphia: Wolters Kluwer Health/Lippincott Williams & Wilkins; 2014b. p. 511–32. isbn:978-1609139568.

American College of Sports Medicine. Special considerations for chronic pain. In: Bayles MP, Swank AM, editors. ACSM's exercise testing and prescription. Philadelphia: Wolters Kluwer; 2018. isbn:9781496338792.

Andrade A, de Azevedo Klumb Steffens R, Sieczkowska SM, Peyré Tartaruga LA, Torres Vilarino G. A systematic review of the effects of strength training in patients with fibromyalgia: clinical outcomes and design considerations. Adv Rheumatol. 2018;58(1):36.

Benedetti MG, Furlini G, Zati A, Mauro GL. The effectiveness of physical exercise on bone density in osteoporotic patients. Biomed Res Int. 2018;2018:4840531.

Bidonde J, Busch AJ, Schachter CL, Overend TJ, Kim SY, Góes SM, Boden C, Foulds HJ. Aerobic exercise training for adults with fibromyalgia. Cochrane Database Syst Rev. 2017;6(6):CD012700.

Brightwell CR, Markofski MM, Moro T, Fry CS, Porter C, Volpi E, Rasmussen BB. Moderate-intensity aerobic exercise improves skeletal muscle quality in older adults. Transl Sports Med. 2019;2(3):109–19.

Frontera WR, Ochala J. Skeletal muscle: a brief review of structure and function. Calcif Tissue Int. 2015;96(3):183–95.

Fukutani A, Herzog W. Current understanding of residual force enhancement: cross-bridge component and non-cross-bridge component. Int J Mol Sci. 2019;20(21):5479.

Heiss R, Lutter C, Freiwald J, Hoppe MW, Grim C, Poettgen K, Forst R, Bloch W, Hüttel M, Hotfiel T. Advances in delayed-onset muscle soreness (DOMS)—part II: treatment and prevention. Sportverletz Sportschaden. 2019;33(1):21–9.

Hessel AL, Lindstedt SL, Nishikawa KC. Physiological mechanisms of eccentric contraction and its applications: a role for the giant titin protein. Front Physiol. 2017;8:70.

Hoffman NJ. Omics and exercise: global approaches for mapping exercise biological networks. Cold Spring Harb Perspect Med. 2017;7(10):a029884.

Hughes DC, Ellefsen S, Baar K. Adaptations to endurance and strength training. Cold Spring Harb Perspect Med. 2018;8(6):a029769.

Joanisse S, Snijders T, Nederveen JP, Parise G. The impact of aerobic exercise on the muscle stem cell response. Exerc Sport Sci Rev. 2018;46(3):180–7.

Lemmey AB. Part VI—Disorders of the bones and joints. In: Ehrman JK, Gordon PM, Visich, PS, Keteyian SJ, editors. Clinical exercise physiology, 4th ed. Human kinetics; 2019. p. 817–72, isbn:9781492546467 (e-book), isbn:9781492546450 (print).

Lewis R, Gómez Álvarez CB, Rayman M, Lanham-New S, Woolf A, Mobasheri A. Strategies for optimising musculoskeletal health in the 21st century. BMC Musculoskelet Disord. 2019;20(1):164.

Montesano P, Palermi S, Massa B, Mazzeo F. From "sliding" to "winding" filaments theory: a narrative review of mechanisms behind skeletal muscle contraction. J Hum Sport Exerc. 2020;15(3proc):S806–14.

Nazmi N, Abdul Rahman MA, Yamamoto S, Ahmad SA, Zamzuri H, Mazlan SA. A review of classification techniques of EMG signals during isotonic and isometric contractions. Sensors (Basel). 2016;16(8):1304.

Nishikawa K. Eccentric contraction: unraveling mechanisms of force enhancement and energy conservation. J Exp Biol. 2016;219(Pt 2):189–96.

Powers SK, Howley ET. Skeletal muscle: structure and function. In: Powers SK, Howley ET, editors. Exercise physiology: theory and application to fitness and performance, 10th ed. McGraw-Hill Education; 2018a. p. 166–92, isbn:9781259870453.

Powers SK, Howley ET. The physiology of training: effect on VO_2 max, performance, and strength. In: Powers SK, Howley ET, editors. Exercise physiology: theory and application to fitness and performance, 10th ed. McGraw-Hill Education; 2018b. p. 293–328. isbn:9781259870453.

Rice D, Nijs J, Kosek E, Wideman T, Hasenbring MI, Koltyn K, Graven-Nielsen T, Polli A. Exercise-induced hypoalgesia in pain-free and chronic pain populations: state of the art and future directions. J Pain. 2019;20(11):1249–66.

Saltin B. Training for anaerobic and aerobic power. In: McArdle WD, Katch FI, Katch VL, editors. Exercise physiology energy, nutrition & human performance, 8th international ed. Wolters Kluwer Health/Lippincott Williams & Wilkins; 2015. p. 461–98. isbn:9781469895246.

Snijders T, Nederveen JP, McKay BR, Joanisse S, Verdijk LB, van Loon LJ, Parise G. Satellite cells in human skeletal muscle plasticity. Front Physiol. 2015;6:283.

Svensson RB, Heinemeier KM, Couppé C, Kjaer M, Magnusson SP. Effect of aging and exercise on the tendon. J Appl Physiol (1985). 2016;121(6):1237–46.

Neural System and Its Adaptation to Exercise

19

Cevher Demirci and Saniye Aydogan Arslan

Abstract

Neural adaptation is the improvements in coordination and learning allowing the involvement and deactivation of relevant muscles during a forceful task. It occurs at the level of the motor cortex, spinal cord, and/or neuromuscular junction following exercise and varies at significant levels with different exercise training. It is already known that the rapid increase in muscle strength, before the development of hypertrophy in the muscle with exercise, is mainly associated with neural adaptations. Optimizing motor control is the focus of many training and rehabilitation programs. Therefore, understanding how neural adaptations occur and their relationship with functional development is crucial for planning exercise programs. Studies investigating the response to exercise in neural system pathologies are insufficient in the literature. To plan an individualized and functional exercise program, it is necessary to know these effects in healthy individuals as well as in patients.

C. Demirci (✉)
Physiotherapy and Rehabilitation, Faculty of Health Sciences, Balikesir University, Balikesir, Turkey
e-mail: cevher.demirci@balikesir.edu.tr

S. Aydogan Arslan
Physiotherapy and Rehabilitation, Faculty of Health Sciences, Kirikkale University, Kirikkale, Turkey
e-mail: saniyearslan@kku.edu.tr

19.1 Introduction

A movement with controlled force can be defined as an activity that requires skill and emerges with the maximum activation of the agonist muscles, minimum activation of the antagonists, and appropriate activation of the synergist and stabilizer muscles. Neural adaptation, on the other hand, is the whole of the changes in the neural system ensuring that the primary muscles are fully activated in specific movements, the activation of the associated muscles is coordinated, and a net force is released in the intended direction of movement. In other words, they are improvements in coordination and learning allowing the involvement and deactivation of relevant muscles during a forceful task.

Neural adaptations occur at the level of the motor cortex, spinal cord, and/or neuromuscular junction following exercise. It is already known that the increase in muscle strength, before the development of hypertrophy in the muscle with exercise, occurs because of neural adaptations. This rapid increase in muscle strength is mainly associated with the increased ability to mobilize the muscles. Although there are studies conducted on neural system adaptations after exercising in the literature, studies investigating the response to exercise in neural system pathologies are insufficient. To plan an individualized and functional exercise program, it is necessary to know these effects in healthy individuals as well as in patients. Understanding how neural adaptations occur and their relationship with functional development is crucial for planning exercise programs because optimizing motor control is the focus of many training and rehabilitation programs. In this section, the anatomy and physiology of the neural system, the adaptations of the neural system to different exercise types, and the factors affecting these adaptations will be explained briefly.

19.2 Anatomy

The nervous system is responsible for perceiving the events in the internal and external environment and for the responses to these events. Receptors perceiving touch, pain, temperature changes, and chemical stimuli send information to the central nervous system (CNS) about the changes in the environment, and the CNS creates an appropriate response to these stimuli. In addition to the adaptation of body activities and control of voluntary movement, the nervous system is responsible for storing experiences (i.e., memory) and forming responses based on previous experiences (i.e., learning). The nervous system is divided into the CNS and the Peripheral Nervous System (PNS).

The CNS consists of the brain and spinal cord, and the brain consists of the cerebrum, cerebellum, and brain stem.

The cerebrum is divided into right and left cerebral hemispheres and its outermost layer is called the cerebral cortex and contains more than eight million neurons. The surface of the cerebral cortex is covered with many indentations and protrusions in humans. The function of the cerebrum is the organization of complex movements, storage of experiences in memory, and the perception of sensory information. The part of the cortex dealing with voluntary movements is called the motor cortex. Although the motor cortex plays an important role in motor control, input from subcortical structures to the motor cortex is also very important for coordinated movements. After the motor cortex collects inputs, the movement is changed and the motor command is sent to the spinal cord. The fine details of this movement can be modified by the subcortical and spinal centers.

The cerebellum is located behind the pons and medulla. The cerebellum is responsible for the coordination of complex movements with connections to the motor cortex, the brain stem, and the spinal cord as well as for maintaining balance, controlling muscle tone, and walking.

The brain stem consists of a complex series of nerve pathways and nuclei (i.e., clusters of neurons) and is responsible for many metabolic functions, cardiorespiratory control, and some complex reflexes. In anatomical terms, it consists of the medulla, pons, and midbrain. Another important structure in the brain stem is **reticular formation**. In this structure, neurotransmitters providing communication and signal transfer among neurons are secreted in the neurons. The reticular formation receives and harmonizes information from all regions of the CNS, working with the upper centers to control muscle activity. Also, there are interneurons between the sensory and motor pathways in the CNS. The tasks of interneurons are processing, storing, and verifying information.

The spinal cord makes a great contribution to the control of any movement to achieve it in the desired manner. Although the upper centers of the motor system deal only with general movement variables, the details of movement are regulated by the interaction of neurons and upper centers in the spinal cord, which acts as a center for spinal reflexes.

The PNS is the part of the nervous system consisting of the nerves outside the CNS. PNS consists of two parts, sensory and motor. The sensory part is responsible for transmitting the stimuli from the sensory receptors to the CNS. These sensory nerve fibers transmitting information to the CNS are called **afferent fibers**. The motor part, on the other hand, is divided into the somatic motor part, which stimulates the skeletal muscles, and the autonomic motor part, which stimulates the smooth muscles surrounding the blood vessels, heart muscle, and effector organs surrounding the glands. Motor nerve fibers transmitting impulses from the CNS are

Fig. 19.1 The structure of the neural system

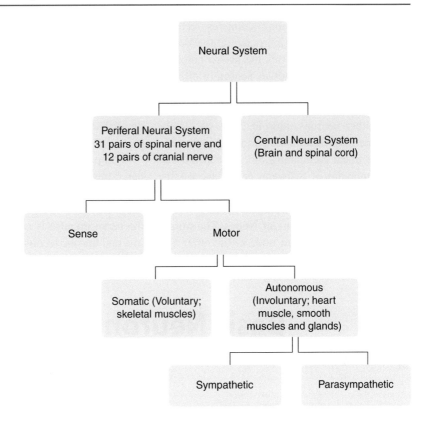

called **efferent fibers**. The structure of the nervous system is shown in Fig. 19.1.

19.3 Physiology

Neurons are the basic cells of the nervous system and are responsible for transmitting and evaluating information. Other cellular elements are glial cells, which are cells that maintain homeostasis, form myelin, and provide support and protection for neurons in the CNS and PNS. Glial cells do not have stimulability. Glial cells in the CNS consist of astrocytes, oligodendrocytes, microglia, and ependymal cells. Astrocytes are responsible for the nutrition of neurons and the formation of the blood-brain barrier. Oligodendrocytes undertake the construction of the myelin sheath around the axons in the CNS. Microglia cells develop from macrophages and clean dead cells by phagocytosis in inflammatory and degenerative lesions of the CNS. Ependymal cells make up the walls of the ventricle and the epithelial layer in the *canalis centralis* and take part in the production of Cerebrospinal Fluid (CSF). The glial cells in the PNS are Schwann cells and satellite cells. Schwann cells are similar to oligodendrocytes and microglia cells in function and provide the myelination to axons in the PNS. They also have phagocytosis characteristics allowing the neurons in the PNS to regrow. Satellite cells are skeletal muscle-specific stem cells between the sarcolemma and endomysium, providing structural support to the neuron within the ganglion. They are also highly susceptible to injury and inflammation and are responsible for the regeneration of the injured muscle.

In anatomical terms, neurons consist of three main parts; cell body, dendrites, and axon. The cell body is the main biosynthetic center of the neuron and contains the neurotransmitters and other organelles necessary to synthesize proteins and chemicals. The neuron body communities in the CNS are called nuclei, and the neuron body communities in the PNS are called ganglions.

Dendrites are extensions acting as receptor sites transmitting the action potential toward the cell body. The axon carries the action potential from the cell body to another neuron or effector organ. Each neuron has only one axon. However, the axon can give off several side branches ending in other neurons, muscle cells, or glands. Axons are covered with a layer of Schwann cells in nerve fibers stimulating the skeletal muscle. The membranes of Schwann cells have a large amount of lipid-protein substance called myelin. The myelin sheath is interrupted every 1–3 mm, which are called the **Ranvier Nodes**. The stimuli are transmitted from one node to the other in a jumping fashion in myelinated nerves. The myelin sheath also insulates the axon from the surrounding tissues speeding up conduction in the nerve. Any damage to myelin causes dysfunction in the nervous system.

Neuron Types: There are different neuron types in the nervous system, which can be classified according to different variables. Neurons are divided into four according to their extensions (Fig. 19.2).

Synapses are connections through which nerve impulses are transmitted from one neuron to the other. There are two types of synapses, chemical and electrical. The neuron transmitting the nerve impulse is called the presynaptic neuron, and the one receiving it is called the postsynaptic neuron. Almost all of the synapses transmitting signals in the nervous system are

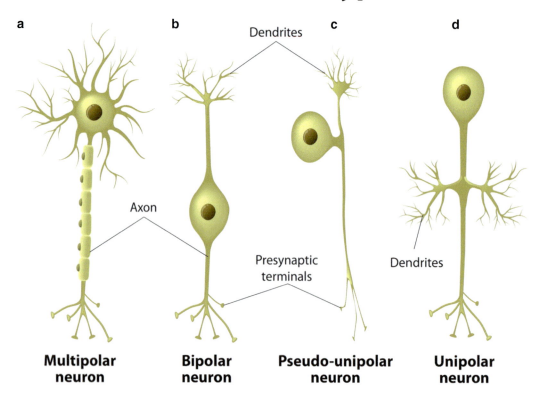

Fig. 19.2 Neuron Types: (**a**) **Multipolar neuron:** it has more than two extensions, dendrite being many, axon is one; (**b**) **Bipolar neuron:** two extensions emerge from the trunk, one acting as a dendrite, and one as an axon; (**c**) **Pseudo-unipolar neuron:** one single extension emerges from the neuron trunk. However, this extension is then divided into two "T" shapes; (**d**) **Unipolar neuron:** one single extension emerges from the trunk (Designua/Shutterstock.com)

chemical synapses. A neuron releases a neurotransmitter that binds to chemical receptors on the target neuron. The combination of neurotransmitter and receptor characteristics brings a change in the membrane permeability with an excitatory, inhibitory, or regulatory effect on the target neuron. For example, the two most common neurotransmitters in the brain (released by 90% of neurons), Glutamate and Gamma-Aminobutyric Acid (GABA), have opposing effects. Glutamate has a highly stimulating effect on the receptors, and the effect of GABA is inhibitory. Other neuron types include excitatory motor neurons releasing Acetylcholine (Ach) and inhibitory spinal neurons releasing glycine in the spinal cord. Synapses are dynamic structures and might show plasticity. New synaptic connections may be formed or unused connections may be removed depending on the requirement of the CNS.

19.3.1 Electrical Activity in Neurons

Neurons are electrically excitable cells with two main functional characteristics as irritability and conductivity. Irritability is the ability of the dendrites and/or neuron cell trunk to respond to a stimulus by converting it into a neural stimulus. Conductivity, on the other hand, refers to the transmission of the stimulus throughout the axon.

19.3.2 Parts of the Action Potential

Polarization: The neuron's plasma membrane is in a polarized state at rest, which means that there are fewer positive ions inside the neuron's plasma membrane than outside. The neuron will remain passive as long as the inside of the membrane is more negative than the outside.

  Depolarization: In the intracellular fluid, there is a high concentration of Potassium (K+) ions, other anions, and low concentrations of Sodium (Na+) and Chlorine (Cl) ions. The equilibrium potential of the membrane is −70 mV. Depolarization takes place when the axon membrane is stimulated. In this way, the Na+ permeability in the membrane increases,

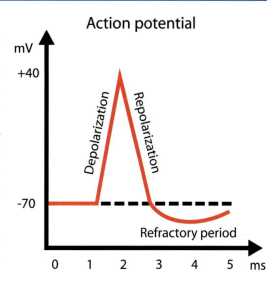

Fig. 19.3 Repolarization: For the cell to be re-stimulated, the membrane potential must return to the resting potential ion distributions. The Na+ ions entering the cell are pumped out with the Na/K pump, and the K+ ions coming out of the cell are pumped in. The makes the nerve cell ready for impulse transmission again. Another impulse above the threshold cannot generate an impulse in the axon within a short time following a nerve impulse. This short period is called the "Absolute Refractory Period" after which action potentials occur only in suprathreshold stimuli. This period is called the "Relative Refractory Period" (Anya Ku/Shutterstock.com)

Na+ is balanced, and the action potential reveals itself, which spreads along with the nerve fiber. The lowest stimulus intensity causing a stimulus to occur in a neuron is called the threshold. When the neuron responds with full strength to stimuli at and above the threshold value but does not respond at all to stimuli below the threshold value, it is called the All-or-None Law. The action potential sections are given in Fig. 19.3.

19.4 Acute Response of the Neural System to Aerobic Exercise

Firstly, some measurements that will be repeated frequently in this section will be briefly mentioned to understand how the neural system adapts to exercise. Electromyographic activity (EMG) is an outcome measure that is employed to evaluate neuromuscular fatigue and adaptations to exercise and is applied by placing electrodes on the relevant muscles to measure the electrical activity (i.e., the sum of action potentials) in the muscles. The increased amplitude of the superficial EMG signals is interpreted as increased efferent motor output from the cortical motor areas. Supramaximal stimulation of the motor nerve shows the compound muscle action potential, in other words, the M-wave, which indicates intramuscular sarcolemmal spread in EMG studies. This recorded motor response provides information on the bioelectrical state of motor axons, neuromuscular junctions, and muscle fibers. Motoneuronal stimulability can be evaluated through the submaximal stimulation of the motor nerve in a relaxed or slightly contracted muscle. The resulting response is called the Hoffmann Reflex (H-Reflex), which can be used to evaluate the stimulability of the spinal alpha-motor neurons and the efficacy of Ia-afferents. However, its use is limited to certain muscles (i.e., soleus, flexor carpi radialis) limiting its interpretation as a technique for measuring motor neuron stimulability because the magnitude of the response is affected by the level of presynaptic inhibition.

Voluntary activation (VA) is the gold standard for evaluating the development of central drive and central fatigue. A stimulus is given to the peripheral nerve or muscle and the resulting contraction response is evaluated during Maximal Voluntary Contraction (MVC). This response provides the simultaneous firing of all motor units in the muscle and enables the clinician to obtain information on the muscular strength. The evaluation of VA with this method gives an idea about central fatigue, and evaluation with Transcranial Magnetic Stimulation (TMS) gives an idea about supraspinal fatigue.

TMS is used to evaluate the cortical (Motor Cortex: M1) stimulability. The magnetic field that is generated by TMS activates the axons of corticospinal and intracortical neurons in the motor cortex. This firing stimulates the alpha motor neuron and Motor Evoked Potential (MEP) emerges. Its size shows the measure of corticospinal stimulability. Silent Period (SP), which is a parameter triggered by TMS, is widely accepted as an indicator of intracortical inhibition.

The V-wave is a measure reflecting the degree of overall efferent motor output from the alpha motor neuron pool. The increased V-wave amplitude following resistance exercise training show increased efferent excitation and increased activation of the motor neuron pool. These increases in motor neuron activation, especially the V-wave changes and the parallel H-Reflex, are characterized as an adaptation at the supraspinal level. Also, the firing rate of motor neurons is affected by the efficiency of the synaptic transmission between motor neurons and group Ia afferents, and by the sensitivity of motor neurons. The methods used to evaluate neural system adaptations are summarized in Fig. 19.4.

19.4.1 Acute Response of the Peripheral Nervous System to Aerobic Exercise

The adaptation of the nervous system to exercise and the mechanisms in this process has been the subjects of studies in recent years. However, most of these studies conducted on this subject have focused on strength training rather than aerobic training. When the literature was reviewed, it was found that although there were not many studies investigating the acute response of the neural system to aerobic exercise, current studies focused on central fatigue occurring especially after an exercise session that involves running or cycling. The knee extensor and plantar flexor muscles, which are more active during cycling and running, were evaluated in these studies and it was emphasized that as the exercise time increased, supraspinal fatigue also increased, and supraspinal fatigue reached 16% levels in exercises that lasted more than 13 h. It was also suggested that there is a decreased motor neuron stimulability, which is characterized by a reduction, in the magnitude of V-wave and H-Reflex responses. The type of aerobic activity is an effective factor in central fatigue, and it is considered that when activities that put less mechanical stress on the muscles are selected, they will cause less fatigue.

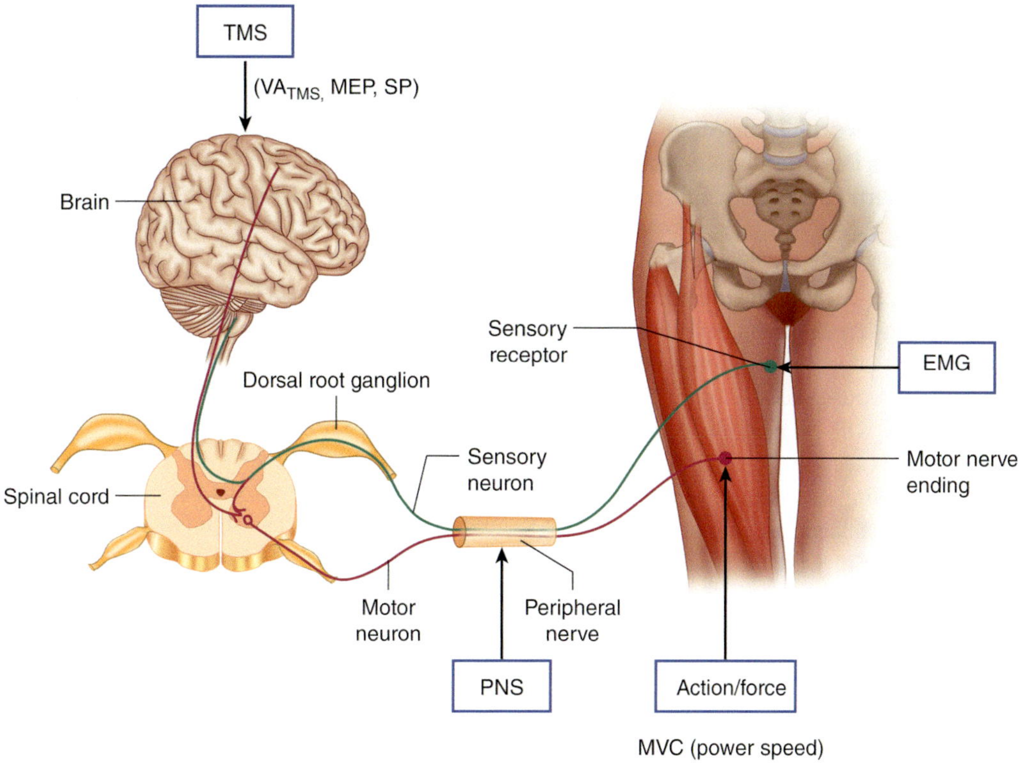

Fig. 19.4 The methods employed in the evaluation of neural system adaptations. *EMG* Electromyography, *TMS* Transcranial Magnetic Stimulation, *VA* Voluntary Activation, *MEP* Motor Evoked Potential, *SP* Silent Period, *MVC* Maximum Voluntary Contraction, *PNS* Peripheral Nerve Stimulation (Blamb/Shutterstock.com)

19.4.2 The Acute Response of the Central Nervous System to Aerobic Exercise

The primary motor cortex is an important center playing a role in motor skills and memory formation. The adaptation and reorganization of the primary motor cortex, which includes strengthening and weakening of the synaptic transmission depending on use, play an important role in the acquisition and maintenance of motor skills. It was reported that aerobic exercise is an approach to stimulating these mechanisms, and in this way, short-term neuroplasticity. It was shown that this is caused by changes in circulating biomarkers (e.g., neurotrophic and growth factors) and catecholamines (e.g., epinephrine, norepinephrine, dopamine, and lactate). Previous studies also showed that the density levels of neurotransmitters such as serotonin, dopamine, glutamate, and G-Aminobutyric Acid (GABA) were regulated by one single session of aerobic training, and the levels of circulating Brain-Derived Neurotrophic Factor (BDNF), Insulin-like Growth Factor 1-IGF-1, and Vascular Endothelial Growth Factor (VEGF) were increased. It is also known that BDNF plays a crucial role in neuroplasticity through proliferation, differentiation, survival, and synaptogenesis of neurons. In this respect, IGF-1 plays a role in brain development and maturation of CNS myelination and VEGF contributes to the development and maintenance of the vascular system, increasing capillary density, and contributing to the mobilization of the circulating angiogenic cells, which provide a suitable vascular medium for the growth of neurons. Although studies conducted on chronic exercise are clearer in the literature, it is considered that an acute aerobic exercise session stimulates these changes, supporting neuroplasticity, facilitating the acquisition and preservation of motor skills, and making motor learning easier.

19.5 The Chronic Response of the Neural System to Aerobic Exercise

19.5.1 The Chronic Response of the Peripheral Nervous System to Aerobic Exercise

Studies conducted on this subject in the literature named aerobic exercises endurance exercises, and used long-term, low-intensity aerobic exercises in which large muscle groups (e.g., cycling and running) were generally used. For this reason, exercises will be mentioned as endurance exercises in this section. The literature agrees that endurance training improves physical health. It is argued that mechanisms such as increased stroke volume because of increased blood volume and increased oxidative capacity of the muscle may explain the improvements in aerobic fitness. It was also shown that strength training, especially plyometric training, can trigger neural adaptations. However, the neural adaptations that are caused by endurance training have not yet been fully understood and are considered to be at smaller levels compared to the neural adaptations occurring after strength training.

VA, which is considered one of the most valid indicators of neural adaptation, does not change after endurance and strength training in healthy individuals. The reason for this is that this measurement is close to the exact value before training in healthy individuals, and therefore, does not improve. For this reason, the evaluation of VA is not sufficient in assessing small increases in central conduction. When the MVC Value and the V-Wave were evaluated, it was found that both increased in strength training, but did not change in endurance training. These results can be explained by the fact that MVC is an isometric measurement and the neural adaptations occur in a short time during strength training. It was shown that the H-Reflex increases after endurance training in the evaluations at the spinal level. For this reason, it was suggested that the stimulability of motor neurons and the response of muscle spindles to stretching increase with endurance training. Also, this increase was associated with an increase in Type I fibers. It was emphasized in previous studies that the activation rates of the selected muscles in the evaluation might be affected by the frequency and type of exercise. For this reason, it was stated that a regular and continuous aerobic exercise program must be maintained to observe the changes in H-Reflex responses. Sports such as running, which put more stress on the muscles, are considered to have stronger impacts on spinal reflex responses compared to cycling sports. It was shown in studies using TMS after aerobic exercises (e.g., running, cycling, continuous or interval training) that endurance increased after a 6- to 8-week training program, but no significant changes were detected in VA, SP, and MEP.

In a study that evaluated the effects of 4-week high-intensity interval training in recreational athletes, it was shown that the H-Reflex was increased and there were no changes in the MVC and V-Wave. It was also observed that motor unit discharge ratios increased after strength training and decreased after endurance training in participants evaluated at 30% MVC after 6-weeks of strength and endurance training. However, it must also be noted that short-term endurance training had no effects on muscle activation or maximal force production ratios at the beginning of the contraction, and the evaluation was made at 30% MVC. For this reason, there is a need for further studies on this topic.

19.5.2 The Chronic Response of the Central Nervous System to Aerobic Exercise

BDNF is a protein in high density in the hippocampus, cerebral cortex, hypothalamus, and cerebellum, and can also be produced by peripheral tissues. It is difficult to determine whether the source of BDNF level changes in serum is central or peripheral because it can also cross the blood-brain barrier. For this reason, animal studies are important in showing that aerobic exercise increases BDNF levels. Such studies, both conducted with animals and humans, show that BDNF increases after chronic aerobic exercise. Increased BDNF levels were associated with increased cognitive and hippocampal functions. A study that examined the level of BDNF in terms of exercise intensity, along with IGF-1, cortisol levels, and working memory compared 4 groups (40% and 55% of maximum oxygen consumption, 3 groups that did 70% aerobic exercise, and a control group that did stretching exercise) and showed that all increased in the high-intensity exercise group after a 12-week aerobic exercise program performed 4 days a week at different intensities.

In brief, aerobic training was shown to increase cognitive and neural plasticity in many regions of the brain, including the cerebellum, hippocampus, and cerebral cortex, and angiogenesis in the motor cortex. Chronic exercise triggers appropriate adaptations in the brain over the synaptic plasticity, which may reduce age-related declines in cognitive functions and the risk of neurodegenerative diseases. Studies conducted on exercise-induced neurogenesis focused mainly on endurance exercise and show that endurance training is a potent stimulator of neurotrophic factors in increasing neurogenesis.

It is not clear whether other types of exercise will produce similar adaptations in the structure and functions of the brain. Long-term exercise programs were shown to be a powerful triggering factor for neurogenesis and vascular plasticity. The optimal duration, intensity, and type of exercise needed to stimulate neurogenesis were not defined clearly in the literature.

19.6 The Adaptation Mechanisms in Different Exercise Types

The neuromuscular system exhibits different adaptations to different strengthening programs. The specific neuromuscular adaptations that are responsible for the increased muscle strength are usually grouped as morphological and neural. The most important morphological adaptation is skeletal muscle hypertrophy. Also, hypertrophy and adaptive changes in more than one region in the nervous system play a role in increased muscle strength occurring with resistance training. The most important of the neural system adaptations is the increased ability to stimulate the motor neuron pool at the maximum level, which may be due to greater stimulation of the descending pathways, a decrease in its inhibition, and/or an increase in facilitation mechanisms.

The neuromuscular system also adapts to resistance exercise training, responding in a way that increases the production of the force. Increased muscle strength during resistance exercise training before hypertrophy develops is the first evidence of neural adaptation. In other words, this rapid increase in muscle strength is associated with an increased ability to mobilize the muscles. It is seen that the neural adaptations occurring in resistant exercise training are at the spinal and supraspinal levels. Spinal adaptations, especially H-Reflex, were shown to change following resistance exercise training. Although one single training was shown to facilitate the H-Reflex, the interpretation of the increased H-Reflex after resistance exercise training remains ambiguous. Increased H-Reflex shows increased motor neuron stimulability. The determinant of motor neuron stimulability is the presence of presynaptic inhibition. The mechanism increasing the H-Reflex still remains unclear because H-Reflex measurement cannot measure the level of presynaptic inhibition directly. There is evidence that resistance exercise training can also trigger alpha motor neuron adaptations (e.g., increased neurotransmitter release at the neuromuscular junction or changes in motor neuron biophysical characteristics).

The changes in the primary motor cortex following resistance exercise training are less clear. Although studies are showing a decreased activation, there are also studies reporting that there are no increases or changes. Although there are also some results showing that resistance exercise training leads to changes in the CNS, which plays an important role in strength development, the nature of the neural responses to resistance exercise training at the CNS level has not yet been clearly proven. Motor learning principles are important in planning exercise training. It was reported that resistance exercise training can trigger some changes in the organization of the cortex because it is now well understood that motor learning accompanies the changes in the functional organization of the cerebral cortex. Studies also show that resistance exercise training changes the functional characteristics of the corticospinal pathway and the organization of synaptic circuits in the spinal cord. It was reported in previous studies that neural activity in the primary motor cortex and additional motor area increases if high-intensity isometric force is applied. If each motor unit is capable of producing more force after training in a muscle, fewer motor neurons fire as a result, and less cortical activation is needed to achieve an equivalent kinetic or kinematic result. It can be argued that there will be an increase in the simultaneous firing tendency of motor units with resistant training and based on this, the connections between corticospinal cells and spinal motoneurons may change.

As a result, the neural mechanisms that underlie the increased force production after resistance exercise training are unclear and inconsistent. The participation of the motor units of a trained muscle and the increased firing rate will increase the force production. Other mechanisms that are considered to contribute to this are increased motor output from the motor cortex, increased spinal motor neuron stimulability, and decreased inhibition in descending motor pathways. Also, there are several studies in the literature reporting that the reduction in the co-activation of the antagonists is also important.

Another exercise form in which the effects of neural adaptations on strength gain can be observed is imagination training (imagined contractions) and contralateral training (cross-over training), which can also be called virtual training. Contralateral training can be defined as an increase in strength in one extremity and strength training given to the other extremity not trained. It is argued that the increase in strength in the non-trained extremity in this type of exercise occurs because of the stabilizing and supporting activity. The extent of such pre-learning depends on the previous level of physical activity and coordination of the individual specific to the exercise done. The effect of contralateral strength training was demonstrated in many muscles, including the hand muscles. Previous studies showed that the effect of contralateral strength training complies with the principle of specificity in that it occurs only in homologous muscle and is strongest when tested in the training method and contraction type. It was shown that imaginative exercise in imagery training increases the stimulability of cortical areas involved in movement and movement planning, increasing muscle strength by stimulating CNS adaptations. Also, the same adaptations were shown for a wide variety of training methods and contraction types, including isometric exercises, isotonic exercises that involve both concentric and eccentric contractions, and isokinetic exercises using purely concentric contractions, and isokinetic exercises using purely eccentric contractions. In addition, mental imagery was proven effective in developing motor skills that are not related to force.

It is seen that the neural adaptations emerging as a result of the Electrical Stimulation (ES) applications that were used for muscle training are similar to other strengthening training types. The increase in MVC strength measured by EMG after electrical stimulation, the increase in muscle strength without hypertrophy as a result of short-term ES, and the increase in strength in the contralateral muscle after unilateral ES application are evidence of increased MVC strength over the neural adaptations following a stimulation. Also, the increase in strength in the contralateral homologous muscle shows that ES and training affect the supraspinal centers and cortical regions.

The hallmarks of the supraspinal neural adaptations are the "drive" changes in neural transmission.

These are the changes brought by increased superficial EMG activity during MVC measurement, contralateral training, task specificity, and increases in the output of the primary motor cortex and associated cortical areas measured with electroencephalography (EEG). Also, the increases in MVC strength may be mediated by spinal adaptations. These include the changes in motor unit activation, motor neuron stimulability that is measured with the H-Reflex and V-Wave, spinal reflex mechanisms such as presynaptic inhibition, reciprocal inhibition, Renshaw Inhibition, and synaptic activity.

When the neural adaptations are evaluated according to the contraction types, cortical stimulability is greater, but motor unit activity is lower in eccentric contractions. It was shown that low motor unit discharge ratios and spinal inhibition limit eccentric force, especially in individuals without training history. Although more studies are needed to determine the exact mechanisms, it was stated that spinal inhibition is primarily responsible for the differences in adaptations.

Another important issue in neural adaptations is central fatigue, which can be considered as the inability of the CNS to activate a muscle to its full capacity. The decreased voluntary muscle activation as the load continues is indicative of central fatigue. MVC and TMS can be used to examine types of fatigue. A related study reported that a TMS applied during the performance of MVC elicits amplitude twitches increasing as fatigue develops. The mechanisms of central and supraspinal fatigue are still not fully elucidated.

19.7 The Factors that Affect Adaptation to Exercise

Adaptation to exercise is affected by age, gender, duration of exercise, intensity, training history, focus, and psychological factors. In the early phase of exercise training, neural adaptations predominate.

Men have a higher rate of force generation compared to women during maximum voluntary contraction. This shows their ability to generate force more quickly. Such gender differences can be associated with many factors (e.g., muscle architectural characteristics, muscle fiber type, muscle biomechanical characteristics, and neural activity during muscle contractions). In contrast, many studies reported that resistance training at a similar intensity in men and women produced similar hypertrophic adaptations, neural drive improvements, and strength gains. In general, women have higher thresholds and lower maximum amplitudes for H and M responses in EMG measurements. The ratios between maximum H and M response amplitudes are smaller in older athletes than in younger athletes, and the amplitude of M responses is higher. The gains in muscle strength with resistance training are the result of both neural and muscular factors. Neural factors account for approximately 90% of the strength gains in the first 2 weeks of a typical 8-week training session and between 40 and 50% of strength gain is related to neural system adaptation over the next 2 weeks. Muscle fiber adaptations become more and more important in the next process. When whether exercise intensity affected neural adaptation was evaluated, studies in the literature report that there was more neural adaptation after high-intensity resistance exercise training. Focusing also affects performance directly. For this reason, long periods of training may be required to avoid the effects of external stimuli on performance, especially in athletes.

19.8 The Side/Undesirable Effects that Might Occur During/After Exercise in Neural System Pathologies and Their Management

Following neural system pathologies, exercise affects many physical and psychosocial areas positively. The side/undesirable effects of exercise must be examined specifically for the pathology in this patient group, just as the exercise program, which is very important in terms of supporting motor learning, providing improvement in daily living activities, and increasing participation, is planned individually. For this reason, three important side/undesirable effects that are faced most frequently during the rehabilitation of neural system pathologies and which are frequently mentioned in the literature will be discussed in this section.

1. One of the most common side/undesirable effects of Central Nervous System pathologies is orthostatic hypotension. Standing up for exercise may cause pooling of blood in the distal lower extremities, triggering coagulation, and/or cerebral hypoperfusion for a patient who is lying for a long time. In such a situation, which is common in many patients, especially in stroke and spinal cord injuries, avoiding prolonged standing or performing periodic lower extremity movements to activate the venous muscle pump can prevent blood pooling, and minimize the activation of coagulation, alleviating cerebral hypoperfusion.
2. Chronic fatigue, which is another important and most common side/undesirable effect, is a typical finding of neurological diseases and is mostly seen in CNS diseases such as multiple sclerosis and stroke. Also, in some neural system pathologies such as neuromuscular junction conduction disorders, muscle pathologies, and peripheral nerve injuries, the inability to sustain muscle contraction force, in other words, peripheral fatigue, occurs. Physical activity levels and the management of fatigue during exercise are important issues in neurological diseases. Patients remain sedentary because of its accompanying symptoms and decreased physical activity levels. However, physical inactivity caused by fatigue causes deterioration of cardiovascular fitness, muscular condition, and various health issues. Excessive physical activity is a condition increasing the symptoms and fatigue complaints in the neurological patient group. For this reason, the intensity of exercise must be well adjusted, planned specifically for the disease and the symptoms of the person, and spread throughout the day. The patients must also be followed carefully with their feedback and evaluations.
3. Another side/undesirable effect, which might occur during exercise, is falling. Although falls after neural pathologies occur depending on many factors, it is a condition jeopardizing exercise safety. For this reason, care must be taken during exercise, a safe environment should be provided, and the patient must not be left alone.

Aside from these, there are also some different side/undesirable effects caused by the nature of each disease. To cope with these effects, the risks that may be faced, particularly for a certain disease, must be analyzed and necessary precautions must be taken before an exercise program is initiated.

19.9 The Comparison of the Adaptation Mechanism of the Neural System to Exercise: a Healthy Individual and a Patient with Stroke

The comparison of the adaptation mechanism of the neural system to exercise in patient with stroke and healthy individual is given in Table 19.1.

The adaptation of the neural system to exercise is summarized in Table 19.2 and the clinical implications of the cases are summarized in Table 19.3.

Table 19.1 The comparison of the treatment programs for healthy individual and patient with stroke

Case 1. Healthy individual	Case 2. Patient with stroke
K.C. (male) 35 years old, 1.80 meters tall, weighs 88 kg, works in a bank K.C. consults a physiotherapist to improve general fitness K.C. reports no regular exercise habits for the last 3 years K.C., who does not have any diagnosed disease, does not smoke	S.A. (female) 58 years old, 1.63 m tall, weighs 75 kg, and is a retired teacher. Diagnosed with stroke about 3 years ago, the patient developed a hemiparesis in the first stroke and was hospitalized twice to receive a physiotherapy and rehabilitation program. The patient can walk independently and has gastrosoleus spasticity of 1. She said that she was an active person before she had a stroke and that she regularly did jogging for 1 h, 3 days a week. However, she also stated that she could not go out especially in the first year after the stroke because she was afraid of falling, therefore her performance decreased, she became tired quickly, had respiratory distress when going up and down the stairs and walking for long distances, and could not walk as long as before
The evaluation of the cases	
Case 1. Healthy individual	**Case 2. Patient with stroke**
– Curriculum Vitae/Family history – Body Mass Index – Exercise habit – Identification of risk factors	– Curriculum Vitae/Family history – Medical history, medications used, surgical history – Affected extremity – Exercise habit – Determining risk factors – Motor and sensory evaluation – Evaluation of balance, functional mobility, and fall risk
The evaluation of the exercise capacity	
Cardiopulmonary exercise test – Field tests (6 min walking, shuttle walking test)	Cardiopulmonary exercise test – Field tests (6 min walking, shuttle walk test)
Assessment of the physical activity level	
International Physical Activity Scale, accelerometer, pedometer	International Physical Activity Scale, accelerometer, pedometer
Fatigue assessment	
–	Fatigue Severity Scale Visual Analog Scale (VAS)
Evaluation of the dyspnea	
During the exercise: Borg Scale Visual Analog Scale (VAS)	During daily activities: Medical Research Council (MRC) Dyspnea Scale During exercise: Borg Scale Visual Analog Scale (VAS)
Treatment program	
Case 1. Healthy individual	**Case 2. Patient with stroke**
Aerobic exercise training program	
Exercise intensity: 70–85% of maximal heart rate **Exercise frequency:** 3–5 days a week **Exercise duration:** At least 30 min 8–12 weeks a week for a total of ≥150 min	>20 min of aerobic exercise sessions are recommended along with a 3–5-min warm-up and cool-down cycle. A gradual progression over time is recommended for patients in poor condition or with significant motor impairments, starting with 5-min rest intervals and lower-intensity exercises. At low severity: <64% maximal heart rate or Borg Scale (6–20) <12 Upper and lower body ergometers, bicycle ergometers, and treadmills (including underwater and robot-assisted treadmills) were proposed as arm ergometers Exercises that involve large muscle groups are preferred (e.g., walking, bicycle ergometer, arm ergometer)

(continued)

Table 19.1 (continued)

Strength and endurance exercises	
Exercises that involve major muscle groups are preferred: **Exercise intensity:** Moderate/High intensity **Exercise frequency:** 2–3 days/week **Exercise duration:** 8–12 repetitions, 2–4 sets	Exercises involving large muscle groups are preferred: **Exercise intensity:** 70–80% of 1 maximum repetition is preferred **Exercise frequency:** 2–5 days/week, 4–12 weeks **Exercise duration:** 3 sets, 8–15 repetitions
Neuromuscular exercises	
	Balance and coordination exercises Neurodevelopmental treatment approaches

Table 19.2 The adaptation of the neural system to exercise

The adaptation of the neural system to exercise	
Case 1. Healthy individual	**Case 2. Patient with stroke**
Acute response to the aerobic exercise	
When the literature was reviewed, it was found that there are few studies on this subject, and fatigue was emphasized in these studies The type of aerobic activity is an effective factor in the resulting central fatigue	When the literature was examined, no study was found on this subject in stroke patients
Chronic response to aerobic exercise	
– Increased stimulability of the H-Reflex – Increase in α motor neuron stimulability – Increase in force production rates – Increase in cognitive and neural plasticity and increase in angiogenesis in the motor cortex	When the literature was reviewed, no study was found on this subject in stroke patients
Acute response to strength exercise training	
It was shown to facilitate the H-Reflex in a single strength training session	There is a need for studies to investigate the acute responses of the neural system to reinforcement training in neurological diseases
Chronic response to strength exercise training	
– Muscle fiber conduction ratio increases – Motor unit discharge ratios increase – H-Reflex increases – CNS activation increases – Motor unit simultaneous activity develops – Neural inhibitory reflexes are reduced – Previous studies suggest that hypertrophy that results from high and low-intensity strength training is similar, but greater strength development is achieved in high-intensity exercise. It was reported that this is the result of more neural adaptation – It was also shown that eccentric training is more effective in neural adaptation	No study was detected on the neural adaptation of strengthening exercise training in stroke It was also shown that muscle strengthening training increases muscle strength and gait speed, and improves functional outcomes and quality of life without causing increased spasticity in post-stroke patients. The benefits and risks of resistance exercises in post-stroke patients still continue to be a matter of debate. Isotonic exercises are the most commonly used. For this reason, more controlled studies are needed to identify the most appropriate variants of strength training in stroke individuals to be used as a resource for personalized treatment

Table 19.3 Clinical inferences from the cases

Do's and don'ts when planning exercise training
No study was detected on neural adaptations that result from aerobic exercise training in stroke. The following should be considered when planning an exercise program with the inferences made from the results of the studies conducted with healthy individuals
1. A personalized exercise program must be planned according to the training history, exercise capacity, and functional level
2. To increase aerobic capacity along with neurodevelopmental treatment approaches used for stroke rehabilitation, aerobic exercises must also be included in the treatment program
3. The exercise program must start from low intensity and progress gradually. Attention must be paid to the fatigue, which might occur in the individual during the process

19.10 Conclusion

Neural adaptations vary at significant levels with different exercise training. Many previous studies show that there are changes in subcortical levels as a result of strength training, most clearly evidenced by increased active H-Reflex. However, the changes in the primary motor cortex are more ambiguous. CNS activation increases, motor unit simultaneous activity improves, and neural inhibitory reflexes decrease with resistance exercise training. Cortical stimulability is greater in eccentric contraction, but motor unit activity is lower. Lower motor unit discharge ratios suggest that spinal inhibition limits eccentric force, especially in individuals with no training. ES increases the force of maximal voluntary contraction in a very short time for muscle hypertrophy. Also, as a result of the ES, it is seen that there is an increased strength in the homologous muscle on the opposite side following unilateral training, which shows that ES increases the force of voluntary contraction over neural adaptations. Although there are not many studies in the literature that investigate the effects of aerobic exercise on neural adaptation, present studies show that central fatigue occurs following an acute exercise session, especially involving running or cycling exercises. The type, intensity, and duration of aerobic activity are effective factors in the resulting central fatigue. For this reason, it is recommended to prefer activities that cause less mechanical stress on muscles.

Further Reading

Akin Ş, Demirel AH. Skeletal muscle satellite cells and role in muscle regeneration. Turkiye Klinikleri J Sports Med-Special Topics. 2017;3:227–32.

Barbosa DD, Trojahn MR, Porto DVG, Hentschke GS, Hentschke VS. Strength training protocols in hemiparetic individuals post stroke: a systematic review. Fisioter Mov. 2018;31:e003127.

Cattagni T, Lepers R, Maffiuletti NA. Effects of neuromuscular electrical stimulation on contralateral quadriceps function. J Electromyogr Kinesiol. 2018;38:111–8.

Centner C, Lauber B. A systematic review and meta-analysis on neural adaptations following blood flow restriction training: what we know and what we don't know. Front Physiol. 2020;11:887.

Chaudhuri A, Behan PO. Fatigue in neurological disorders. Lancet. 2004;363:978–88.

Dornowski M, Kolosova YV, Gorkovenko AV. Gender and age-related peculiarities of the H-reflex indices in sportsmen. Neurophysiology. 2017;49:458–61.

Douglas J, Pearson S, Ross A, McGuigan M. Eccentric exercise: physiological characteristics and acute responses. Sports Med. 2017;47:663–75.

Folland JP, Williams AG. Morphological and neurological contributions to increased strength. Sports Med. 2007;37:145–68.

Guillaume YM, John T. Neural adaptations to endurance training. In: Schumann M, Rønnestad BR, editors. Concurrent aerobic and strength training. Scientific basics and practical applications. Springer; 2019. p. 35–50.

Hall JE, Hall ME. Guyton and Hall textbook of medical physiology e-Book. Elsevier Health Sciences; 2020.

Hedayatpour N, Falla D. Physiological and neural adaptations to eccentric exercise: mechanisms and considerations for training. Biomed Res Int. 2015;2015:193741.

Hortobágyi T, Maffiuletti NA. Neural adaptations to electrical stimulation strength training. Eur J Appl Physiol. 2011;111:2439–49.

Hughes DC, Ellefsen S, Baar K. Adaptations to endurance and strength training. Cold Spring Harb Perspect Med. 2018;8:a029769.

Jenkins ND, Miramonti AA, Hill EC, Smith CM, Cochrane-Snyman KC, Housh TJ, et al. Greater neural adaptations following high-vs. low-load resistance training. Front Physiol. 2017;8:331.

MacKay-Lyons M, Billinger SA, Eng JJ, Dromerick A, Giacomantonio N, Hafer-Macko C, et al. Aerobic exercise recommendations to optimize best practices in care after stroke: AEROBICS 2019 update. Phys Ther. 2020;100:149–56.

Marzolini S, Robertson AD, Oh P, Goodman JM, Corbett D, Du X, et al. Aerobic training and mobilization early post-stroke: cautions and considerations. Front Neurol. 2019;10:1187.

McArdle WD, Katch FI, Katch, VL. Neural control of human movement. In: McArdle WD, Katch FI, Katch VL, editors. Essentials of exercise physiology. 4th ed. Lippincott Williams & Wilkins; 2011. p. 338–374.

Minetto MA, Botter A, Gamerro G, Varvello I, Massazza G, Bellomo RG, et al. Contralateral effect of short-duration unilateral neuromuscular electrical stimulation and focal vibration in healthy subjects. Eur J Phys Rehabil Med. 2018;54(6):911–20.

Peterson CR. Acute neural adaptations to resistance training performed with low and high rates of muscle activation. 2009.

Scott KP, Edward TH. The nervous system: structure and control of movement. In: Powers SK, Howley E.T, editors. Exercise physiology theory and application to fitness and performance. 10th ed. New York: McGraw-Hill Education. 2018. p. 140–165.

Siddique U, Rahman S, Frazer AK, Pearce AJ, Howatson G, Kidgell DJ. Determining the sites of neural adaptations to resistance training: a systematic review and meta-analysis. Sports Med. 2020;50:1107–28.

Škarabot J, Brownstein CG, Casolo A, Del Vecchio A, Ansdell P. The knowns and unknowns of neural adaptations to resistance training. Eur J Appl Physiol. 2020;121:675–85.

Bioenergetics and Metabolism

20

Ozge Ozalp

Abstract

A continuous supply of chemical energy is needed to sustain many complex functions in the human body. For this reason, thousands of chemical reactions occur in the body every minute of the day. These reactions are collectively called *metabolism*. Metabolism is broadly defined as the sum of all cellular reactions and includes chemical pathways that cause the synthesis of molecules (anabolic reactions) and the breakdown of molecules (catabolic reactions).

Since energy is necessary for all cells, nutrients (fats, proteins, carbohydrates) are converted into a form of energy that can be used biologically by chemical pathways. This metabolic process is called *bioenergetics*. During physical activities such as walking, running, throwing, jumping, or swimming, skeletal muscle cells need to constantly provide energy from nutrients. In the field of bioenergetics, studies are carried out on topics such as exercise intensity, performance, fatigue, lactate accumulation and differences between individuals, and energy use. Given the importance of cellular energy production during exercise, comprehensive knowledge of bioenergetics is essential. This chapter examines the concepts of bioenergetics and cellular metabolism and their adaptation to exercise.

20.1 Adenosine Triphosphate: Energy Unit

The energy obtained through nutrients is not transferred directly to the cells for biological work. Energy from the oxidation of macronutrients is harvested and transferred via the energy-rich compound adenosine triphosphate (ATP). The potential energy in this nucleotide molecule powers all the energy-requiring processes of the cell. The role of ATP in giving and receiving energy ensures that potential energy from nutrients is stored in bonds within ATP, and the chemical energy in ATP is used to power biological work.

The structure of ATP consists of three main parts (Fig. 20.1):

1. Adenine
2. Ribose
3. Three phosphates

Adenine and ribose in the biochemical structure of ATP are collectively called adenosine. Adenine is a nitrogen-containing base and ribose is a five-carbon sugar. Three phosphate groups

O. Ozalp (✉)
Physiotherapy and Rehabilitation, Faculty of Health Sciences, Cyprus International University, Nicosia, Cyprus
e-mail: oozalp@ciu.edu.tr

Adenosine triphospate (ATP)

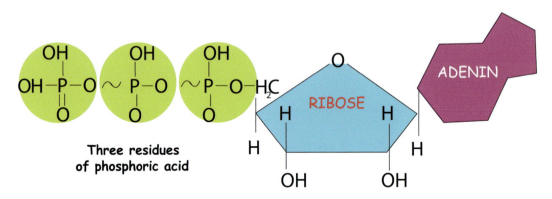

Fig. 20.1 Structure of adenosine triphosphate (Zvitaliy/Shutterstock.com)

are formed by adding energy to the combination of adenosine diphosphate (ADP) and inorganic phosphate (Pi). Some of this energy is stored in the chemical bond that joins ADP and Pi. Accordingly, this bond is called *a high-energy bond*. When the enzyme ATPase breaks this bond, energy is released and this energy can be used to do work. The energy produced when a phosphate is removed from ATP acts as a unit to enable muscles to move, synthesize molecules, or actively transport or excrete against a concentration gradient. A cellular energy-requiring process always uses ATP as its main energy source. As ATP is broken down and formed, it is hydrolyzed by enzymes called ATPase, which causes the formation of ADP and Pi (Fig. 20.2).

$$\text{Adenosine diphosphate}(\text{ADP}) + \text{Inorganic phosphate}(P_i)$$
$$+ \text{Energy}(7.3 \text{kcal}/\text{mole}) \overset{\text{ATP}_{ase}}{\leftrightarrow} \text{Adenosine triphosphate}(\text{ATP})$$

The above process can be performed bi-directionally. The ATP molecule can be regenerated from ADP as long as the energy required to restore the remaining Pi molecule to ADP is available.

ATP is often called the universal energy donor. It preserves the energy released from the breakdown of nutrients as a usable form of energy needed by all cells. Inside the cell, ATP can then be used to drive energy-requiring processes in the cell. Inside the cell, ATP can then be used to sustain energy-requiring processes in the cell. Therefore, energy-releasing reactions are associated with energy-requiring reactions such as gear wheels.

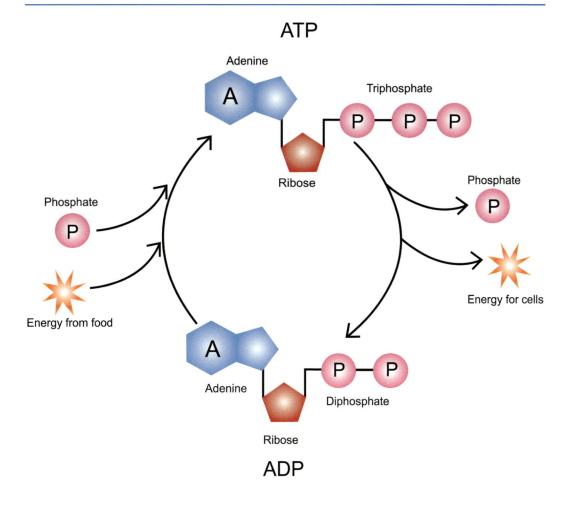

Fig. 20.2 ATP and ADP energy conversion (Kicky_princess/Shutterstock.com)

20.2 Energy Systems in the Body

The amount of ATP that muscle cells can store is limited. There are metabolic pathways that ensure the continuous production of ATP in the cell to provide the energy needed for muscle contraction during exercise. The total amount of ATP in a muscle cell is about 80–100 g. This amount is sufficient to provide 3–5 s of vigorous physical activity. This amount is sufficient to provide 3–5 s of vigorous physical activity. Since this is not a large amount, adequate amounts of ATP must be resynthesized for exercise to take place.

Muscle cells produce ATP using a combination of three metabolic pathways that are activated from the onset of contractions (Fig. 20.3):

1. Phosphagen system (ATP-PCr system): Formation of ATP by the breakdown of phosphocreatine
2. Glycolysis (short-term energy system): Formation of ATP through the breakdown of glucose or glycogen
3. Aerobic energy system (long-term energy system): The formation of ATP in the presence of oxygen

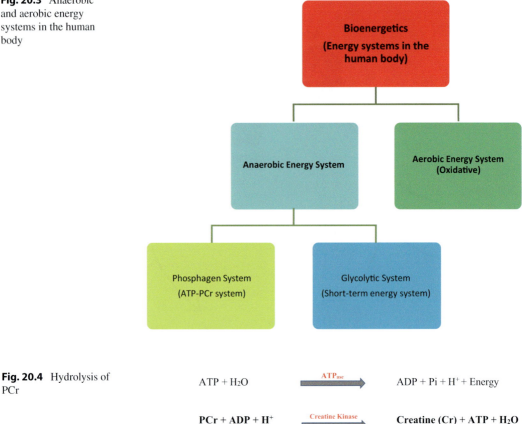

Fig. 20.3 Anaerobic and aerobic energy systems in the human body

Fig. 20.4 Hydrolysis of PCr

$$ATP + H_2O \xrightarrow{ATPase} ADP + Pi + H^+ + Energy$$

$$PCr + ADP + H^+ \xrightarrow{Creatine\ Kinase} Creatine\ (Cr) + ATP + H_2O$$

There are two basic energy systems in the body, the aerobic pathway (oxidative) that works in the presence of oxygen and the anaerobic pathway that works without oxygen. The anaerobic pathway is divided into two the phosphagen system and the glycolytic system (lactate system). Oxidative formation of ATP in the presence of oxygen is called aerobic metabolism. All of these systems are involved in the production of ATP.

20.2.1 Phosphagen System (ATP-PCr System)

The fastest and simplest way to create ATP is the phosphagen system. This pathway consists of two components: storage ATP molecules within the cell and phosphocreatine or creatine phosphate (PCr). Hydrolysis of PCr is carried out by the enzyme creatine kinase (CK). The phosphagen system generates ATP through a series of events which is shown in Fig. 20.4.

ADP levels increase as a result of the hydrolysis of ATP catalyzed by ATPase, especially with the onset of activity in high-intensity exercises. The increase in ADP levels within the cell activates the enzyme creatine kinase, which is responsible for facilitating the hydrolysis of PCr to Cr and Pi. The structure of this system provides very fast energy production to meet the ATP requirement. The maximum rate of ATP production from the phosphagen system is more than twice as fast as in glycolysis. However, the skeletal muscle concentration of PCr is limited, and resting PCr stores are rapidly depleted within a period of about 10 s during movements requiring near-maximal effort.

The energy continuity during movement is determined by the use of energy sources according to the intensity and duration of the exercise.

At the start of an activity, the first source of energy is ATP stores in the muscle cross bridges. PCr quickly becomes the next main energy source to replace ATP. After PCr, the anaerobic breakdown of muscle glycogen via glycolysis predominates to generate ATP, while aerobic processes predominate at about 60 s and beyond. For example, at the 20th second of maximal intensity exercise, approximately 40% of the energy comes from PCr, 50% from glycolysis, and 10% from aerobic processes, while at the 40th second the contribution is approximately 5, 80, and 15% for PCr, glycolysis, and aerobic system, respectively.

Pole vaulting, chopping wood, running 100 m, jumping rope, and other high-intensity exercises repeated in more than one round for a short time can be given as examples of movements that produce ATP predominantly through the phosphagen system. Studies report that it may take 5–15 min for PCr levels to fully recover after vigorous exercise, in which the phosphagen system is completely depleted. It has also been shown that active recovery after exercise facilitates PCr refill compared to passive recovery, and higher cardiorespiratory fitness levels accelerate recovery due to improved oxygen delivery. In addition, PCr levels are restored more rapidly in slow-twitch muscle fibers than in fast-twitch muscle fibers.

Considering that the total capacity for the phosphagen system, which acts as the immediate energy system, is limited to a period of approximately 10 s, there is a need for an alternative route that can rapidly regenerate ATP for the continuation of high-intensity exercises.

20.2.2 Glycolysis (Short-Term Energy System)

The phosphagen system has a limited ATP production capacity, which takes only a few seconds for energy. A second metabolic pathway for rapid ATP production without the participation of O_2 is *glycolysis*. Glycolysis can be defined as the metabolic pathway that breaks down glucose ($C_6H_{12}O_6$) or muscle glycogen into a three-carbon two pyruvate or two-lactate structure. Glycolysis is the anaerobic pathway used to produce ATP by recombining Pi and ADP with the bond energy obtained from glucose. This process involves a series of enzymatically catalyzed, paired reactions. Glycolysis occurs in the sarcoplasm of the muscle cell and produces a net gain of two molecules of ATP and two molecules of pyruvate or lactate per molecule of glucose. Although pyruvate is technically the end-product of glycolysis, when there is not enough oxygen it is converted to lactate or, if there is enough oxygen, it is sent to the mitochondria for aerobic reactions.

Glycolysis consists of 10 reactions to produce 2 pyruvate structures. It uses energy to complete certain steps in glycolysis and also produces ATP molecules. Additionally, during this process, NADH+H$^+$ is formed by transferring hydrogen atoms to an electron carrier called nicotinamide adenine dinucleotide (NAD$^+$). The steps involved in glycolysis and the electron carrier system that transfers hydrogen atoms out of the glycolysis pathway are shown in Fig. 20.5. There are generally 10 steps in the glycolytic process, and ultimately two or three molecules of ATP are produced depending on whether glucose or glycogen is used as the initial substrate.

Compounds formed in glycolysis also provide entry and exit points for other substances into glycolysis. For example, the dihydroxyacetone phosphate produced in step 5 is an input or production source for glycerol formed by the breakdown of triglycerides. Glycolysis can be studied by dividing it into two phases. The first phase of glycolysis represents the energy expenditure phase and the second phase represents the energy production phase.

In order for glycolysis to complete 10–12 steps, one or two ATP molecules must be consumed in the first phase. The difference between one or two ATP expenditures at the start of glycolysis is explained by whether the carbohydrate source used as fuel is glucose or glycogen. Before glucose or glycogen can be used, it must be converted to a compound called glucose-6-phosphate. Although the purpose of glycolysis is to release ATP, converting one glucose molecule to glucose-

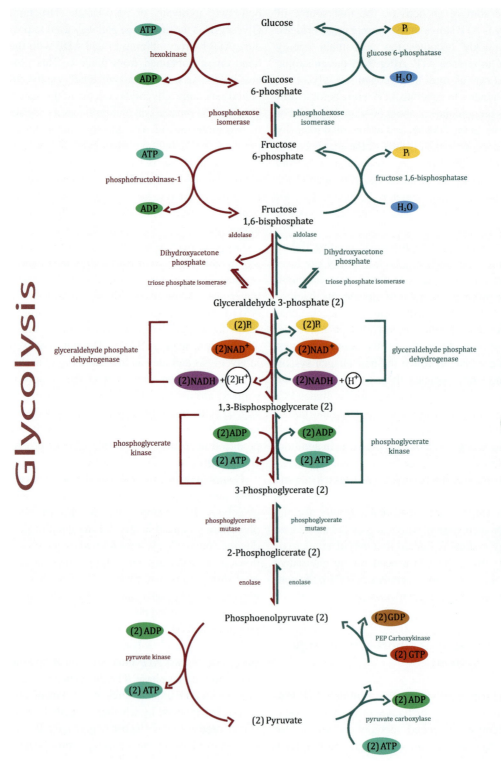

Fig. 20.5 Glycolytic reactions (Borbely Edit/Shutterstock.com)

6-phosphate requires the expenditure of one ATP molecule. When glycogen stored in the muscle is used, glucose-6-phosphate is formed from glucose-1-phosphate without this energy expenditure. Since glucose is transported from the blood to the muscle cell via a specific protein carrier, it costs as much energy as one molecule of ATP. Glycolysis mainly starts when the glucose-6-phosphate compound is formed.

In the second phase of glycolysis, four moles of ATP molecules are produced (in steps 7 and 10), and in the final step, two pyruvate molecules are formed. As shown in Fig. 20.5, the net gain of glycolysis is calculated as 3 moles of ATP when the first substrate is glycogen, and 2 moles of ATP if glucose is used instead of glycogen, since 1 mole of ATP is used to convert glucose to glucose-6-phosphate. Also, during the second phase, two NAD^+ molecules are reduced to $NADH+H^+$. These reduced carrier molecules then move to the electron transport chain (ETS) to produce ATP. In summary, the process of glycolysis taking place within the sarcoplasm in muscle cells produces two pyruvate molecules, two $NADH+H^+$, and two or three net ATP molecules.

This energy system does not produce large amounts of ATP. However, the combination of ATP-PCr and a glycolytic system allows the muscles to generate force when the oxygen supply is limited. These two systems predominate in the first minutes of high-intensity exercise. Under steady-state exercise conditions, the ions carried by $NADH+H^+$ are transferred to the mitochondria, where they are used to generate ATP. *Steady-state exercise* is defined as exercise intensity where energy needs are met aerobically at relatively constant exercise intensity. In non-steady-state exercise conditions, $NADH+H^+$ transfers ions to pyruvate to form lactate via lactate dehydrogenase enzyme (Fig. 20.6). During steady-state exercise, ions transported in $NADH+H^+$ formed by glycolysis pass to the mitochondria, but this cannot occur at higher exercise intensities. As a result, $NADH+H^+$ begins to accumulate in the cytosol, while NAD^+ utilization is limited and hydrogen ions begin to accumulate in the cell or blood. If NAD^+ is not reused in the lactate dehydrogenase reaction, the glycolytic flow is affected and ATP production is reduced.

20.2.2.1 Lactate Production and Utilization

Lactate is not a metabolic waste product formed as a result of glycolysis, but a compound that plays an important role in energy pathways. Lactate is constantly produced in the human body. Since lactate can be used as a substrate by cells such as the heart, liver, and muscle, it is converted back to pyruvate during rest and under steady-state exercise conditions, thus providing a balance between lactate production and removal.

During glycolysis, blood sugar or muscle glycogen either enters the mitochondria to continue the aerobic system or is converted to pyruvate, which will be converted to lactate, depending on the intensity of the exercise and the availability of oxygen. Both uses can occur simultaneously but at different rates. At rest or during low-intensity exercise, almost all pyruvate enters the mitochondria. However, if the capacity of the aerobic system is exceeded during exercise at higher intensities, most of the pyruvate is converted to lactate. The lactate can then be used as fuel elsewhere in the body (e.g., heart, liver, non-exercising muscles).

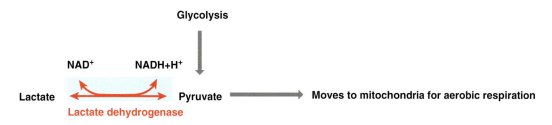

Fig. 20.6 Pyruvate forms lactate

Lactate molecules produced in skeletal muscle are transported out of the cell via a carrier protein called the *monocarboxylate transporter (MCT)* found in the muscle cell. The primary route of lactate utilization is as metabolic fuel by the heart, liver, kidneys, and less active skeletal muscle. Especially during exercise, lactate produced in the skeletal muscle is transported to the liver through the blood after being taken out of the muscle cell. Lactate contributes to the production of glucose in the liver, known as gluconeogenesis. This glucose produced can then be released back into the bloodstream and transported back to the exercising skeletal muscle and used as fuel. This lactate-glucose cycle between skeletal muscle and liver is known as the Cori cycle and is an efficient pathway for blood lactate removal and utilization.

20.2.2.2 Lactate Threshold and Onset of the Blood Lactate Accumulation (OBLA)

Although there is always a small amount of lactate in our blood, a significant increase occurs during exercise. As exercise intensity increases, the use of carbohydrates becomes more efficient in producing energy. Therefore, there is a gradual transition from fats to carbohydrates as the primary fuel. At the same time, a shift occurs from the use of type I muscle fibers with a higher aerobic capacity to type II fibers with greater anaerobic capacity. This means a slight but stabilized increase in lactate levels and a balance exists between lactate production and removal.

The initial accumulation of blood lactate above the resting concentration is defined as *the lactate threshold.* Basically, this point indicates the level at which carbohydrates now become the body's primary fuel source. This also represents the point at which aerobic efficiency begins to lose and anaerobic systems begin to speed up to aid energy production.

If exercise intensity increases, blood lactate levels continue to rise. As a result, the balance between lactate production and excretion is disrupted, resulting in a disproportionate increase in blood lactate. The point at which the ability to sustain high-intensity exercise cannot be sustained for longer is known as *the onset of blood lactate accumulation (OBLA).* Physiologically, this marker can be considered as an inability to balance the rate of increase in blood lactate produced in muscle cells. From a performance standpoint, approaches to improve OBLA or to increase the body's capacity to buffer lactate so that it can tolerate a greater release of lactate into the blood are crucial.

20.3 Aerobic Energy System (Oxidative System)

The third pathway for ATP production is the aerobic energy system (Fig. 20.7). It is the most efficient chemical route in which the most ATP molecules are produced in total. However, the rate of ATP production is significantly slower than the phosphagen system or glycolysis. Another benefit of this system is that all three macronutrients (fats, carbohydrates, and proteins) can be utilized as substrates for energy production. Low-to-moderate exercise, such as walking, running, or cycling, generally uses aerobic metabolism. However, in sports branches such as basketball and football, systems are generally used together by switching between aerobic and anaerobic metabolism between short-term-vigorous and long-term-low-intensity physical activities.

Carbohydrates in the form of glucose or glycogen are converted to pyruvate or lactate after entering glycolysis, or to acetyl-coenzyme A (CoA) if they move into the mitochondria. Triglycerides are composed of free fatty acids and glycerol and enter the bioenergetic pathways via beta-oxidation and glycolysis, respectively. Proteins contain nitrogen atoms in addition to carbon, hydrogen, and oxygen. Therefore, they must first undergo deamination, the process of removing the nitrogen group from the amino acid. The remaining amino acid skeleton is either converted to acetyl-CoA or intermediates of the Krebs cycle or converted to pyruvate. Proteins are mostly used as energy

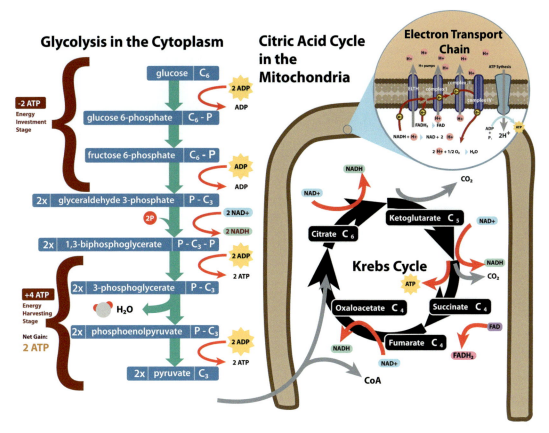

Fig. 20.7 ATP synthesis process of glycolysis and aerobic system (gstraub/Shutterstock.com)

fuel during prolonged fasting or long and intense exercise conditions. Since proteins are not the main energy source in the body, the use of their as a substrate will not be given in detail in the section.

20.3.1 Entrance to the Aerobic System

The end-product of glycolysis is two pyruvate molecules that move through the sarcoplasm and enter the mitochondria for further oxidation. Carbohydrates undergo two additional pathways to complete aerobic metabolism after anaerobically undergoing glycolysis. These are the aerobic energy mechanisms called the *Krebs cycle (Citric acid cycle)* and the *Electron Transport Chain (ETS)* (Fig. 20.8).

The Krebs cycle and the use of ETS occur in the presence of sufficient oxygen and when the rate of pyruvate production in glycolysis does not exceed the capacity to take up pyruvate in the mitochondria. With the effect of the pyruvate dehydrogenase enzyme, pyruvate, a three-carbon structure, moves towards the mitochondria, and in this process, it is converted to a two-carbon structure acetyl-CoA. With this reaction, a molecule of NADH+H$^+$ is produced simultaneously and a molecule of carbon dioxide (CO_2) is released. One of the most important features of this step is that the reaction is not bidirectional. This means that the process cannot be reversed when pyruvate is converted to acetyl-CoA. This means that if acetyl-CoA is composed of fats or certain proteins, it cannot be used to form glucose. Only substrates that enter the bioenergy pathway as pyruvate or as an intermediate of gly-

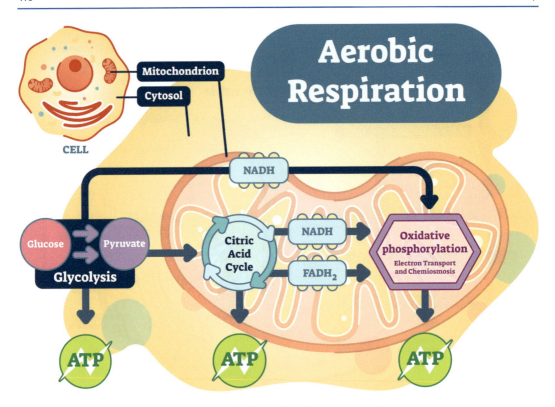

Fig. 20.8 Krebs cycle and ETS scheme in the cell (VectorMine/Shutterstock.com)

colysis (e.g., glycerol) can form glucose. The free fatty acids portion of fats and some proteins enter the energy pathways as acetyl-CoA and therefore cannot be converted to carbohydrates. Acetyl-CoA represents the common substrate to which all three macronutrients are converted before entering the aerobic pathway.

20.3.2 Krebs Cycle (Citric Acid Cycle)

The Krebs cycle is the second stage of aerobic respiration after glycolysis, and the last is the electron transport chain. The Krebs cycle completes the oxidation of pyruvate, which is formed at the end of glycolysis. The Krebs cycle includes a series of enzymatically catalyzed reactions shown in Fig. 20.9. This cycle begins by combining a two-carbon structure, acetyl-CoA, with a four-carbon structure, oxaloacetate, to form citrate, a six-carbon structure.

Before entering the enzymatically controlled 10-step Krebs cycle, pyruvate combines with 2-coenzyme A (CoA) to form the two-carbon compound acetyl-CoA. The two hydrogens that are also liberated as a result of this reaction transfer their electrons to NAD^+ to form a molecule of carbon dioxide (CO_2).

$$Pyruvate + NAD^+ + CoA \rightarrow Acetyl\ CoA + CO_2 + NADH^+ + H^+$$

Acetyl-CoA molecules entering the Krebs cycle then go through one full turn of this cycle to form ATP, CO_2, $FADH_2$, and $NADH+H^+$ molecules. The main function of the Krebs cycle is to remove hydrogen and use the energy trapped within these molecules in other parts of the cycle. NAD^+ and flavin adenine dinucleotide (FAD^+) molecules are reduced to $NADH+H^+$ and $FADH_2$ to remove hydrogen. Glycolysis, the conversion of pyruvate to acetyl-CoA, and the $NADH+H^+$ and $FADH_2$ molecules produced during the Krebs cycle are all transported to the ETS, where substantial amounts of ATP are produced.

Acetyl-CoA combines with oxaloacetate to form citrate at the beginning of the Krebs cycle.

Citric acid cycle – Krebs cycle

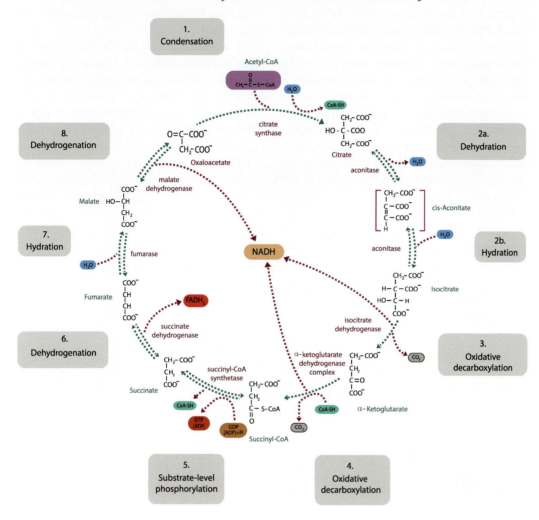

Fig. 20.9 Krebs cycle (Borbely Edit/Shutterstock.com)

Each acetyl-CoA molecule entering the Krebs cycle releases two carbon dioxide molecules and four pairs of hydrogen atoms and one ATP molecule. Considered from glycolysis, a glucose molecule splits into two pyruvate molecules, both forming acetyl-CoA molecules, which then enter the Krebs cycle. One turn of the Krebs cycle is shown in Fig. 20.9 consists of an acetyl-CoA. The primary function of the Krebs cycle is to generate electrons (H^+) to be transported by NAD^+ and FAD^+ in the respiratory chain. Two $NADH+H^+$ and two or three ATPs from one glucose molecule are formed during the conversion of pyruvate to acetyl-CoA. In the Krebs cycle, a total of six $NADH+H^+$ and two $FADH_2$ are formed.

20.3.3 Electron Transport System

The aerobic production of ATP also called oxidative phosphorylation, takes place in the mitochondria. The main pathway responsible for this process is the electron transport system. $FADH_2$ and $NADH+H^+$ molecules produced from glycolysis and the Krebs cycle transport the ions obtained from the hydrogen atom to the ETS (Fig. 20.10). $NADH+H^+$ and $FADH_2$ molecules do not react directly with oxygen. Instead, electrons removed from hydrogen atoms carried by $NADH+H^+$ and $FADH_2$ are passed through a series of iron-containing electron carriers known as cytochromes, which are attached to the inner mitochondrial membrane. Each cytochrome alternately accepts and releases an electron at a slightly lower energy level as cytochrome b, cytochrome c_1, cytochrome c, cytochrome a, and cytochrome a_3, respectively.

Two different electron carriers entering the ETS produce different amounts of ATP. NAD^+ begins to release its electrons at the beginning of the chain, whereas FAD^+ does not release its electrons until it reaches the second cytochrome along the chain. This difference causes less potential energy to be produced to phosphorylate ATP molecules. As a result, each $NADH+H^+$ molecule available for passage through ETS produces three ATP molecules, while each $FADH_2$ molecule produces two ATP molecules.

As electrons pass through the cytochrome chain, sufficient energy is released to rephosphorylate ADP and generate ATP. This process, driven by the coupling of oxidation of compounds in ETS and phosphorylation of ATP, is called *oxidative phosphorylation*. Eventually, electrons passing through cytochromes at the end of ETS are transferred to molecular oxygen and combined with hydrogen to form the final product water molecule. Oxygen consumption in the aerobic energy system occurs only at this stage. Since oxygen is the last acceptor of electrons in the chain, if there is a decrease in the amount of oxygen to accept electrons at the end of ETS, the entire oxidative phosphorylation process is delayed and ATP formation in the cell tends to occur through anaerobic metabolism.

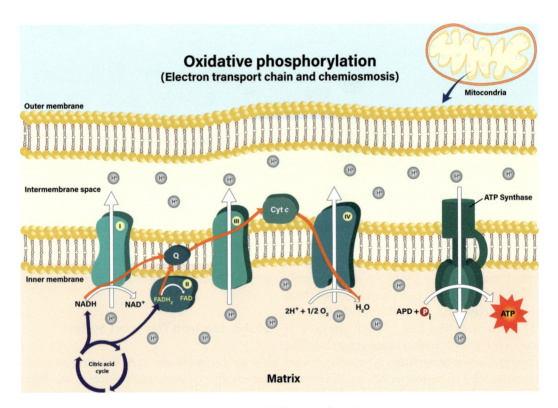

Fig. 20.10 Electron transport system (Kallayanee Naloka/Shutterstock.com)

20.3.4 Total Amount of ATP from Carbohydrates

Two or three ATP molecules are formed by the anaerobic energy system from glycolysis. However, total efficiency should be calculated on the total amount of ATP obtained from the aerobic system (Table 20.1).

20.3.5 Lipid Oxidation

In addition to carbohydrates, the oxidation of lipids also contributes significantly to muscle's energy needs. In addition, storage lipids can provide more energy than glycogen sources stored in the muscle and liver. Fats are stored in muscle fibers and adipose tissue cells in the body. The primary lipid source is free fatty acids (FFA), which are released from the breakdown of triglycerides (glycerol + three fatty acids) supplied from inside or outside the cell. This process is called lipolysis and is controlled by enzymes known as lipases.

Activation of the sympathetic nervous system (SNS) provides a signal that initiates the breakdown of stored triglycerides in muscle or adipose tissue. SNS activation occurs in response to the stress applied to the body, and greater stressors (e.g., moderate-to-vigorous exercise) trigger the release of a major SNS hormone, epinephrine, and activate the lipase enzyme. Activation of the sympathetic nervous system (SNS) provides a signal that initiates the breakdown of stored triglycerides in muscle or adipose tissue. SNS activation occurs in response to the stress applied to the body, and greater stressors (e.g., moderate-to-vigorous exercise) trigger the release of a large SNS hormone, epinephrine, and activate the lipase enzyme. FFAs formed by the breakdown of triglycerides in adipose tissue enter the circulation and most of them bind to albumin, a protein carrier. Albumin is a large water-soluble protein found in blood plasma where particles are suspended. FFA coming from outside the cell pass through the cell membrane and reach the cytosol by certain transporters.

Before FFAs can be used for energy production, they must be converted to acetyl CoA in the mitochondria. This process is called beta-oxidation (β-oxidation). Acetyl-CoA is the common intermediate through which all substrates enter the Krebs cycle for oxidative metabolism. β-oxidation is a series of steps in which two-carbon acyl units are separated from the carbon chain of FFA. The acyl units are then converted to acetyl-CoA, which enters the Krebs cycle for ATP formation. The number of steps depends on the number of carbons in FFA and is usually between 14 and 24 carbons. For example, in palmitate, a 16-carbon FFA, eight molecules of acetyl-CoA are formed by β-oxidation. At the same time, hydrogen electrons are removed and NAD^+ and FAD^+ are reduced to form seven $NADH+H^+$ and seven $FADH_2$. These carriers then enter the ETS. The different FFAs can vary in size, but all that enter the Krebs cycle undergo β-oxidation and the system splits into two carbons to break down into acetyl-CoA. Once they enter the muscle fiber, their FFA must be activated enzymatically by energy from ATP and prepare them for degradation within the mitochondria. As in glycolysis, the input energy of two ATPs is required for activation in β-oxidation. But unlike glycolysis, it does not directly produce ATP.

Table 20.1 Total amount of ATP from carbohydrates

Source	Amount of ATP
Glycolysis	2–3 ATP
2 **NADH+H⁺**: produced during the glycolysis	4–6 ATP
2 **NADH+H⁺**: produced during the conversion of two pyruvate molecules to acetyl-CoA	6 ATP
6 **NADH+H⁺**: produced during the Krebs cycle	18 ATP
2 **FADH₂**: produced during the Krebs cycle	4 ATP
Produced directly in the Krebs cycle	2 ATP
Total	36–39 ATP

20.4 Integrated Function of Energy Systems

It is important to highlight the interaction of anaerobic and aerobic metabolic pathways in ATP production during exercise. While it is common to talk about aerobic and anaerobic exercise, the energy required to perform most types of exercise comes from a combination of the anaerobic and aerobic systems. In fact, ATP production by the ATP-PCr system in contracting skeletal muscles occurs simultaneously with glycolysis and oxidative phosphorylation. However, during periods of very short exercise periods of 1–3 s, the overall contribution of aerobically produced ATP to this movement is low due to the longer time required for the reactions involved in the Krebs cycle and electron transport chain. While the contribution of ATP obtained by the anaerobic system is higher in short-term high-intensity activities, it is seen that aerobic metabolism is dominant in longer activities. For example, about 90% of the energy required to perform a 100-meter sprint comes from anaerobic sources, and most of the energy comes from the ATP-PCr (phosphagen) system. Similarly, the energy in the 400 m run will be largely anaerobic (70–75%). However, ATP and PCr stores are limited and therefore glycolysis provides most of the ATP during such movements.

On the other hand, most of the energy needed in exercises such as marathons is obtained by the aerobic production of ATP. Both anaerobic and aerobic energy systems contribute to energy at different rates for activities of medium length, that is, lasting between 2 and 30 min. In summary, the normal functioning of our energy pathways supports all physical activities in daily life. All our daily activities require energy, whether training as an athlete or doing housework. This energy is collectively provided by three energy systems. Providing the energy required for exercise is not simply a product of the switching on and off of a series of energy systems, but is achieved as a result of the integrated functioning of the three energy systems. Energy systems can contribute to different participation rates depending on the intensity and duration of the movement. The shorter the duration and the higher the intensity of the energy-demanding movement, the greater the contribution of anaerobic energy production; conversely, the longer the duration and the lower the intensity, the greater the contribution of aerobic energy production.

20.5 Capacity of Energy Systems and Effects of Training

Each of the three energy systems undergoes various adaptations in response to exercise training. Short-term high-intensity sprint training or long-term submaximal endurance training, which are two of the most widely applied exercise training types, were examined in detail.

20.5.1 Short-Term, High-Intensity Exercise Training

A significant portion of the ATP demanded during short-duration-high-intensity exercise is met by the phosphagen system and glycolysis. As a result of the effect of high-intensity training, these two systems can increase their capacity and generate ATP more quickly. Resting concentrations of PCr stores in skeletal muscle increase significantly after short-term high-intensity exercise training. The activity of creatine kinase, the rate-limiting enzyme of the phosphagen system, increases. Glucose delivery to working muscles increases and resting concentrations of muscle glycogen increase. The activity of the two rate-limiting enzymes of glycolysis, phosphorylase and phosphofructokinase, increases. To improve the body's capacity to tolerate and remove proton accumulation, the activity of the lactate dehydrogenase enzyme is increased, which allows rapid conversion of pyruvate to lactate when pyruvate production exceeds mitochondrial uptake capacity.

High-intensity interval training (HIIT) has recently been used in clinical and research applications due to its high efficiency in improving cardiovascular endurance and various other physiological parameters. HIIT is generally based on performing periods of high-intensity exercise (20 s–5 min) with alternating periods of rest or mild recovery workloads throughout an exercise session. In general, it is frequently used in sports branches such as athletics or team sports that need both aerobic and anaerobic capacity.

In many published guidelines, 150 min of moderate-intensity exercise per week is recommended for adults in order to provide the target physical activity level and thus contribute to health. However, most of people are not able to implement this recommendation due to time constraints. Studies suggest that HIIT can be a time-efficient strategy to improve the health of all groups if appropriate follow-up is provided.

20.5.2 Long-Term, Submaximal Endurance Training

During prolonged submaximal exercise, the need for ATP is predominantly provided by the aerobic system. After endurance training, the capacity of the aerobic system to produce ATP increases. One of the most important adaptations is the increase in the mass and number of mitochondria, also known as mitochondrial density. Thus, it also increases the enzymatic activities in the beta-oxidation and Krebs cycle.

Endurance training also causes an increase in glucose and FFA delivery for energy production and in resting concentrations of muscle glycogen. It increases the capacity of carbohydrate and lipid metabolism and thus improves performance. Increased muscle glycogen content means that glycolysis can continue at optimum rates for longer. Moreover, increased pyruvate uptake and oxidation capacity provide the potential to increase ATP production through aerobic energy and maintain balanced levels of exercise at higher intensities. Endurance training raises the lactate threshold.

However, physiological adaptations to endurance training are not limited to events within the skeletal muscle cell. Increased blood volume, left ventricular volume, and capillary density in the cardiovascular system; other system adaptations, such as the development of respiratory muscles in the pulmonary system and the exhalation of larger volumes of air, all together with cellular adaptations increase overall metabolic efficiency.

20.6 Conclusion

Both anaerobic and aerobic metabolic pathways provide energy in the form of ATP to muscle cells to perform physical activity. Intramuscular storage ATP, PCr (phosphagen system), and glycolysis are anaerobic energy pathways, and they are the predominant energy sources for short-term high-intensity physical activities. Carbohydrates, lipids, and proteins can be metabolized aerobically in the mitochondria by the Krebs cycle and the electron transport system. Normally, carbohydrates and triglycerides are the predominant nutrients for the aerobic system, while proteins in amino acid form are minimally metabolized as a source of energy. Aerobic metabolism is the predominant source of ATP for prolonged low-intensity physical activities. However, many physical activities used during activities of daily life and exercise occur with the important interaction of aerobic and anaerobic metabolism. Both aerobic and anaerobic energy systems adapt to exercise training with various adaptations such as increasing enzyme activity and substrate availability. Knowing these characteristics is important for optimizing physical performance and developing exercise training strategies.

Further Reading

Birch K, George K, McLaren D. Energy sources and exercise. In: Birch K, McLaren D, George K, editors. BIOS instant notes in sport and exercise physiology. Taylor & Francis; 2005. p. 11–16.

Kenney WL, Wilmore JH, Costill DL. Fuel for exercise: bioenergetics and muscle metabolism. In: Kenney WL, Wilmore JH, Costill DL, editors. Physiology of sport and exercise. Human Kinetics Publishers; 2020. p. 162–215.

Kraemer WJ, Fleck SJ, Deschenes MR. Bioenergetics and meeting the metabolic demand for energy. In: Kraemer WJ, Fleck SJ, Deschenes MR, editors. Exercise physiology: integrating theory and application. Lippincott Williams & Wilkins; 2012. p. 26–66.

McArdle WD, Katch FI, Katch VL. Energy transfer in the body. In: McArdle WD, Katch FI, Katch VL, editors. Exercise physiology: nutrition, energy, and human performance. Lippincott Williams & Wilkins; 2015a. p. 134–61.

McArdle WD, Katch FI, Katch VL. Energy for physical activity. In: McArdle WD, Katch FI, Katch VL, editors. Exercise physiology: nutrition, energy, and human performance. Lippincott Williams & Wilkins; 2015b. p. 162–77.

Powers SK, Howley ET, Quindry J. Energy transfer in the body. In: Powers SK, Howley ET, Quindry J, editors. Exercise physiology: theory and application to fitness and performance. New York: McGraw-Hill Education; 2018a. p. 134–61.

Powers SK, Howley ET, Quindry J. Energy transfer during exercise. In: Powers SK, Howley ET, Quindry J, editors. Exercise physiology: theory and application to fitness and performance. New York: McGraw-Hill Education; 2018b. p. 162–77.

Porcari J, Bryant C, Comana F. Bioenergetics of exercise and energy transfer. In: Porcari J, Bryant C, Comana F, editors. Exercise physiology. F.A. Davis Company; 2015. p. 64–96.

Saghiv MS. Metabolism. In: Saghiv MS, editor. Basic exercise physiology: clinical and laboratory perspectives. Springer; 2020. p. 33–74.

Respiratory System and Its Adaptations to Exercise

21

Dilara Saklica

Abstract

It is essential to know the anatomy and the physiology of the respiratory system to be able to observe, evaluate, and interpret possible physiological responses during exercise training. When planning exercise training for respiratory system pathologies, acute and chronic adaptation mechanisms that vary according to the type of exercise guide us to eliminate ventilatory failure. Predicting situations that may arise during exercise training reduces possible risks and helps the patient get the maximum benefit.

This section will explain the anatomy and the physiology of the respiratory system, acute and chronic adaptations to exercise training, factors affecting the adaptation, possible complications that may occur during or after exercise for respiratory system pathologies, and ways to deal with them.

21.1 Anatomy

The anatomy of the respiratory system includes all the structures involved in the process necessary for the continuation of life: bringing in oxygen, converting it into carbon dioxide, and flushing it out.

21.1.1 Nose

The nose is the starting point of the respiratory system and is responsible for warming, moistening, and filtering the inhaled air. It consists of two main parts: the external nose or "Nasus Externus" and the nasal cavity or "Cavitas Nasi." The nasal septum separates cavitas nasi into two cavities: nares or the nostrils are the openings to the outside, while choanae lead to the nasopharynx. The nasal cavity is divided into three parts according to its functions: nasal vestibule, respiratory region, and olfactory region. The nasal vestibule filters the air through the hair inside. The mucosa of the respiratory region is covered with multilayered, ciliated, prismatic epithelium cells, and this area moistens and warms up the air inhaled. The olfactory region is the area concerning the sense of smell. There are three convexes in the lateral wall of the nasal cavity called superior nasal concha, middle nasal concha, and inferior nasal concha (Fig. 21.1).

21.1.2 Larynx

The larynx, located between the C3-C6 vertebrae, is a structure consisting of cartilage, ligaments,

D. Saklica (✉)
Faculty of Physical Therapy and Rehabilitation, Hacettepe University, Ankara, Turkey
Email: dilarasaklica@hacettepe.edu.tr

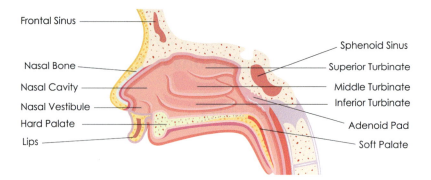

Fig. 21.1 Nose (stockshoppe/Shutterstock.com)

NOSE

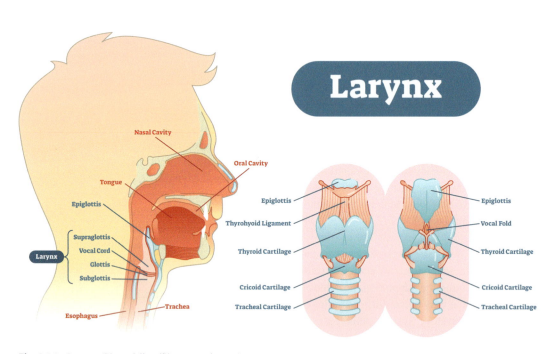

Fig. 21.2 Larynx (VectorMine /Shutterstock.com)

membranes, and muscles. The essential function of the larynx for the respiratory system is to protect the lower respiratory tract during foreign body aspiration. It is located below the hyoid bone and above the trachea. The unpaired cartilages of the larynx are called thyroid cartilage, cricoid cartilage, and epiglottis, while the paired cartilages are named arytenoid cartilage, corniculate cartilage, and cuneiform cartilage (Fig. 21.2).

21.1.3 Thorax

The thorax (rib cage) is a formation of bones and cartilage structure between the neck and the abdomen. Thorax consists of the sternum, costal cartilages, and front ends of ribs on the anterior, while T1-T12 vertebrae and back ends of ribs make up the posterior. The upper aperture is named superior thoracic aperture (sternum on the

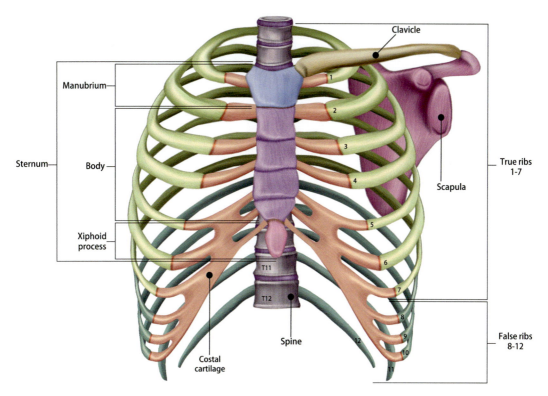

Fig. 21.3 Thorax (studiovin/Shutterstock.com)

anterior, 1st ribs on the sides, T1 vertebra at the posterior), while the lower aperture is named inferior thoracic aperture (xiphoid process on the anterior, costal margin, and 11-12th ribs on the sides, T12 vertebra at the posterior). There are a total of 12 pairs of ribs. The last two pairs at the front are floating ribs (Fig. 21.3).

The cavity between two ribs is named intercostal space, and this cavity includes muscles named external intercostal muscles, internal intercostal muscles, and innermost intercostal muscles. There are also other muscles such as transversus thoracis muscle (inserts into the costal cartilage behind the sternum), levatores costarum muscles (located like external intercostal muscles), and subcostal muscles (fibers of which are parallel to internal intercostal muscles fibers). The most essential function of the thorax is to participate in breathing, in addition to protecting the heart, lungs, and some abdominal structures.

21.1.4 Trachea

The trachea extends from the larynx and is related to respiratory function. All sides of the trachea are covered in membrana elastica tracheae, and this membrane becomes thicker between two adjacent cartilages (18–20 pieces of C-shaped rings) and makes up the annular ligament. The up and down movement of the trachea during breathing is possible as a result of the elasticity of these ligaments. Its inner face is covered with multilayered, ciliated epithelium (Fig. 21.4).

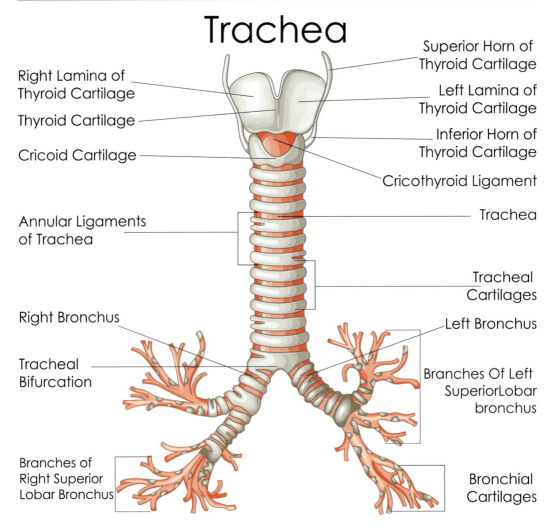

Fig. 21.4 Trachea (Vecton/Shutterstock.com)

The trachea begins at the level of the C6 vertebra; at the level of the C5 vertebra and the point of the tracheal bifurcation, it divides into two parts named the right primary bronchus and the left primary bronchus. The right primary bronchus divides into three parts called the right superior lobar bronchus, middle lobar bronchus, and the right inferior lobar bronchus. The primary left bronchus divides into two parts called the left superior lobar bronchus and the left inferior lobar bronchus. Since the lower respiratory tract is associated with trees because of its branching, it is also called the bronchial tree. The area in the airways up to the distal of terminal bronchioles is named conductive airways. Gas exchange does not occur in this section. The respiratory bronchioles, the alveolar duct, the alveolar sac, and the pulmonary alveolus are named the pulmonary acinus as it is where gas exchange takes place.

21.1.5 Lungs

The lungs, located in the thoracic cavity, are the organs responsible for the gas exchange between the air and blood. Its uppermost part or the apex pulmonis extends from the back of the clavicle to the neck. Its lowermost point or the basis pulmonis is located above the diaphragm. Lungs divide into lobes with fissures. The right lung consists of the superior lobe, the middle lobe, and the inferior lobe, while the left lung consists of the superior lobe and the inferior lobe (Fig. 21.5). If you examine the projection of the lungs on the thorax, you can see that its anterior lower edges end at the level of the T6 and T8 vertebrae, and the posterior edge ends at the level of the T10 vertebra.

The vessels that feed the lung tissue and the vessels that transport blood from and to the heart and the lungs are different. Bronchial arteries nourish lung tissues, and bronchial veins collect venous blood. Vessels that carry blood from the heart to the lungs to nourish the blood with oxygen are pulmonary arteries, and the vessels that carry the oxygen-rich blood from the lungs to the heart are pulmonary veins (Fig. 21.6).

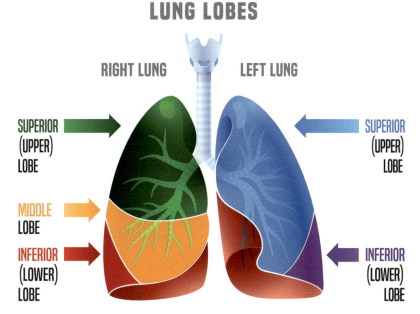

Fig. 21.5 Pulmonary lobes (Double Brain/Shutterstock.com)

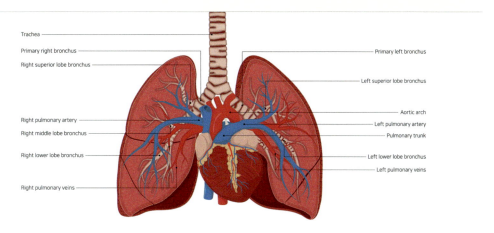

Fig. 21.6 Pulmonary arteries and veins (cono0430/Shutterstock.com)

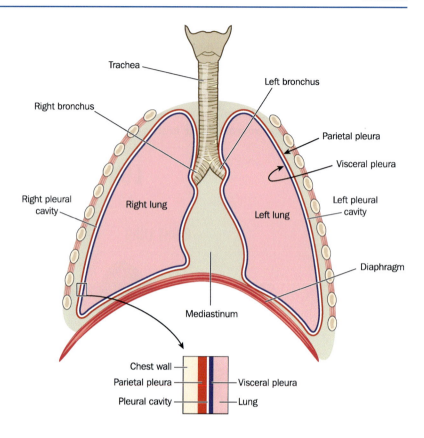

Fig. 21.7 Pleura (Blamb/Shutterstock.com)

21.1.6 Pleura

The pleura is a serous membrane that surrounds the lungs, and consists of two layers called the parietal pleura and the visceral pleura. The visceral pleura adheres to the lung tissue and tightly lines each lobe. It then continues as the parietal pleura. The parietal pleura lines the inner side of the ribs, forming the pleural cavity. The liquid in this cavity prevents friction between the two membranes (Fig. 21.7).

21.1.7 Diaphragm

The diaphragm is the fibromuscular structure that separates the thorax and the abdominal cavity. It serves as a respiratory muscle. When it contracts, it gets straight towards the abdomen and reduces the pressure in the thoracic cavity, increasing its volume. When it relaxes, it returns to its dome shape and increases the thoracic pressure, reducing its volume. It consists of three parts called the sternal diaphragm, the costal diaphragm, and the lumbar diaphragm. The cavities on the diaphragm allow the passage of some formations. These are aortic hiatus (at the T12 level, aorta current), esophageal hiatus (at the T10 level, esophagus, and vagus nerve current), and vena cava foramen (at the T8-T9 level, inferior vena cava and right the phrenic nerve current). It is innerved by the phrenic nerve (C3-C5).

21.2 Physiology

The purpose of the respiratory system is to maintain the concentration of O_2, CO_2, and H^+ ions at optimal levels. Respiration has four main functions. These are air conduction between the atmosphere and the alveoli (pulmonary ventilation), O_2-CO_2 diffusion between the alveoli and the blood, carrying O_2-CO_2 in the blood and body fluids, and the regulation of respiration. To better understand the physiology of the respiratory system, it is necessary to learn some concepts and understand their importance for the respiratory system.

Ventilation: The process of the air's mechanical entry to and exit from the lungs.

Pulmonary ventilation: Inspiring air in the atmosphere and exchanging it with air in the lung.

Inspiration: Inhaling, breathing. Inspiration at rest occurs by the contraction of the diaphragm. This way, the thoracic volume increases, the intrathoracic pressure decreases, and the air enter the lungs. During inspiration, the external intercostal muscles contract alongside the diaphragm, and the internal intercostal muscles relax. Ribs move upwards, increasing the anterior-posterior diameter of the thorax (bucket handle movement); with the contraction of the diaphragm, the vertical diameter increases. As a result, air fills the lungs.

Expiration: Exhalation. Expiration at rest occurs passively due to the relaxation of the diaphragm and the elastic retraction of the lungs. The internal intercostal muscles pull lower ribs towards the diaphragm. This condition causes the anterior-posterior diameter to decrease, and the air leaves the lungs.

In abnormal situations, other muscles along with the above-mentioned muscles come into play during inspiration or expiration. These muscles are called accessory respiratory muscles (Table 21.1).

Cough reflex: Rapidly removing the air inhaled after a quick inspiration, using all the expiratory muscles.

Respiratory rate: The number of breaths a person takes in a minute. The resting respiratory rate of an adult is 12 breaths per minute.

Work of breathing: The energy expended on respiration. In a healthy individual, the energy expended for inspiration corresponds to 3–5% of the total energy. With respiratory diseases, this rate increases.

Valsalva maneuver: The forced expiration against a closed glottis. Intrathoracic pressure is compressed to the vein walls—the blood returning to the heart decreases. Arterial blood pressure decreases. Cerebral blood flow decreases. In cases where it is repeated several times in a row, dizziness or fainting may occur.

Diffusion: The transition of molecules from a dense environment to a lower density environment without expending energy. In the respiratory system, since the amount of oxygen in the air inhaled is higher than the amount of oxygen in the venous blood of the lungs, oxygen tends to diffuse into the blood inside the vessel. Similarly, carbon dioxide in the veins diffuses into the lungs.

Elastic recoil: The negative pressure between the two pleural membranes (the thoracic wall and the lung) creates a suction force. This condition causes the lung to move as if it is attached to the inner wall of the thorax. With inspiration, the pressure in the pleura decreases (-5 cmH$_2$O → -7.5 cmH$_2$O). Meanwhile, the glottis is open, and when the airflow entering the lungs stops, the alveolar pressure equalizes to atmospheric pressure (the moment before the completion of inhalation and the transition to exhalation). The difference between the alveolar and the pleural pressure (also called transpulmonary pressure) forms the elastic recoil. At the beginning of inspiration, the alveolar pressure decreases by one cmHg, creating negative pressure that allows air to fill the lungs.

Pulmonary compliance: The amount of expansion in the volume of the lungs in response to each one-unit increase in the transpulmonary pressure. In an average adult, the volume of air corresponding to the change of 1 cmH$_2$O in transpulmonary pressure is 200 mL. While compliance decreases in restrictive lung diseases, it increases in obstructive lung diseases.

Table 21.1 Accessory respiratory muscles

	Inspiration	Expiration
Accessory respiratory muscles	Sternocleidomastoid (lifts the sternum upwards) Pectoral muscles Serratus anterior (lifts the ribs upwards) Serratus posterior superior Iliocostalis (upper)	Abdominal muscles (brings the ribs closer to the diaphragm) Iliocostalis (lower) Longissimus (lower) Serratus posterior inferior

Alveolar-capillary membrane: The structure consisting of the fluid on the surface of the alveolar mucosa, the alveolar epithelial cell, the alveolar basement membrane, the interstitial space, the capillary endothelial cell, and the capillary basement membrane (Fig. 21.8).

Surfactant: Secreted from the type II cells in the alveoli. Surfactant helps to prevent an end-expiratory collapse of the alveoli by reducing the surface tension.

Alveolar ventilation: The rate at which the fresh air enters the gas exchange areas in the lungs. Alveolar ventilation depends on the tidal volume, respiratory rate, and dead space volume.

Collateral ventilation: Gas exchange by diffusion occurs between the alveoli and the capillaries located side by side. This area is a diffusion zone where oxygen and carbon dioxide exchange occur. Gas exchange also occurs between the neighboring alveoli through the pores of Kohn in the alveolar structure. This way, ventilation can occur indirectly in damaged or restricted alveoli (e.g., emphysema). This type of ventilation is named collateral ventilation.

Anatomical dead space: The volume of areas without gas exchange, such as the nose, the larynx, and the trachea, which serve as conductive airways in the respiratory system. The air that circulates in these areas during inspiration is the air that leaves the body first during expiration without undergoing any exchange. The anatomical dead space is about 150 mL for an adult.

Physiologic dead space: The volume of air that fills the alveoli which have damaged capillaries or structures for some reason, plus the anatomical dead space. Since these regions are damaged, they cannot participate in the gas exchange. If the alveoli or capillaries are not damaged, the anatomical dead space and the physiologic dead space are equivalent in a healthy individual.

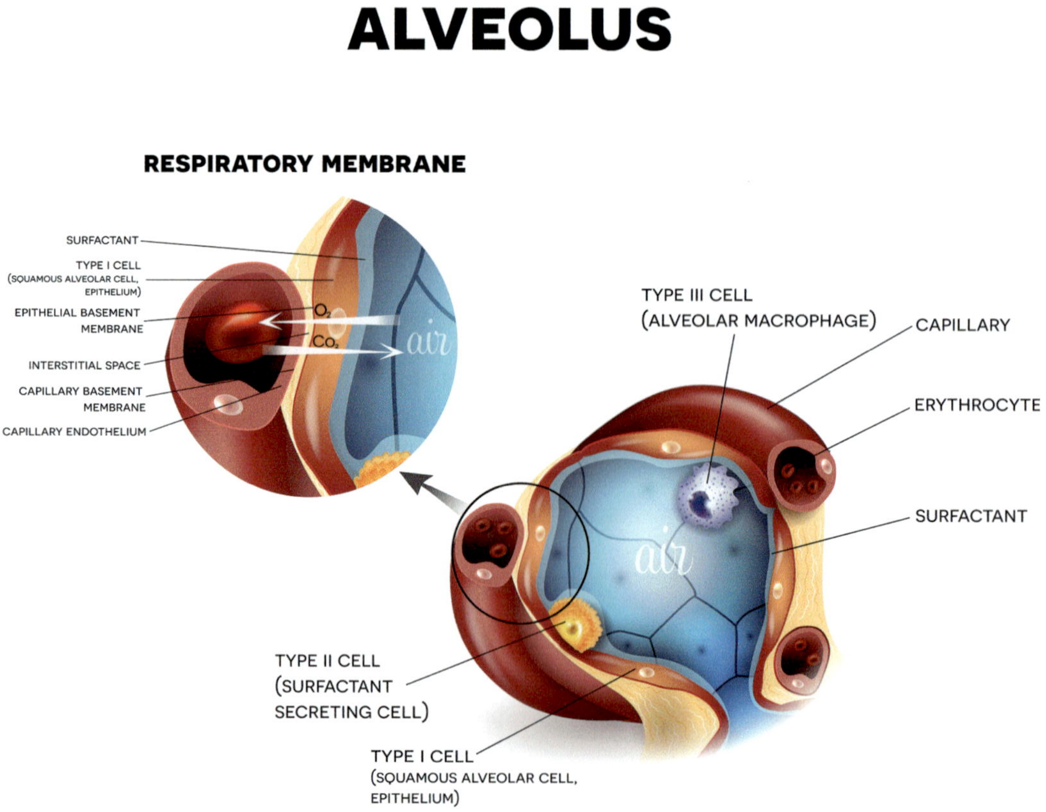

Fig. 21.8 Structure of the alveoli (TimeLineArtist/Shutterstock.com)

Ventilation/perfusion ratio (V_A/Q): While some parts of the lung are well ventilated, other parts are insufficiently ventilated. Similarly, while perfusion is at a sufficient level in some alveolar capillaries, it is insufficient in other areas. The alveolar ventilation and perfusion relationship are called the ventilation/perfusion ratio. In a healthy individual at rest, ventilation is 4–5 L per minute, while perfusion is 5 L per minute. In this case, the standard V_A/Q ratio is 1. When the physiologic dead space increases, even if enough air reaches the alveoli, perfusion is insufficient due to alveolar/capillary damage. Thus, the V_A/Q ratio increases, and ventilation efficiency decreases.

Physiological shunt: As a result of insufficient ventilation of the alveoli (e.g., bronchial obstruction), oxygenation is insufficient even though the blood flow in the capillaries is sufficient. This condition reduces the amount of oxygen in the blood in the venous circulation through the pulmonary capillaries. Thus, the V_A/Q ratio decreases. The abnormal V_A/Q ratio in patients with COPD (chronic obstructive pulmonary disease) is due to the physiological shunt with bronchial obstruction in some places and physiological dead space with alveolar wall damage caused by emphysema in other places. This is the most common cause of lung failure.

Minute ventilation: The respiratory rate multiplied by the tidal volume equals the minute ventilation (V_E). If we take the tidal volume as 500 mL and the respiratory rate as 12 breaths per minute, the minute ventilation is 6 L. Minute ventilation does not always reflect alveolar ventilation.

The ventilatory equivalent for oxygen: The ratio of minute ventilation to oxygen consumption (V_E/VO_2). A healthy young adult corresponds to the level at which 1 L of oxygen is taken from approximately 25 L of air in a submaximal exercise (55% VO_{2max}).

a-V O_2 difference: The muscle tissue's need for oxygen is named the arteriovenous oxygen difference. a-V O_2 in 100 mL of blood is 4–5 mL at rest.

21.2.1 Lung Volumes and Capacities

Lung volume and capacity vary depending on age, sex, height, and body weight. Lung volumes measured without a time limit are called static lung volumes, while those measured under a time limit are called dynamic lung volumes.

21.2.1.1 Static Lung Volumes

In normal respiration, the total volume of air entering the lung (inspired air) plus the air leaving the lung (expired air) is called the tidal volume (TV). On average, tidal volume is 500 mL in a healthy adult. The anatomical dead space increases with the tidal volume. The volume of air a person can breathe as deeply as possible after a regular inspiration while resting is called the inspiratory reserve volume (IRV) and is about 1.5–3 L. The sum of the inspiratory reserve volume and the tidal volume is the inspiratory capacity (IC). The maximum amount of air a person can exhale after a normal expiration, while resting is named the expiratory reserve volume (ERV) and is about 1–1.5 L. The total volume of the maximum expiration after the maximum inspiration is called the vital capacity (VC). This value is 3–4 L for women and up to 5–6 L for men. While this value is higher in taller people, the level of physical activity also affects the vital capacity. It is at higher levels for White people than for Asians or Black people. This difference is due to the ratio of body and height length varying in different ethnic groups, differences in the ratio of fat-free mass, and various factors such as respiratory muscle strength. No matter how deep the expiration is, some air remains in the lungs. This air volume is called the residual volume (RV). This prevents the collapse of the alveoli, and the gas exchange between the alveoli and the blood is not interrupted. The residual volume on average is 1 L for women and 1.2 L for men. As a result of the elasticity loss of the lung tissue with age, the inspiratory and the expiratory volumes decrease, and in turn, the residual volume increases. The sum of the expiratory reserve volume and the residual volume is the functional residual capacity (FRC). Total lung capacity (TLC) is the sum of vital capacity and residual volume (Fig. 21.9).

$$IRV + ERV + TV = VC$$

$$ERV + RV = FRC$$

$$VC + RV = TLC$$

Regular TLC, FRC, and RV limits are 80–120%. TLC drops below 80% in restrictive lung diseases; when pulmonary hyperinflation develops in obstructive diseases, the volumes increase above 120%. An increase in lung volumes occurs in diseases accompanied by airway obstruction (e.g., COPD). This increase occurs primarily in RV and FRC, but TLC is also affected in the following periods. In all diseases that cause a restrictive respiratory defect, TLC decrease occurs, often accompanied by a decrease in VC. In interstitial lung diseases, RV is stable while TLC decreases; thus, the RV/TLC ratio increases. TLC may be an indicator of survival in interstitial lung diseases. In neuromuscular diseases, VC often decreases when respiratory muscle weakness occurs. While inspiratory muscle weakness obstructs maximal inspiration, expiratory muscle weakness obstructs deep expiration, as a result of which RV increases. A decrease in the chest wall and lung compliance also further decreases VC.

21.2.1.2 Dynamic Lung Volumes

Forced expiratory volume (the air exhaled) in 1 s is FEV_1. FEV_1 value indicates expiratory strength and resistance to air movement in the lung. Its average value is 80%. In obstructive pulmonary diseases such as emphysema or bronchial asthma, FEV_1 can decrease down to 40% of vital capacity. Forced vital capacity (FVC) is measured by rapid and forced expiration after maximal inspiration. The maximum flow during the FVC maneuver is called the peak expiratory flow (PEF). Maximum voluntary ventilation (MVV) is assessed by having a person breathe fast and regularly for 15 s, and this value is calculated based on 1 min. On average, it is 140–180 L/min for an adult man and 80–120 L/min for an adult woman (Fig. 21.10). In healthy people, the time to empty 80% of the lung volume is 6 s or less. In people with severe obstruction, this period can last up to 20 s. In the presence of obstructive disease, the MVV value barely reaches 40% of what it should be. The decrease in FEV_1/FVC ratio indicates obstruction, while FEV_1 indicates the severity of obstruction.

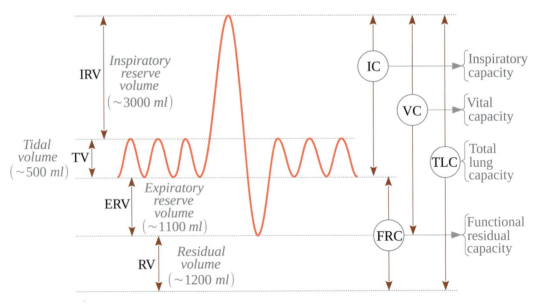

Fig. 21.9 Lung volumes and capacities (ScientificStock/Shutterstock.com)

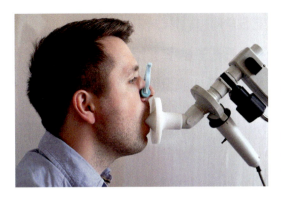

Fig. 21.10 Spirometry (RealPeopleStudio/Shutterstock.com)

Breathing reserve index: The ratio of minute ventilation in maximal exercise ($V_E$max) to the voluntary ventilation at rest is called the breathing reserve index (BRI). The MVV needs to be measured for 12 s to calculate the BRI. The BRI can also be estimated by multiplying the FEV_1 value by 40. While a regular person can maintain 15 min of exercise in 70% of the BRI, sedentary people cannot reach values above 75%. This condition indicates that the VO_{2max} of regular people is limited by cardiac factors instead of ventilatory factors. Patients with parenchymal lung disease typically have low BRI.

21.2.2 Respiratory Gas Exchange and Transport

Under normal conditions, room air contains nitrogen (79.04%), oxygen (20.93%), carbon dioxide (0.03%), and water vapor. Partial pressures (the percentage of concentration in the environment multiplied by the total pressure of the gas mixture) of these gases in the alveoli, tissues, and blood differ. The partial pressure of oxygen in the alveoli (P_AO_2) is 103 mmHg, and partial pressure of carbon dioxide in the alveoli (P_ACO_2) is 39 mmHg. The partial pressure of oxygen in the arterial blood (PaO_2) is 95 mmHg, and partial pressure of carbon dioxide in the arterial blood ($PaCO_2$) is 40 mmHg. The partial pressure of oxygen in the tissue or the muscle (PO_2) is 40 mmHg, and the partial pressure of carbon dioxide in the tissue or the muscle (PCO_2) is 40 mmHg.

The regeneration duration of air in the alveoli is relatively long. This condition requires the respiratory control mechanisms to be stable. Alveolar ventilation is adjusted according to metabolic needs. Even when breathing is interrupted for short periods, the respiratory control mechanisms can tolerate O_2, CO_2, and pH changes in the tissues. For emphysema, diffusion is insufficient because the surface area of the respiratory membrane (caused by the junction of the alveoli) decreases. O_2 diffusion in the pulmonary capillaries occurs according to the partial oxygen pressure (PO_2). Since the oxygen pressure in the tissue is low at the arterial end of the circulation, oxygen molecules tend to diffuse into the tissue. At the venous end, carbon dioxide molecules are removed from the tissue since the partial pressure of carbon dioxide in the tissue (PCO_2) increases (Fig. 21.11). As the diffusion rate of carbon dioxide is higher, it can be easily removed from the tissue even at a low-pressure change.

While 99% of oxygen in the blood is carried through hemoglobin, 1% of it is found in plasma as dissolved (PaO_2). Hemoglobin levels are 15–16 g/100 mL of blood for men, while 14 g/100 mL of blood for women. The essential task of hemoglobin is to keep the oxygen pressure in the tissues stable. As long as PO_2 is high, hemoglobin does not release the oxygen it is bound to. In cases where oxygen demand increases, such as exercise (when PO_2 decreases), oxygen is released (Fig. 21.12). Thanks to this, in situations where the partial oxygen pressure in the atmosphere changes, such as high altitude or deep diving, PO_2 is stable. A decrease in the erythrocyte iron levels (iron deficiency anemia) reduces the O_2-carrying capacity of the blood.

In blood, 70% of carbon dioxide is transported in the form of bicarbonate ions (HCO_3^-), 20% in the form of carbaminohemoglobin (CO_2Hgb), and 10% as dissolved.

$$CO_2 + H_2O \rightarrow H_2CO_3 \rightarrow HCO_3^- + H^+$$

If this reaction does not occur, the partial pressure of carbon dioxide in the tissue (PCO_2)

External respiration gas exchange between alveoli and capillaries

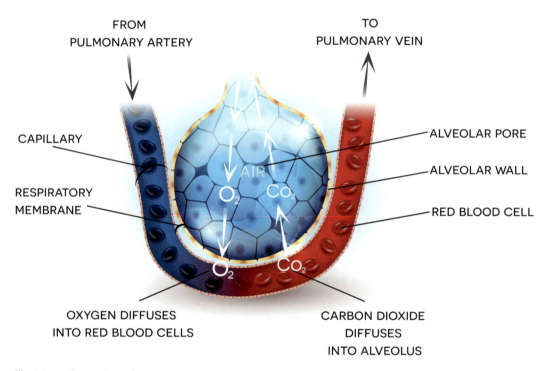

Fig. 21.11 Gas exchange between the alveoli and pulmonary capillaries (TimeLineArtist/Shutterstock.com)

increases too much, causing acidosis in the tissue.

The Bohr effect is when the affinity of hemoglobin changes from CO_2 to O_2. This occurs directly or by H^+. Hemoglobin's change of affinity for CO_2 depending on the saturation of O_2 is called the Haldane effect. The relationship between PO_2 and O_2 attaching to the hemoglobin in the oxygen is named the oxygen-hemoglobin (or oxyhemoglobin) dissociation curve.

The ratio of the speed of carbon dioxide removed from the body to the speed of oxygen taken into the body is called the respiratory exchange ratio (R). If the metabolism uses carbohydrates as the energy source, then $R \cong 1$; if it uses fat, $R \cong 0.7$.

The protein that binds oxygen in the skeletal and heart muscles is called myoglobin. It serves as storage for intramuscular oxygen. Even at low oxygen partial pressures, it easily binds O_2 to itself (its affinity is high). It is found in large quantities in muscle fibers with high aerobic capacity (slow-twitch or type I).

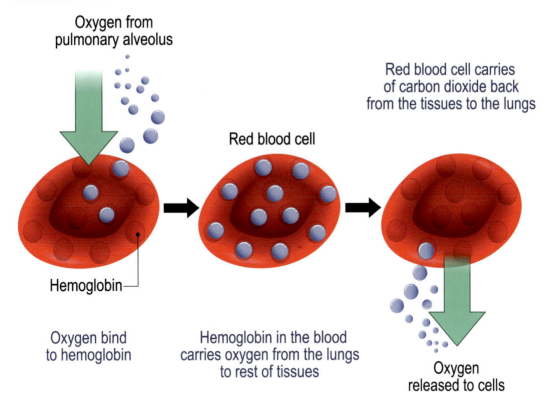

Fig. 21.12 Hemoglobin carrying O_2 (Designua/Shutterstock.com)

21.2.3 Regulation of Respiration

21.2.3.1 Central Control of Respiration

The respiratory center comprises bilateral neurons in the medulla oblongata and pons (central control). There are dorsal and ventral respiratory group neurons in the medulla oblongata. The dorsal respiratory group neurons are located in the nucleus tractus solitarius. These neurons are responsible for inspiration. The inspiratory signal is a ramp signal. The firing rate of the signal to the diaphragm starts slowly and increases gradually. Then, it abruptly stops. When the signal stops, the diaphragm relaxes while the lung is slowly expanding. Respiration accelerates by a short expiration after a short inspiration. Also, the peripheral chemoreceptors, baroreceptors, and sensory fibers of the vagus and the glossopharyngeal nerves that carry the sensory impulses to the respiratory center end in the nucleus tractus solitarius. (Fig. 21.13).

The ventral respiratory group neurons are located in the nucleus retroambiguus. They are inactive during restful breathing. In case of a high need for pulmonary ventilation, the impulses coming from the dorsal group spread to the ventral group neurons. Stimulation of some of the ventral group neurons supports inspiration, while some neurons support expiration by causing the contraction of the abdominal muscles.

The pneumotaxic center in the pons transmits incoming signals to inspiration-related areas. It is responsible for controlling the sudden switch-off of the inspiration ramp. The pneumotaxic center also limits inspiration through the vagus nerve. The limitation of inspiration leads to a rapid expiration. In this case, the respiratory rate increases. While a strong pneumotaxic signal increases the respiratory rate, a weak one decreases it.

In addition to the centers in the brain stem, the stress receptors in the lung tissue also can switch off the inspiration ramp when the lungs are overstretched. When the tidal volume increases above

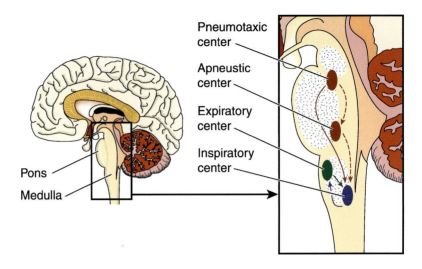

Fig. 21.13 Respiratory centers (Blamb/Shutterstock.com)

1 L, the receptors are stimulated, and the inspiration ramp is switched off by the vagus nerve and dorsal respiratory neurons. A rapid expiration occurs after a rapid inspiration. The breathing depth decreases, and the respiratory rate increases. This reflex is called the Expansion reflex or the Hering–Breuer reflex.

21.2.3.2 Chemical Control of Respiration

Central chemoreceptors located in the medulla oblongata are susceptible to changes in CO_2 and H^+ ion concentration. It is worth noting that none of the previously mentioned ventral, dorsal, or pneumotaxic centers are affected by these ions. A decrease or increase in O_2 in the blood does not stimulate the respiratory centers of the brain. It is necessary to remember this principle when providing oxygen support to patients. Another chemoreceptor area is the aorta and carotid bodies, where peripheral chemoreceptors are located. These areas are sensitive to oxygen exchange.

$$CO_2 + H_2O \rightarrow H_2CO_3 \rightarrow H^+ + HCO_3^-$$

When the level of carbon dioxide in the arterial blood increases, two things occur: (1) Acute strong effect: Increased level of carbon dioxide in the cerebrospinal fluid (CSF) stimulates respiration in seconds. The buffer effect is minimal. The ventilation rate increases. (2) Chronic weak effect: The kidneys increase HCO_3^- in the blood, causing the buffer of H^+ ions generated as a result of the reaction mentioned above. The effect declines due to the concentration of H^+ ions. The patient adapts.

When the level of oxygen in the arterial blood decrease, two things occur: (1) Acute weak effect: Acutely reduced oxygen pressure stimulates peripheral chemoreceptors. Ventilation increases by 70%—$PaCO_2$ decreases. Peripheral chemoreceptor activity decreases. (2) Chronic strong effect: HCO_3^- in CSF decreases. HCO_3^- in the kidneys decreases. Ventilation increases (by 400–500%). After 2–3 days, the patient adapts to low oxygen pressure.

Other factors regulating respiration:

Pulmonary irritant receptors: These are sensory nerve endings in the epithelium of the trachea, the bronchi, and the bronchioles. They cause a cough or sneeze against irritants.

Pulmonary J receptors: They are located near the pulmonary capillaries. They are stimulated when the capillaries expand or in cases of pulmonary edema in heart failure. It causes dyspnea. Rapid and shallow breathing develops.

Bronchopulmonary C-fibers: They are stimulated by histamine. It increases mucus secretion.

21.2.3.3 Neural Control of the Bronchi

Smooth muscles in the walls of the bronchi are stimulated by norepinephrine/epinephrine secreted from the adrenal gland instead of being directly stimulated by sympathetic fibers. Epinephrine stimulates the beta-adrenergic receptors and causes dilatation of the bronchial walls. Parasympathetic nerve fibers originating from the vagus nerve secrete acetylcholine, which causes vasoconstriction in the bronchioles.

21.3 Acute Response of the Respiratory System to Aerobic Exercise

From the moment of transition from rest to exercise, body systems adapt to the changes in cardiorespiratory needs. These adaptations may be limited to the moment of exercise (acute) or may become permanent as a result of exercise training (chronic).

During exercise, alveolar ventilation increases so that appropriate gas concentrations can be maintained. The respiratory rate and the tidal volume (both or alone) lead to an increase in minute ventilation (Fig. 21.14). If the nervous impulses are insufficient for the regulation of breathing during exercise, chemical factors come into play. The change in partial pressures of oxygen and carbon dioxide in the muscles and the blood and the H+ ion concentration causes the stimulation of chemoreceptors, regulating breathing according to changing needs. Another reason for increased ventilation is that the brain simultaneously stimulates the respiratory center while signaling muscles to contract (Golgi tendon organs). Thus, an increase in ventilation occurs without the need. This is the reason behind a small amount of decrease in $PaCO_2$ at the start of the workout. $PaCO_2$ returns to its average level with carbon dioxide passing through the muscles into the blood. While the number of H+ ions decreases with skeletal muscle exercise, it also causes an increase of potassium ions outside the cell. The increased potassium levels also act as a stimulant for chemoreceptors. Ventilation does not limit aerobic capacity in a healthy individual. However, in the presence of a respiratory system pathology, the ability to breathe decreases, and the consumption of oxygen and pulmonary ventilation are inconsistent with each other. This condition causes a decrease in the ventilatory equivalent for oxygen.

In high-intensity exercise, while the respiratory frequency measurement is 35–45 breaths/min for healthy young adults, it is 60–76 breaths/min for elite athletes with the same type of exercise. While the tidal volume during exercise can reach 2 L and above, the minute ventilation can go up to 100 L or even 17 times more than the resting value. An increase in the tidal volume and the respiratory rate causes more respiratory muscles to participate in the work of breathing. The increase in tidal volume occurs due to the inspiratory and expiratory reserve volumes. This increases the oxygen expenditure in ventilation. Respiratory muscles are skeletal muscles, and

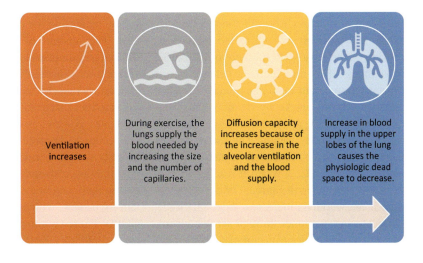

Fig. 21.14 Respiratory system's acute response to aerobic exercise

Ventilation increases

During exercise, the lungs supply the blood needed by increasing the size and the number of capillaries.

Diffusion capacity increases because of the increase in the alveolar ventilation and the blood supply.

Increase in blood supply in the upper lobes of the lung causes the physiologic dead space to decrease.

they are functionally similar to locomotor muscles. Although the first studies in this field defined the respiratory muscles as *"fatigueless,"* later studies have shown that prolonged or high-intensity exercise can cause fatigue in the respiratory muscles. High-intensity exercise causes deterioration in the V_A/Q ratio.

The increase in ventilation while exercising is both neural and due to the interaction of chemoreceptors with the respiratory control center.

With exercise, increased heat in the contracting muscles causes the oxyhemoglobin dissociation curve to shift to the right. An increase of H^+ ions in the blood causes acidosis. Acidosis facilitates the separation of oxygen from hemoglobin.

While the participation of dormant capillaries in the circulation and the tension in the pulmonary arteries reduce pulmonary vascular resistance, it also increases the pulmonary artery blood flow. Thus, the circulation improves in the upper lobes of the lungs, which receive relatively little blood. The physiologic dead space shrinks.

21.4 Chronic Response of the Respiratory System to Aerobic Exercise

Static lung volumes cannot improve by exercise training. However, with regular exercise, it is possible to cope with the effects caused by age or other environmental factors on the lungs.

The maximal oxygen consumption (maximal oxygen uptake or VO_{2max}) calculated during aerobic exercise, which indicates the body's capacity to use and transport oxygen to the muscles, is considered the most valid measure of cardiovascular fitness. This measurement determines the capacity to maintain maximal exercise. You get maximal oxygen uptake by dividing the maximum volume of oxygen consumed in one minute (in mL) by the body weight. The use of oxygen increases in direct proportion to the workload until it reaches VO_{2max}. When it reaches VO_{2max}, there is no change in the amount of oxygen used, even if the workload increases. After this stage, physical work continues through aerobic glycolysis. Lactic acid begins to accumulate. It becomes difficult to continue the exercise. However, it is necessary to remember that not everyone can reach this point. While pH decreases with training, the level of lactic acid is obtained much more later.

VO_{2max} depends on the cardiorespiratory system's ability to meet the oxygen needs of the muscle and the ability of the muscle to use oxygen and produce ATP aerobically. Although genetic factors determine VO_{2max}, it can be increased through exercise training. Eight to twelve weeks of aerobic exercise training can lead to an improvement of 15–20% in VO_{2max}. People who start the exercise with low VO_{2max} measurements achieve higher levels of increase. When deciding on the severity of aerobic exercise training, an exercise test at the beginning of the training and a percentage of VO_{2max} measurements come into play. In people with cardiac or respiratory pathologies, VO_{2max} measurements are below 20 mL/kg/min.

The increase in the a-V O_2 difference is the increase in muscles' use of oxygen. The density of capillaries and the mitochondrial volume increase in the muscle with exercise. Higher capillary density slows down the passage of erythrocyte through the vessel, allowing time to the muscle fiber for oxygen diffusion.

In addition, regular exercise provides the brain with the signals that help keep PCO_2 levels within normal limits.

The myoglobin in the skeletal muscle increases, and the ability of the muscles to retain oxygen improves with exercise training.

Exercise training reduces the work of breathing by increasing the oxidative capacity of muscles. The amount of air inhaled at the same oxygen consumption levels decreases. Ventilatory competence increases. This increase allows respiratory muscles to consume less oxygen during activities that need to be done for a long time. It enables oxygen transport to the necessary muscle groups to become easier. In addition to the benefits for the cardiorespiratory system, exercise training also reduces oxygen consumption during daily activities. This is especially important for patients with respiratory diseases such as COPD. Exercise training for these patients who have ventilatory limitations also contributes to the recovery of problems such as dyspnea, increased ventilatory load, respiratory muscle weakness, hypoxia, and dynamic hyperinflation.

21.5 Adaptation Mechanisms in Different Types of Exercises

There are various ventilatory adaptations for different types of exercises. Thus, the ventilatory requirements of individuals should also be taken into account when planning exercise training.

The exercise minute ventilation drops by 20–25% after submaximal endurance training compared to the pre-training levels. Although the cause of this effect has not yet been fully explained, it can be associated with an increase in the oxidative capacity of the muscles. This effect is even more pronounced at exercise levels where the lactate threshold is crossed. At the end of submaximal exercise training, the ventilatory equality of oxygen decreases—the tidal volume increases. Individuals make better use of oxygen in the inhaled air.

With maximal exercise, alveolar ventilation increases. Oxygen demand and carbon dioxide production increase. Blood lactate levels equivalent to VO_{2max} are lower in elite athletes compared to sedentary individuals. With the effect of training, the blood lactate level of a sedentary individual who has participated in endurance training decreases.

There is no direct effect of resistant exercise training on COPD patients' respiratory functions. It has been shown that resistance exercise training during the COPD exacerbation period prevents skeletal muscle dysfunction and does not cause any side effects. If COPD patients who are scheduled for long-term pulmonary rehabilitation are not able to participate in aerobic exercise due to dyspnea, resistance exercise training may be a choice.

It has been shown that some components of upper extremity resistance exercise training reduce dyspnea. While the ventilatory equality for oxygen is higher while training, it significantly drops as a training effect. Thus, there is a need for randomized controlled resistance exercise training studies to be performed on COPD patients.

Station training is another type of exercise used in respiratory system diseases. While higher exercise intensities can be achieved during exercise training, dyspnea, and ventilatory limitation decrease.

Recently, new exercise approaches have been used in respiratory system diseases. These are high-intensity training (HIT), water, eccentric, downhill, single-limb training, Nordic walking (Fig. 21.15), whole-body vibration, calisthenics, balance and coordination exercises, and mind-body unity approaches.

The desired VO_{2max} percentage can be achieved with water exercises at lower heart rates. Resistance to exposure to water affects the perception of exertion. In a study, it was shown that in-water exercises increase the maximum inspiratory (MIP) and expiratory pressure (MEP) values in COPD patients. Single-limb exercises in patients with COPD reduce the dyspnea perception while increasing VO_{2max}. Studies show that eccentric training reduces the ventilatory load and heals the dyspnea perception. Similarly, it is known that Nordic walking also benefits in tolerating higher

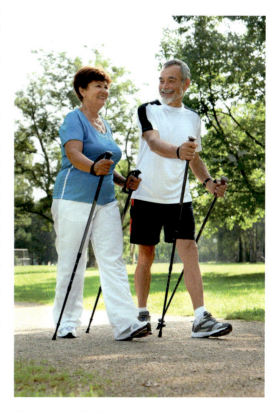

Fig. 21.15 Nordic walking (Alexander Raths/Shutterstock.com)

intensity exercise and thus increases oxygen consumption. There is yet no evidence that proves it improves pulmonary function. Yoga exercises with breathing exercises improve respiratory muscle strength and endurance and FEV_1 value.

21.6 Factors Affecting Adaptation to Exercise

The exercise adaptation is influenced by age, sex, muscle fiber type, exercise type, exercise intensity and frequency, exercise duration, suitability to the person (customization), and genetic factors.

21.6.1 Age

The age of the individual training is important in terms of VO_{2max} since VO_{2max} varies according to age. VO_{2max} values drop for sedentary people over 40 years old. The ventilatory equivalent for oxygen is higher for children.

21.6.2 Sex

Women and men may have different responses to the same exercise training. Men have higher hemoglobin values in the blood, and this makes their aerobic capacity higher than that of women. New evidence has revealed that men have wider airways than women. Smaller airways cause greater resistance to airflow. This causes women to perform more work of breathing during exercise while limiting their maximum ventilatory capacity. Increased work of breathing causes fatigue. This difference in aerobic capacity caused by sex also affects body mass and body fat ratio.

21.6.3 Exercise Type

Different types of exercise cause different adaptations in the respiratory system (see Sect. 21.5). Thus, it is recommended to organize an exercise training program for the specific needs of individuals.

21.6.4 Exercise Intensity

For aerobic exercise training (rhythmic movements aimed at large muscle groups) to have a curative effect on the cardiorespiratory system, the exercise intensity should be adjusted according to a certain workload measured by an exercise test or VO_{2max} percentage. In pathologies of the respiratory system, training should be performed at 30–40% of the maximal workload for low-intensity exercise training and at 60–80% of the maximal workload for high-intensity exercise training. Resistance exercise training should be carried out at 50–85% of one-maximum repetition, 2–4 sets, 6–12 reps, and rest intervals of 1–2 min between sets.

"The higher the intensity of exercise, the more gains a person makes."

21.6.5 Exercise Duration

Each session of exercise can go on for 20–60 min, depending on the individual's condition and tolerance. Short periods of exercise may not have the desired effect on the cardiorespiratory system. Prolonged exercise periods, on the other hand, can cause fatigue in respiratory muscles and cardiac stress.

21.6.6 Exercise Frequency

Aerobic exercise training can be carried out 3–5 days a week. On the other hand, resistance training can be carried out 2–3 days a week. In the presence of a pathological condition, exercising on consecutive days is not recommended.

21.6.7 Exercise Suitability (Customization)

The question of whether the exercise is suitable for the person should be considered when planning exercise training. For example, in dyspneic patients who cannot tolerate constant endurance training (severe respiratory tract obstruction, $FEV_1 <40\%$) or experience severe oxygen desaturation during exercise (SpO$_2$ <85%), intermittent exercise training may be the right choice. When choosing resistant exercises in the presence of osteoporosis or cardiovascular disease, necessary modifications should be made to exercise training.

21.6.8 Genetic Factors

Capacities such as the distribution of muscle fibers, VO$_{2max}$, lactic acid systems, and static lung volumes can be improved to the extent the genetic structure tolerates. For example, the ratio between fast-twitch fibers and slow-twitch fibers differs depending on the person. This brings about differences in exercise compliance and performance between people.

21.7 Possible Complications During/After Exercise in Respiratory System Pathologies and Their Management

Some factors may limit exercise in respiratory system pathologies, such as dyspnea, fatigue, a decline in ventilatory capacity, expiratory airflow restriction, dynamic hyperinflation, increase in respiratory rate, hypoxemia, impaired tissue oxygenation, circulatory disorders, circulatory limitations, change in diffusion capacities, pulmonary hypertension, low lactate threshold, changes in respiratory and peripheral muscles. When planning and during exercise training, patients should be very well observed, and their needs, obstacles they come across, and possible risks should be well calculated. Extreme caution should be exercised in evaluating individuals with low resting saturation or desaturation during exercise before exercise training. Other systemic diseases besides respiratory diseases should be taken into account, and modifications should be made to the exercise training program if necessary.

Those with lung disease are at increased risk of obesity due to physical inactivity and side effects of oral glucocorticoids prescribed for exacerbations. It should be considered that the work of breathing will increase during exercise in obese people. On the contrary, cachexia is observed in patients with cystic fibrosis. The physiotherapist should be careful in exercise overload for muscle weakness.

Arm exercise without support can disorganize breathing and create an asynchronous breathing pattern.

Patients who need oxygen while exercising can exercise with proper oxygen support. These patients and their physiological responses should be monitored. A bicycle ergometer may be preferred for these patients since desaturation is rarely seen.

Patients who experience excessive dyspneic or peripheral muscle fatigue during exercise can use a non-invasive mechanical ventilator.

When exercising, the Valsalva maneuver should be prevented. For this, counting out loud or pursed-lip breathing may be preferred.

It is recommended that asthma patients be monitored for the risk of bronchospasm during exercise. PEF and FEV$_1$ values before and after exercise training their values should be monitored. For an exercise in cold and dry weather, the face can be covered with a mask. The guidelines recommend using inhalers 5–20 min before exercise training in patients whose disease is under control but who have frequent asthma attacks. A slower warm-up period in exercise training in athletes who have asthma can prevent bronchospasm.

21.8 Comparison of the Adaptation Mechanism of the Respirator System to Exercise: A Healthy Individual and a Patient with COPD

The comparison of the adaptation mechanism of the respiratory system to exercise in a patient with COPD and a healthy individual is given in Table 21.2. The adaptation of the respiratory system to exercise is summarized in Table 21.3. The clinical implications of the cases are summarized in Table 21.4.

Table 21.2 Comparison of treatment programs for healthy individuals and patients with COPD

Case 1. Healthy individual	Case 2. Patient with COPD
K.C. (male) is 55 years old, 1.80 cm in height, and weighs 88 kg. He works at a bank. He consults a physiotherapist to improve his overall fitness. K.C. notes that he has not done regular exercise for the last three years. K.C. does not have any diagnosed disease and does not smoke.	L.A. (male) is 66 years old, 1.68 cm in height, and weighs 70 kg. He is a retired government official. He consulted a physiotherapist after he experienced shortness of breath while playing in the park with his grandchild. He was hospitalized for a week due to an acute exacerbation five months ago. He smoked 40 packs of cigarettes a year. However, he quit smoking six years ago.
Assessment of the cases	
Case 1. Healthy individual	**Case 2. Patient with COPD**
Normal joint range of motion	**Subjective assessment:**
Right and left shoulder flexion 180°	• Dyspnea: chronic, progressive, and increases with exertion
Right and left shoulder extension 60°	• Cough: productive, more at night, not severe
Right and left shoulder abduction 180°	• Sputum: a tablespoon per day, white, purulent
Hip flexion 120°	• Wheezing: At night (+)
Right and left knee flexion 135°	• Chest pain: Burning sensation in the middle of the chest when coughing (tracheitis)
Right and left ankle dorsiflexion 20°	• Medications used: Salbutamol, Tiotropium
Right and left lateral body flexion 80°	**Objective assessment:**
	• Inspection: Frog eyes, Central cyanosis, Auxiliary respiratory muscle activity, Pursed lip breathing, Redness of the skin, Flapping tremor, Pectus excavatum, Kyphosis
	• Palpation: Trachea in midline, Chest: Ventilation is even, Vocal fremitus: In the upper left zones, decrease in resonance, Percussion resonance increase in the middle left and lower, and middle right lobes.
	• Auscultation: Decrease in respiratory sounds in general, Ronchi in the left basal
	Laboratory findings:
	• Respiratory Function Test: $FEV_1\% = 29\%$ $FVC\% = 55\%$ $FEF_{25-75}\% = 14\%$ $PEF = 33\%$ $FEV_1/FVC = 55\%$
	• Complete blood count: Hb: 17.1 g/dL Hematocrit (Hct): 50.7% Leukocytes (WBC): 11.8/mm^3 Thrombocytes: 401,000/mm^3
	• Arterial blood gases: pH = 7.432 PaO_2 = 64.7 mmHg $PaCO_2$ = 34 mmHg SaO_2 = 93% HCO_3 = 22.2 mEq/L
	Thoracic CT: Increased number of lymph nodes not at pathological levels in the mediastinum, areas with low density in places suggestive of small airway disease in both lungs.

Table 21.2 (continued)

Case 1. Healthy individual	Case 2. Patient with COPD
Muscle strength assessment	
Quadriceps femoris right and left: 5 Gross flexion and extension of the upper limb: 5 Anterior deltoid right and left: 4+ Middle deltoid right and left: 4+	Quadriceps femoris right and left: 4 Gross flexion and extension of the upper limb: 5 Anterior deltoid right and left: 3+ Middle deltoid right and left: 3+ Handgrip: 22 kgF
Posture analysis	
Anterior: shoulder asymmetry Lateral: kyphosis, rounded shoulder, head tilt anteriorly Posterior: no feature	Anterior: Pectus excavatum Lateral: kyphosis, rounded shoulder, head tilt anteriorly Posterior: no feature
Physical fitness assessment	
Senior Fitness Test	–
	Respiratory muscle strength
–	MIP: 85 cmH$_2$O MEP: 140 cmH$_2$O
Assessment of functional capacity	
6-min walk test: 525 m.	Assessment of functional capacity 6-min walk test: 224 m, rested two times for 90 s.
Aerobic capacity assessment	
CPET (Cardiopulmonary exercise testing) VO$_{2max}$: 30.2 mL/kg/min	CPET (Cardiopulmonary exercise test) VO$_{2max}$: 14.3 mL/kg/min
	Dyspnea assessment mMRC→ 2
	Evaluation of daily life activities The London Chest Activity of Daily Living Test
Quality of life assessment	
SF-36	St. George's Respiratory Questionnaire
Treatment Program	
Case 1. Healthy individual	**Case 2. Patient with COPD**
Aerobic exercise training:	**Aerobic exercise training:**
An exercise training recommendation of 3 days a week, 5-min warm-up, 5-min cool-down, and 30 min of walking on the treadmill at a workload equivalent to 65% of VO$_{2max}$.	An exercise training recommendation of 3 days a week, 10-min warm-up, 10-min cool-down, and 20 min of walking on the treadmill at a workload equivalent to 60% of VO$_{2max}$.
Posture exercises are recommended for kyphotic posture. TID every day	Posture exercises are recommended for kyphotic posture. TID every day
One-maximum repetition for upper extremity muscle strength training (10 kg) 10 reps in 3 sets in 70% (1–2 min rest between sets) *chest press, vertical hanging*	One-maximum repetition for upper extremity muscle strength training (10 kg) 10 reps in 3 sets in 70% (1–2 min rest between sets) shoulder flexion, extension, and abduction with free weight
	For respiratory muscle training, 15 min at 40% of the MIP, two times a day, five days a week

Table 21.3 Adaptation of the respiratory system to exercise

Adaptation of the respiratory system to exercise	
Case 1. Healthy individual	**Case 2. Patient with COPD**
Acute response to aerobic exercise	
An increase in the tidal volume and respiratory frequency is observed.	An increase in the tidal volume and respiratory frequency is observed. Work of breathing increases. Dyspnea may be observed.
Chronic response to aerobic exercise	
There is an increase in the ability of O_2 use. Capacity to transport O_2 increases due to the increased gas exchange in the peripheral muscle. VO_{2max} increases. It improves the functional exercise capacity by increasing the oxidative capacity of skeletal muscle. The ventilatory requirement decreases at the same workloads. There is an improvement in the quality of life.	There is an increase in the ability of O_2 use. Capacity to transport O_2 increases due to the increased gas exchange in the peripheral muscle. VO_{2max} increases. The severity of dyspnea and the need for ventilation decrease at the same workloads. Dynamic hyperinflation decreases. It improves the functional exercise capacity by increasing the oxidative capacity of skeletal muscle. The activity of daily living improves. The quality of life improves.
Acute response to strength training	
Pulmonary ventilation increases—the amount of lactate production by the muscle increases. H^+ levels increase.	Pulmonary ventilation increases—the amount of lactate production by the muscle increases. H^+ levels increase.
Chronic response to strength training	
Muscle mass increases. Muscle strength and bone mineral density improved. The muscle endurance increases. Exercise capacity increases. Exercise peripheral muscle fatigue and exercise dyspnea decrease.	Muscle mass increases. Muscle strength and bone mineral density improved. The muscle endurance increases. Exercise capacity increases. Exercise peripheral muscle fatigue and exercise dyspnea decrease. The support of the muscles of the upper extremities to breathing decreases. The breathing pattern improves.

Table 21.4 Clinical inferences from the cases

Do's and don'ts when planning the exercise training
A healthy individual: The person should be taught to count heart rate during exercise and interpret the Modified Borg Scale (m.Borg) for fatigue and shortness of breath. In cases where VO_{2max} cannot be measured, exercise can be done at 60–80% of the maximum heart rate. The importance of warm-up and cool-down periods should be explained, and its necessity should be emphasized. They should know to avoid the Valsalva maneuver during resistance training. Physical activity counseling should be provided since the working environment (the bank) during the day feeds sedentary behavior. The person's sitting time should be shortened, and their movement should be encouraged as much as possible. Directing them to an activity that they can enjoy other than aerobic exercise training (swimming, cycling, tennis) supports lifestyle modifications.
An individual with COPD: Dyspnea reduction positions and energy conservation techniques should be taught. During exercise training, the patient's vitals (saturation and heart rate) should be evaluated well, and in case of an adverse condition, the exercise training plan should be reviewed and suited to the patient. Oxygen support can be provided if necessary. Do not forget that exercise can be limited mainly due to leg pain/fatigue/dyspnea in diseases of the respiratory system. In cases where VO_{2max} cannot be measured, exercising so that the perception of dyspnea is according to m.Borg 4–6 degrees would lead to better results. Exercise training should be planned in such a way that at least 2 sessions per week are supervised. They should know to avoid the Valsalva maneuver during resistance training. If during exercise training a person is hospitalized for acute exacerbation, training should start at lower intensities after their discharge.

21.9 Conclusion

The physiology of the respiratory system consists of mechanisms that allow it to maintain the concentration of O_2, CO_2, and H^+ ions at appropriate levels. In respiratory pathophysiology in lung diseases, it is essential to understand the disease to plan a relaxing/therapeutic rehabilitation program for symptomatic relief. Acute and chronic responses of the respiratory system during exercise training determine the effectiveness of the training program. Considering that the mechanisms of adaptation to various types of exercise training in diseases of the respiratory system will differ, it is recommended to add it to the pulmonary rehabilitation program.

Further Reading

Banzett RB, O'Donnell CR, Guilfoyle TE, Parshall MB, Schwartzstein RM, Meek PM, et al. Multidimensional dyspnea profile: an instrument for clinical and laboratory research. Eur Respir J. 2015;45:1681–91.

Bonini M, Di Mambro C, Calderon MA, Compalati E, Schünemann H, Durham S, et al. Beta2-agonists for exercise-induced asthma. Cochrane Database Syst Rev. 2013;10

Camillo CA, Osadnik CR, Burtin C, Everaerts S, Hornikx M, Demeyer H, et al. Effects of downhill walking in pulmonary rehabilitation for patients with COPD: a randomised controlled trial. Eur Respir J. 2020:(56).

Cramer H, Haller H, Klose P, Ward L, Chung VC, Lauche R. The risks and benefits of yoga for patients with chronic obstructive pulmonary disease: a systematic review and meta-analysis. Clin Rehabil. 2019;33:1847–62.

de Castro LA, Felcar JM, de Carvalho DR, Vidotto LS, da Silva RA, Pitta F, et al. Effects of land- and water-based exercise programmes on postural balance in individuals with COPD: additional results from a randomised clinical trial. Physiotherapy. 2020;107:58–65.

Evans RA, Dolmage TE, Mangovski-Alzamora S, Romano J, O'Brien L, Brooks D, et al. One-legged cycle training for chronic obstructive pulmonary disease. A pragmatic study of implementation to pulmonary rehabilitation. Ann ATS. 2015;(12):1490–7.

Gallo-Silva B, Cerezer-Silva V, Ferreira DG, Sakabe DI, Kel-Souza LD, Bertholo VC, et al. Effects of water-based aerobic interval training in patients with COPD: a randomized controlled trial. J Cardiopulm Rehabil Prev. 2019:(39).

Gonzalez-Bartholin R, Mackay K, Diaz O, Jalon M, Peñailillo L, Nickel R, et al. Physiological response to eccentric and concentric cycling in patients with chronic obstructive pulmonary disease. Appl Physiol Nutr Metab. 2020;45(11):1232–7.

Grünig E, Eichstaedt C, Barberà JA, Benjamin N, Blanco I, Bossone E, et al. ERS statement on exercise training and rehabilitation in patients with severe chronic pulmonary hypertension. Eur Respir J. 2019;53:1800332.

Hall JE, Hall ME. Respiration. In: Hall JE, Hall ME, editors. Guyton and Hall textbook of medical physiology. 14th ed. Elsevier Health Sciences; 2020. p. 490–549.

Kruel LFM, Beilke DD, Kanitz AC, Alberton CL, Antunes AH, Pantoja PD, et al. Cardiorespiratory responses to stationary running in water and on land. J Sports Sci Med. 2013;12:594–600.

Maltais F, Simard AA, Simard C, Jobin J, Desgagnés P, LeBlanc P. Oxidative capacity of the skeletal muscle and lactic acid kinetics during exercise in normal subjects and in patients with COPD. Am J Respir Crit Care Med. 1996;153:288–93.

McKeough ZJ, Velloso M, Lima VP, Alison J. Upper limb exercise training for COPD. Cochrane Database Syst Rev. 2016;11:CD011434.

Ochman M, Maruszewski M, Latos M, Jastrzębski D, Wojarski J, Karolak W, et al. Nordic walking in pulmonary rehabilitation of patients referred for lung transplantation. Transpl Proc. 2018;50:2059–63.

Parsons JP, Hallstrand TS, Mastronarde JG, Kaminsky DA, Rundell KW, Hull JH, et al. An official american thoracic society clinical practice guideline: exercise-induced bronchoconstriction. Am J Respir Crit Care Med. 2013;187:1016–27.

Puhan MA, Gimeno-Santos E, Cates CJ, Troosters T. Pulmonary rehabilitation following exacerbations of chronic obstructive pulmonary disease. Cochrane Database Syst Rev. 2016;12:CD005305.

Ribeiro F, Oueslati F, Saey D, Lépine P-A, Chambah S, Coats V, et al. Cardiorespiratory and muscle oxygenation responses to isokinetic exercise in chronic obstructive pulmonary disease. Med Sci Sports Exerc. 2019;51:841–9.

Sallis R, Franklin B, Joy L, Ross R, Sabgir D, Stone J. Strategies for promoting physical activity in clinical practice. Prog Cardiovasc Dis. 2015;57:375–86.

Powers SK, Howley ET. Respiration during exercise. In: Powers SK, Howley ET, McGraw, editors. Exercise physiology: theory and application to fitness and performance. 10th ed. New York: Hill Education; 2018. p. 224–55.

Sharman JE, La Gerche A, Coombes JS. Exercise and cardiovascular risk in patients with hypertension. Am J Hypertens. 2015;28:147–58.

Sheel AW, Dominelli PB, Molgat-Seon Y. Revisiting dysanapsis: sex-based differences in airways and the mechanics of breathing during exercise. Exp Physiol. 2016;101(2):213–8.

Vonbank K, Strasser B, Mondrzyk J, Marzluf BA, Richter B, Losch S, et al. Strength training increases maximum working capacity in patients with COPD—randomized clinical trial comparing three training modalities. Respir Med. 2012;106:557–63.

Circulatory System and Its Adaptation to Exercise

22

Filiz Erdem Eyuboglu

Abstract

When faced with stress, living things respond to stress within their current state and try to adapt to the new situation. Our body responds to the stress caused by exercise with adaptations in the circulatory system, respiratory system, musculoskeletal system, renal system, and endocrine system. Depending on the type, duration, intensity, frequency, and the current capacity of the person, both immediate and long-term changes occur in the circulatory system to rebalance. Understanding the effect of exercise on the circulatory system will guide the assessment and exercise program planning in patients, healthy individuals, or elite athletes. In this chapter, the anatomy and physiology of the circulatory system, the acute and chronic effects of exercise on the circulatory system, the factors affecting exercise adaptation, and the side effects that may occur during exercise in patients with pathologies affecting the circulation and their management will be discussed.

22.1 Introduction

When faced with stress, living things respond to stress within their current state and try to adapt to the new situation. Our body responds to the stress caused by exercise with adaptations in the circulatory system, respiratory system, musculoskeletal system, renal system, and endocrine system. Depending on the type, duration, intensity, frequency, and the current capacity of the person, both immediate and long-term changes occur in the circulatory system to rebalance. Understanding the effect of exercise on the circulatory system will guide the assessment and exercise program planning in patients, healthy individuals, or elite athletes. In this chapter, the anatomy and physiology of the circulatory system, the acute and chronic effects of exercise on the circulatory system, the factors affecting exercise adaptation, and the side effects that may occur during exercise in patients with pathologies affecting the circulation and their management will be discussed.

22.2 Anatomy of the Circulatory System

The circulatory system consists of the cardiovascular system and the lymphatic system. The cardiovascular system consists of four main structures: the heart, which is the driving force

F. Erdem Eyuboglu (✉)
Physiotherapy and Rehabilitation, Faculty of Health Sciences, Üsküdar University, Istanbul, Turkey
e-mail: filiz.eyuboglu@uskudar.edu.tr

for pumping blood; the arterial system, which works under high pressure to transport blood to the tissues; the capillaries, which carry out substance and gas exchange in the tissue; and the venous system, which allows blood to return to the heart.

22.2.1 Heart

The heart is a pyramidal muscular organ approximately 14 cm long and 9 cm wide, located in the center of the thorax. It is located in a lateral recumbent position with 2/3 of its main body on the left side of the body's midline. The average weight is 326 g for men and 275 g for women. Less than half a kilogram, this four-chambered muscular organ is very strong. The heart is located between the two lungs in the mediastinum in a double-layered fibrous sac called the "pericardium" and is innervated by the autonomic nervous system. It consists of four chambers: the upper two chambers are called "atria" and the lower two chambers are called "ventricles." The right and left ventricle and the right and left atrium are separated from each other by a wall structure called the septum.

From the inside out, the heart consists of three layers: the endocardium, myocardium, and epicardium. Between the parietal and visceral leaves of the pericardium, which serves as the outermost protective layer, there is a serous fluid ranging from 10 to 50 mL. This fluid allows the two membranes to move around each other as the heart contracts and relaxes, minimizing friction. The characteristics and functions of each layer are shown in Table 22.1.

The heart's blood supply is the heart's own circulatory network, called the "coronary circulation." The left and right coronary arteries terminate on the surface of the heart. They are located just above the semilunar valve in the aorta. The left coronary artery supplies the left atrium and ventricle and a small part of the right ventricle, while the right coronary artery supplies the right atrium and ventricle. The branching capillaries surround the myocardium like a net. Blood leaves the left ventricle via the coronary sinus and exits the right ventricle via the anterior cardiac veins. Per minute, 5% of cardiac output flows into the myocardium.

Table 22.1 Layers, properties and function of the heart

Layers of the heart	Characteristics of the heart layers	Function of the heart layers
Epicardium	It is a layer of mostly connective tissue containing blood and lymph capillaries and nerve fibers.	It acts as a protective layer.
Myocardium	Muscle tissue contains blood and lymph capillaries, nerve fibers.	It pumps blood through the heart by raising blood pressure to a certain level through muscle contractions.
Endocardium	It is composed of cells resembling vascular endothelium that secrete agents that allow the myocardium to contract and relax. It is a thin tissue and is in direct contact with the blood. It also contains blood vessels and especially cardiac muscle fibers known as Purkinje fibers.	It protects the myocardium in a thin layer. It is like a heart-blood barrier surrounding cardiac muscle cells.

22.2.1.1 Heart Muscle

The heart muscle, or "myocardium," is a striated muscle like skeletal muscle. But there are some differences between heart muscle and skeletal muscle. Skeletal muscle is innervated by the somatic nervous system, while cardiac muscle is innervated by the autonomic nervous system. The mitochondria of cardiac muscle are large and numerous, contain more myoglobin, have a single nucleus, are shorter than in skeletal muscle, and have a relatively longer action potential. Smooth muscle, skeletal muscle, and cardiac muscle are shown in Fig. 22.1. Cardiac muscle fibers are composed of a large number of cells connected in parallel. There are low-resistance physical connections between two neighboring cells of the heart muscle that allow the passage of

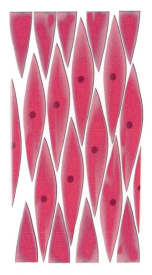 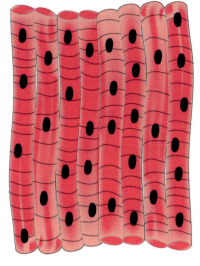 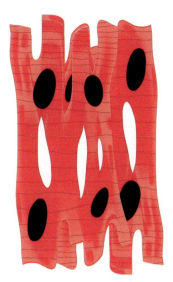

Smooth Muscle Tissue   Skeletal Muscle Tissue   Cardiac muscle tissue

Fig. 22.1 Smooth muscle, skeletal muscle, cardiac muscle (K.K.T Madhusanka/Shutterstock.com)

amino acids, ions, sugars, and nucleotides. These connections between cells, called *gap junctions*, also allow electrical impulses to be transmitted from one cell to another. When one cell is stimulated, the action potential spreads from cell to cell. So, when one muscle fiber depolarizes to contract, other fibers depolarize and the myocardium works as a whole. This is called "functional syncytium." The muscle cells in the atrium and ventricle are separated by a connective tissue that does not allow electrical stimulation to pass through. This is why atrial and ventricular contraction are different.

22.2.2 Peripheral Vascular System

The peripheral vascular system includes all blood vessels located outside the heart. The peripheral vascular system consists of arteries, arterioles, capillaries, venules, and veins that return blood to the heart. Each part of the peripheral vascular system has a different function and structure. Veins and arteries (large and medium diameter arteries, arterioles) have the following three layers. Capillaries consist only of the tunica intima (Fig. 22.2).

Tunica externa (Adventitia, outer layer): The outer layer that provides structural support and shape to the vessel.

Tunica media (middle layer): The middle layer of elastic and muscular tissue that regulates the inner diameter of the vessel.

Tunica intima (inner layer): The inner layer of endothelial lining that provides a frictionless pathway for the movement of blood.

The amount of muscle and collagen fibrils in each layer varies depending on the size and location of the vessel.

22.2.2.1 Arterial System

Arteries play an important role in supplying organs with blood and nutrients. Arteries are always working under high pressure and have plenty of elastic tissue and less smooth muscle to meet this stress. When an artery reaches a particular organ, it divides into smaller vessels with more smooth muscle and less elastic tissue. As blood vessels become smaller in diameter, the rate of blood flow decreases. About 10–15% of the total blood volume is found in the arterial system.

There are two main types of arteries found in the body: (1) elastic and (2) muscular. The aorta and arteria pulmonalis, which carry blood away

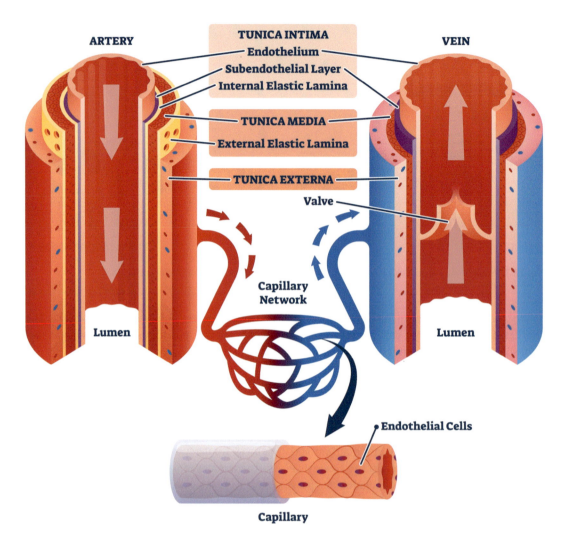

Fig. 22.2 Blood vessels (VectorMine/Shutterstock.com)

from the heart, are elastic arteries. Elastic arteries contain much more elastic tissue in the tunica media than muscular arteries. This allows them to soften the pressure waves generated during the outflow of blood from the heart.

Muscular arteries include the brachial artery, radial artery, and femoral artery, which have smaller diameters than elastic arteries and contain more smooth muscle cells in the tunica media layer.

Arterioles provide blood flow to the organs and are mainly composed of smooth muscle. The autonomic nervous system allows the size and diameter of these vessels to change. Thus, they respond to the tissue's need for more nutrients and oxygen. Because arterioles have less elastic tissue in their walls, they play an important role in systemic vascular resistance.

22.2.2.2 Capillary System

Capillaries are thin-walled vessels composed of a single layer of endothelium. Due to the thin walls of the capillary, the exchange of nutrients and metabolites occurs mainly by diffusion. Capillaries have a smooth muscle ring called the precapillary *sphincter*, which regulates the diameter of the capillary opening. During exercise, the *sphincter* opens and closes, allowing blood flow to be reorganized to meet metabolic demand. The capillary system opens into venules or small veins.

22.2.2.3 Venous System

Blood is transported from the periphery to the heart through the venous system, which has valves that allow one-way flow of blood. The venous system is composed of thin-walled and less elastic veins that, with their high resistance, can accommodate large volumes of blood at relatively low pressures. At any given time, about three-quarters of the volume of circulating blood are held in the venous system. Blood arriving at the heart via the vena cava inferior and vena cava superior is transported to the lungs via the pulmonary artery. After gas exchange in the alveoli, the blood returns to the left side of the heart via the pulmonary vein and enters the systemic circulation. In the lower limbs, skeletal muscle contractions help blood flow in the veins (Fig. 22.3).

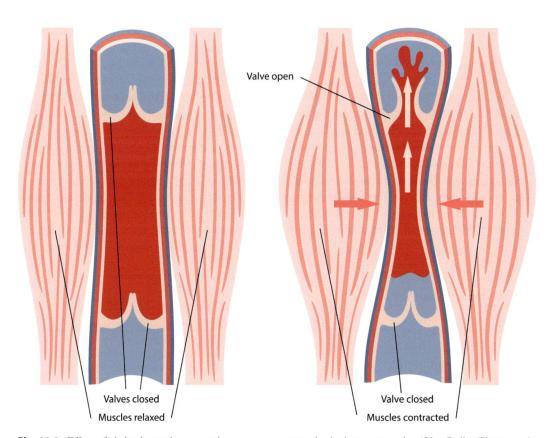

Fig. 22.3 Effect of skeletal muscle contraction on venous return in the lower extremity (Olga Bolbot/Shutterstock.com)

Forward blood flow from the lower limbs to the heart is also affected by respiratory changes that affect the pressure difference between the abdominal and thoracic cavity.

22.2.2.4 Lymphatic System

The lymphatic system consists of anatomical parts such as lymph capillaries and vessels, lymph nodes, lymphocytes, tonsils, thymus gland, and spleen. The main function of the lymphatic system is to regulate fluid balance in tissues. The lymphatic system as a whole is very large and complex, with lymph vessels and lymph nodes located in specific areas. The wall of the lymph capillaries is composed of an endothelial layer and, similar to blood capillaries, they surround the tissue like a network. However, they are more permeable than blood capillaries.

Large molecules (such as protein) that can hardly pass through blood capillaries can easily enter lymph capillaries. The lymph vessel pathways are occasionally interrupted by lymph nodes (lymph glands) to allow filtration of the lymph fluid. Some of the lymph vessels show rhythmic contractions. These contractions help the lymph to move forward. The lymph follows a long path through the lymph vessels and returns to the circulatory system by being transported to the venous system at certain points. The lymphatic system is part of the immune system and plays an important role in the body's defense against bacteria and toxins. It also helps to absorb fats and other substances from the digestive system.

22.2.3 Hemodynamics

From an anatomical and histological point of view, blood is considered a specialized tissue. Blood is a tissue with cells originating from the bone marrow and proteins in its plasma. Physiologically, blood is a specialized body fluid. An adult human being has about 8% of his or her body weight in blood. A 70-kg person has about 5.5 L of blood. Of this amount, about 3 L is plasma and the rest is the volume of the shaped elements of the blood. Having discussed the general physical properties of blood, it is necessary to take a closer look at plasma and blood cells. Blood plasma is 92% water, 6% plasma proteins, and 2% others. The ratio of the shaped elements of blood to the total blood volume is called the **hematocrit** value. This ratio is around 45% in men and 40% in women.

22.3 Circulatory System Physiology

The circulatory system is a set of functions that enable blood to be transported to the extremities of tissues and/or organs. The circulatory system is very important for maintaining homeostasis within the body. The primary function of the circulatory system is to deliver oxygen and nutrients to the tissues and to remove residual metabolites and carbon dioxide from the tissues. It also ensures the transfer of nutrients, regulation of body temperature, pH balance, and transport of hormones to the relevant organs.

The right ventricle for the pulmonary system and the left ventricle for the systemic circulation act as a pump to send blood from the heart. The blood leaving this pumping mechanism is completed by a closed-circuit system of arteries and arterioles, a capillary network for gas and nutrient exchange, and venules and veins that carry blood back to the heart. The capillaries merge into larger venules and the blood collected in the veins is brought back to the heart. The components of the cardiovascular system are shown in Table 22.2.

Table 22.2 Components of the cardiovascular system

Components of the cardiovascular system	
Pulmonary circulation	Blood is collected into the right atrium via the vena cava inferior (trunk and legs) and vena cava superior (head, neck, chest and collar) and sent to the lungs via the pulmonary artery.
Systemic circulation	Oxygenated blood comes from the lung into the left atrium via the pulmonary vein and is distributed throughout the body by the systemic circulation via the aorta.

22.3.1 Dynamic Physiology of the Heart

Unidirectional blood flow to the heart is mediated by atrioventricular valves (bicuspid-mitral, tricuspid) located between the atrium and ventricles and semilunar valves (aortic and pulmonary) outside the heart that control the outflow of blood from the ventricles (Table 22.3). These valves are composed of a thin fibrous structure. They open and close passively in response to changes in chamber pressure. The valves open when chamber pressure increases during myocardial contraction and close when contraction decreases and chamber pressure decreases. These valves provide one-way blood flow to the heart.

22.3.1.1 Cardiac Cycle

The entire sequence of events from the beginning of one heart beat to the beginning of the next heart beat is called the "cardiac cycle." The cardiac cycle consists of the repetition of the contraction and relaxation pattern of the heart. The contraction phase is called "systole" and the relaxation phase is called "diastole." When these terms are used alone, ventricular contraction and relaxation come to mind. But the atrium also has phases of contraction and relaxation. Atrial contraction occurs during ventricular diastole and atrial relaxation during ventricular systole.

The right and left atria contract together to send blood to the ventricles. Up to 70% of the blood entering the atria is delivered to the ventricles before the atria even contract. The remaining blood is delivered to the ventricles as the atria contract. Immediately after atrial contraction, the ventricles contract. The diastole phase consists of isovolemic relaxation, rapid filling, slow filling (diastasis) and atrial systole, while the systole phase consists of isovolemic contraction, rapid ejection and slow ejection. The pressure/volume exchange during the phases of the cardiac cycle is summarized in Table 22.4.

The value that shows what percentage of the incoming blood the heart pumps during systole is called **the ejection fraction**. Ejection fraction increases during exercise and decreases in conditions where the force of contraction is impaired, such as cardiomyopathy.

The heart muscle is capable of producing rhythmic contractions without any stimulation from the nervous system. In a healthy heart, the sinoatrial (SA) node is a natural "*pacemaker*" and controls the electrical impulses that cause contractions. When the action potential from the SA node propagates into the atrium and a depolarization wave is generated, the cardiac cycle begins. The impulses are collected in the atrioventricular (AV) node, amplified and passed to the ventricles via the atrioventricular bundles.

It divides into branches and terminates in Purkinje fibers in the subendocardium. The electrical fields generated by action potentials generated by myocardial cells are transmitted through electrolyte-containing fluids in the body and recorded on the body surface by electrocardiogram (ECG). Deviations on the ECG are called P, Q, R, S and T waves (Fig. 22.4).

P wave Atrial depolarization

Table 22.3 Location and functions of heart valves

Heart valve	Location of heart valves	Function of heart valves
Tricuspid valve	It is located between the right atrium and the right ventricle.	During ventricular systole, it blocks the passage of blood from the right ventricle to the right atrium.
Pulmonary valve	It is located at the point where the pulmonary artery connects to the right ventricle.	During ventricular diastole, it blocks the passage of blood pumped into the pulmonary artery into the right ventricle.
Mitral (bicuspid) valve	It is located between the left atrium and the left ventricle.	During ventricular systole, it blocks the passage of blood from the left ventricle to the left atrium.
Aortic valve	It is located at the point where the aorta connects to the left ventricle.	During ventricular diastole, it blocks the passage of blood pumped in the aorta to the left ventricle.

Table 22.4 Pressure/volume variation during the phases of the cardiac cycle

Phases of the heart cycle	Pressure/volume change
Isovolemic relaxation	Ventricular diastole begins. When the ventricular pressure falls below the atrial pressure, the mitral and tricuspid valves open and the ventricles begin to fill.
Fast filling	As ventricular pressure falls to diastole, the high pressure in the atria opens the atrioventricular valves, allowing blood to fill the ventricles rapidly.
Slow filling (Diastasis)	During the second 1/3 of diastole, very little blood passes into the ventricles. This second 1/3 of diastole, when the flow of blood into the ventricles almost stops, is called **diastasis**.
Atrium systole	During the last 1/3 of diastole, the atria contract, giving a new speed to the flow of blood to the ventricles. This period, called **atrial systole**, is responsible for about 30% of the filling of the ventricles.
Isovolemic contraction	The mitral valve and aortic valve are closed. Ventricular pressure increases, ventricular volume remains unchanged.
Fast ejection period	It starts when the aortic and pulmonary valves open. Aortic pressure and ventricular pressure peak. Two thirds of the blood in the ventricle passes into the aorta.
Slow ejection period	Aortic pressure, pulmonary artery pressure and ventricular pressure decrease. When the ventricular pressure falls below the aortic and pulmonary artery pressure, the aortic and pulmonary valves close.

QRS complex: Ventricular depolarization

T wave Ventricular repolarization

*Atrial repolarization is covered/obscured by the QRS complex.

The two factors that affect **heart rate** are the ability of the SA nodule to act as a pacemaker and the autonomic nervous system. At rest, the vagus nerve releases acetylcholine as a neurotransmitter, creating a strong parasympathetic activity on the heart; this neurotransmitter directly affects the SA node and AV node and decreases the heart rate. In a state of rest, the heart rate is reduced to less than 100 beats per minute by the action of the parasympathetic nervous system. **The stroke volume** is the difference between end-diastolic and end-systolic volumes. With each beat, the heart pumps about 60% (70 mL) of the blood in the ventricle.

$$\text{Stroke Volume} = \text{Enddiastolic Volume} - \text{Endsystolic Volume}$$

Cardiac output is the amount of blood pumped by the heart into the aorta in one minute. Heart rate and stroke volume are the two factors that affect it and its unit is mL/min.

$$\text{Cardiac Output Rate}\,(\text{mL}/\text{min}) = \text{Heart Rate}\,(\text{beats}/\text{min}) \times \text{Stroke Volume}\,(\text{mL})$$

Assuming an average heart rate of 72 beats/min and a stroke volume of 0.07 L, the heart pumps 5 L of blood in one minute.

$$\text{Cardiac Output} = 72 \times 0.070 = 5\,\text{L}/\text{min}$$

Blood pressure is heard as a pulse in a superficial artery of the body during the cardiac cycle, when the arterial wall stretches and recovers. The maximum pressure produced by the heart during

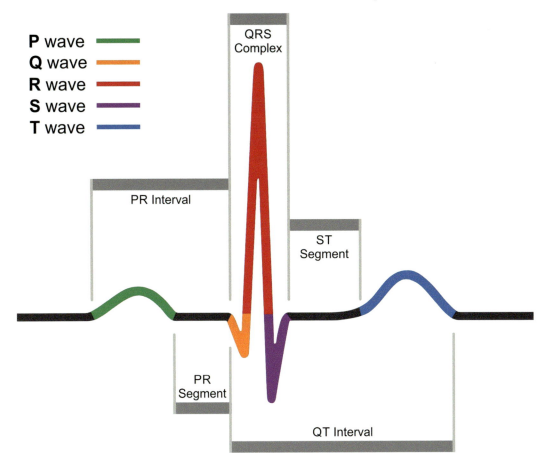

Fig. 22.4 Normal sinus rhythm (udaix/Shutterstock.com)

systole of the left ventricle is called systolic blood pressure.

After the aortic and pulmonary valves close during diastole, diastolic blood pressure is the pressure that ensures uninterrupted blood flow thanks to the elastic components of the vessels.

Since the duration of diastole is greater than the duration of systole, the mean arterial pressure is calculated by the following equation. When the heart rate increases, the mean arterial pressure approaches the average of the systolic and diastolic pressures because the duration of diastole is shorter.

$$\text{Mean Blood Pressure} = \text{Diastolic Pressure} + \left[0.333\left(\text{Systolic} - \text{Diastolic Pressure}\right)\right]$$

22.3.1.2 The Relationship Between Pressure, Resistance, and Flow

Pressure is the force exerted by a fluid and is usually measured in mmHg in physiology. Resistance is a measure of the friction resisting flow and is how hard blood flows between two points of pressure difference. If resistance increases while pressure remains the same, cardiac output decreases. There are three factors that cause resistance: (1) Blood viscosity (volume and number of red blood cells affect it), (2) Total blood vessel length (constant), (3) Blood vessel diameter (relaxed vessels decrease resistance, narrowed vessels increase it; this is the greatest help for minute control of resistance in the vascular system. The basic connection between these variables:

$$\text{Total Peripheral Resistance} = \frac{\text{Vessel length} \times \text{Viscosity}}{(\text{Vessel Radius})^4}$$

Hormonal and neural mechanisms regulate blood pressure by influencing cardiac output and peripheral resistance.

The main factors determining blood flow are the viscosity of the blood, defined as "Poiseuille's Law," the pressure difference between the two ends of the vessel, the length of the vessel, and the radius of the vessel.

$$Q = \frac{\Delta P \pi r 4}{8 \eta l}$$

Q: Blood flow, ΔP: Pressure difference between the two ends of the vessel, r: Radius of the vessel, η: Viscosity coefficient, l: Length of the vessel

22.4 Acute Effects of Exercise on the Circulatory System

During exercise, skeletal muscles require more oxygen than at rest. The increased oxygen demand is met in two ways (1) increased cardiac output and (2) redistribution of blood flow from inactive organs to working muscles. For these two mechanisms, the circulatory system regulates heart rate, stroke volume, total peripheral resistance and local blood flow during exercise to meet the oxygen demand of active muscles. Acute effects include the changes that occur to adapt to a single bout of exercise. The acute adaptation mechanisms of the circulatory system to meet the increased oxygen demand of the tissues during exercise and to restore the balance will be explained in this chapter.

22.4.1 Cardiac Output, Stroke Volume, and Heart Rate During Exercise

During exercise against an increased workload, cardiac output also increases as the oxygen demand of active muscles increases 15–20 times compared to rest. Because cardiac output and maximal oxygen uptake percentage are directly proportional. During exercise performed in an upright position (e.g., bicycle, treadmill), cardiac output increases with an increase in both heart rate and stroke volume. Up to 40–60% of VO_{2max} in both trained and untrained individuals, cardiac output increases with an increase in both heart rate and stroke volume. At workloads above 40–60% of VO_{2max}, cardiac output increases only with an increase in heart rate.

22.4.1.1 Stroke Volume During Exercise

The stroke volume is the amount of blood pumped from each of the ventricles in each systole. It is regulated by preload (end-diastolic volume), afterload (mean aortic pressure) and myocardial contractility (strength of ventricular contraction) both at rest and during exercise.

Pre load: Increased venous return to the heart increases the stroke volume. The main reason for this is that the heart has a mechanism that automatically pumps all the blood coming into the right atrium via the veins. Within physiologic limits, the more the myocardium is stretched during diastole, the more forcefully it contracts. The greater the amount of blood pumped to the periphery and to the lungs. This feature of the heart is called the "Frank Starlink mechanism." Although the right and left ventricle pump different amounts of blood when they contract at the same time, they pump equal amounts of blood per unit time. This mechanism is called "heterometric autoregulation," so that the amount of blood coming from the venous circulation and going to the lung is the same as the amount of blood coming from the lung and joining the peripheral circulation. The increased venous blood returning from the peripheral muscles during exercise pumps more blood to the periphery during systole. There are three factors that cause increased venous return during exercise: skeletal muscle pump, respiratory and abdominal pumps, and venoconstriction.

The skeletal muscle pump constricts the surrounding veins during the contraction of the skeletal muscle and the rhythmic contractions create a mechanical effect that directs blood to the heart through one-way valves that prevent the backward flow of blood in the veins. When the muscle relaxes, the veins fill with blood again and when the skeletal muscle contracts, blood returns to the heart. The skeletal muscle pump is especially active in exercises where skeletal muscles work rhythmically, such as walking and running. In isometric exercises involving prolonged contraction of the muscle, the skeletal muscle pump cannot work and venous return to the heart decreases.

Respiratory and abdominal pumps are a mechanical pump whose rhythmic pattern of breathing facilitates venous return. During inspiration, intrathoracic pressure decreases, abdominal pressure increases, thoracic veins empty. There is a pressure difference between the region of the vena cava inferior entering the right atrium and exiting through the diaphragm into the thorax. The blood in the vena cava accelerates and moves towards the right atrium. The flattening of the diaphragm during inspiration also increases the abdominal pressure and the blood in the abdominal veins drains towards the heart. During expiration, thoracic pressure increases, abdominal pressure decreases and the opposite happens to inspiratory pressure, filling the thoracic veins. The increase in respiratory frequency and depth during exercise leads to a greater increase in venous return by respiration and abdominal pump. In deep inspiration, venous return to the right atrium increases, while venous return to the left atrium decreases.

Venoconstriction, the contraction of smooth muscles in the wall of veins is called venoconstriction. During exercise, the release of neurotransmitter of the sympathetic nervous system, norepinephrine, causes venoconstriction. When the veins contract, blood volume decreases and more blood enters the circulation, adding to the preload of the heart.

After load: Another factor affecting stroke volume is aortic pressure, also known as mean arterial pressure. For blood to be pumped into the aorta, the pressure generated by the left ventricle must exceed the aortic pressure. Therefore, aortic pressure (afterload) acts as a barrier to ejection of blood from the ventricles. The stroke volume is therefore inversely proportional to aortic pressure. An increase in aortic pressure leads to a decrease in stroke volume. However, arteriolar dilatation in the working muscles during exercise reduces the afterload and facilitates the pumping of large volumes of blood from the heart.

Myocardial contractility: During exercise, the increase in circulating catecholamines (epinephrine, norepinephrine) and increased contraction of the ventricles with the direct effect of sympathetic stimulation allow more blood to be pumped. Especially epinephrine and norepinephrine increase extracellular calcium entry into cardiac muscle fibers and cross-bridge activation.

22.4.1.2 Heart Rate During Exercise

During exercise, changes in both the autonomic nervous system and blood biochemistry affect heart rate. The ventricles are dominated by sympathetic innervation and the atria by both sympathetic and parasympathetic innervation. Increased sympathetic stimulation and decreased parasympathetic activity due to activation of the motor center and higher centers cause an increase in heart rate even before exercise begins.

The initial increase in heart rate occurs in the first few minutes of activity due to the withdrawal of parasympathetic activity and the activation of the sympathetic nervous system. At the beginning of exercise during low-intensity exercise, the increase in heart rate up to 100 beats/min is due to a decrease in parasympathetic tone. Acetylcholine released from the neurons of the parasympathetic nervous system decreases sinus discharge and therefore heart rate. At higher workloads, the action of the sympathetic nervous system on the SA and AV nodule increases the heart rate. If the exercise intensity is constant and below the lactate threshold, the heart rate reaches a plateau and remains relatively constant. This point indicates that the circulatory system is supplying blood, oxygen and nutrients to the working skeletal muscles. If the intensity of the exercise increases towards the maximum, the heart rate will increase to meet the increased oxygen demand.

Finally, changes in body temperature can affect heart rate. Above normal body temperature increases the heart rate and vice versa, below normal body temperature decreases the heart rate. Exercising in a hot environment causes an increase in both body temperature and heart rate compared to exercising in a cool environment.

22.4.2 Blood Pressure and Total Peripheral Resistance

During exercise at a constant workload at a constant speed, vasodilatation of the vessels in the working muscles reduces total peripheral resistance and thus facilitates blood flow. The decrease in total peripheral resistance is directly proportional to the mass of the muscles used during exercise. This is because the rhythmic contraction and relaxation of large muscle groups during aerobic exercise further facilitates the return of blood to the heart. For example, total peripheral resistance decreases more in exercises using the muscles of the lower extremities than in the upper extremities.

During aerobic exercise, there is an increase in systolic blood pressure despite a decrease in peripheral resistance. The reason for the increase in blood pressure at the beginning of exercise is that the cardiovascular system is trying to supply sufficient blood to the tissues. The brain activity that sends motor signals to the muscles also sends simultaneous signals to the autonomic centers that stimulate circulatory activity, causing constriction of the great veins and an increase in heart rate and contractility. All of these changes acting together increase arterial pressure above normal level, which results in more blood supply to active muscles. Systolic blood pressure (SBP) also plateau (stable) as the stroke volume plateau during balanced levels of submaximal exercise.

During exercise, SBP is expected not to exceed 160–220 mmHg. Exercise should be terminated when it exceeds these values. While SBP increases, diastolic blood pressure (DBP) increases minimally or does not change. The reason for the minimal change in DBP is that the vessels in the working muscles decrease the total peripheral resistance during exercise. Therefore, there is a moderate increase in mean arterial pressure. An increase in DBP of more than 15 mmHg is considered an abnormal blood pressure response. A detailed evaluation of the cardiovascular system is required.

After the end of exercise, blood pressure may drop even below the pre-exercise value. This decrease in blood pressure after exercise is called "post-exercise hypotension." Post-exercise hypotension is thought to be caused by the triggering of vasodilation in skeletal muscle by nitric oxide-mediated processes. The magnitude of this hypotension, which we see in the early stages of recovery, can vary between 2 and 12 mmHg in magnitude and 4–16 h in duration. The greater the duration and intensity of the exercise, the greater the decrease in blood pressure after exercise. Acute changes in blood pressure after a single session of aerobic exercise demonstrate the importance of physical activity in helping to control blood pressure in hypertensive patients. Therefore, regular participation in aerobic exercise is one of the strategies to prevent hypertension. Because it has the effect of lowering both diastolic and systolic blood pressure. However, it is important to remember that the response of the circulatory system varies according to the type and intensity of exercise.

22.4.3 Blood Flow and Oxygen Distribution During Exercise

The balance between vasodilation and vasoconstriction ensures blood redistribution during exercise.

Nerve impulses, which become more active during exercise, affect the smooth muscle in the arteriolar wall and change the vessel diameter. The task of the myogenic mechanism is to maintain tissue blood flow in the event of changes in perfusion pressure. Vascular smooth muscle will contract when the pressure in the vessel wall increases and relax when the pressure decreases.

During exercise, a redistribution of blood occurs to meet the demand for oxygen needed by skeletal muscles. More blood flows to active muscles and less to organs that need less, such as the kidneys and liver. The narrowing and widening of blood vessels allow blood to redistribute. Sympathetic system-mediated neural and hormonal effects cause vasoconstriction of arterioles supplying blood to the digestive tract and kidneys. Local autoregulatory factors such as temperature, CO_2, H^+, K^+, and endothelium-derived nitric oxide cause vasodilation of arterioles and capillary blood flow in working muscles increases to meet metabolic demand. During rest, 15–20% of the cardiac output goes to skeletal muscle, while during exercise this rate increases up to 80–85%. The brain and heart activate their internal mechanisms to ensure uninterrupted oxygen supply. Coronary blood flow increases 4–6 times with the increase in workload. Skin blood flow increases during mild and moderate exercise and decreases during maximal exercise. As body temperature increases, more blood is sent to the skin. With prolonged exercise, especially in a hot and humid environment, more and more of the cardiac output will be redistributed to the skin to counteract the increased body temperature, thus limiting both the amount to skeletal muscle and exercise endurance.

22.4.4 Arteriovenous Oxygen Difference During Exercise

How much oxygen is used in tissues can be explained by the concept of arteriovenous oxygen difference. This is determined by the difference in the amount of oxygen in the blood coming into and leaving the tissue. At rest, the arteriovenous oxygen difference is 4–5 mL of O_2 for every 100 mL of blood, while this ratio reaches 15–16 mL as the exercise approaches the maximum. The amount of oxygen used per unit time by the tissues depends on the arteriovenous oxygen difference and cardiac output.

$$\text{Oxygen uptake}\left(VO_{2max}\right)\left(mL/kg/min\right) = \text{Cardiac Output} \times \left(a - vO2\right)$$

22.4.5 Autonomic Control of Heart Rate and Blood Pressure During Exercise

During rest, the balance between parasympathetic tone and sympathetic activity is maintained by the cardiovascular control center in the medulla oblangata. The cardiovascular control center receives impulses from various parts of the circulation and sends motor impulses to the heart through the sympathetic and parasympathetic nervous system in response to cardiovascular needs.

- Mechanoreceptors provide information about muscle length, tension, force of contraction and joint angle during exercise. When stimulated, these receptors send signals to the cardiovascular control center regarding the intensity of the movement.
- Peripheral chemoreceptors called carotid and aortic bodies regulate both respiration and the tone of arteries and veins during exercise due to a decrease in arterial blood pH and an increase in CO_2 partial pressure.
- Baroreceptors in the heart, carotid sinus, aortic arch and major circulating arteries regulate blood pressure. As blood pressure increases, the tension of the arterial vessels activates these baroreceptors, causing reflex slowing of the heart and compensatory dilation of the peripheral vessels.

All these mechanisms play an important role in rebalancing blood pressure changes during exercise.

22.5 Chronic Effects of Exercise on the Circulatory System

Regular aerobic exercise at a certain intensity, frequency and duration causes permanent changes in the circulatory system. These effects, which occur at rest and during exercise, are defined as chronic adaptations.

22.5.1 Effect on Heart Rate, Stroke Volume, and Cardiac Output

Aerobic exercise training reduces heart rate due to the effect of the autonomic nervous system on the SA nodule. This change in heart rate is due to an increase in parasympathetic activity (vagal tone) and a decrease in sympathetic nervous system activity.

Although the heart rate decreases at rest, the stroke volume increases to maintain cardiac output. Following aerobic exercise training, at rest and during submaximal exercise, heart rate decreases, stroke volume increases and cardiac output remains unchanged. This decrease in heart rate provides more time for the ventricles to fill and the chamber width of the ventricles increases, which is the main reason for the higher resting stroke volume in endurance athletes. In trained individuals, the increase in heart rate during exercise is lower. This is because the blood demand can be met at a slower heart rate because the stroke volume is higher. After aerobic exercise training, maximal heart rate remains unchanged or decreases slightly in elite athletes, while maximal stroke volume and maximal cardiac output increase. Factors that cause maximal stroke volume to increase:

(1) Left ventricular chamber enlargement and increased plasma volume greatly increase end-diastolic volume, (2) Increased end-diastolic volume increases preload and myocardial contractility, (3) Training promotes ventricular emptying by decreasing total peripheral resistance and improves diastolic filling so that the ventricles fill more and faster, maintaining end-diastolic volume even at high heart rates. After training, an increase in maximal stroke volume also increases maximal cardiac output. These adaptations increase cardiac output during exercise, leading to increased maximal oxygen consumption. At rest, while a person who has been aerobic exercising for a long time meets a cardiac output of 5.00 L with a heart rate of 50 beats/min and a stroke volume of 100 mL, non-exercises person meets the same cardiac output with 72 beats/min and a stroke volume of 70 mL.

22.5.2 Cardiac Hypertrophy

Aerobic exercise training causes eccentric hypertrophy and increases the size of the heart. During aerobic exercise, the heart is subjected to hemodynamic stresses such as pressure and volume increases. To meet such stresses and increased blood demand, it morphologically adapts to repetitive exercise by enlarging its ventricular chamber. This increase in heart size is mainly due to an increase in the size of cardiac myocytes. The remodeling of the heart in response to exercise ensures the maintenance and recovery of contractile function. That is, regular aerobic exercise increases the end-diastolic volume of the heart. End-diastolic volume increases during exercise due to increased peripheral venous return, whereas at rest it increases due to decreased heart rate and prolonged duration of diastole. The increase in end-diastolic volume leads to an increase in stroke volume. Hypertrophy occurs in two ways: enlargement of the ventricular

cavity and thickening of the ventricular wall. The type of exercise is very important in cardiac hypertrophy. Hypertrophy occurs in two ways: enlargement of the ventricular cavity and thickening of the ventricular wall. Thickening of the left ventricular wall of the heart (muscular hypertrophy) is seen in sports with static muscular activities such as hammer throwing, shot put, weightlifting. The ventricular volume does not change or increases only slightly. The ventricular cavity increases in the hearts of athletes who perform dynamic activities such as swimming, cycling and running. When athletes perform both static and dynamic activities, both types of car-

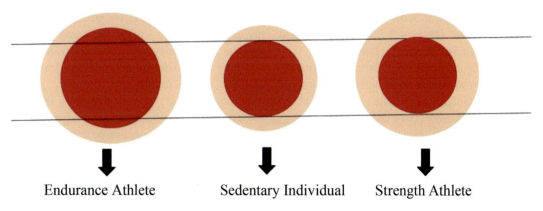

Endurance Athlete   Sedentary Individual   Strength Athlete

Fig. 22.5 Comparison of left ventricular hypertrophy in sedentary, endurance athletes and weightlifting athletes. Red color: represents the ventricular cavity (space) and yellow color: represents the ventricular wall

diac hypertrophy may be seen together. A comparison of left ventricular hypertrophy in sedentary, endurance, and weightlifting athletes is shown in Fig. 22.5.

22.5.3 Effect on Endothelial Function and Capillary Density

It has been reported that exercise improves epicardial coronary vessels and vascular endothelial function. The endothelial layer in the vessel maintains vascular homeostasis and regulates vascular tone. It is an active organ that plays paracrine, endocrine and autocrine roles and provides active transport of substrates. The endothelium is composed of specialized cells that can secrete endothelium-derived hyperpolarizing factors, prostacyclin and nitric oxide (NO), which regulate vascular tone. Increased NO production with exercise training increases endothelium-dependent vasodilation. NO also plays an important role in myocardial repair, regeneration and regulation of myocardial oxygen consumption. It increases the capillary to muscle fiber ratio in skeletal muscles and the heart.

Regular exercise increases coronary flow reserve, coronary collateral circulation, tolerance to ischemia, myocardial capillary density, epicardial coronary artery size, and reduces atherosclerosis, morbidity, and mortality. Abnormal endothelial dysfunction increases the risk of cardiovascular events.

22.5.4 Effect on Blood Pressure

Exercise training regulates blood pressure and reduces peripheral resistance, mostly through its effect on vascular function and structure. Increased NO production and improvements in its bioavailability are important factors contributing to improved endothelium-dependent vasodilation following exercise training. This decreases peripheral vascular resistance and thus blood pressure at rest. In addition to NO-mediated decreases in vascular tone, decreased sympathetic nervous system activity and increased parasympathetic nervous system activity also have a blood pressure-lowering effect. The chronic effect of aerobic exercise on blood pressure;

- Reduction in resting blood pressure
- Lower blood pressure during submaximal exercise
- Reduction risk of hypertension
- Reduction in blood pressure in hypertensive individuals

Hypertension is a major risk factor for many adverse cardiovascular events, including heart failure, stroke, myocardial infarction, and kidney failure. In addition to medication, regular physical activity and exercise are considered essential in the prevention and management of hypertension. Long-term exercise can produce a net reduction in blood pressure at rest. In a meta-analysis of normo/hyper-tensive patients, prolonged exercise was shown to reduce SBP by 3.3 mmHg and DBP by 3.5 mmHg. Although these reductions may seem relatively small, they are clinically very important. Because a 2 mmHg reduction in blood pressure can reduce the risk of myocardial infarction by 6% and the risk of developing coronary artery disease by 4%.

22.5.5 Effect on Blood Volume and Plasma

The oxygen-carrying capacity of the blood, determined by the number of circulating erythrocytes and their associated intracellular hemoglobin density, is an important determinant of exercise performance and resistance to fatigue. Blood volume and hemoglobin content increase with exercise. While the amount of hemoglobin increases, hemoglobin density does not change or may even decrease slightly due to the increase in plasma volume. Athletes with high endurance often have "athlete's anemia" due to erythrocyte loss or low hematocrit secondary to increased plasma volume. However, in athletes, especially those training at high altitude, the overall total erythrocyte mass increases.

22.5.6 Effect on Blood Lipids

Regular aerobic exercise lowers low-density lipoprotein cholesterol (LDL-cholesterol) levels and increases high-density lipoprotein cholesterol (HDL-cholesterol) levels. Although the mechanism of exercise-induced lipid changes is not clear, it is thought to be caused by increased lipoprotein lipase activity in exercise.

22.5.7 Effect on Arteriovenous Oxygen Difference

Biochemical changes that occur in skeletal muscle with regular exercise increase the arteriovenous oxygen difference.

Increases in mitochondria size and number, myoglobin density, Krebs cycle and electron transport system enzyme activity, glycogen stores and fatty acid oxidation increase oxygen availability in skeletal muscle.

In aerobic exercise with gradually increasing exercise intensity, maximal oxygen uptake increases in direct proportion to exercise intensity, and after a certain point it does not increase even if exercise intensity increases. The amount of oxygen use recorded at this point is the maximal oxygen consumption. Maximal oxygen consumption, which is an indicator of aerobic capacity, increases due to chronic adaptations. Maximal oxygen consumption increases due to changes in cardiac output and arteriovenous difference caused by regular exercise.

22.5.8 Effect on Lactic Acid Tolerance

Anaerobic glycolysis is the dominant energy system in muscle metabolism during high intensity exercise. During this type of exercise, the amount of lactic acid in the blood and muscle increases significantly. Lactic acid, which is a very strong acid, decomposes into lactate and H^+ ions, causing a decrease in pH (metabolic acidosis) and fatigue. Regular exercise delays lactic acid accumulation and improves sustained activity at high lactate levels. This is called lactate tolerance. As lactate tolerance increases, fatigue occurs at a later time.

22.5.9 Effect on Post-Exercise Recovery

After a maximal exercise, it takes time for changes such as increase in heart rate, increase in stroke volume, increase in blood pressure to return to resting levels and for the increase in lactic acid to decrease. In people who exercise regularly, these values can return to the initial value in a much shorter time.

22.6 Adaptation Mechanisms in Different Exercise Types

Circulatory system adaptations may also differ in different exercise methods such as high intensity intermittent exercise, eccentric exercise, and strength training. High-intensity intermittent exercise (HIIT) consists of alternating periods of short-term/high-intensity exercise and long-term/low-intensity exercise. Its advantage over moderate-intensity continuous aerobic exercise (MCAE) is that more benefit can be obtained in a shorter exercise period. Recent studies have proven the positive effects of HIIT on cardiovascular and metabolic functions both in healthy individuals and in chronic patient groups such as diabetes, heart failure, and hypertension, which increases the interest even more.

Therefore, HIIT is considered as an alternative exercise method to improve aerobic capacity and cardiac function. It can be better applied in people with coronary artery disease and heart failure as it causes less dyspnea and leg fatigue compared to MCAE.

It has been shown that the cardiovascular adaptations of the HIIT are similar to, and in some cases superior to, the MCAE. In a study comparing the HIIT and MCAE in patients with chronic heart failure, it was found that VO_2max increased by 11.2% in the HIIT group and 8.3% in the MCAE group. Compared to MCAE performed at 70% of maximal heart rate three times a week for eight weeks, HIIT performed at 90–95% of maximal heart rate for 4 min, exercise, 3 min active rest 4 repetitions provided 10% more increase in stroke volume. In another study, high-intensity aerobic training at 90–95% of VO_2max was shown to increase left ventricular heart mass by 12% and cardiac contraction by 13%. HIIT also provides a significant increase in capillarization compared to MCAE. Although the reason for the greater increase in capillarization cannot be fully elucidated, it is thought that capillarization is increased in the HIIT to ensure the return of oxygen-dependent metabolic processes in anaerobic energy production and the rapid removal of metabolic wastes and/or selective rapid electrical stimulation of glycolytic fast-twitch fibers may increase capillarization.

At the same workload, metabolic demand is lower during eccentric exercise than during concentric exercise. Regardless of anaerobic metabolism, eccentric exercise results in 4–5 times less oxygen consumption, lower cardiac output and lower heart rate than concentric exercise. Therefore, less oxygen is consumed during downhill walking and running than during uphill walking and running at the same speed. At the same mechanical workload, the degree of difficulty felt, lactate accumulation in the blood, energy expenditure and carbohydrate oxidation were lower and fat oxidation was higher during eccentric cycling compared to concentric cycling. To reach a VO_2 above a certain threshold (e.g., >1 L/min), cardiac output can increase by 27% and heart rate by 17% more, accompanied by a greater perceived degree of exertion during eccentric exercise. Eccentric and concentric cycling at similar metabolic intensities below this threshold results in a similar heart rate response. In summary, eccentric exercise is metabolically less expensive at the same workload. A significantly higher workload is required to achieve a comparable VO_2 during downhill running and eccentric cycling.

There are significant differences in dynamic resistance upper and lower body exercise, especially in blood pressure.

Generally, SBP is higher in lower body dynamic resistance exercises than in upper body. DBP may decrease in both dynamic exercises. However, since larger muscle groups are used during lower body dynamic resistance exercises, more vasodilation and larger decreases can be observed. In fact, in most individuals, SBP and DBP values similar to the response to aerobic exercise are obtained during dynamic resistance exercise training. Compared to dynamic resistance exercise, the acute hemodynamic response to isometric exercise is an increase in SBP and DBP. During isometric exercise, the accumulation of metabolites activates mechanoreceptors and chemoreceptors in skeletal muscle that cause an increase in blood pressure and heart rate. Even sustained isometric contractions performed at a relatively low load, such as 20% maximal voluntary contraction (MVC), can cause rapid increases in heart rate during contraction. Individuals engaged in heavy resistance exercise training often unknowingly perform what is known as the "Valsalva maneuver," which involves exhaling against a closed glottis that does not allow air to be expelled through the mouth and nose. The increase in intrathoracic pressure caused by the Valsalva maneuver can lead to a further increase in blood pressure. This response can be dangerous for patients with cardiovascular disease by increasing myocardial work and pressure in blood vessels. The greater the intensity of isometric exercise (duration of contraction and muscle mass), the greater the heart rate and blood pressure response. Chronic dynamic resistance exercise training lowers resting SBP, DBP, and MAP (mean arterial pressure) compared to pre-training. Isometric exercise training, when performed correctly at the appropriate intensity, also has a lowering effect on SBP and DBP at rest. Resistance exercise training is a type of exercise that can be safely performed in elderly people with cardiovascular disease without causing more stress to the cardiovascular system than aerobic exercise.

22.7 Factors Affecting Adaptation to Exercise

Age: Children and adults have similar metabolic demands and oxygen needs during exercise. But the way they meet these needs is different. For example, for the same workload on a bicycle ergometer, children's hearts are smaller than adults' and therefore have a lower stroke volume. The heart rate increases to compensate for the stroke volume. But cardiac output still remains low. Physical function changes with ageing. This change is accompanied by inactivity. Maximal heart rate and maximal stroke volume decrease, and therefore cardiac output also decreases. This results in lower VO_{2max} in the elderly compared to the young. According to data from cross-sectional studies, the decline in VO_{2max} is about 0.40–0.50 mL per kilogram per year in men. This rate of decline is smaller in women. With exercise training, both older men and women can increase their VO2max by approximately the same percentage.

Gender: There are gender differences that affect the adaptation of the circulatory system to exercise. Because women have smaller right and left ventricular chamber sizes than men, end-diastolic volume is generally lower in women. However, despite lower end-diastolic volumes, *ejection fraction* tends to be slightly higher in women. Because women generally have a smaller body size than men, their total blood volume is also smaller. Because of these differences, women have lower stroke volume and cardiac output at rest and during exercise and have lower cardiorespiratory fitness than men.

Environmental conditions: Basic physiological responses during exercise are significantly altered by changes in environmental conditions. To compensate for the increased body temperature during exercise, blood vessels in the skin dilate to transport more blood to the body surface. Evaporation of water from the surface of the skin aids heat loss. As long as the ambient temperature does not exceed the body temperature, body heat is transferred to the environment. If humidity increases, evaporation becomes more difficult. Greater blood flow to the skin can limit blood flow to active muscles during exercise. If body temperature is not stabilized during prolonged exercise, stroke volume decreases due to dehydration. To maintain cardiac output, the heart rate may increase significantly, compromising cardiovascular function.

A short or long stay at high altitude causes a number of adaptations. For oxygen demand, the first adaptation in the first 24 h is an increase in cardiac output both at rest and during submaximal exercise. Red blood cells (hemoconcentration) also increase in plasma volume for more oxygen molecules.

Fitness level: The magnitude of the response to exercise training depends on the person's initial fitness level. People with low cardiorespiratory fitness have a larger magnitude of improvement, while people with high cardiorespiratory fitness have a relatively smaller magnitude of improvement. One study showed that the same exercise training increased VO_{2max} by 50% in sedentary, middle-aged men with heart disease and by 10-15% in active healthy adults. It is important to remember that a 5% increase for elite athletes represents as significant a change as a 40% increase in a sedentary person.

Duration, intensity, frequency of exercise: The intensity and duration of exercise are important determinants of physiological adaptations in response to training. The same intensity of exercise may be a significant stressor for one person, while for another it may be below the threshold required for adaptation to occur. Therefore, exercise programs should be tailored to the individual. In aerobic exercise training, aerobic capacity can be increased if the exercise intensity is at least between 55 and 70% of HRmax and between 45 and 55% of VO_{2max}. Some patients, for example, a patient with heart failure, can start an exercise program with daily exercise cycles of 3–5 min. Optimal results are achieved when the intensity of an exercise session of 20–30 min in duration reaches at least 70% of HR_{max}. In higher intensity training, significant improvements can also be achieved with 10 min of exercise.

It is not clear whether exercise produces different effects if the frequency of exercise is changed but the duration and intensity are kept constant. Some researchers report that exercise frequency significantly influences cardiovascular improvements, while others argue that this factor contributes less than the intensity or duration of exercise. Aerobic exercise training programs are usually performed 3 days per week with an intermittent rest day between exercise days. If the duration and intensity of exercise is low, increasing the frequency of exercise will be beneficial for cardiovascular adaptations.

Trainability and genes: While a good exercise training program increases aerobic and anaerobic capacity regardless of a person's genetic background, the limits to the development of these capacities are closely linked to genetic endowment. For two people undertaking the same exercise program, one person may improve 10 times more than the other. Genetic research suggests a genotype dependence for much of our sensitivity to respond to maximal aerobic and anaerobic power training, including adaptations of most muscle enzymes.

22.8 Side/Unwanted Effects that May Occur During/After Exercise in Circulatory System Pathologies and Management

Exercise offers numerous benefits to individuals with peripheral vascular and cardiovascular disease. Improving physical function, providing independence in activities of daily living, prolonging life expectancy and improving quality of life are some of the benefits of exercise. Increased cardiovascular functional capacity has an important role in the primary/secondary prevention of cardiovascular diseases. In circulatory system pathologies, attention should be paid to side effects such as sudden increases in heart rate, blood pressure, arrhythmias and chest pain that may occur with exercise. People with cardiovascular disease (CVD) should be evaluated in detail before being enrolled in an exercise program and a limited exercise test should be performed. Heart rate, blood pressure, symptoms, ECG changes and hemodynamic changes should be monitored and recorded before, during and after the exercise test.

Variables such as the patient's clinical status, exercise tolerance, patient's interest, and ability should be taken into consideration when creating an exercise program. Individuals with CVD can better tolerate dynamic types of exercise in which large muscle groups participate, such as walking, jogging, running, swimming, and cycling. Aerobic exercise sessions should include a warm-up, exercise and cool-down period. Warm-up and cool-down periods have a protective effect against angina. When exercising, environmental factors such as humidity, temperature, high altitude should be taken into account and adequate water should be drunk. A hot shower after exercise may increase heart rate and arrhythmia. Therefore, hot showers should be avoided for at least 15 minutes after exercise.

When creating an exercise prescription, the intensity and frequency of exercise should be determined specifically for the patient. Exercise intensity should be calculated in such a way that it can create positive adaptations but at the same time does not cause cardiovascular symptoms and fatigue. Exercise intensity can be between 55 and 80% of maximal heart rate in most patients, 12–14 on the Borg scale (6-20) or 3-7 METs per week. Exercise intensity should be below the point of onset of symptoms. For example, if the patient's symptoms start at 132 beats/min, it would be beneficial to exercise between 110 and 120 beats/min. Maximum increases of 10% per week are recommended. If the patient's exercise capacity is less than 5 METs, exercise at a lower intensity of 40–50% can be started. It has also been stated that 2–3 METs or 20–30 beats/min more than the resting heart rate can be used as exercise intensity in these patients. The duration of exercise is recommended between 30–60 min and 3–5 days a week. Again, the duration and frequency of exercise can be reduced according to the clinical condition of the patient. If there is a change in the clinical condition of the patient during the rehabilitation process, the exercise prescription should be changed.

Some heart patients may develop arrhythmias during or after exercise. For this reason, warm-up and cool-down periods of 10–15 min should not be neglected, and the desired exercise intensity should be reached with gradual increases.

Exercise is contraindicated in recent myocardial ischemia, unstable ischemia, decompensated heart failure, exercise-induced and uncontrollable arrhythmia, and diseases in which symptoms and side effects occur with exercise (hypertrophic cardiomyopathy, severe aortic stenosis, arrhythmogenic heart disease, etc.).

If the heart rate is less than 40 beats/min or greater than 130 beats/min, SBP is greater than 180 mmHg, DBP is greater than 110 mmHg, the patient should not be included in exercise training that day. If the blood glucose level is below 100 mg/dL, exercise should be started after carbohydrate supplementation.

If the blood glucose level is greater than 250 mg/dL, exercise should not be performed if there is ketosis, and above 300 mg/dL even if there is no ketosis.

Exercise should be stopped if chest pain (angina), nausea, dizziness, shortness of breath, abnormal increase or decrease in blood pressure, and heart rate occur during exercise. The patient should be referred back to medical control and the exercise program should be rearranged or interrupted according to the results. Exercise should never be terminated abruptly. There must be a cooling down period of at least five minutes.

People with circulatory pathologies may experience various side effects during exercise. The most important point for this is that the patient should be subjected to an exercise test before being included in the exercise program and vital signs should be monitored before, during, and after exercise. It should not be forgotten that the exercise program prepared specifically for the patient is a "medicine."

22.9 Comparison of Circulatory System Adaptation Mechanism to Exercise: Healthy Individual and Patient with Heart Failure

The comparison of the adaptation mechanism of the circulatory system to exercise in patients with heart failure and healthy individuals is given in Table 22.5. Adaptation of the circulatory system to exercise is summarized in Table 22.6. Clinical implications of the cases are summarized in Table 22.7.

Table 22.5 Comparison of treatment programs of healthy individuals and patients with heart failure

Case 1. Healthy individual	Case 2. Patient with heart failure
K.Ç (Male), 35 years old, 1.80 m tall, weighing 88 kg, works in a bank. K.Ç. is consulting a physiotherapist to improve his general fitness. K.Ç. states that he has not had a regular exercise habit for the last 3 years. K.Ç. does not have any diagnosed disease and does not smoke.	52-year-old A.D. She is 164 m tall, weighs 75 kg and is a housewife. Five years ago, she was diagnosed with hypertensive dilated cardiomyopathy and started to be monitored by the cardiology department. Echocardiography revealed global hypokinesia and systolic dysfunction, mitral and aortic valve regurgitation. Ejection fraction was 38%. According to the congestive heart failure classification of the New York Heart Association, she is in stage 3. A.D. is a non-smoker.
Case evaluation	
Case 1. Healthy individual	**Case 2. Patient with heart failure**
Before being enrolled in the program, the individual was asked to complete **the Physical Activity Readiness Questionnaire (PAR-Q).** He was included in the program because he did not have a health problem that would prevent him from participating in a regular exercise program. **Determination of exercise capacity** • He was evaluated with cardiopulmonary exercise test. • The Treadmill/Bruce protocol was used. VO2max was measured as 37 mL/kg/min. Peak heart rate was recorded as 164 beats/min. • The VO2max value indicated a low exercise capacity for his age. In the exercise test, 87% of maximal heart rate was reached.	**Determination of exercise capacity** • Functional aerobic capacity was evaluated with a 6-min walk test. The patient walked 175 m and completed 32% of the expected values calculated according to weight, age and height. • She was evaluated with cardiopulmonary exercise test. • Upper extremity aerobic exercise capacity was assessed using an arm ergometer by increasing the workload by 5 watts every 2 min. The patient asked to stop the test due to fatigue and dyspnea. • The patient reached 45% of maximal heart rate. Oxygen saturation decreased by 3%. • She showed a lower exercise capacity than a healthy person of the same age.
Peripheral muscle strength test • The 1-maximal repetition (1-RM) was calculated with lying barbell lifts (bench- press), leg press, pull-down. • He had intermediate muscle strength and endurance for age and gender.	**Peripheral muscle strength test** • Peripheral muscle strength assessment was performed by calculating the muscle strength of large muscle groups with 1 maximum repetition method. • Muscle strength was reduced compared to healthy individuals of the same age.
	Respiratory muscle strength assessment • Respiratory muscle strength was evaluated with an intraoral pressure measuring device. • MIP was evaluated as 60% and MEP as 70%. • The patient had decreased inspiratory and expiratory muscle strength.
Posture assessment Anterior: shoulder asymmetry Lateral: kyphosis, rounded shoulder, anterior head tilt Posterior: no feature	**Posture assessment** Anterior: Pectus excavatum Lateral: kyphosis, rounded shoulder, anterior head tilt Posterior: no feature
	Dyspnea assessment • The "Modified Medical Research Council" (MMRC) dyspnea assessment was used to evaluate shortness of breath during activities of daily living. • The patient's score on the scale was 4.
	Assessment of fatigue • Fatigue Severity Scale (40/63). The patient complained of severe fatigue. Fatigue was affecting her physical and psychosocial functioning.

(continued)

Table 22.5 (continued)

Case 1. Healthy individual	Case 2. Patient with heart failure
	Assessment of quality of life • Health-related quality of life was assessed with the Nottingham health profile. • It was observed that health-related quality of life decreased especially in the dimensions of sleep, social isolation, physical activity and activities of daily living.
Treatment program **Case 1. Healthy individual** **Type of exercise:** Moderate intensity aerobic with treadmill **Exercise intensity:** Exercise was started at 40–59% of VO2max **Duration:** 5–10 min warm-up 20–60 min load 5–10 min cool down **Frequency:** 5 days a week After 3 weeks, switched to vigorous exercise training (60–89% of VO2max) 3 days per week.	**Case 2. Patient with heart failure** **Type of exercise:** Aerobic exercise on an arm ergometer **Exercise intensity:** Perceived exertion intensity according to the Borg scale at the 3–5 level **Duration:** O W at 25 RPM for 5–10 min warm-up, 4 W at 35 RPM for 15–20 min load, 0 W at 25 RPM for 5–10 min cool down **Frequency:** 3 days a week
Peripheral muscle strength training type of exercise: Resistance exercise **Intensity of exercise:** Started at 70% of 1 maximum repetition. **Duration**: 3 sets of 10 repetitions Frequency 3 times a week	**Peripheral muscle strength training** After the first 3 weeks of aerobic exercise training was completed, resistance exercise training was started. **Type of exercise:** Resistance exercise **Intensity of exercise:** Started at 40% of 1 maximal repetition for upper extremity muscles and 50% for lower extremity muscles. **Duration:** 2 sets of 8–12 repetitions **Frequency** 2 times a week
Posture exercises Posture exercises were recommended three times a day, three days a week for kyphotic posture.	**Posture exercises** Posture exercises were recommended three times a day, three days a week for kyphotic posture.
	Respiratory muscle strength training **Type of exercise:** Respironics Threshold IMT, **Intensity of exercise:** At 30% of MIP **Duration:**15 min/session **Frequency** 2 times a day, 5 days a week
	Energy conservation techniques and dyspnea reduction positions were taught.

Table 22.6 Adaptation of the circulatory system to exercise

Case 1. Healthy individual	Case 2. Patient with heart failure
Acute response to aerobic exercise	
Cardiac output is increased by an increase in both heart rate and stroke volume. SBP increases, DBP increases minimally or remains unchanged. More blood flows to active muscles and less to organs that need less, such as the kidneys and liver. The arteriovenous oxygen difference increases.	Cardiac output is mostly increased by an increase in heart rate. SBP increases, DBP increases minimally or does not change. It should be kept in mind that sudden changes in heart rate and blood pressure may occur depending on the clinical condition of the patient. More blood flows to active muscles and less to organs that need less, such as the kidneys and liver. The arteriovenous oxygen difference increases.
Chronic response to aerobic exercise	
Cardiac output is mostly increased by an increase in stroke volume. Cardiac hypertrophy maintains and improves the contractile function of the heart. NO production increases endothelium-dependent vasodilation. Blood pressure is regulated. LDL → cholesterol → decreases, → while → HDL cholesterol increases. Lactic acid tolerance increases. Recovery after exercise is accelerated.	Cardiac output is mostly increased by an increase in stroke volume. Cardiac hypertrophy maintains and improves the contractile function of the heart. NO production increases endothelium-dependent vasodilation. Blood pressure is regulated. LDL → cholesterol → decreases, → while → HDL cholesterol increases. Lactic acid tolerance increases. Recovery after exercise is accelerated. The patient performs daily life activities with less shortness of breath and fatigue.
Acute response to strengthening exercise training	
SBP increases, DBP decreases.	SBP increases, DBP decreases.
Chronic response to strengthening exercise training	
Loss of muscle strength decreases, blood pressure decreases, bone mineral density increases	Existing muscle strength is maintained and increased, blood pressure is reduced, bone mineral density is increased

Table 22.7 Clinical inference from cases

Do's and don'ts when planning exercise training
- Exercise is contraindicated in recent myocardial ischemia, unstable ischemia, decompensated heart failure, exercise-induced and uncontrollable arrhythmia, exercise-induced symptoms and side effects (hypertrophic cardiomyopathy, severe aortic stenosis, arrhythmogenic heart disease, etc.).
- People with cardiovascular disease and peripheral vascular disease should be evaluated in detail before being enrolled in an exercise program and a symptom-limited exercise test should be performed.
- It is safer to adjust the intensity of aerobic exercise according to perceived exertion intensity rather than heart rate in patients on beta-blockers.
- Combined exercise training using aerobic and resistance training is more effective in improving physical function.
- Drink enough fluids during and after exercise.
- Heart rate, blood pressure, symptoms, ECG changes, and hemodynamic changes should be monitored and recorded before, during, and after the exercise test.
- Some heart patients may develop arrhythmias during or after exercise. For this reason, warm- up and cool-down periods of 10–15 min should not be neglected, and the desired exercise intensity should be reached with gradual increases.
- If the heart rate is less than 40 beats/min or greater than 130 beats/min, SBP is greater than 180 mmHg, DBP is greater than 110 mmHg, the patient should not be included in exercise training that day.
- If the blood glucose level is below 100 mg/dL, exercise should be started after carbohydrate supplementation. If the blood glucose level is greater than 250 mg/dL, exercise should not be performed if there is ketosis, and should not be performed even if there is no ketosis above 300 mg/dL.
- The patient should be informed that if he/she experiences any of the following conditions during exercise, he/she should stop exercising:
    - Significant shortness of breath and fatigue,
    - Pallor, sweating, confusion
    - Nausea or vomiting
    - Sudden headache or dizziness
    - Sudden weakness in the arms or legs
    - Muscle cramps or joint pain

22.10 Conclusion

Depending on the type, duration, intensity, and frequency of exercise and the person's current capacity, both acute and chronic changes occur in the circulatory system to rebalance. Understanding the anatomy and physiology of the circulatory system and the effect of exercise on the circulatory system is instructive when assessing and designing exercise programs in patients, healthy individuals, and elite athletes. Exercise prescription should be prepared by taking into account the adaptations to different exercise methods in circulatory system diseases, the patient's current clinical status, and tolerance.

Further Reading

American College of Sports Medicine. Preliminary section: background materials functional anatomy. In: Swain DP, Brawner CA, Chambliss HO, Nagelkirk PR, Paternostro-Bayles M, Swank AM, editors. ACSM's resource manual for guidelines for exercise testing and prescription. 7th ed. Philadelphia: Wolters Kluwer Health/Lippincott Williams & Wilkins; 2014. p. 2–31. ISBN: 978-1609139568.

American College of Sports Medicine. Exercise prescription for patients with cardiac, peripheral, cerebrovascular, and pulmonary disease. In: Bayles MP, Swank AM, editors. ACSM's exercise testing and prescription. Philadelphia: Wolters Kluwer; 2018. p. 379–416. ISBN: 9781496338792.

Anonymous. Tolga Saka Koroner Kalp Hastalığı ve Egzersiz. Spor Hekimliği Dergisi. 2016;51(2):56–68. https://doi.org/10.5152/tjsm.2016.007.

Arıkan H, Sağlam M, Çalık Kütükçü E, Vardar Yağlı N. "Kardiyovasküler Sistem Fizyolojisi". In Fizyoterapi ve Rehabilitasyon Cilt 3. Nörolojik Rehabilitasyon ve Kardiyopulmoner Rehabilitasyon, Editors Karaduman A, Yılmaz Ö. Ankara, Hipokrat Publishing House, 1st Edition, Page: 305-316, 2017, ISBN: 978-605-9160-26-1

Chrysant SG. Current evidence on the hemodynamic and blood pressure effects of isometric exercise in normotensive and hypertensive persons. J Clin Hypertens (Greenwich). 2010;

Da Silva CA, Mortatti A, Silva RP, Silva GB Jr, Erberelli VF, Stefanini F, Lima MR. Acute effect of isometric resistance exercise on blood pressure of normotensive healthy subjects. Int J Cardiol. 2013;168(3):2883–6. https://doi.org/10.1016/j.ijcard.2013.03.104. Epub 2013 May 2.

Douglas J, Pearson S, Ross A, McGuigan M. Eccentric exercise: physiological characteristics and acute responses. Sports Med. 2017;47(4):663–75. https://doi.org/10.1007/s40279-016-0624-8.

Ehrman KJ, Kerrigan JD, Keteyian JS 'Kardiyovasküler Sistem: Fonksiyon ve Kontrol'. In:'İleri Egzersiz Fizyolojisi-Temel Kavramlar ve Uygulamalar' Translation Editor: Baltaci G. (2018) Ankara, Turkey 1st Edition, Pages 51-83, ISBN: 978-6059160803

Evans DL. Cardiovascular adaptations to exercise and training. Vet Clin North Am Equine

Pract. 1985;1(3):513–31. https://doi.org/10.1016/s0749-0739(17)30748-4.

Fagard RH. Exercise characteristics and the blood pressure response to dynamic physical training. Med Sci Sports Exerc. 2001;33(6 Suppl):S484–92; discussion S493-4. https://doi.org/10.1097/00005768-200106001-00018.

Hellsten Y, Nyberg M. Cardiovascular adaptations to exercise training. Compr Physiol. 2015;6(1):1–32. https://doi.org/10.1002/cphy.c140080.

Hughes DC, Ellefsen S, Baar K. Adaptations to endurance and strength training. Cold Spring Harb Perspect Med. 2018;8(6):a029769.

Janot JM, Van Guilder GP. Cardiovascular system. In: Porkari J, Bryant C, Comana F, editors. Exercise physiology. 1st ed. Philadelphia: F.A. Davis Company; 2015. p. 162–88. ISBN: 978-0803625556.

Lavie CJ, Arena R, Swift DL, Johannsen NM, Sui X, Lee DC, Earnest CP, Church TS, O'Keefe JH, Milani RV, Blair SN. Exercise and the cardiovascular system. Circ Res. 2015;117(2):207–19. https://doi.org/10.1161/CIRCRESAHA.117.305205.

Lemmey AB. Part VI - Disorders of the bones and joints. In: Ehrman JK, Gordon PM, Visich PS, Keteyian SJ, editors. Clinical exercise physiology. 4th ed. Human Kinetics; 2019. p. 817–72, ISBN: 9781492546467 (e-book), ISBN: 9781492546450.

M. Istanbul, Istanbul Medical Bookstore, 1st ed.; 2019, pp. 167–182. ISBN: 978-605-9528-85-6.

Powers SK, Howley ET. Physiology of exercise: circulatory responses to exercise. In: Powers SK, Howley ET, editors. Exercise physiology: theory and application to fitness and performance. 10th ed. New York: McGraw-Hill Education; 2018a. p. 193–223: ISBN: 9781259870453.

Powers SK, Howley ET. The physiology of training: effect on VO2 max, performance, and strength. In: Powers SK, Howley ET, editors. Exercise physiology: theory and application to fitness and performance. 10th ed. New York: McGraw-Hill Education; 2018b. p. 293–328. ISBN: 9781259870453.

Powers SK, Howley ET. Exercise for special populations. In: Powers SK, Howley ET, editors. Exercise physiology: theory and application to fitness and performance. 10th ed. McGraw-Hill Education, New York; 2018c. p. 396–411. ISBN: 9781259870453.

Rognmo Ø, Hetland E, Helgerud J, Hoff J, Slørdahl SA. High intensity aerobic interval exercise is superior to moderate intensity exercise for increasing aerobic capacity in patients with coronary artery disease. Eur J Cardiovasc Prev Rehabil. 2004;11(3):216–22. https://doi.org/10.1097/01.hjr.0000131677.96762.0c.

Gary P. Van Guilder, Jeffrey M. Janot. "Acute and chronic cardiorespiratory responses to exercise'. In Exercise physiology. Porkari J, Bryant C, Comana F., editors. F.A. Davis Company; 1st ed (2015) Philadelphia, 1st ed, 196-228, ISBN: 978-0803625556.

Endocrine System and Its Adaptations to Exercise

Cemile Bozdemir Ozel

Abstract

The function of the endocrine system is to regulate body functions by maintaining the internal balance of the body. The hormones released from endocrine glands regulate body functions by activating enzyme systems, changing cell permeability, triggering muscle contraction or relaxation, stimulating protein, carbohydrate, and fat metabolism, and determining how the body will respond to physiological and psychological stresses from inside and outside. Exercise is one of the most important factors affecting the endocrine system and body metabolism. This chapter explains the acute and chronic responses of exercise to the endocrine system and their associated mechanisms.

23.1 Anatomy of Endocrine System

Endocrine glands are structures that take part in the metabolism and physiological events occurring in an organism. Secretions from endocrine glands are released into the blood to bind to the surrounding extracellular space or specific body receptors. Besides glands with only internal secretion, there are also glands with internal and external secretions. Endocrine glands include six main glands: pineal gland, pituitary gland, thyroid gland, parathyroid gland, thymus gland, and adrenal glands.

The pineal gland consists of the corpus pineal and the pineal stalk. In its structure, there are pituitary and gonads, pinealocytes that cause rhythmic changes in the secretions of the hypothalamus, and glial cells that support the pinealocytes.

The pituitary gland is anatomically divided into anterior pituitary (adenohypophysis) and posterior pituitary (neurohypophysis). The anterior pituitary, a tissue of three different epithelial origins, consists of the distal lobe, the intermediate lobe, and the tuberous lobe. The posterior pituitary consists of the neural lobe, pituitary stalk, and infundibulum.

The thyroid gland is a brown and red gland located between C5 and T1 and has high vascularization. The thyroid gland consists of two lobes (lobus dexter and sinister) and a part called isthmus glandulae thyroidea that connects them.

The parathyroid gland is a small oval-shaped gland located behind the thyroid gland. The structure usually has four glands, and a connective tissue capsule surrounds each parathyroid gland.

The adrenal glands, one on the right and one on the left, are yellowish glands located in the poles

C. Bozdemir Ozel (✉)
Physiotherapy and Rehabilitation, Faculty of Health Sciences, Eskisehir Osmangazi University, Eskisehir, Turkey
e-mail: cozel@ogu.edu.tr

superior to the kidneys. These are separated from the kidneys by fibrous connective tissue. The anatomical locations, sizes, and weights of the endocrine glands are summarized in Table 23.1.

Besides the endocrine glands, there are organs that directly produce hormones such as the pancreas, gonads (ovary and testis), hypothalamus, and adipose tissue (Fig. 23.1). Some organs have

Table 23.1 Endocrine glands

Endocrine gland	Anatomical location	Size/weight	
Pineal gland	The posterior wall of the third ventricle	Size: $5–8 \times 3–5 \times 3–5$ mm^3 Weight: 100–200 mg	
Pituitary gland	In the fossa of the sphenoid bone	Size: $13 \times 10 \times 6$ mm^3 Weight: 500 mg	
Thyroid gland	Lateral to the trachea, near the base of the laryngeal cartilage, below the sternohyoid and sternothyroid muscles	Size: $5–6 \times 2–2.5 \times 2$ cm^3 Weight: 15–25 g	

Table 23.1 (continued)

Endocrine gland	Anatomical location	Size/weight	
Parathyroid gland	In the posterior connective tissue of the thyroid gland	Size: $3–6 \times 2–4 \times 0.5–2$ mm^3 Weight: 40 mg	
Adrenal gland	In the upper layer of the kidneys	Size: $5 \times 3 \times 1$ cm^3 Weight: 8–13 g	

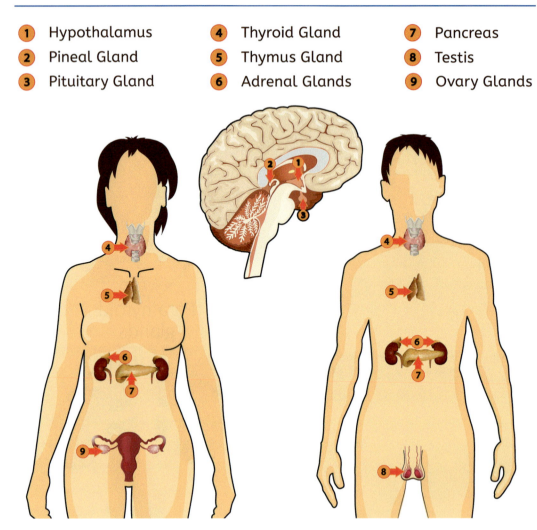

Fig. 23.1 Endocrine system *1* Hypothalamus, *2* Pineal gland, *3* Pituitary gland, *4* Thyroid gland, *5* Thymus, *6* Adrenal glands, *7* Pancreas, *8* Testis, *9* Ovary glands (Double Brain/Shutterstock.com)

pockets in their walls that produce hormones such as the stomach, kidneys, small intestine, and myocytes. All of them play a role in regulating body functions.

23.2 Physiology of Endocrine System

The endocrine system responds to the changing conditions of the internal and external environment of the body through chemical receptors called hormones and controls metabolism, energy balance, growth, and development of the body.

Hormones are classified into four categories according to molecular structures: amino acid derivatives (epinephrine, noradrenaline, and thyroxine), small peptides (encephalin and vasopressin), proteins [insulin, growth hormone, and thyroid-stimulating hormone (TSH)], and steroids (cortisol, progesterone, and testosterone).

The release of hormones is adjusted by the nervous system activity according to the body's needs. The plasma levels of hormones can vary depending on the amount synthesized in the gland, the amount released and catabolized into the blood, and the changes in plasma volume and especially the number of carrier proteins for some hormones. The plasma levels of hormones fluctuate throughout the day. Negative and positive feedback mechanisms control this fluctuation. The negative feedback mechanism has a suppressive feature that slows down the secretion of hormones when the activity of the target tissue reaches a certain level to prevent the excessive release of hormones and the effect of their excess on the target tissues. In the positive feedback mechanism, the biological effect of the hormones increases their release. Besides, hormone secretion is affected by circadian rhythms such as seasonal changes, different stages of growth and aging, daily cycle, and sleep. The onset and end times of the effect of each hormone differ. While some hormones are released within a few seconds after the stimulation of the relevant gland and show their effect immediately, some hormones can show their effects for a long time.

Hormones are transported in different ways. Water-soluble hormones such as peptides and catecholamines are transported to the target tissue in plasma by dissolving. In tissues, hormones reach the target tissue by passing the intercellular fluid through diffusion from the capillaries. Steroid and thyroid hormones are transported in the blood by binding to plasma proteins.

Hormones show their effects by binding to the hormone-specific receptors located in the cell membrane, cytoplasm, or nucleus of the target organ. The activation of the target cell depends on the hormone concentration in the blood, the number of target cell receptors, and the strength or sensitivity of the binding between the hormone and the receptors. The hypothalamus is located at the top of the hormone production system in the organization of the endocrine system. Its secretions have a substantial effect on the cerebral cortex. The pituitary gland is responsible for controlling the secretion of many endocrine glands. Adrenocorticotropic hormone (ACTH), TSH, growth hormone, prolactin, luteinizing hormone (LH), and follicle-stimulating hormone (FSH) are released from the anterior pituitary.

There is an overproduction of one or more hormones in the case of hyperpituitarism, usually caused by anterior lobe tumors. Giganticism and acromegaly, which are seen as a result of excessive secretion or irregularity in the secretion of growth hormone, and Cushing's syndrome observed in cases of increased secretion of ACTH are among the anterior lobe pathologies. Oxytocin and antidiuretic hormones (ADH vasopressin) are secreted from the posterior pituitary. Diabetes insipidus is seen as a deficiency in ADH secretion. Thyroid hormone is released from the thyroid gland, and its production/secretion is regulated by the hypothalamic, pituitary, and adrenal axis pathways and a negative feedback mechanism.

The iodide is required for the synthesis of the hormones. Primary hypothyroidism is observed due to an autoimmune disease, and secondary hypothyroidism is observed in cases where thyroid secretion is decreased due to the hypothalamus or pituitary. Hyperthyroidism occurs as a result of the over-activation of the thyroid gland. Parathyroid hormone (PTH) is released from the parathyroid gland. Hyperplasia of the parathyroid gland, hyperparathyroidism in tumoral conditions, hypoparathyroidism associated with surgical removal of the parathyroid gland, neoplasia, or some endocrinological system diseases are pathologies affecting parathyroid glands. Cortisol hormone (which follows the circadian rhythm sensitive to light, stress, sleep, and diseases) and aldosterone hormone (which plays a role in body fluid balance) are released from the adrenal cortex. Depending on the deterioration in the functions of the adrenal gland, glucocorticoid deficiency (Addison's disease) and hypoaldosteronism are observed.

Excessive aldosterone secretion causes Conn's disease, while excessive cortisol production occurs in Cushing's syndrome. Epinephrine and norepinephrine are produced from the adrenal medulla. In pheochromocytoma (pheochromocytoma), which develops due to a tumor of the adrenal medullary tissue, hypertension, headache, sweating, and palpitations can be seen due to the overproduction of catecholamines. Insulin and glucagon hormones are released from the pancreas, which has an essential role in nutrition, digestion, usage, and energy storage. Insulin is involved in regulating the glucose entry into cells, especially in muscle and adipose tissue, outside the brain. In the case of deficiency, impaired glucose metabolism and diabetes mellitus are observed. The hormones testosterone, estrogen, and progesterone are released from the gonadal cells. Endocrine system secretions, target tissue, and main effects are shown in Table 23.2.

Table 23.2 Secretions, target tissue, and main effects of the endocrine system

Anatomic part	Gland/cell	Hormone	Structure	Target tissue	Main effect
Adipose tissue	Cell	Leptin and adiponectin (resistin)	Peptide	Hypothalamus and other tissues	Suppresses appetite, stimulates thermogenesis, and plays a role in metabolism and reproduction
Adrenal cortex	Gland	Aldosterone	Steroid	Kidney	Stimulates sodium reabsorption and potassium secretion
Adrenal cortex	Gland	Glucocorticoid (cortisol and corticosterone)	Steroid	Mainly tissue	Supports protein and fat metabolism, raises the blood glucose level, and adapts the body to stress
Adrenal medulla	Gland	Epinephrine (adrenaline) and norepinephrine (noradrenaline)	Amino	Mainly tissue	Stimulates sympathetic activity, increases cardiac output, regulates blood vessels, increases glycogen catabolism, and releases fatty acids
Stomach	Cell	Gastrin	Peptide	Parietal cells	Stimulates the release of hydrochloric acid from parietal cells
Small intestine	Cell	Secretin	Peptide	Pancreas	Stimulates the release of water and bicarbonate from pancreatic cells
Small intestine	Cell	Cholecystokinin	Peptide	Gallbladder and pancreas	Stimulates the contraction of the gallbladder and the release of enzymes in the pancreas
Heart	Cell	Atrial natriuretic peptide	Peptide	Kidney tubules	Prevents the reabsorption of sodium and lowers blood pressure
Kidney	Cell	Erythropoietin	Peptide	Bone marrow	Increases erythrocyte production
Kidney	Cell	1,25-Dihydroxy-vitamin D3 (calciferol)	Steroid	Intestine	Increases the absorption of calcium from the intestines and bone mineralization
Kidney	Cell	Renin	Peptide	Kidney	Catalyzes the conversion of angiotensinogen into angiotensin 1
Liver	Cell	Angiotensinogen	Peptide	Adrenal cortex, blood vessels, and brain	Increases aldosterone secretion and blood pressure
Liver	Cell	IGF-1	Peptide	Mainly tissues	Stimulates growth
Muscle	Cell	IGF-1 and IGF-2 and myogenic regulatory factor	Peptide	Mainly tissues	Stimulates growth

Table 23.2 (continued)

Anatomic part	Gland/cell	Hormone	Structure	Target tissue	Main effect
Pancreas	Gland	Insulin	Peptide	Mainly tissues	Lowers blood glucose levels and supports protein, lipid, and glycogen synthesis
Pancreas	Gland	Glucagon	Peptide	Mainly tissues	Increases blood glucose level and supports glycogenolysis and gluconeogenesis
Pancreas	Gland	Somatostatin	Peptide	Mainly tissues	Inhibits the secretion of pancreatic hormones and regulates the digestion and reabsorption of nutrients
Hypothalamus	Neuron assemblage	Thyrotropin-releasing hormone	Peptide	Anterior pituitary	Stimulates the secretion of TSH and prolactin
Hypothalamus	Neuron assemblage	Corticotropin-releasing hormone	Peptide	Anterior pituitary	Releases ACTH
Hypothalamus	Neuron assemblage	Growth-hormone-releasing hormone	Peptide	Anterior pituitary	Stimulates the release of growth hormone
Hypothalamus	Neuron assemblage	Growth-hormone-suppressant hormone (somatostatin)	Peptide	Anterior pituitary	Suppresses the release of growth hormone
Hypothalamus	Neuron assemblage	Gonadotropin-releasing hormone	Peptide	Anterior pituitary	Releases LH and FSH
Hypothalamus	Neuron assemblage	Dopamine- and prolactin-suppressing hormone	Peptide	Anterior pituitary	Suppresses the release of prolactin
Pineal gland	Gland	Melatonin	Amino	–	Controls the circadian rhythm
Pituitary anterior lobe	Gland	Growth hormone	Peptide	Mainly tissues	Stimulates growth and bone and soft tissue growth and regulates protein, lipid, and carbohydrate metabolism
Pituitary anterior lobe	Gland	ACTH	Peptide	Adrenal cortex	Stimulates corticoid release
Pituitary anterior lobe	Gland	TSH	Peptide	Thyroid gland	Stimulates the release of thyroid hormones
Pituitary anterior lobe	Gland	Prolactin	Peptide	Breast	Stimulates milk secretion
Pituitary anterior lobe	Gland	FSH	Peptide	Gonads	Female: stimulates growth, follicle development, and estrogen synthesis Male: stimulates sperm production
Pituitary anterior lobe	Gland	LH	Peptide	Gonads	Female: stimulates ovulation, estrogen, and progesterone synthesis Male: stimulates testosterone synthesis
Pituitary posterior lobe	Extensions of peptide hypothalamic neurons	Oxytocin	Peptide	Breast and uterus	Stimulates uterine contractions and milk ejection in women
Pituitary posterior lobe	Extensions of peptide hypothalamic neurons	ADH (vasopressin)	Peptide	Kidney	Reduces urine output from the kidneys and promotes the contraction of blood vessels

(continued)

Table 23.2 (continued)

Anatomic part	Gland/cell	Hormone	Structure	Target tissue	Main effect
Thyroid	Gland	Triiodothyronine (T3) and thyroxine (T4)	Iodinized amine peptide	Mainly tissues	Increases metabolic rate and stimulates physical development
Thyroid	Gland	Calcitonin	Iodinized amine peptide	Bone	Increases calcium storage in the bone and lowers the blood calcium level
Parathyroid	Gland	PTH	Peptide	Bone and kidney	Stimulates the release of calcium from the bone and the absorption of calcium from the kidneys and intestines, increases the level of calcium in the blood, and stimulates the synthesis of vitamin D3
Thymus	Gland	Thymosin and thymopoietin	Peptide	Lymphocytes	Stimulates the proliferation and function of T lymphocytes
Ovary	Gland	Estrogen	Steroid	Mainly tissues	Responsible for egg production and secondary characteristics
Ovary	Gland	Progesterone	Steroid	Uterus	Supports endometrial growth to prepare the uterus for pregnancy
Ovary	Gland	Ovary inhibin	Peptide	Anterior pituitary lobe	Inhibits the release of FSH
Testis	Gland	Androgen	Steroid	Most textures	Sperm production is responsible for secondary characteristics
Testis	Gland	Inhibin	Peptide	Anterior pituitary lobe	Inhibits the release of FSH
Skin	Cell	Vitamin D_3	Steroid	Intermediate hormone form	1,25-Dihydroxy-vitamin D3 precursor
Placenta (pregnancy)	Gland	Estrogen and progesterone	Steroid	Mainly tissues	Plays a role in fetal and maternal development
Placenta (pregnancy)	Gland	Chorionic somatomammotropin	Peptide		Plays a role in the regulation of metabolism
Placenta (pregnancy)	Gland	Chorionic gonadotropin	Peptide	Mainly tissues	Ensures the growth of the corpus luteum and the secretion of estrogen and progesterone from there

ACTH Adrenocorticotropic hormone, *ADH* Antidiuretic hormone, *FSH* Follicle-stimulating hormone, *IGF-1* Insulin-like growth factor 1, *IGF-2* Insulin-like growth factor 2, *LH* Luteinizing hormone, *PTH* Parathyroid hormone. *[Adapted from Guyton et al. (2017) and McArdle et al. (2015).]*

23.3 Acute Response of the Endocrine System to Aerobic Exercise

Exercise affects the response of the endocrine system by influencing the pathways involved in hormone secretion. The release and amount of growth hormone are increased during exercise. With the increase in growth hormone response, glucose use decreases during exercise, free fatty acid mobilization increases, and thus plasma glucose concentration is preserved. A moderate-intensity continuous submaximal exercise increases growth hormone secretion with training in sedentary individuals. However, growth hormone response is higher in sedentary individuals. The growth hormone response increases with an increase in exercise intensity. Although the growth hormone is generated in 10 min from the start of aerobic exercise, its response reaches a peak within 25–30 min of starting the exercise. The levels of insulin-like growth hormones 1 and 2 (IGF-1 and IGF-2) released from the liver due to growth hormone stimulation also increase with acute exercise. TSH levels also increase with exercise. The ACTH release increases with exercise intensity and duration after exceeding 25% of aerobic capacity. At the same time, high-intensity physical activity and prolonged exercise trigger factors that suppress ACTH secretion.

Although it is difficult to determine the effect of exercise on FSH and LH, the levels of LH increase with exercise. Exercise has a strong stimulating effect on ADH secretion. The thyroid hormone secretion increases with exercise owing to increased body temperature. The levels of adrenal medulla hormones vary depending on the intensity of exercise. Although norepinephrine increases with exercise, exceeding 50% of the maximum oxygen consumption, the increase in epinephrine levels is observed at 75% and above the maximum oxygen consumption. During maximum exertion, the increase in norepinephrine levels is doubled. The cortisol levels increase during heavy exercise and decrease during light exercise. The level of increase remains high for about 2 h after exercise. This situation is vital for tissue recovery and tissue repair. Although the level of insulin hormone, which plays an important role in regulating glucose metabolism, decreases with exercise, an increase in the amount of glucagon is observed. The levels of interleukin-6, interleukin-10, interleukin-15, and irisin released from the muscle tissue, which it acts as an endocrine organ, increase with exercise. The adiponectin levels increase with exercise, while leptin levels decrease as hormones are released from adipose tissue. Table 23.3 shows the responses of major hormones in the endocrine system to acute exercise.

Table 23.3 Chronic response of the endocrine system to aerobic exercise

Hormone	Response
Growth hormone	↑
TSH (IGF-1 and IGF-2)	↑
TSH	↑
ACTH	↑
Prolactin	↑
FSH and LH	↑↔
ADH (vasopressin)	↑
Oxytocin	Unknown
Thyroid hormones (T3 and T4)	↑
Parathyroid	↑
Epinephrine and norepinephrine	↑
Cortisol	↑,↓ (Depends on intensity)
Aldosterone	↑
Testosterone	↑
Estrogen and progesterone	↑
Insulin	↓
Glucagon	↑

↓: decreased; ↑: increased; ↔: unchanged. *ACTH* Adrenocorticotropic hormone, *ADH* Antidiuretic hormone, *FSH* Follicle-stimulating hormone, *IGF-1* Insulin-like growth factor 1, *IGF-2* Insulin-like growth factor 2, *TSH* Thyroid-stimulating hormone. [Adapted from McArdle et al. (2015).]

23.4 Chronic Response of the Endocrine System to Aerobic Exercise

The chronic effect of exercise varies according to the characteristics of exercise training. An examination of the chronic effect of exercise on growth hormone shows that exercise does not affect the resting plasma level of growth hormone, an increase in growth hormone levels is observed after exercise training. ACTH secretion, which provides free fatty acid mobilization, increases with exercise training, especially at high intensities and during long periods. The levels of FSH and LH are affected by the menstrual cycle. Although their oscillations decrease in trained individuals, the levels of progesterone and LH increase during the follicle phase of the cycle. The prolactin level is proportional to the exercise intensity in continuous exercise training. As the duration increases, the magnitude of the prolactin response increases.

Although the level of ADH does not change with prolonged submaximal and near-maximal exercise training, no long submaximal exercise training leads to a decrease in the ADH level. The TSH level increases with exercise lasting more than 20 min, and the intensity is 60% or more of the maximum oxygen consumption as a response to exercise training on thyroid hormones. Exercise training does not affect the resting plasma level of thyroid hormones. An increased TSH level leads to an increase in T4 hormone levels and causes a decrease in T3 levels. The effect of submaximal exercise training on thyroid hormones varies. While prolonged submaximal (60 min and above) exercise does not affect thyroid function, some evidence shows that steady-state exercise lasting 40 min increases T4 levels. T4 levels increase with maximal exercise. Besides, the peripheral sensitivity of thyroid hormones increases with exercise training. The cortisol hormone levels increase less at the same workload intensity after exercise training. Insulin and glucagon hormone levels are close to resting levels during exercise training. The insulin level shows less difference at the same exercise load. The chronic response of the endocrine system to aerobic exercise is shown in Table 23.4.

Table 23.4 Chronic response of the endocrine system to aerobic exercise

Hormone	Response
Growth hormone	↑
TSH	↑
ACTH	↑
Prolactin	↑
FSH and LH	↓
ADH (vasopressin)	↓
Oxytocin	Unknown
Thyroid hormones (T3 and T4)	T3 ↓, T4 ↑
Parathyroid	↑
Epinephrine and norepinephrine	Resting time and similar exercise intensity ↓
Cortisol	↑
Aldosterone	No training adaptation
Testosterone	↓
Insulin	↓
Glucagon	↑

↓: decreased; ↑: increased; ↔: unchanged. *ACTH* Adrenocorticotropic hormone, *FSH* Follicle-stimulating hormone, *LH* Luteinizing hormone, *TSH* Thyroid-stimulating hormone. [Adapted from McArdle et al. (2015).]

23.5 Adaptation Mechanisms in Different Types of Exercises

23.5.1 Resistance Training

The remodeling of the muscle seen after strength training occurs with different hormonal responses and the production of new contractile mechanisms. This change in the muscle is affected by many factors such as exercise intensity, frequency, volume, mode, and recovery time. Resistance training adaptation differs with the change in hepatic and extrahepatic hormone clearance rates, cell fluid in receptor sites, hormone secretion rate, and receptor site interaction with neurohumoral control. Testosterone and growth hormone are primarily affected by resistance training adaptations. Testosterone and growth hormone interact with the nervous system to increase muscle strength. A single session of resistance exercise training has been shown to increase testosterone levels for a short time and decrease cortisol levels. As exercise intensity increases, testosterone levels also increase. The testosterone level in the chronic exercise response remains constant as long as the exercise intensity and volume do not change. The plasma levels of growth hormone increase depending on the exercise intensity after resistance training. Its levels do not change after moderate resistance training but increase with high-intensity exercise training. The insulin response to strength training does not change, or the plasma levels of insulin decrease. Insulin response to resistance training is affected by the individual's dietary habits. The release of catecholamines also increases in high-intensity exercise training protocols.

23.5.2 High-Intensity Interval Training

High-intensity interval training (HIIT) is exercise training where periods of intense exercise are alternated by low-intensity exercise and rest. It causes a high rate of physiological response on metabolism. Since the physiological stress on the metabolism and the demand of the metabolism differ according to the exercise and rest interval, the hormonal responses may be different. For example, a single supramaximal sprint exercise session (4 × 30 s) can result in a higher growth hormone response than continuous moderate-intensity aerobic exercise. Researchers stated an increase in plasma total T4 levels and a decrease in the peripheral conversion of T4 to T3 after HIIT. Testosterone levels are higher at the end of the HIIT session compared with moderated exercise. A study showed that plasma ACTH, cortisol, and growth hormone levels increased while plasma insulin levels decreased after HIIT. A greater increase in adrenal hormone levels is observed in sprint exercise training than in aerobic activity.

23.5.3 Whole-Body Vibration

The repetitive muscle contractions with low-amplitude and high-frequency vibration exercise affect metabolism. Whole-body vibration training increases the levels of growth hormone, testosterone, and norepinephrine. Besides, a study showed an increase in the levels of growth hormone, testosterone, cortisol, and interleukin-6 after whole-body vibration training.

23.6 Factors Affecting Exercise Adaptations

Exercise response and adaptation of the endocrine system are affected by physiological and environmental factors such as sex, age, ethnicity and race, body composition, mental health, circadian cycle, nutrition, cold environment, and brown adipose tissue.

23.6.1 Sex

Sex-specific differences exist in hormonal response to exercise. An elevation in testosterone levels during exercise is both earlier and higher in men. The growth hormone response is greater in women before exercise. The response of sex-specific hormones in women varies according to the phase and condition of the menstrual cycle. Besides, the hormones involved during the menstrual cycle change the effects of other hormones and their response to exercise. No sex-specific differences exist between the response of some hormones to exercise, such as aldosterone and vasopressin.

23.6.2 Age

Exercise response can change before and after puberty, postmenopausal or andropause, and plasma hormone levels. For example, the levels of growth hormone and testosterone decrease with age, while the levels of cortisol and insulin increase with age.

23.6.3 Ethnicity and Race

Hormonal components differ between different races and ethnic groups. The resting level of parathyroid hormone tends to be higher in blacks than in Caucasian individuals. Caucasian women may have higher estrogen levels than Asian women. Although not many studies are available investigating the effect of race and ethnicity on the hormonal system response to exercise, it is thought that the differences in plasma levels affect the training response.

23.6.4 Body Composition

Endocrinal responses resulting from cytokines released by adipose tissue affect metabolism, reproduction, and inflammatory function. Some cytokines directly increase hormone levels (interleukin-6 increases cortisol levels). An increase in the hormonal level can be greater with obesity. Obese people have higher levels of insulin and leptin. The acute and training response of the exercise can change as body weight increases compared with people with normal body weight. The catecholamine and growth hormone response to exercise is reduced in obese individuals. With exercise, the cortisol levels increase in some obese individuals and decrease in others. The hormonal response is normalized as a result of the decrease in body weight with exercise training.

23.6.5 Mental Health

High levels of anxiety or other mental health-related conditions cause changes in the activation of the sympathetic nervous system and the activity of the hypothalamic–pituitary–adrenal pathway. The levels of catecholamine, ACTH, and cortisol in circulation vary in individuals with anxiety. Depression has adverse effects on the hypothalamic–pituitary–adrenal pathway activity.

23.6.6 Circadian Rhythm

The levels of many hormones fluctuate throughout the day (24-h cycle). The spontaneous release of some hypothalamic hormones plays a role in regulating the endocrine system; behavioral and environmental factors cause this fluctuation. The cortisol levels are twice as high in the morning than in the daytime. The levels of hormones such as ACTH, growth hormone, melatonin, prolactin, and testosterone increase in the early part of the day and decrease in the afternoon. The levels of hormones such as aldosterone and parathyroid hormone are lower in the morning than in the afternoon. The levels of hormones according to the circadian rhythm are also affected by factors such as sleep and menstrual cycle. Besides, circadian rhythm has a direct effect on exercise performance. In particular, internal body temperature has a significant effect on physical performance and biological processes. Increasing the body temperature affects the performance by triggering carbohydrate burning and the establishment of actin–myosin cross-bridges in the musculoskeletal system; therefore, performance may be higher in the afternoon and early evening hours. It has also been stated that circadian gene expression may be dissimilar during different types of exercise training. This difference can be seen clearly in strengthening exercises. The highest performance in the strength training is seen in the afternoon and evening time. Like strength training, the peak performance in short-duration high-intensity exercise training is higher in the afternoon and evening hours than in the morning. Performance during moderate- continued exercise training is equal in all hours of the day.

23.6.7 Nutrition

Hormones such as insulin, glucagon, epinephrine, growth hormone, insulin-like growth factor, and cortisol play a role in the mobilization and usage of energy substrates and meet the energy metabolism demands during exercise. The levels of glucagon, epinephrine, growth hormone, and cortisol are higher in low-carbohydrate diets.

23.6.8 Cold Environment

Environmental temperature changes the exercise response by affecting cortisol. The cortisol levels increase more in exercise performed in a cold environment.

23.6.9 Brown Adipose Tissue

Brown adipose tissue, which is a thermogenic tissue, leads to the use of significant amounts of glucose and fatty acids for energy metabolism and thermogenesis. Increased brown adipose tissue activity is associated with a decrease in glucose levels. Especially, exercise performed in a cold environment results in higher glucose uptake, improved insulin sensitivity, increased glucose transporter proteins, and decreased free fatty acid usage.

23.7 Possible Complications During/After Exercise in Endocrine System Pathologies and Their Management Pathologies

Obesity, type 2 diabetes, and metabolic syndrome are the most common endocrinological conditions resulting from impaired glucose metabolism. During exercise, attention should be paid to the presence of micro- and macrovascular complications in a population with diabetes. Exercise type and duration should be planned considering these complications in the case of coronary artery disease, peripheral artery disease, nephropathy, retinopathy, and neuropathy. The loss of sensation may cause foot ulcerations in peripheral neuropathy, and necessary precautions should be taken for this. Prolonged and weight-bearing exercises should be avoided, and appropriate shoes should be used by patients with foot ulceration and advanced neuropathy. In autonomic neuropathy, heart rate response to exercise may be impaired (low heart rate response to exercise, inappropriate heart rate increase, and resting tachycardia). When planning an exercise program for this population, perceived effort, heart rate reserve, and maximum oxygen uptake are used for calculating the exercise intensity. Jumping activities in individuals with retinopathy and exercises that may cause sudden blood pressure elevation in those with nephropathy should be avoided. Hypoglycemia is the most important complication in individuals exercising at high intensity using insulin and exercising. The blood glucose levels should be measured before starting exercise to prevent the risk of hypoglycemia. If the blood glucose level is less than 90 mg/dL, additional carbohydrates should be taken. If the exercise time is more than 30 min, the blood sugar level should be rechecked, and additional carbohydrates should be taken if necessary. Insulin intake and exercise time should be considered, especially in individuals using short-acting insulin derivatives. Besides, exercise should not be done actively in the area where insulin is applied in that session.

Body weight–supported exercise should be preferred to prevent joint degeneration in individuals with obesity. Since thermoregulation mechanisms may be affected in these individuals, adequate hydration should be ensured during exercise and at ambient temperature. It should be considered that there may be sudden blood pressure elevation in some endocrine pathologies, especially in cases with affected adrenal glands.

23.8 Comparison of the Adaptation Mechanism of the Endocrine System to Exercise: A Healthy Individual and a Patient with Type 2 Diabetes

Comparison of the adaptation mechanism of the endocrine system to exercise in a patient with type 2 diabetes and a healthy individual is given in Table 23.5. The clinical implications of the cases are summarized in Table 23.6.

Table 23.5 Comparison of adaptations to exercise in healthy individuals and patients with type 2 diabetes

Case 1. Healthy individual	Case 2. Patient with type 2 diabetes
K.Ç (male)	A.S. (male)
Age: 35 years	Age: 50 years
Height: 1.80 m	Height: 1.84 m
Weight: 88 kg	Weight: 102 kg
K.C. consulted a physiotherapist to improve his general fitness. He said that he had been doing regular exercise for the last 3 years. He was not diagnosed with any disease. He did not smoke. He worked at the bank.	He was diagnosed with type 2 diabetes 3 years ago. He used long-acting insulin (dosage: 24 units) every evening. He did not smoke.

(continued)

Table 23.5 (continued)

Case 1. Healthy individual	Case 2. Patient with type 2 diabetes
Assessment	
Case 1. Healthy individual	**Case 2. Patient with type 2 diabetes**
Laboratory parameters	
Parameters that can provide information about the patient's glucose profile should be examined in the follow-up of individuals with diabetes	
Fasting blood glucose (normal range: 70–100 mg/dL) and glycated hemoglobin (HbA1c) <6.4%)	
Fasting blood glucose: 85 mg/dL	Fasting blood glucose: 185 mg/dL
Glycated hemoglobin: 5.4%	Glycated hemoglobin: 7.2%
Vital parameters at the beginning of the exercise test	
Heart rate: 82 beats/min	Heart rate: 90 beats/min
Systolic and diastolic blood pressure: 120/70 mmHg	Systolic and diastolic blood pressure: 130/80 mmHg

Exercise capacity

Before performing an exercise program, the patient's cardiorespiratory fitness level should be examined. For this, the cardiopulmonary exercise test and field tests should be used. Individuals should perform the symptom-limited cardiopulmonary exercise test using the Bruce protocol on a treadmill.

Speed/incline/time	Case 1. Healthy individual Heart rate (beats/min)/systolic and diastolic blood pressure (mmHg)	Case 2. Patient with type 2 diabetes Heart rate (beats/min)/systolic and diastolic blood pressure (mmHg)
2.7 km/h/10%/3 min	108/120–80	118/140–80
4 km/h/12%/3 min	120/136–80	134/150–85
5.5 km/h/14%/3 min	136/145–85	155/160–90
6.8 km/h/16%/3 min	153/150–88	Test terminated due to fatigue [Borg scale (0–10): 8]
8.0 km/h/18%/3 min	185/170–90	–
Peak heart rate values reached during the test (beats/min)/percentage of maximum heart rate	185/100%	160/94%
Peak maximum oxygen consumption reached during the test [mL/(kg / min)]	31	20

The exercise test was terminated because the maximum heart rate was reached in a healthy person, while it was finished earlier due to fatigue in the patient with type 2 diabetes (94% of the maximal heart rate).
The maximum oxygen consumption at the end of the exercise test decreased in a patient with diabetes while it was at a normal level in a healthy person.

Continuous moderate-intensity aerobic exercise training and moderate-intensity resistance training were planned for both cases.

Case 1. Healthy individual	Case 2. Patient with type 2 diabetes
Aerobic exercise training	**Aerobic exercise training**
Intensity: 80% of predicted maximum heart rate	Intensity: 80% of predicted maximum heart rate
Frequency: 5 days of the week	Frequency: 5 days of the week
Type: Treadmill	Type: Treadmill
Time: 45 min	Time: 45 min
Resistance training	**Resistance training**

Table 23.5 (continued)

Case 1. Healthy individual	Case 2. Patient with type 2 diabetes
Intensity: 70% of one repetition maximum Frequency: 5 days per week Nine resistance exercises (including big muscle groups) 10–20 repetition/2 sets	Intensity: 70% of one repetition maximum Frequency: 5 days per week Nine resistance exercises (including big muscle groups) 10–20 repetition/2 sets
Endocrine system to exercise adaptations	
Case 1. Healthy individual	**Case 2. Patient with type 2 diabetes**
Acute response to aerobic resistance	
Insulin: Decrease Glucagon: Increase	Insulin: Decrease Glucagon: Increase
Chronic response to aerobic resistance	
Insulin: Decrease Glucagon: Increase	Insulin: Decrease Glucagon: Increase
Acute response to resistance training	
Insulin: Unchanged	Insulin: Decrease
Chronic response to resistance training	
Insulin: Unchanged	Insulin: Unchanged

Table 23.6 Clinical inferences from the cases

Do's and don'ts when planning the exercise training
• The patient's complication, glucose profile, and drug used should be considered when planning the exercise training. Individuals with uncontrolled glucose profile, fluctuating glucose levels, and frequent hypoglycemia attacks should be treated after the controlling the glucose profile.

23.9 Conclusion

Exercise has varying effects on the endocrine system. These physiological changes differ according to the intensity and duration of exercise training. Exercise training is one of the most treatment approaches in managing type 2 diabetes and obesity due to its beneficial effects on the endocrine system.

Further Reading

Ball D. Metabolic and endocrine response to exercise: sympathoadrenal integration with skeletal muscle. J Endocrinol. 2015;224(2):R79–95.

Becic T, Studenik C, Hoffmann G. Exercise increases adiponectin and reduces leptin levels in prediabetic and diabetic individuals: systematic review and meta-analysis of randomized controlled trials. Med Sci. 2018;6(4):1–18.

Colberg SR, Sigal RJ, Yardley JE, Riddell MC, Dunstan DW, Dempsey PC, et al. Physical activity/exercise and diabetes: a position statement of the American Diabetes Association. Diabetes Care. 2016;39(11):2065–79.

Deemer SE, Castleberry TJ, Irvine C, Newmire DE, Oldham M, King GA, et al. Pilot study: an acute bout of high intensity interval exercise increases 12.5 h GH secretion. Physiol Rep. 2018;6(2):1–10.

Di Giminiani R, Rucci N, Capuano L, Ponzetti M, Aielli F, Tihanyi J. Individualized Whole-body vibration: neuromuscular, biochemical, muscle damage and inflammatory acute responses. Dose-Response. 2020;18(2):1–12.

Forkin KT, Huffmyer JL, Nemergut EC. Endocrine physiology. In: Hugh CH, Egan TD, editors. Pharmacology and physiology for anesthesia. Elsevier; 2019. p. 693–707.

Hackney AC, Saeidi A. The thyroid axis, prolactin, and exercise in humans. Curr Opin Endocrine Metab Res. 2019;9:45–50.

Hackney AC, Smith-Ryan AB. Methodological considerations in exercise endocrinology. In: Constantini N, Hackney AC, editors. Endocrinology of physical activity and sport. Humana Press; 2013. p. 1–19.

Gabriel BM, Juleen RZ. Circadian rhythms and exercise—re-setting the clock in metabolic disease. Nat Rev Endocrinol. 2019;15(4):197–206.

Giunta M, Cardinale M, Agosti F, Patrizi A, Compri E, Rigamonti AE, et al. Growth hormone-releasing effects of whole body vibration alone or combined with squatting plus external load in severely obese female subjects. Obes Facts. 2012;5(4):567–74.

Guyton AC, Hall JE. Guyton and hall textbook of medical physiology. 14th ed. Elsevier Health Sciences; 2020.

McArdle W, Katch FI, Katch VL. The endocrine system: organization and acute and chronic responses to physical activity. In: McArdle W, Katch FI, Katch VL, editors. Exercise physiology nutrition, energy and human performance. Wolters Kluwer; 2015. p. 407–49.

La Perle KMD, Dintzis SM. Endocrine system. In: Treuting PM, Dintzis SM, Montine KS, editors. Comparative anatomy and histology. Academic Press; 2018. p. 251–73.

Leal LG, Lopes MA, Batista LM. Physical exercise-induced myokines and muscle-adipose tissue crosstalk: a review of current knowledge and the implications for health and metabolic diseases. Front Physiol. 2018;9(1307):1–17.

Lowe JS. Endocrine system. In: Lowe JS, Anderson PG, editors. Human histology. Elsevier Mosby; 2015. p. 263–85.

Izawa S, Kim K, Akimoto T, Ahn N, Lee H, Suzuki K. Effects of cold environment exposure and cold acclimatization on exercise- induced salivary cortisol response. Wilderness Environ Med. 2009;20(3):239–43.

Kraemer RR, Castracane VD. Endocrine alterations from concentric vs. eccentric muscle actions: a brief review. Metabolism. 2015;64(2):190–201.

Peake JM, Tan SJ, Markworth JF, Broadbent JA, Skinner TL, Cameron-Smith D. Metabolic and hormonal responses to isoenergetic high-intensity interval exercise and continuous moderate-intensity exercise. Am J Physiol Endocrinol Metab. 2014;307(7):E539–52.

Valgas P, da Silva C, Hernández-Saavedra D, White JD, Stanford KI. Cold and exercise: Therapeutic tools to activate brown adipose tissue and combat obesity. Biology. 2019;8(1):1–29.

Teo W, Newton MJ, McGuigan. Circadian rhythms in exercise performance: implications for hormonal and muscular adaptation. J Sports Sci Med. 2011;10:600–6.

Wahl P. Hormonal and metabolic responses to high intensity interval training. J Sports Med Doping Stud. 2013;3(1):e132.

Renal System, Fluid Balance, and Its Adaptations to Exercise

24

Selda Gokcen

Abstract

The renal system, especially its primary organ, the kidney, plays an essential role in protecting body homeostasis. Acute exercise creates stress on the body and disrupts homeostasis. On the other hand, chronic exercise can cause the body to develop beneficial adaptations in the renal system as well as other parts of the body. Therefore, it is essential and necessary to analyze the renal response to exercise so that the safety limit and the profitable outcomes can be understood in both healthy individuals and renal failure patients. In this section, the renal system and its adaptation to exercise and fluid balance will be explained.

24.1 Anatomy

The renal system (urinary system) consists of two kidneys, two ureters, a bladder, and a urethra. Kidneys are responsible for producing urine while the other structures transfer it and act as a temporary reservoir (Fig. 24.1).

S. Gokcen (✉)
Physiotherapy and Rehabilitation, Faculty of Health Sciences, Kutahya Health Sciences University, Kutahya, Turkey

24.1.1 Kidneys

Lying between the T_{12} and L_3 vertebrae, kidneys are dark red bean-shaped organs. They have an average length of 12 cm and a weight of 150 g each. The right kidney is located slightly lower than the left due to the location of the liver superior to it.

Kidneys consist of two parts: the cortex and the medulla. Cortex structures produce urine and the medulla is comprised of collector ducts.

The arterial sources of the kidneys are the renal arteries. Renal artery branches are aligned with the intervertebral disks of L_1 and L_2, and they originate from the abdominal aorta. Renal arteries carry a quarter of the cardiac output to the kidneys, which is an indication of how well the kidneys are perfused.

24.1.2 Ureters

The urine produced in the kidneys then consecutively goes to the minor renal calyx, the major renal calyx (which consists of a few minor renal calyxes), and the renal pelvis before it enters the ureters. Ureters act as a urine transporter from the kidneys to the bladder and they are each approximately 27–30 cm in length and 1–5 mm in diameter. After entering the pelvic cavity, the ureters open into the bladder.

Fig. 24.1 Anatomy of the urinary system (Olga Bolbot/Shutterstock.com)

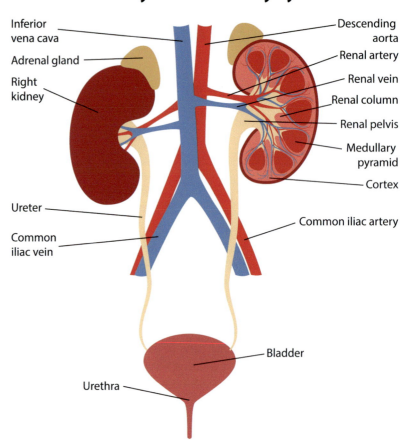

24.1.3 Bladder

The bladder temporarily stores urine until it is discharged through the urethra. The bladder can store up to 500 mL of urine, but its normal volume is around 220 mL. It is located intraperitoneally between the pubic diaphragm and the pelvic diaphragm.

24.1.4 Urethra

The urethra is the conduit for urine excretion from the bladder. Both structure and length are different in men and women.

The male urethra is divided into three parts: prostatic urethra (pars prostatica), membranous urethra (pars membranacea), and penile urethra (pars spongiosa). The widest part, the prostatic urethra, is about 3 cm in width. Here the urinary and semen tracts join. The narrowest part is the membranous urethra, which measures 2 cm. The penile (spongy) urethra is the part that passes through the penis and opens out. The penile urethra is about 15 cm long.

The female urethra consists of two parts called the pelvic urethra and perineal urethra. Its total length is 3–5 cm.

24.2 Physiology

The renal system is the body's excretory system, which includes the kidneys that produce the urine, ureters that transfer it, a bladder that stores it, and a urethra that is the outlet. The kidneys are mainly responsible for the removal of toxins, metabolic waste, and excess ions from the body as well as for regulation of the liquid–electrolyte balance. The kidneys have many more vital functions in addition to those mentioned above (Fig. 24.2).

24.2.1 Elimination of Metabolic Waste from the Body

Kidneys filter an average of 1200 mL of blood a minute, which is 20% of the cardiac output. This filtration is done in the smallest functional part of the kidney: a nephron. An adult has approximately 1–2.5 million nephrons in their body and each nephron can create urine as an output. The formation of urine occurs in three steps:

1. *Glomerular Filtration*: Glomerular filtration is the passage of plasma from the capillaries into the Bowman's space. The glomeruli are balls of capillaries in the renal cortex that are responsible for the filtration of blood. A significant part of the blood plasma in the glomerulus is filtered through the glomerular membrane into the tubular system.
2. *Tubular Reabsorption*: The essential materials get reabsorbed from the filtrate.
3. *Tubular Secretion*: Unwanted substances are excreted, and urine is formed.

As a result, 1700 L of blood are cleaned in a day by this mechanism. An average of 1 L of urine is produced (Fig. 24.3).

24.2.2 Regulation of Fluid–Electrolyte Balance

In a healthy body, the volume and composition of fluids are kept in balance. In this mechanism called the fluid–electrolyte balance, the kidneys play a vital role. An adult person takes approximately 1600 mL of liquid by mouth in 1 day. In addition, 700 mL of fluid is gained through the absorption of food from the gastrointestinal system and another 200 mL is produced through cell

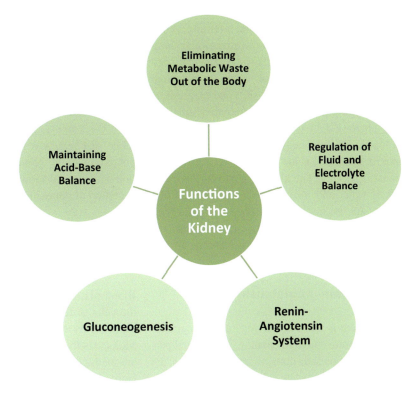

Fig. 24.2 Vital functions of the kidney

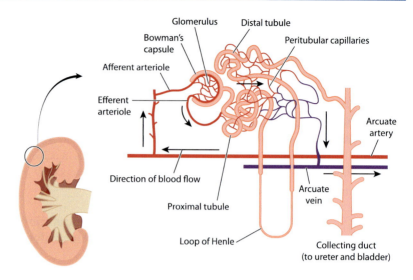

Fig. 24.3 Function of the nephron (Blamb/Shutterstock.com)

metabolism. Consequently, a daily average of 2500 mL of liquid is taken into the body. About 100 mL of liquid is excreted with feces, 600 mL of liquid evaporates from the skin, and 300 mL of liquid is lost through the respiratory tract in the process of breathing. Kidneys eliminate about 1500 mm of liquid ensuring an equal amount of fluid intake and outtake.

An adult male's body weight consists of approximately 60% water while a female's body consists of about 50% water. Intracellular compartments contain 2/3 of this water. The main cations (positive ions) of the intracellular compartment are potassium (K^+) and magnesium (Mg^{++}), while its main anions (negative ions) are phosphate (PO_4^{3-}) and proteins. The main cation of the extracellular compartment is sodium (Na^+), and its main anions are chlorine (Cl^-) and bicarbonate (HCO_3^-). The kidneys perform the transfer of water and ions between the extracellular space and the intracellular space through retention or excretion of water, ensuring that the amount of sodium in the body is stable.

24.2.3 Renin–Angiotensin System

This system is a hormonal system that regulates blood pressure and fluid balance. When renal perfusion is decreased, juxtaglomerular cells in the kidneys (smooth muscle cells located in the afferent arterioles of the kidney, which are responsible for the synthesis and storage of renin) secrete a hormone called renin. The main determining factor in the secretion of renin is the reduced intake of sodium into the body. Another substance called angiotensinogen is a hormone synthesized in the liver. After renin is secreted, it stimulates the formation of angiotensin I from angiotensinogen. Angiotensin I is converted to angiotensin II. Angiotensin II increases the volume of plasma by stimulating the absorption of water and sodium through the kidneys. Angiotensin II causes vasoconstriction in the vascular bed, which increases blood pressure. Angiotensin II also stimulates the release of aldosterone, which is another factor that increases the absorption of water and sodium from the kidneys. Aldosterone is a steroid hormone that regulates the balance of sodium and potassium in the blood. It ensures the reabsorption of water and sodium from the tubules and the excretion of potassium into the urine.

24.2.4 Maintaining Acid–Base Balance

Blood pH should be between 7.36 and 7.44 for the cells to function normally. The blood pH is sustained by the balance between acids and bases. Molecules that give an H^+ ion to the environment are acids, and molecules that receive an H^+ ion from the environment are bases. In the body, there are physiological buffer systems and respiratory mechanisms for the regulation of the acid–base balance. The kidneys are the most important organs that ensure the acid–base balance by performing the excretion of H^+ (acid) and the reabsorption of filtered HCO_3^- (base). Kidneys prevent acidity by the reabsorption of HCO_3^- when the blood PCO_2 is high, hypokalemia is present, there is an excess filtration of HCO_3^-, or the H^+ secretion from the proximal tubules is increased. In contrast, HCO_3^- reabsorption is reduced when the filtration of HCO_3^- is decreased, the plasma PCO_2 is low, the body is hypervolemic, or the secretion of H^+ from the proximal tubules is decreased.

The HCO_3^- buffer system is associated with the lungs. Increased plasma levels of HCO_3^- or decreased plasma levels of CO_2 cause alkalosis, while a decrease in plasma HCO_3^- levels or an increase in plasma CO_2 levels causes acidosis. Metabolic acidosis, which occurs when the plasma HCO_3^- levels decrease, is corrected by reducing the plasma CO_2 levels through an enhanced ventilation rate. This mechanism is called respiratory compensation. When the plasma HCO_3^- levels increase, metabolic alkalosis occurs. In this case, the ventilation rate is decreased so that an increase in the plasma CO_2 levels can be achieved.

24.2.5 Gluconeogenesis

Gluconeogenesis is the process of making glucose from amino acids and glycerol when carbohydrate stores decrease in the body. Even though gluconeogenesis happens mainly in the liver, the renal medulla can also carry out gluconeogenesis. Especially in acidosis, renal gluconeogenesis is increased whereas hepatic gluconeogenesis is decreased. This suggests that the kidney is an important source of glucose, especially after prolonged fasting.

24.3 Acute Response of the Renal System to Exercise

The kidneys have an important role in maintaining the body's homeostasis. Similar to other parts of the body, exercise creates stress on the renal system. The kidneys form several responses to exercise stress in order to maintain homeostasis. Acute changes in the renal system in response to exercise are usually associated with the autonomic nervous system, the endocrine system, and the hemodynamic system.

24.3.1 Renal Hemodynamic Responses

Factors such as renal blood flow (RBF) and glomerular filtration rate (GFR) are associated with renal hemodynamics.

With the activation of the sympathetic nerves and the increase in noradrenaline during exercise, RBF decreases due to vasoconstriction in the renal vessels. Even though there is no consensus as to what exercise intensity causes decreased RBF, studies indicate that the RBF declines when the lactate threshold is exceeded.

At rest, the renal system uses 20% of the cardiac output. During exercise, this rate decreases to 3–5%. But if it is considered that with exercise, the cardiac output increases by about five times, the decreased percentage in renal blood flow is actually negligible in healthy people. Consequently, intense exercise in patients with renal insufficiency can worsen the already existing renal dysfunction, albeit temporarily.

Renal vasoconstriction has an important role in blood pressure control in exercise. During exercise, vasodilation occurs in the respective arteries in order to provide more blood flow to the working skeletal muscles. The powerful vasoconstriction in the renal blood vessels stabilizes vasodilation in the body, preventing a rapid decrease in total peripheral resistance. Thus, the blood pressure is controlled and a sudden decline is prevented.

The change in GFR during exercise is not parallel to the change in RBF. GFR is an important diagnostic tool for evaluating renal function. Its normal value in healthy adults is in the range of 120–130 mL/min/1.73 m^2. GFR stays almost the same during mild and moderate exercise. However, in severe exercise, it drops. When the severity of the exercise is increased, the GFR declines because the body tries to minimize the urinary sodium loss to balance out the increased salt loss through sweating.

The filtration fraction, which shows the ratio of GFR/RBF, is an indicator reflecting renal hemodynamics and renal function. Its rate at rest is about 20%. When the lactate threshold is exceeded, the RBF drops considerably more than the GFR, so the filtration fraction value increases significantly.

After exercise, blood pressure decreases due to lessened total peripheral resistance. Hypotension, which lasts up to an hour after exercise, is more often a result of vascular vasodilation in skeletal muscles. Renal, splenic, and cutaneous vessels return to their pre-exercise state within an average of 20 min after exercise. After dynamic exercise, orthostatic intolerance might be seen. The main cause of this is the blood that is in stasis in the vessels due to vasodilation that occurs in the vascular beds of the skeletal muscles. The increase in resistance of renal vascularity, which is provided by about 20% of the cardiac output, plays an important role in restoring orthostatic tolerance.

24.3.2 Endocrine Responses

The kidneys release certain hormones into the circulation in response to exercise. The sympathetic nervous system is activated during exercise, and this contributes to the stimulation of renal nerves. In turn, renal nerves stimulate the synthesis of plasma norepinephrine, epinephrine, and atrial natriuretic peptide (ANP).

24.3.2.1 Renin and Angiotensin

Renin is a hormone secreted by the juxtaglomerular cells of the kidney when blood pressure is low. As the intensity of exercise increases, the amount of renin secretion also increases. The renin–angiotensin system (RAS) exerts its physiological responses with two opposite systems:

The Classical Pathway
Renin stimulates the formation of angiotensin I. Angiotensin I is converted into angiotensin II, a potent vasoconstrictor, by the angiotensin-converting enzyme (ACE). The increased levels of angiotensin II, which are significantly above the lactate threshold, cause lower renal blood flow and higher blood pressure. The increased blood pressure during exercise is an unwanted situation in patients with chronic renal failure (chronic kidney disease, CKD). Therefore, it is appropriate to limit the continuous aerobic exercise (CAE) severity below the lactate threshold for the CKD patient.

Angiotensin 1–7 Axis
An ACE homologous enzyme called ACE-2 is a regulatory enzyme comprised of the angiotensin 1–7 heptapeptide and its G-protein-bonded Mas receptor. In contrast to the classical pathway, the second pathway has anti-inflammatory and vasodilator effects. Therefore, it has a protective effect on the heart and kidneys. Continuous moderate aerobic exercise activates this branch of the RAS and prevents a sudden rise in blood pressure during exercise.

24.3.2.2 Prostaglandins
For kidneys, the function of prostaglandins, which are compound lipids produced in the body, is to regulate vascular tone and salt–water homeostasis. Prostaglandin E2 (PGE2) and prostacyclin (PGI2) are vasodilators that block sodium transport. They increase during exercise. Although there is not enough evidence, non-steroidal anti-inflammatory drugs (NSAIDs) may suppress the synthesis of renal prostaglandins. The renal prostaglandins have vasodilator and natriuretic effects; hence, it is thought the suppression of prostaglandins by NSAIDs may cause vasoconstriction and sodium retention. Although this does not cause problems in short exercise durations, it should be kept in mind that NSAID use during long sports such as marathons and triathlons may impair renal hemodynamics.

24.3.2.3 Nitric Oxide
Nitric oxide is a potent vasodilator secreted from the vascular endothelium. The increase in nitric oxide synthesis during acute exercise stabilizes renal vasoconstriction because nitric oxide balances the renal sympathetic activity.

24.3.2.4 Norepinephrine

Renal sympathetic activity increases in accordance with the severity of the exercise. Norepinephrine, which is usually associated with severe exercise, is released from the adrenal glands into circulation. Norepinephrine levels are increased in the blood during acute exercise, and norepinephrine affects the cardiovascular system, increasing heart rate and blood pressure.

24.3.2.5 Atrial Natriuretic Peptide

Atrial natriuretic peptide (ANP) is a powerful vasodilator released by heart muscle cells. There is a positive relationship between exercise and ANP levels. With increased sympathetic activation and venous return during exercise, ANP release is stimulated. ANP reduces the volume of plasma by enhancing the excretion of salt and water from the kidneys. Therefore, it takes on a balancing role for kidney function by lowering blood pressure.

24.4 Chronic Response of the Renal System to Aerobic Exercise

Long-term continuous exercise training has curative effects on renal function. Trained individuals show more moderate renal responses to exercise than sedentary people because a trained person had already developed some adaptations to exercise.

One of the most important adaptations that occur with exercise is a decrease in the activity of the sympathetic nervous system. With a decrease in renal sympathetic activation, changes in hemodynamic responses, such as RBF, GFR, and renin, are also seen. Compared to sedentary CKD patients, those who participate in regular exercise programs show an increase in their GFR levels, which is associated with an improvement in renal function. However, GFR levels can be lower due to increased serum creatinine levels caused by muscle hypertrophy. Therefore, the increased muscle mass might mask some of the improvement in renal function making it seem lower than it is.

Endothelial dysfunction is the first step of atherosclerosis. It is observed even in the early stages of chronic kidney disease (CKD). Renal arteriole vasoconstriction occurs in response to endothelial damage, and this leads to a further deterioration in GFR. Exercise training can produce increases in antioxidant factors and blood volume, thus repairing kidney blood flow and slowing down the process of renal dysfunction.

Moderate aerobic exercise training inhibits the classical branch of the RAS and activates the angiotensin 1–7 pathway, providing vasodilation of the renal arterioles. The decline in angiotensin II-induced vasoconstriction is a positive acquisition for patients with hypertension. In response to regular exercise, an average drop of 4–7 mmHg in systolic blood pressure is observed in hypertensive patients. Since even a 2 mmHg drop in systolic blood pressure reduces the mortality risk of ailments such as coronary artery disease or stroke, a drop of 4–7 mmHg is of huge importance. The effect of exercise on blood pressure is more prominent in hypertensive patients than normotensive individuals. The underlying mechanisms of the adaptation to exercise are vascular remodeling of the renal arterioles, the suppression of the sympathetic nervous system, and the inhibition of the RAS. This adaptation to exercise training plays an important role in the regulation of blood pressure and is vital for protecting kidney function.

With aerobic exercise training, the plasma volume increases. This adaptation is facilitated by a decrease in sodium excretion from the kidneys, which leads to an increase in extracellular sodium levels. The extracellular sodium content and plasma volume are linked. With an increase in extracellular sodium, an increase in plasma volume also occurs in order to restore balance.

Obesity is an independent risk factor for the conditions of diabetes and hypertension, which are also causes of CKD. Long-term aerobic exercise training provides a decrease in adipose tissue mass and waist circumference. Because visceral fat is burned faster than subcutaneous fat as an energy source, the loss of fat mass mostly originates from the visceral fat. An increase in the amount of visceral fat is associated with atherosclerosis, inflammation, and insulin resistance in dialyzed and non-dialyzed CKD patients. Visceral adiposity is also a risk factor for cardiovascular events in patients with CKD. For this reason, visceral fat loss is very important in the prevention of cardiovascular diseases in CKD. Low- to moderate-intensity aerobic exercise training is sufficient to achieve this effect.

24.5 Adaptation Mechanisms in Different Exercise Types

There are also different renal system adaptations to different methods of exercise such as high-intensity interval training (HIIT), intradialytic training, and strength training.

High-intensity interval training (HIIT) consists of consecutive short-term/high-intensity exercise periods and long-term/low-intensity exercise periods. It is an exercise type that has more positive effects on the body and is considered less monotonous by the patients than continuous aerobic exercise (CAE). HIIT's biggest advantage over CAE is that it provides more improvement in a shorter amount of time. HIIT's effectiveness and reliability have been shown both in healthy people and in patients with chronic metabolic syndrome, heart failure, as well as CKD.

High blood pressure is often observed in people with impaired renal function. HIIT and CAE have similar effects on lowering resting blood pressure. For this reason, HIIT might be seen as a more efficient exercise to control blood pressure compared to CAE timewise. Moderate CAE prevents sudden increases in blood pressure by activating the angiotensin 1–7 pathway of RAS. However, when the long-term effects of HIIT and CAE are observed, there is no significantly superior method for lowering blood pressure. The exercise method that should be avoided in patients with CKD is high-intensity resistance training (HIRT), which is a type of strengthening exercise. Even a single HIRT session can cause muscular and renal damage. After a session, the levels of creatine kinase (CK), myoglobin, creatinine, and microalbumin in the blood can become elevated as well as the indicators in urine. Those parameters all show signs of renal tubular damage. Because these indicators increase after HIRT even in healthy and young individuals, this type of exercise can cause more kidney damage in patients with CKD.

HIIT is more effective in inhibiting sympathetic nervous activity than CAE. Improvements in baroreflex sensitivity after HIIT are thought to be associated with advanced autonomic functions. HIIT supplies more fat oxidation and fat mass loss compared to CAE. Even though fat mass loss is associated with sympathetic inhibition, especially in hypertensive patients, it is not clear how much fat loss would improve autonomic functions.

Aerobic exercise is an effective way to repair vascular structures in patients with endothelial dysfunction. HIIT enhances the availability of nitric oxide and improves the antioxidant capacity. Therefore, it is more effective in restoring endothelial functions than CAE. The vascular adaptations as a result of CAE and HIIT are different. HIIT increases flow-mediated dilation (FMD), which is the dilative response of blood vessels to tensile stress caused by increased flow. FMD demonstrates that the endothelium can synthesize nitric oxide. On the other hand, CAE shows its healing effects on vascular structures by the dilation of arteries and increase in endothelial capacity.

Another important problem seen in patients with end-stage renal failure or kidney transplantation is osteoporosis. Along with immobilization during these periods, the drugs used during end-stage renal failure or the early stages of renal transplantation cause decreased bone mineral density. Exercise is an effective non-drug treatment approach to preventing bone loss. Regular exercise diminishes the muscle loss caused by corticosteroid use, improves glucose metabolism, and lowers blood pressure. In addition to these effects, exercise also has a significant contribution to increasing bone mineral density in patients with CKD or renal transplants.

Due to factors such as oxidative stress, inflammation, and physical inactivity, muscle loss is observed from the early stages of CKD. The loss of muscle mass in end-stage renal failure patients has been associated with mortality. However, in patients receiving hemodialysis treatment, mortality is associated more with a loss in muscle strength. In CKD patients who never exercised before, an acute cytokine response is seen after one session of moderate resistance training exercise. The synthesis of inflammatory cytokines such as interleukin (IL)-6 and tumor necrosis factor (TNF)-α increases, while anabolic cytokines such as IL-15 are suppressed. After the exercise is finished, this inflammatory effect disappears. With regular moderate resistance training, muscle hypertrophy is stimulated by regulating the acute response of IL-15.

Compared to the same-age healthy population, the functional capacity and health-related quality of life are significantly lower in end-stage renal failure patients who need hemodialysis treatment. Exercise has positive effects on functional capacity and life quality in these patients. However, hemodialysis is a time-consuming treatment, and it may be difficult for the patients to create extra time to exercise. For this reason, intradialytic exercise, i.e., exercise during hemodialysis, is a feasible alternative for end-stage CKD patients. Carrying out hemodialysis and exercise simultaneously also increases the adaptation of patients to the exercise. Peak VO_2 is a powerful predictor of survival in this patient group. An increase in peak VO_2 by 3.5 mL/kg/min (1 metabolic equivalent of task, 1 MET) is associated with a 15–25% increase in survival rate. Therefore, improvement in aerobic capacity in end-stage renal failure patients is very important. The combination of resistance and aerobic exercises during dialysis increases aerobic capacity and controls blood pressure better than just aerobic or just resistance training. Physical function, which is a health-related quality of life parameter in hemodialysis patients, is one of the most powerful predictors of mortality in this group. An integrated training where aerobic and resistance training are adopted together is the best method to improve physical function. HIIT is also a training that can be safely applied during dialysis. Intradialytic exercise would be a better choice to improve aerobic endurance as soon as possible because it is more easily adapted to and complied with by the patients.

24.6 Factors Affecting Adaptation to Exercise

Aging is a natural biological process that is characterized by decreased cellular function and progressive structural changes in organ systems. Old age affects the basic structure and function of renal cells, too. This leads to changes in glomerular capillary permeability and regressions in RBF, GFR, and sodium excretion. GFR, the main indicator of kidney function, is decreased primarily because of functional glomerulus loss and progressive nephrosclerosis. The decrease in GFR during exercise is less prominent in the elderly. Previous research shows that exercise does not cause abnormal reactions of glomerular function in non-dehydrated elderly individuals. In fact, the acute decrease in GFR is less in elderly people who receive exercise training. Nevertheless, the decrease in GFR is associated with the severity of exercise. GFR decreases might be less pronounced in the elderly because many older people do not exercise at a high-intensity level.

Dietary composition affects the acid–base balance of the body. Digesting meat, grains, and dairy increases the acid load of the body, but fruits and vegetables lower it. Dietary acid load should be monitored in the elderly because, with age, renal functions decrease, and the acid load negatively affects the already impaired kidney functions. High endogenous acid production accelerates the decrease in GFR. This decrease in GFR is more pronounced in the elderly than in young people, and in women than in men. Better renal functions are associated with a lower acid load. A low acid load can reduce exercise-related acidosis and boost maximum aerobic performance. In other words, a decrease in blood alkalinity negatively affects aerobic performance.

24.7 Possible Complications During/After Exercise in Renal System Pathologies and Their Management

Exercise has numerous benefits for CKD patients. Improving physical function, prolonging life expectancy, providing independence in daily life activities, and improving quality of life are only some of those benefits. However, CKD is a complicated disease and close attention should be paid to complications such as hypotension, proteinuria, and acute renal failure that may occur with exercise.

24.7.1 Proteinuria

Proteinuria means increased protein volume in urine. In healthy individuals, only a small amount of protein passes through the glomerular capillary membrane to the urine because of the size and electrical charge of proteins. In physiological conditions, this amount is less than 150 mg. If protein filtration is increased and/or protein reabsorption is decreased, the amount of protein in the urine increases. Detection of protein above 150 mg indicates kidney damage.

Proteinuria can be seen in a healthy person as well as in a person with CKD. In renal pathologies, a damaged glomerular membrane lets the protein through, and this causes proteinuria. In the case of healthy people, acute exercise causes glomerular membrane permeability to increase. Proteinuria that occurs with exercise is temporary. Within approximately 24–48 h, the amount of protein in the urine decreases. This does not constitute a big problem in healthy individuals. But in a damaged kidney, proteinuria caused by exercise can disrupt kidney function. It is known that intense exercise can contribute to the onset or escalation of proteinuria. Moderate exercise does not lead to proteinuria in people with CKD. Therefore, moderate exercise can be safely prescribed to CKD patients.

24.7.2 Acute Renal Failure

The higher the amount of sodium reabsorbed in the kidneys, the higher the oxygen consumption of the kidneys. Increased oxygen demand during exercise does not harm the kidneys. However, after long-term exercise, acute renal failure (i.e., acute kidney injury, AKI) may develop in healthy people or hypouricemia patients. Acute kidney injury (AKI) is a sudden kidney dysfunction caused by a severe acute decrease in GFR. Conditions that reduce renal blood flow, such as increased renal sympathetic nerve activity, increased angiotensin II, and hypovolemia, can cause AKI. The heightened levels of serum creatine phosphokinase (CPK) and serum myoglobin, caused by rhabdomyolysis (skeletal muscle lysis) after heavy exercises such as marathons or mountain climbing, damage renal functions and cause AKI. In addition, AKI may develop due to myolysis of Type II muscle fibers after anaerobic exercises such as 200 m of running.

The probability of AKI after exercise is low in healthy individuals. In athletes, dehydration due to intense exercise and sympathetic responses caused by the competition can temporarily impact renal functions. Exercise-induced AKI generally occurs after high-intensity anaerobic exercise in mostly hypouricemic people. Avoiding such exercises, and getting enough fluid during and after exercise, reduces the risk of developing AKI.

Apart from these, other rare exercise-related side effects that are observed in CKD patients include:

- Fatigue
- Leg cramps
- Hypotension
- Autonomic dysregulation

Hypotension and autonomic dysregulation are side effects often observed in diabetic kidney disease because diabetes itself affects many organ systems.

24.8 Comparison of the Adaptation Mechanism of the Respiratory System to Exercise: A Healthy Individual and an Individual with Chronic Renal Failure

Because it was thought that decreased renal blood flow during exertion could have negative effects on kidney function, exercise was not recommended for patients with CKD in the past. However, since it is known today that inactivity leads to the progression of kidney disease and even mortality, exercise has become a very important part of CKD rehabilitation. CKD is a risk factor for cardiovascular diseases. Hypotension, dyslipidemia, and diabetes mellitus are often observed in patients with CKD. Regular physical activity has many beneficial effects on the renal system, cardiovascular system, cognitive function, general mood, and health-related quality of life in renal failure patients.

The exercise capacity of patients with renal failure is quite low. The reduced bioavailability of nitric oxide and endothelial dysfunction lead to insufficient vasodilation during exercise. Therefore, renal failure patients have exercise intolerance. Because exercise tolerance is an indicator of survival in renal failure patients, developing exercise tolerance and increasing exercise capacity are very important in CKD. Both aerobic and resistance exercises decrease arterial resistance and increase peak VO_2 by 2.38 mL/kg/min on average. The minimal clinical significance of a VO_2 rise is 2 mL/kg/min in CKD and heart diseases. Therefore, the increase in VO_2 via exercise (2.38 mL/kg/min) is very important for CKD patients. The improvement of endothelial function in patients with CKD is possible with a long-term (on average, 12 months) exercise program. Short-term exercise training may not be enough to reduce arterial resistance. In healthy people, the endothelial function response can be observed after short-term (on average, eight weeks) training. The increase in antioxidant factors gained through exercise can prevent progressive fibrosis in kidneys. The increased levels of antioxidant enzymes and nitric oxide also have positive effects in healthy individuals. Nitric oxide and antioxidants act as protective factors against chronic diseases.

From the early stages of CKD, the glomeruli narrow in response to endothelial damage. This contributes to a drop in GFR. A drop in GFR in response to acute exercise is more prominent in CKD patients than in the healthy population. The drop in GFR increases the risk of mortality associated with cardiovascular diseases. This risk increases especially in end-stage kidney failure patients. Exercise training increases plasma volume, RBF, and antioxidant factors causing a beneficial effect on GFR and slowing the progression of CKD. Although GFR decreases during acute exercise in CKD patients, the GFR is higher in exercise-trained patients than in sedentary individuals without CKD. Exercise training should be continued for a long time (on average, 12 months) for the GFR to increase.

Hypertension is the most common comorbid condition in chronic renal failure patients. In addition to accelerating the progression of kidney disease, hypertension also sets a base for cardiovascular diseases. Water–salt retention, sympathetic nerve activity, and RAS play key roles in the development of hypertension. In hypertensive renal failure patients, endothelial function improvement, sympathetic nerve activity inhibition, and the downregulation of RAS can be achieved through aerobic exercise. In fact, these changes are observed more prominently in hypertensive CKD patients (providing a greater reduction in blood pressure) than in healthy individuals.

There are no big differences in renal adaptation mechanisms developed with exercise between CKD patients and healthy people. However, since adaptation may occur later in patients with CKD, a longer training period is required to see the effects of exercise training. In addition, CKD patients may not reach a similar functional level as healthy individuals of the same age. The comparison of the adaptation of the renal system to exercise between a patient with CKD and a healthy individual is given in Table 24.1. The adaptation of the renal system to exercise in chronic renal failure is summarized in Table 24.2. The clinical implications of the cases are summarized in Table 24.3.

Table 24.1 Comparison of adaptations to exercise in healthy individual and patient with CKD

Case 1. Healthy individual	Case 2. Patient with CKD
A 55-year-old male patient K.Ç. has a height of 180 cm, weighs 88 kg, and works at a bank. The patient applies physiotherapy to enhance his general condition. He states that he has not had a regular exercise routine for the last three years. He does not have any diagnosed illnesses, and he does not smoke.	A 62-year-old female patient M.A. has a height of 162 cm, weighs 75 kg, and is a retired teacher. She has hemodialysis treatment 3 days a week. The patient is directed to physiotherapy by her physician. She does not have a regular exercise routine. She does not smoke.
Assessment of the cases	
Before participating in the program, the patient was asked to fill out the Physical Activity Readiness Questionnaire (PAR-Q). The patient was included in the program after ensuring that he had no health issues prohibiting regular exercise.	
Assessment of exercise capacity • Cardio-pulmonary exercise test was administered. • Treadmill/Bruce protocol was used. • Peak VO_2 was measured as 37 mL/kg/min. • Peak heart rate was 164 bpm. • Peak VO_2 showed that his exercise capacity was low compared to his age group. • He reached 87% of the maximal heart rate during the exercise test.	**Assessment of exercise capacity** • Cardio-pulmonary exercise test was administered. • Bicycle ergometer was used. • Warm-up was 20–25 W. • 10–30 W increase was applied every 1–3 min. • The test was concluded due to over-fatigue (17/20 in Borg Scale). • Peak VO_2 was measured as 17 mL/kg/min. • Peak heart rate was 120 bpm. • Peak VO_2 showed that her exercise capacity was lower than a healthy person of her age. • She reached 76% of the maximal heart rate during the exercise test.
Assessment of the one-repetition maximum (1-RM) • 1-RM was calculated with "Bench-press," "Leg-press," and "Pull-down." • Endurance was evaluated with push-ups. • He had moderate muscle strength and moderate endurance for his age and sex.	**Assessment of the one-repetition maximum (1-RM)** • Considering the spontaneous avulsion fracture risk, a 10-RM test was used, and an estimated 1-RM was calculated. • Muscle strength was considerably low compared to the same-age healthy group.
Flexibility evaluation • Shoulder flexibility was evaluated with back scratch test. Right: +3 cm Left: +2 cm was recorded. • Hamstring and lumbar flexibility were evaluated with supine to long sit test. Right: −1 Left: −1 was recorded. • Hamstring–lumbar flexibility was low.	**Flexibility evaluation** • Shoulder flexibility was evaluated with back scratch test. Right: −7 cm Left: −9 cm was recorded. • Hamstring and lumbar flexibility were evaluated with supine to long sit test on a chair. Right: −3 Left: −2 was recorded. • Hamstring–lumbar flexibility was low.
	Assessment of daily life activities • Barthel Activities of Daily Life Index was 95/100. • She was found minimally dependent.

Table 24.1 (continued)

Case 1. Healthy individual	Case 2. Patient with CKD
	Assessment of fatigue • Fatigue severity scale: 37/63. • Fatigue impact scale: 60/160. • The patient had complaints of severe fatigue. Fatigue was affecting her physical and psychosocial functioning.
	Assessment of the quality of life • Kidney Disease Quality of Life Instrument was used to evaluate the health-related life quality (score was 60/100). • Especially in aspects of physical activity and daily life activities, the health-related life quality was considerably low.

Aerobic exercise
Type:
• Moderate aerobic exercise with a treadmill
Intensity:
• Started at 40–59% of peak VO_2 (perceived exertion according to the Borg Scale was 13–14)
Time:
• 5–10 min warm-up
• 20–60 min workout
• 5–10 min cool-down
Frequency:
• 5 days a week
• After 3 weeks, it was switched to intense exercise training 3 days a week
• The intensity of exercise was at 60–89% of the peak VO_2 (perceived exertion rate was 16–17 according to Borg Scale)
	Aerobic exercise
	Type:
	• Low-intensity intradialytic aerobic exercise with an exercise bike
	Intensity:
	• Started at 30–39% of peak VO_2 (Borg Scale Perceived Exertion Rate was 9–11)
	• After 4 weeks, the exercise was continued at 40–59% of peak VO_2 with 30–60 min of exercise training (Borg Scale Perceived Exertion Rate was 13–14)
	Time:
	• Started with 10 min periods.
	• Increased by 3–5 min per week.
	• The intensity of the exercise was increased when 30 min of continuous exercise could be performed
	  – 5–1 min warm-up
	  – 20–60 min workout
	• 5–10 min cool-down
	Frequency:
	• 3 days a week (during dialysis)

Resistance (strengthening) training Type: • Multiple joint strengthening exercises (multi-joint) with weight machines Intensity: • 60–70% of 1-RM (moderate to high severity) Time: • 8–12 repetitions/2–4 sets (2–3 min rest between sets) Frequency: • 2–3 days a week (provided there are no consecutive days)	**Resistance training** Type: • Single joint strengthening exercise with free weight (single joint) Intensity: • 50–65% of 1-RM (low to moderate severity) Time: • 10–15 repetitions/1–2 sets (2–3 min rest between sets) • A total of 6 exercises from the muscles of the hip, leg (quadriceps, hamstring), chest, back, shoulder, triceps, biceps, waist, and abdomen • It was aimed to increase the number of exercises to 8–10 after 2–3 months Frequency: • 2–3 days a week (provided there are no consecutive days)

(continued)

Table 24.1 (continued)

Case 1. Healthy individual	Case 2. Patient with CKD
Flexibility exercises Type: • Static stretching exercise (after aerobic exercise) Intensity: • It was explained that a slight feeling of tension and discomfort should be felt Time: • 10–30 s • 2–4 repetitions Frequency: • 2–3 days per week	**Flexibility exercises** Type: • Static stretching exercise (after a light warm-up period) Intensity: • It was explained that a slight feeling of tension and discomfort should be felt Time: • Initially 10 s, an increase to 30–60 swas aimed • 2–4 repetitions Frequency: • 2–3 days per week

Table 24.2 Adaptation of the renal system to exercise in chronic renal failure

Acute Response to Aerobic Exercise
- RBF decreases.
- GFR remains almost the same with mild and moderate exercise but decreases in severe exercise.
- Filtration fraction increases.
- Blood pressure drops.
- The secretion of renin increases.
- Prostaglandins increase.
- The synthesis of nitric oxide increases.
- The secretion of norepinephrine increases.
- With an increase in the level of ANP, blood pressure decreases.

Chronic Response to Aerobic Exercise
- Renal sympathetic activation is reduced.
- GFR increases.
- With an increase in antioxidant factors and blood volume, a slowdown in the progression of renal dysfunction is achieved.
- A decrease in systolic blood pressure is observed with a decrease in the vasoconstrictive response caused by angiotensin II.
- As a result of reduced excretion of sodium from the kidneys, there is an increase in plasma volume.

Acute Response to Resistance Exercise Training
- An increase in the secretion of inflammatory cytokines such as IL-6 and TNF-α is observed.
- IL-15, which is known to have anabolic effects on the skeletal muscles, is suppressed.

Note: These inflammatory responses seen in sedentary patients stop with the end of exercise and damage to kidney function does not occur.

Chronic Response to Resistance Exercise Training
- Muscle strength loss decreases.
- Blood pressure drops.
- Bone mineral density increases.
- A more pronounced improvement in kidney function is observed when combined with aerobic exercise.
- The risk of cardiovascular diseases, which are often seen as comorbidities in CKD, also decreases.

Table 24.3 Clinical inferences from the cases

Do's and don'ts when planning the exercise training
- Moderate-intensity (40–59% of peak VO_2) exercise with a duration of 20–60 min is targeted for patients with CKD. In patients with low aerobic capacity, it is safe to start with periods of low intensity for 10–15 min (30–39% of peak VO_2).
- Exercise can be done on the days of dialysis or the other days. If exercise is to be performed on dialysis days (intradialytic exercise), the exercise must be performed during the first two hours of dialysis to prevent hypotension.
- Exercise should not be done immediately after dialysis, as it can cause hypotensive attacks.
- It is safer to adjust the intensity of aerobic exercise according to the perceived exertion rate rather than the heart rate.
- Integrated training, in which aerobic training and resistance training are used together, is more effective in improving physical capacity.
- High-intensity interval training can be safely performed during dialysis.
- Sufficient fluids should be taken during and after exercise.
- Hypotension may occur during exercise in patients with CKD. Blood pressure should be monitored from the non-arteriovenous fistula arm.
- The patient should be informed that they should stop the exercise if they encounter one of the following conditions during the exercise:
  – Muscle cramps or joint pain
  – Nausea or vomiting
  – Pain in the upper part of the body, including the face and jaw
  – Problems with vision, speech, or swallowing
  – An abnormal shortness of breath
  – Sudden headache or dizziness
  – Sudden weakness in the arms or legs

24.9 Conclusion

The response of the renal system to exercise is quite complex. The hemodynamic and functional responses to exercise play a big part in slowing the progression of CKD as well as preventing or rehabilitating the biggest comorbid condition, cardiovascular disease. The once-avoided exercise training in CKD, because of the supposed safety reasons, now has a big part in the treatment of patients with renal diseases. Now it is understood that it is not only safe but it also improves renal function, increases daily functional capacity, and reduces the risk of mortality. When safety limits are well established, exercise has numerous benefits for renal failure patients.

Further Reading

Afsar B, Siriopol D, Aslan G, Eren OC, Dagel T, Kilic U, et al. The impact of exercise on physical function, cardiovascular outcomes and quality of life in chronic kidney disease patients: a systematic review. Int Urol Nephrol. 2018;50(5):885–904.

Baria F, Kamimura MA, Aoike DT, Ammirati A, Leister Rocha M, De Mello MT, et al. Randomized controlled trial to evaluate the impact of aerobic exercise on visceral fat in overweight chronic kidney disease patients. Nephrol Dial Transplant. 2014;29(4):857–64.

Clark T, Morey R, Jones MD, Marcos L, Ristov M, Ram A, et al. High-intensity interval training for reducing blood pressure: a randomized trial vs. moderate-intensity continuous training in males with overweight or obesity. Hypertens Res. 2020;43(5):396–403.

Costa EC, Hay JL, Kehler DS, Boreskie KF, Arora RC, Umpierre D, et al. Effects of high-intensity interval training versus moderate-intensity continuous training on blood pressure in adults with pre-to established hypertension: a systematic review and meta-analysis of randomized trials. Sports Med. 2018;48(9):2127–42.

Denic A, Glassock RJ, Rule AD. Structural and functional changes with the aging kidney. Adv Chronic Kidney Dis. 2016;23(1):19–28.

Eatemadololama A, Karimi MT, Rahnama N, Rasolzadegan MH. Resistance exercise training restores bone mineral density in renal transplant recipients. Clin Cases Miner Bone Metab. 2017;14(2):157.

Ellison D, Farrar FC. Kidney influence on fluid and electrolyte balance. Nurs Clin North Am. 2018;53(4):469–80.

Heiwe S, Jacobson SH. Exercise training in adults with CKD: a systematic review and meta-analysis. Am J Kidney Dis. 2014;64(3):383–93.

Hietavala EM, Stout JR, Frassetto LA, Puurtinen R, Pitkänen H, Selänne H, et al. Dietary acid load and renal function have varying effects on blood acid-base status and exercise performance across age and sex. Appl Physiol Nutr Metab. 2017;42(12):1330–40.

Kawakami S, Yasuno T, Matsuda T, Fujimi K, Ito A, Yoshimura S, et al. Association between exercise intensity and renal blood flow evaluated using ultrasound echo. Clin Exp Nephrol. 2018;22(5):1061–8.

Lima PS, Campos A, Corrêa CS, Dias CJM, Mostarda CT, Amorim CEN, et al. Effects of chronic physical activity on glomerular filtration rate, creatinine, and the markers of anemia of kidney transplantation patients. Transplant Proc. 2018;50(3):746–9.

Magalhães DM, Nunes-Silva A, Rocha GC, Vaz LN, de Faria MHS, Vieira ELM, et al. Two protocols of aerobic exercise modulate the counter-regulatory axis of the renin-angiotensin system. Heliyon. 2020;6(1):e03208.

Namasivayam-MacDonald AM, Slaughter SE, Morrison J, Steele CM, Carrier N, Lengyel C, et al. Inadequate fluid intake in long term care residents: prevalence and determinants. Geriatr Nurs. 2018;39(3):330–5.

Nilsson BB, Bunæs-Næss H, Edvardsen E, Stenehjem AE. High-intensity interval training in hemodialysis patients: a pilot randomized controlled trial. BMJ Open Sport Exerc Med. 2019;5(1)

Sawyer BJ, Tucker WJ, Bhammar DM, Ryder JR, Sweazea KL, Gaesser GA. Effects of high-intensity interval training and moderate-intensity continuous training on endothelial function and cardiometabolic risk markers in obese adults. J Appl Physiol. 2016;121(1):279–88.

Scapini KB, Bohlke M, Moraes OA, Rodrigues CG, Inácio JF, Sbruzzi G, et al. Combined training is the most effective training modality to improve aerobic capacity and blood pressure control in people requiring haemodialysis for end-stage renal disease: systematic review and network meta-analysis. J Physiother. 2019;65(1):4–15.

Schlader ZJ, Chapman CL, Benati JM, Gideon EA, Vargas NT, Lema PC, et al. Renal hemodynamics during sympathetic activation following aerobic and anaerobic exercise. Front Physiol. 2019;9:1928.

Scott RP, Quaggin SE. The cell biology of renal filtration. J Cell Biol. 2015;209(2):199–210.

Spada TC, Silva JM, Francisco LS, Marçal LJ, Antonangelo L, Zanetta DMT, et al. High intensity resistance training causes muscle damage and increases biomarkers of acute kidney injury in healthy individuals. PloS One. 2018;13(11):e0205791.

Tsukiyama Y, Ito T, Nagaoka K, Eguchi E, Ogino K. Effects of exercise training on nitric oxide, blood pressure, and antioxidant enzymes. J Clin Biochem Nutr. 2017;16-108

Vanden Wyngaert K, Van Craenenbroeck AH, Van Biesen W, Dhondt A, Tanghe A, Van Ginckel A, et al. The effects of aerobic exercise on eGFR, blood pressure and VO2peak in patients with chronic kidney disease stages 3-4: a systematic review and meta-analysis. PloS One. 2018;13(9):e0203662.

Villanego F, Naranjo J, Vigara LA, Cazorla JM, Montero ME, García T, et al. Impact of physical exercise in patients with chronic kidney disease: systematic review and meta-analysis. Nefrología (English Edition). 2020;40(3):237–52.

Watson EL, Viana JL, Wimbury D, Martin N, Greening NJ, Barratt J, et al. The effect of resistance exercise on inflammatory and myogenic markers in patients with chronic kidney disease. Front Physiol. 2017;8:541.

Zambraski EJ. The renal system. In: Farrell PA, Joyner MJ, Caiozzo V, editors. Acsm's advanced exercise physiology. 2nd ed. Wolters Kluwer; 2012. p. 551–63.

Immune System and Its Adaptation to Exercise

25

Ozden Ozkal

Abstract

It is well known that exercise has an effect on the functioning of the immune system. Aging, the increase in chronic diseases, and the coronavirus disease-2019 (COVID-19) epidemic, which started in Wuhan, China, in 2019 and spread all over the world, have led to an intense increase in research related to how to strengthen the immune system. Studies are in agreement that moderate-intensity regular exercise has positive effects on the immune system, whereas high-intensity/long-term exercise suppresses the immune system temporarily. The most important factor affecting the adaptation of the immune system to acute and chronic exercise is the dosage of exercise. It is necessary to know the acute and chronic responses of the immune system to exercise in order to create an individual-specific exercise prescription in health and disease conditions. In this chapter, the immune system structure and functions, immune system adaptations to aerobic and resistance exercise training, and the factors affecting these adaptations will be explained.

O. Ozkal (✉)
Physiotherapy and Rehabilitation, Faculty of Health Sciences, Bursa Uludag University, Bursa, Turkey
e-mail: ozdenozkal@uludag.edu.tr

25.1 Immune System Structure and Functions

The main function of the immune system is to maintain health by protecting the body against foreign agents such as viruses and bacteria. The immune system has an important role in different physiological processes such as tissue repair, metabolism, thermoregulation, sleep/fatigue, and cognitive health. The immune system is the body's most basic defense tool against infection and infectious diseases.

There are two main defense systems used by the immune system.

Innate immunity (non-specific immunity) serves as the first line of defense. The innate immune response occurs within the first four hours after exposure to the foreign agent, but long-term immunity cannot be achieved. As there is no memory in the response, when the same foreign agent is encountered again, the response formed is of the same intensity.

Long-term immunity is obtained through antibodies and lymphocytes formed by *acquired immunity (specific immunity)*. B-lymphocytes are responsible for humoral immunity while T-lymphocytes are responsible for cellular immunity. A unique response is created to foreign agents in acquired immunity, and, because of the memory feature, a stronger response is formed when the same agent is encountered again. Acquired immunity consists of *active* and *pas-*

sive immunity. *Active immunity* is acquired by vaccination or experiencing the disease. *Passive immunity* is formed by the transfer of serum and cells from an immune individual to a non-immune individual. Active immunity provides longer-term protection, whereas passive immunity provides shorter-term protection.

The structures involved in this system are summarized in Fig. 25.1.

25.1.1 Lymphoid Organs

Lymphoid organs and tissues within the immune system structures and elements have different functions in the defense system. Bone marrow, thymus, lymph nodes, spleen, and mucosa-associated lymphoid tissues are included in the classification of lymphoid organs (Fig. 25.2).

25.1.1.1 Bone Marrow
There are two types of bone marrow; red and yellow. Red bone marrow is the production site of all blood cells in the body, whereas yellow bone marrow is richer in fat cells than red bone marrow. Since the bone marrow is the stem cell center, it plays an important role in the defense mechanism of the immune system.

25.1.1.2 Thymus
The thymus, which lies behind the sternum, in the anterior mediastinal space, consists of two main lobes and the capsule surrounding these lobes. Each lobe is divided into smaller lobules, which consist of the two parts of the medulla and the cortex. The thymus is the organ where T-lymphocytes mature. In addition to lymphocytes, there are also epithelial cells and macrophages. The thymus acts as an important lymphoid organ in the response of the immune system with these features,

25.1.1.3 Lymph Nodes
These are small communities located along lymphatic vessels in different parts of the body. Lymph nodes contribute to the formation of an immune response by removing the foreign agent entering the body before it enters the bloodstream. The lymph nodes are bean-shaped, surrounded by a capsule on the outside, and contain T- and B-lymphocytes and many macrophages.

25.1.1.4 Spleen
The spleen, which is surrounded by a capsule on the outside, consists of worn/aged red pulp containing abundant erythrocytes and white pulp containing abundant T- and B-lymphocytes and

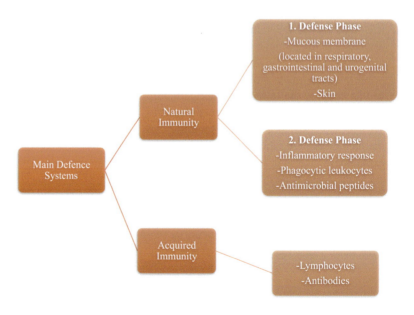

Fig. 25.1 Defense mechanisms of the immune system

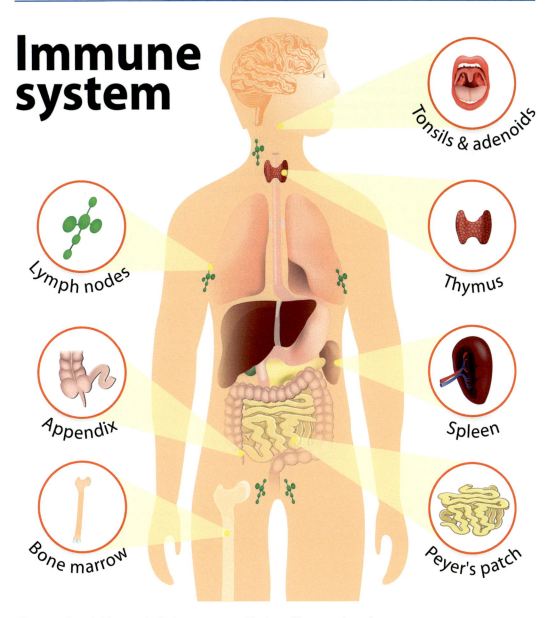

Fig. 25.2 Lymphoid organs in the immune system (Designua/Shutterstock.com)

macrophages. The spleen protects the blood from foreign micro-organisms by filtering it and plays a role in the formation of a systemic immune response.

25.1.1.5 Mucosa-Associated Lymphoid Tissues

These are located in the inner parts of the digestive, respiratory, and urogenital tracts. Lymphoid tissues can be found as follicles in bulk or scattered. These tissues contain all the cells involved in creating an immune response, and thus play a role in the protection of internal organs.

25.1.2 Cells

Macrophages/monocytes, lymphocytes, and natural killer (NK) cells together with other cells such as neutrophils, basophils, eosinophils, and platelets involved in the immune system have different functions. These cells are involved in the formation of the immune response and their functions are summarized in Table 25.1. Some information is provided in the bottom line of the table for a better understanding of the subject.

25.1.3 Immunoglobulins

Immunoglobulins in the body and their functions are summarized in Table 25.2. In the bottom line of the table, some information is provided for a better understanding of the subject.

25.1.4 Cytokines

The main cytokines involved in the formation of the immune response and their properties are summarized in Table 25.3. At the end of the table, some information is provided for a better understanding of the subject.

Table 25.1 Cells involved in the immune response and their functions

Immune system cells		Function
Macrophages/Monocytes		• They are immune system cells responsible for phagocytosis. • They function in cytokine secretion and antigen presentation.
Lymphocytes	T-lymphocytes	• These are one of the main immune cells of the body. • Lymphocytes, a type of leukocyte, are responsible for the formation of a cellular-type immune response. *Helper T-cells (CD4+ Lymphocytes)*: • Helper T-cells are responsible for cytokine release, and the activation and regulation of B-lymphocytes, monocytes, macrophages, and other immune cells. *T-cytotoxic CD8+ Lymphocytes*: • These participate in the destruction of cells infected with viruses/bacteria, etc.
	B-lymphocytes	These are responsible for antibody production and humoral immunity.
Natural killer cells		These have the ability to kill virus-infected cells and tumor cells. They kill cells with a direct cytotoxic effect without the need to recognize the antigen.
Other cells	Neutrophils	These have phagocytosis abilities.
	Basophils and mast cells	These participate in allergic reactions (anaphylactic type).
	Eosinophils	These participate in allergic reactions.
	Platelets	These are responsible for blood coagulation.

Antibody: Molecules produced by the body against foreign substances entering the body. *Antigen*: A protein-made substance such as bacteria and viruses that cause the formation of antibodies in the body. *Cytokine*: A group of proteins that provide intercellular communication. *Cytotoxic*: A substance that stops the function of the cell/kills the cell. *Phagocytosis*: The ingestion/digestion of a foreign substance/other substance by a cell

Table 25.2 Immunoglobulins and their functions

Immunoglobulin	Function
IgA	It is mainly found in the mouth. The main function is to protect mucous membranes. It constitutes about 15% of immunoglobulins.
IgE	It takes part in allergic reactions and forms a very small part of immunoglobulins.
IgD	It is located on the surface of B-lymphocytes and constitutes a very small proportion of the immunoglobulins.
IgG	It is found in blood and other body fluids. It protects the body against bacterial and viral infections. It constitutes about 75% of immunoglobulins.
IgM	It is the first immunoglobulin produced after encountering the antigen. It has an important role in acute responses and constitutes about 10% of immunoglobulins.

Ig: Immunoglobulin; *Immunoglobulin (antibody)*: A molecule produced in the body against antigens/immunogens

Table 25.3 Cytokines and their characteristics

Cytokine	Characteristics
IL-1-α and β	These are pro-inflammatory cytokines, responsible for providing natural immunity. They activate TNF-α and IL-6 release and modulate the acute-phase response of inflammation.
IL-1 receptor antagonist (ra)	It is anti-inflammatory, and an antagonist of IL-1.
IL-2	It is pro-inflammatory and responsible for providing acquired immunity. It is a growth factor for T-lymphocytes.
IL-4	It is anti-inflammatory and is responsible for providing acquired immunity. It is a growth factor for T-lymphocytes and mast cells.
IL-5	It is anti-inflammatory and is responsible for providing acquired immunity. It is involved in the production of antibodies (IgA).
IL-6	It is pro/anti-inflammatory and is responsible for providing natural immunity. It is responsible for the production of acute-phase proteins.
IL-10	It is anti-inflammatory and is responsible for providing natural immunity. It inhibits IL-1, IL-6, and TNF-α production.
IL-12	It is pro-inflammatory and is responsible for providing natural immunity. It increases NK cell activation and stimulates IFN release.
IL-13	It is anti-inflammatory and is responsible for providing acquired immunity. It inhibits IL-1, IL-6, and TNF-α production.
TNF-α	It is pro-inflammatory and plays a role in providing natural immunity.
TGF-β	It is anti-inflammatory and is responsible for providing acquired immunity. It inhibits leukocyte and lymphocyte activation.

Anti-inflammatory: Fighting infection; *Interleukin*: A group of cytokines, effective on leukocytes; *Pro-inflammatory*: Causes inflammation
IFN Interferon, *IL* Interleukin, *NK* Natural killer, *TGF* Transforming growth factor, *TNF* Tumor necrosis factor

25.2 The Immune System and Exercise

The effect of exercise on the immune system is one of the most popular research topics in recent years. A decrease in symptoms related to upper respiratory tract infections in individuals who do moderate-intensity aerobic exercise was first revealed in studies in the 1990s by David C. Nieman, the pioneer of exercise immunology.

There is a consensus that regular, moderate-intensity aerobic exercise strengthens the immune system and reduces mortality and morbidity from viral/respiratory tract infections. Organs and cells in the structure of the immune system do not respond in the same way to acute/chronic exercise. The most important factor affecting the response of the immune system to exercise is the dosage of exercise. The nervous system and the endocrine system play a role together in the regulation of the immune system's response to exercise (Fig. 25.3).

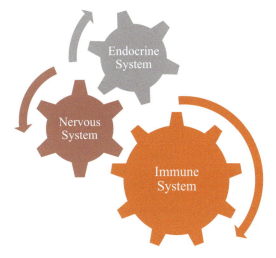

Fig. 25.3 The relationship of the immune system with other systems in response to exercise

25.2.1 Acute Response of the Immune System to Aerobic Exercise

The most important factor affecting the response of the immune system to a single session of aerobic exercise is the intensity and duration of the exercise. A single session of moderate-intensity aerobic exercise creates a cellular response and temporarily strengthens the immune system. The acute response of the immune system to a single session of aerobic exercise is similar to the response to trauma and infection. As in trauma and infection, an increase in the number of leukocytes is observed. The occurrence of exercise-induced leukocytosis is a transient event, and the leukocyte count returns to baseline within 6–24 h after exercise. Despite the rapid decrease in lymphocyte count during the early recovery period after exercise (the first 30–60 min after exercise), the rate of neutrophil increase is maintained. The occurrence of exercise-induced lymphocytopenia during this period may make the individual vulnerable to infections. In addition, it is known that there is an increase in pro-inflammatory cytokines such as tumor necrosis factor (TNF)-α, interleukin (IL)-1β, and anti-inflammatory cytokines such as IL-6, IL-10, and IL-1-receptor antagonist (IL-1ra) and acute-phase proteins. The acute response of the immune system to a single session of moderate-intensity aerobic exercise is summarized in Table 25.4.

25.2.2 Chronic Response of the Immune System to Aerobic Exercise

Low/moderate-intensity regular aerobic exercise reduces the risk of infection by strengthening the individual's immune system. Since exercise has an anti-inflammatory effect on the immune system, low/moderate-intensity aerobic exercise is recommended for chronic inflammatory diseases. The anti-inflammatory effects of aerobic exercise training emerge after 2–12 weeks of regular, supervised exercise training. There are different mechanisms related to the systemic anti-inflammatory effect of exercise. The first mechanism is based on the relationship of regular exercise to abdominal fat mass. Abdominal fat is an important risk factor for systemic

Table 25.4 Acute immune response to a single session of moderate-intensity aerobic exercise

Immune system element	The response of the immune system
Leukocytes	The number of leukocytes increases 2–3-fold during exercise, then returns to baseline within 24 hours after exercise.
Neutrophils	These are primarily responsible for the increase in leukocytes in the blood. This increase continues for a while after exercise.
Lymphocytes	*T-lymphocytes*: The number of T-cells increases during exercise, but falls below the baseline level within 1 hour after exercise. However, T-cell proliferation decreases during and after exercise. Cytotoxic T-cells (CD8+) and helper T-cells (CD4+) increase. The rate of increase of CD8+ cells is higher than CD4+ cells. *B-lymphocytes*: Although there is a slight increase in the number of B-cells, it returns to the baseline level after exercise.
NK cells	NK cells increase transiently after light to moderate aerobic exercise and return to the baseline level within 24 hours after exercise.
Monocytes/ Macrophages	After exercise, the number and activity of monocytes increases. This increase continues up to 6 hours after exercise.
Cytokines	During exercise: • Pro-inflammatory cytokine (TNF-α, IL-1β) secretion increases. • Release of anti-inflammatory cytokines (IL-6, IL-10, and IL-1ra) and acute-phase protein (C-reactive protein) increases. • IL-6 is the most studied cytokine in exercise immunology. • IL-6 usually increases during exercise as it is released from skeletal muscles and creates an anti-inflammatory response.

inflammatory diseases because it causes an increase in pro-inflammatory adipokine production. Regular exercise reduces abdominal fat mass and prevents its accumulation. The second mechanism is associated with both acute and chronic exercise increasing the release of anti-inflammatory cytokines. The increase in IL-6 released from the muscles during exercise contributes to the reduction in systemic inflammation by stimulating the release of anti-inflammatory cytokines such as IL-10 and IL-ra. The last mechanism is based on the fact that the hormones released during exercise are related to the immune system. Cortisol hormone acts as an anti-inflammatory mediator. Adrenaline reduces the release of inflammatory cytokines such as IL-1β and TNF. In addition to these mechanisms, regular exercise enables the conversion of M1 (inflammatory) macrophages to M2 (anti-inflammatory) macrophages and reduces the infiltration of macrophages into adipose tissue. This process results in some reduction in pro-inflammatory cytokine production. It has been shown that individuals who do moderate-intensity aerobic exercise regularly have decreased levels of leukocytes, monocytes, and neutrophils at rest. The anti-inflammatory effect of exercise is associated with the balance between pro- and anti-inflammatory cytokines.

The response of the immune system to regular moderate-intensity aerobic exercise is summarized in Table 25.5.

While regular moderate-intensity aerobic exercise training strengthens the immune system and protects against infections, high-intensity and long-term (>2–3 h) aerobic exercise training suppresses the immune system and increases the risk of infection. The period in which the individual becomes susceptible to infections after high-intensity and prolonged exercise is called the "*open window*" period (Fig. 25.4).

Upper respiratory tract infection symptoms are frequently encountered in the open window period following high-intensity and long-lasting training periods in athletes.

There is a temporary decrease in the number of immune cells and IgA levels in the blood in the open window period. It takes at least 24 h to return to pre-exercise levels, and, depending on the dose of exercise, this process may take up to 72 h. If the exercise is repeated without adequate rest time, the suppression of the immune system may become chronic, the return to the pre-exercise period is prolonged, and the risk of infection increases (Fig. 25.5).

The response of the immune system to high-intensity and long-term aerobic exercise is summarized in Table 25.6.

Table 25.5 Immune system response to moderate-intensity regular aerobic exercise

Immune system element	The response of the immune system
Leukocytes	Leukocyte counts tend to decrease at rest in individuals who exercise regularly.
Neutrophils	Neutrophil counts tend to decrease at rest in individuals who exercise regularly. The phagocytic activity of neutrophils increases.
Lymphocytes	*T-lymphocytes*: T-cell proliferation and activity increase. They reverse the helper T-cells (CD4+)/cytotoxic T-cells (CD8+) ratio, and strengthen the immune system by increasing the number of CD4+ cells. *B-lymphocytes*: There is a slight increase or no change in B-cell count. There are studies showing that they increase the synthesis of immunoglobulin.
NK cells	NK cell count and activation increase.
Monocytes/Macrophages	The monocyte counts of individuals who exercise regularly tend to decrease during the resting period.
Cytokines	• The release of pro-inflammatory cytokines (TNF-α and IL-1β) is suppressed. • The release of anti-inflammatory cytokines (such as IL-4, IL-10, and TGF-β) increases. • IL-6 (anti-inflammatory) release increases.

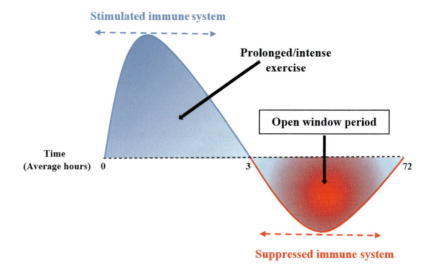

Fig. 25.4 Open window period

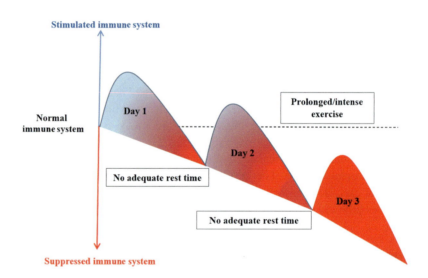

Fig. 25.5 The chronic "open window" period

Table 25.6 Response of the immune system to high-intensity and long-term aerobic exercise

Immune system element	The response of the immune system
Leukocytes	Although they increase during exercise, they do not decrease/change after exercise.
Neutrophils	The activity of neutrophils is reduced.
Lymphocytes	*T-lymphocytes*: T-cell number and proliferation are reduced. The CD4+/CD8+ T-cell ratio is reduced. *B-lymphocytes*: The main effect is on immunoglobulin synthesis. The most researched serum IgA level has been shown to decrease especially in athletes.
NK cells	NK cell count and activation is reduced.
Monocytes/Macrophages	Activation of monocytes is reduced.
Cytokines	The release of pro-inflammatory cytokines (TNF-α and IL-1β) increases. The release of anti-inflammatory cytokines (IL-1ra, IL-10) also increases. IL-6 (pro- and anti-inflammatory) release increases.

25.3 Adaptation Mechanisms in Different Exercise Types

Adaptation of the immune system to exercise is one of the most researched topics in recent years. The effects on the immune system of acute/chronic aerobic exercise training, which are generally performed at different intensities, have been investigated in studies conducted in healthy individuals, athletes, and people with chronic inflammatory diseases. Although resistance exercise training is an essential component of exercise prescription, little is known about its mechanism of action on the immune system.

The adaptation mechanism of the immune system to a single session of resistance exercise is similar to its response to a single session of aerobic exercise. However, the response of the immune system to aerobic exercise training is stronger compared to resistance exercise training. The increases in immune system cells during resistance exercise training are less than increases seen during aerobic exercise. These increases continue for a while after aerobic exercise training and it takes about 24 h to return to the pre-exercise period levels, whereas after resistance exercise training, the immune system cell counts return to the initial level in a very short time.

There are few studies that have investigated the effects of long-term resistance exercise training on the immune system, and there is no consensus on how long resistance exercise training should be continued for an anti-inflammatory effect. However, the most important factor affecting the immune response is the intensity of exercise training. The acute and chronic responses of the immune system to low/moderate strength training are summarized in Table 25.7.

Table 25.7 Acute and chronic immune system responses to strength exercise training

Immune system element	Acute response of the immune system	Chronic response of the immune system
Leukocytes	They increase slightly during exercise. After exercise, they return to the initial level.	There is no significant effect on the leukocyte count measured during the resting period.
Neutrophils	The neutrophil count increases during exercise. This increase is maintained for 60–120 min after exercise.	There is no significant effect on the neutrophil count measured during the resting period.
Lymphocytes	*T-lymphocytes*: CD4+ T-cell and CD8+ T-cell counts increase during exercise. Lymphocyte counts may decrease to the baseline level or below the baseline level 15–30 min after exercise. The count definitely returns to baseline level 3 h after exercise. *B-lymphocytes*: Minimal increase in B-cell count/no change is seen. This increase returns to the initial level within 120 min after exercise.	*T-lymphocytes*: The number of T-cells is increased/unchanged. *B-lymphocytes*: The number of B-cells increases/does not change.
NK cells	NK cell count increases during exercise. This increase continues until 15 min after exercise. NK cell count starts to decrease 30–45 min after exercise and returns to the baseline level. The cell count may fall below that level 2 h after exercise.	The number of NK cells increases/does not change.
Monocytes/Macrophages	The number of monocytes increases during exercise. This increase is maintained for a while after exercise and returns to the initial level within 2 h after exercise.	There is no significant effect on the number of monocytes measured during the resting period.
Cytokines	Pro-inflammatory cytokine (TNF-α, IL-1β) secretion increases. The release of anti-inflammatory cytokines (IL-6, IL-10, and IL-1ra) also increases.	The release of pro-inflammatory cytokines (TNF-α and IL-1β) is suppressed. The release of anti-inflammatory cytokines (e.g., IL-4, IL-10, and TGF-β) increases.

25.4 Factors Affecting Adaptation to Exercise

The most important factor affecting adaptation to exercise is the intensity of exercise. Together with the intensity, the duration of the exercise also affects both the innate and the acquired immune responses. While low/moderate exercise training strengthens the immune system, high-intensity/long-term exercise suppresses the immune system.

Aging is a natural physiological phenomenon that affects all organs and systems. Especially after the age of 50 years, individuals become more susceptible to infections with the decrease in immune system function. Studies have shown that when exercising, individuals aged >50 years sustain losses in the response abilities of leukocytes and their subgroups, and a decrease in T-cell number and proliferation, compared to younger individuals. The inclusion of older individuals in lower-intensity exercise training programs compared to younger individuals can cause confounding factor affecting immune adaptation other than aging. The influence of other systems such as reduction in cardiac output and infection are other age-related factors that affect immune system adaptation.

Diet, especially carbohydrate intake, has a significant effect on immune system adaptation. It has been shown that suppression of the immune system, characterized by an increase in the catecholamine/glucocorticoid response and leukocyte count, occurs after exercise training following low-carbohydrate diets.

The main factor shaping the response mechanism of the immune system is the pathogens transmitted to the individual. The fact that the presence of previous infection may affect the response of the immune system to exercise is a newly studied subject in recent years. It is thought that past/occult infections may cause some changes in the acute response of the immune system to exercise by affecting the exercise-sensitive cellular response. Studies on this subject are needed.

25.5 Possible Complications During/After Exercise in Immune System Pathologies and Their Management

The most common complication for the immune system following acute/chronic aerobic exercise is the "open window" period. The immune system may be suppressed following high-intensity and long-term exercise training. During this suppression period, the individual becomes vulnerable to infections. If exercise training is repeated during this period, suppression of the immune system may become chronic and result in serious infectious diseases. It is recommended to avoid vigorous and strenuous exercise before/during acute infection, as the effect on immune system responses could trigger serious diseases or exacerbate the present disease. Vigorous and strenuous activity/exercise can suppress the immune system by disrupting the pro/anti-inflammatory cytokine balance, and make the individual vulnerable to secondary infections. Low/medium-intensity exercise training suitable and appropriate to the exercise capacity of the patient should be preferred to manage any adverse side-effects that may occur during and after exercise in chronic inflammatory/autoimmune diseases, healthy individuals, and athletes. The exercise program should be progressed gradually and sufficient rest time should be given after high-intensity/long-term exercise training.

25.6 Comparison of the Adaptation Mechanism of the Immune System to Exercise: A Healthy Individual and a Patient with Rheumatoid Arthritis

Comparisons of the adaptation mechanism of the immune system to exercise in a patient with rheumatoid arthritis and a healthy individual is shown in Table 25.8. Adaptation of the immune system to exercise is summarized in Table 25.9. The clinical implications of the cases are summarized in Table 25.10.

Table 25.8 Comparison of adaptations to exercise in healthy individual and patient with rheumatoid arthritis

Case 1. Healthy individual	Case 2. Patient with rheumatoid arthritis (RA)
K.Ç (male), 35 years old, works in a bank, height of 1.80 m and weight of 88 kg.	N.Y (female), 61 years old, retired teacher, height of 1.65 m and weight of 77 kg.
K.C. consults a physiotherapist to improve his general fitness.	This patient was diagnosed approximately 15 years ago and is receiving pharmacological treatment.
K.C. states that he has not undertaken regular exercise for the last 3 years.	She received physical therapy under observation at regular intervals and in the early period after diagnosis.
K.C. has no diagnosed disease and does not smoke.	The physiotherapist stated that the patient did not follow the home program recommendations regularly. The patient had complaints of shortness of breath and fatigue, which had increased during the last year when going up and down stairs, walking uphill, and walking for a long time.
	The patient does not smoke, and has a sedentary life due to the increasing complaints over the last year.

Assessment of Cases

Case 1. Healthy individual	Case 2. Patient with RA
History	
– Patient information/Family history	– Patient information/Family history
– Habits	– Medical history, medications, surgical history
– Evaluation of risk factors	– Habits
	– Evaluation of risk factors
Assessment of body composition	
– Anthropometric measurements	– Anthropometric measurements
– Bioelectrical impedance measurement	– Bioelectrical impedance measurement
Assessment of exercise capacity	
– Cardiopulmonary exercise testing (CPET)	– Cardiopulmonary exercise testing (CPET)
– Field tests (6-min walking, shuttle-walking test)	– Field tests (6-min walking, shuttle-walking test)
Assessment of muscular strength	
– Isokinetic dynamometer	– Isokinetic dynamometer
– Manual muscle test	– Manual muscle test
Assessment of muscular endurance	
– McGill trunk muscle endurance tests	– McGill trunk muscle endurance tests
– Push-up test	– Push-up test
Assessment of the physical activity level	
– Questionnaires	– Questionnaires
– Activity sensors	– Activity sensors
Assessment of the joint normal range of motion	
– This assessment is usually not needed in healthy individuals.	– Active range of motion in the required joints is evaluated with a goniometer according to the symptoms of the disease in a patient with a diagnosis of RA.
Flexibility assessment	
– General flexibility assessment	– General flexibility assessment
– Sit and reach flexibility test	– Sit and reach flexibility test
– Muscle shortening tests	– Muscle shortening tests
Functionality assessment	
– This assessment is usually not needed in healthy individuals.	– Functional Independence Measure
	– Self-Efficacy Scale in Arthritis
	– Disability of Arm, Shoulder, and Hand (DASH) Questionnaire
	– Duruöz Hand Index
Pain assessment	
Pain-related questionnaires are not used in people who do not present with any symptoms or complaints of pain.	**Pain intensity**: Visual Analog Scale, Numerical Analog Scale.
	Localization, severity, type of pain: McGill Pain Questionnaire.
	In illiterate patients: Faces Pain Scale.

(continued)

Table 25.8 (continued)

Case 1. Healthy individual	Case 2. Patient with rheumatoid arthritis (RA)
Fatigue, anxiety, and depression assessment	
The relevant questionnaires are not used in people who do not have any symptoms or complaints related to fatigue, anxiety, and depression.	– Bristol Rheumatoid Arthritis Fatigue Multidimensional Questionnaire – Hospital Anxiety and Depression Scale – Beck Depression Inventory – State-Trait Anxiety Inventory
Sleep quality assessment	
– Pittsburgh Sleep Quality Index	– Pittsburgh Sleep Quality Index
Quality of life assessment	
– SF-36 – Nottingham Health Profile	– Rheumatoid Arthritis Quality of Life Scale – KıSF-36sa Form-36 – Nottingham Health Profile
Treatment Programme	
Case 1. Healthy individual	Case 2. Patient diagnosed with RA
Aerobic exercise training program	
Exercise intensity: Moderate intensity **Exercise frequency**: 5 days a week **Exercise duration**: ≥30 min per day total ≥150 min per week	**Exercise intensity**: Low/moderate exercise Exercise frequency: 3–5 days per week **Exercise time**: 20–30 min Aqua-exercise, cycling, dance-based exercises, and walking are often recommended.
Strength exercise training program	
Comprising the major muscle groups: **Exercise intensity**: Moderate/high intensity **Exercise frequency**: 2–3 days/week (non-consecutive days) **Exercise duration**: 8–12 reps/2–4 sets	Comprising the major muscle groups: **Exercise intensity**: Low/moderate intensity **Exercise frequency**: 2–3 days/week (non-consecutive days) Exercise duration: 8–10 reps/1–3 sets – The exercise program is designed appropriately to the pain tolerance level of the patient.
Flexibility exercise program	
Exercise type: Static stretching **Exercise intensity**: There should be a slight feeling of tension and discomfort. **Exercise frequency**: 2–3 days/week **Exercise duration**: 10–30 s/2–4 reps	Flexibility exercises **Exercise intensity**: It should be at an intensity that does not cause pain. **Exercise frequency**: 2–3 days/week **Exercise duration**: 10–30 s/2–4 reps
	Other treatments – Cognitive exercise therapy in accordance with the biopsychosocial model approach can be included in the treatment program for patients with RA. Yoga, Clinical Pilates, Tai Chi, and relaxation exercises treatment can be added to the program

Table 25.9 Adaptation of the immune system to exercise

Case 1. Healthy individual	Case 2. Patient with RA
Acute response to aerobic exercise	
– There is a temporary increase in the number of cells/elements of the immune system (see Table 25.4). This increase returns to baseline within 24 h after exercise. – A single session of moderate-intensity aerobic exercise temporarily strengthens the immune system.	– There is a need for studies investigating the acute responses of the immune system to a single session of aerobic exercise in patients with a diagnosis of RA.

Table 25.9 (continued)

Case 1. Healthy individual	Case 2. Patient with RA
Chronic response to aerobic exercise	
– Moderate-intensity regular exercise improves the immune system response. – It is known that regular exercise suppresses pro-inflammatory cytokine release and increases anti-inflammatory cytokine release (for detailed information, see Table 23.5).	– There are studies showing that long-term aerobic exercise alleviates disease severity by suppressing the inflammatory process. – Studies have generally investigated the effects of aerobic exercise on cardiovascular fitness, pain, fatigue, functional level, and quality of life. It has been shown that aerobic exercise has positive effects on these parameters.
Acute response to strength exercise training	
– Responses are similar to those given to a single session of aerobic exercise (see Table 23.7). – Although there is an increase in the number of immune system cells/elements, these increases return to the initial level within 24 h after exercise.	– There is a need for studies investigating the acute responses of the immune system to one-session strengthening exercise training in patients with a diagnosis of RA.
Chronic response to strength exercise training	
– Immune response to strengthening exercises is not as strong as the response to the aerobic system (see Table 23.7). – While there is no change in immune system cells/elements, there are studies showing that strengthening training involving major muscle groups has an anti-inflammatory effect.	– There is a need for studies investigating the chronic responses of the immune system to strengthening exercise training in patients with a diagnosis of RA. – Regular strengthening exercise training has been shown to have a positive effect on muscle strength, muscle mass, functionality, exercise capacity, and fatigue.

Table 25.10 Clinical interferences from the cases

Do's and don'ts when planning the exercise training

- Exercise prescription for RA patients should be designed individually in accordance with the individual's initial cardiorespiratory fitness level, functional level, disease severity, and symptoms.
- A combined training program including aerobic and strengthening exercise training is recommended in order to increase aerobic capacity, muscular strength, and functionality in RA patients.
- For RA patients with low exercise capacity, it is recommended to start the aerobic exercise training program at low/moderate intensity and gradually progress the program.
- It is recommended to start strengthening exercise training at low/moderate intensity and gradually increase it in RA patients.
- It is recommended that the intensity of the strengthening exercise training be in the "safe range" that will not cause an increase in the patient's pain.
- There are studies showing that high-intensity strengthening exercises can also be applied safely in RA patients.
- It is recommended to continue regular exercise in RA patients during the active period of the disease.

25.7 Conclusion

In conclusion, the acute and chronic responses of the immune system to exercise vary. The most important factor affecting these responses is the dosage of exercise. Regular moderate-intensity aerobic exercise strengthens the immune system, while high-intensity long-term aerobic exercise suppresses the immune system. With the COVID-19 epidemic that started in Wuhan, China, in 2019 and spread all over the world, exercise became a priority in the list of recommendations to strengthen the immune system. Regular aerobic exercise has been shown to improve the inflammatory profile in chronic inflammatory diseases. Exercise training is currently recommended as a basic building block of the treatment program in chronic inflammatory diseases. Personalized exercise training in chronic inflammatory diseases has a positive effect on many different criteria such as disease symptoms, cardiorespiratory fitness, functionality, and quality of life. However, there remains a need for further studies to investigate the specific effects of exercise on the immune system in chronic inflammatory diseases.

Further Reading

Batatinha HAP, Biondo LA, Lira FS, Castell LM, Rosa-Neto JC. Nutrients, immune system, and exercise: Where will it take us? Nutrition. 2019;61:151–6.

Cerqueira E, Marinho DA, Neiva HP, Lourenço O. Inflammatory effects of high and moderate intensity exercise: a systematic review. Front Physiol. 2020;10:1550.

Forti LN, Van Roie E, Njemini R, Coudyzer W, Beyer I, Delecluse C, et al. Effects of resistance training at different loads on inflammatory markers in young adults. Eur J Appl Physiol. 2017;117:511–9.

Goh J, Lim CL, Suzuki K. Effects of endurance-, strength-, and concurrent training on cytokines and inflammation. In: Schumann M, Cham RB, editors. Concurrent aerobic and strength training. Switzerland: Springer International Publishing; 2019. p. 125–38.

Lakier SL. Overtraining, excessive exercise, and altered immunity: is this a T helper-1 versus T helper-2 lymphocyte response? Sports Med. 2003;33:347–64.

Lewis DE, Blutt SE. Organization of the immune system. In: Rich RR, Fleisher TA, Shearer WT, Schroeder HW, Frew AJ, Weyand CM, editors. Clinical immunology. 5th ed. Elsevier; 2019. p. 19–38.

Liu D, Wang R, Grant AR, Zhang J, Gordon PM, Wei Y, et al. Immune adaptation to chronic intense exercise training: new microarray evidence. BMC Genomics. 2017;18:29.

Metsios GS, Stavropoulos-Kalinoglou A, Kitas GD. The role of exercise in the management of rheumatoid arthritis. Expert Rev Clin Immunol. 2015;11:1121–30.

Mohamed AA, Alawna M. Role of increasing the aerobic capacity on improving the function of immune and respiratory systems in patients with coronavirus (COVID-19): A review. Diabetes Metab Syndr. 2020;14:489–96.

Mondal A, Chatterjee S. Exercise and immunity: A correlated mechanism. Int J Health Sci Res. 2018;8:284–94.

Nicholson LB. The immune system. Essays Biochem. 2016;60:275–301.

Nieman DC, Wentz LM. The compelling link between physical activity and the body's defense system. J Sport Health Sci. 2019;8:201–17.

Peake JM, Neubauer O, Walsh NP, Simpson RJ. Recovery of the immune system after exercise. J Appl Physiol. 2017;122:1077–87.

Scheffer DDL, Latini A. Exercise-induced immune system response: Anti-inflammatory status on peripheral and central organs. Biochim Biophys Acta Mol Basis Dis. 2020;1866:165823.

Schlagheck ML, Walzik D, Joisten N, Koliamitra C, Hardt L, Metcalfe AJ, et al. Cellular immune response to acute exercise: Comparison of endurance and resistance exercise. Eur J Haematol. 2020;105:75–84.

Shaw DM, Merien F, Braakhuis A, Dulson D. T-cells and their cytokine production: The anti-inflammatory and immunosuppressive effects of strenuous exercise. Cytokine. 2018;104:136–42.

Shirvani H. Exercise and COVID-19 as an infectious disease. Iran J Med Sci. 2020;45:311–2.

Simpson RJ, Campbell JP, Gleeson M, Krüger K, Nieman DC, Pyne DB, et al. Can exercise affect immune function to increase susceptibility to infection? Exerc Immunol Rev. 2020;26:8–22.

Simpson RJ, Kunz H, Agha N, Graff R. Exercise and the Regulation of Immune Functions. Prog Mol Biol Transl Sci. 2015;135:355–80.

Szlezak AM, Szlezak SL, Keane J, Tajouri L, Minahan C. Establishing a dose-response relationship between acute resistance-exercise and the immune system: Protocol for a systematic review. Immunol Lett. 2016;180:54–65.

Walsh NP, Samuel JO. Exercise, immune function and respiratory infection: an update on the influence of training and environmental stress. Immunol Cell Biol. 2016;94:132–9.

Wang J, Liu S, Xiao J. Exercise regulates the immune system. In: Xiao J, editor. Physical exercise for human health, advances in experimental medicine and biology. Springer Nature Singapore Pte Ltd; 2020. p. 395–408.

Part IV

Miscellaneous

Balance, Coordination, and Proprioception

26

Oznur Buyukturan

Abstract

The two most basic features that distinguish human beings from other living species are the ability to reason and the ability to perform bipedal tasks in daily life activities. A precise and efficient combination of balance, coordination, and proprioception is a requirement for a stable and controlled movement on two legs. In this section, the definition of balance, coordination, and proprioception, as well as evaluation methods and some treatment options will be discussed.

26.1 Balance

Despite several definitions of balance in the relevant literature, the following is the most accepted and widely used. Balance is an individual's ability to keep the body's center of gravity within the limits of the base of support. In addition, the term "balance" is commonly used by healthcare professionals in a wide variety of clinical specialties. Despite the widespread use of the term, there is no universally accepted definition of human balance. Yet, therapists should have an intuitive understanding of the term. The word balance is often used in conjunction with terms such as stability and postural control. The ability of a person to maintain and/or regain a certain state of balance is called stability. While balance and stability terms are mostly used for static and mechanical definitions, the term postural control refers to the ability of human beings to maintain balance in different situations and conditions and to keep the body's center of gravity in different directions in line with gravity. Postural control is defined as the act of achieving, maintaining, or restoring a state of balance during any posture or activity. Postural control strategies are divided into predictive or reactive strategies and include proper responses to either stable or changing base of support. Although the terms balance, stability, and postural control are often used interchangeably, the term balance is generally used in clinical practice (Fig. 26.1).

Postural control, defined as the ability to control body position in space, consists of a combination of postural orientation and postural stability. Automatic responses to visual, vestibular, and proprioceptive information are crucial for postural control. Postural orientation is the ability to maintain an efficient relationship between body segments on the one hand and between the body and the environment on the other hand during a specific task. It requires active alignment of the head and trunk with respect to gravity, the base of support, visual environment, and internal

O. Buyukturan (✉)
School of Physical Therapy and Rehabilitation, Kırşehir Ahi Evran University, Kirsehir, Turkey
e-mail: obuyukturan@ahievran.edu.tr

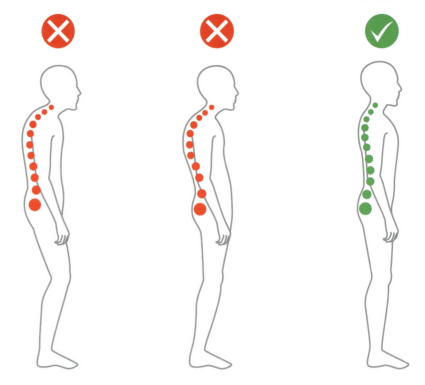

Fig. 26.1 Good posture and postural control (solar22/Shutterstock.com)

references. Posture and postural tone significantly contribute to postural orientation. Postural stability, also known as balance, is the body's ability to keep the center of gravity within the limits of the base of support. Coordination of movement strategies across internal and external perturbations is an indispensable element for balance.

Six basic resources are required for postural stability and orientation:

1. *Sensory strategies:* Visual, vestibular, and somatosensory information are integrated and processed to create an optimal response for adaptation to the complex sensory environment. On a stable surface, healthy individuals rely 70% on somatosensory, 20% on vestibular, and 10% on visual information. On an unstable surface, however, relying on somatosensory information decreases and an individual uses more vestibular and visual data. Vision provides information about the position and movement of the head relative to the surrounding objects. In other words, vision provides a reference for verticality using the surrounding objects and determines the direction of head movement. When moving, objects appear to go in the opposite direction of the movement direction. This is how our visual system realizes the direction of movement of the head. The visual system further supports the sensory data from the vestibular and somatosensory systems. The somatosensory system consists of specialized peripheral receptors in the skin, muscles, and joints, posterior cord conduction system and spinocerebellar tracts, and upper centers where sensory information is processed and integrated. Somatosensory data and particularly proprioception are very important for postural control. While the somatosensory system can provide accurate data for the verticality of the body on stable, even, and horizontal surfaces, it falls short in cases of unstable and/or uneven surfaces (such as a sailing ship or a ramp) and needs help from the vestibular system. The vestibular system provides information to the central nervous system about head movement and position. With the information provided by the vestibular system alone, the central

nervous system cannot distinguish a simple head movement (e.g., forward tilt of the head while the trunk is stable) from the forward movement of the head together with the body (e.g., while walking). This necessitates the simultaneous and precise collaboration of the vestibular and the visual system.

2. *Spatial orientation:* The orientation of body parts with respect to the center of gravity, the base of support, visual field, and internal references is very important for postural control. In healthy individuals, the nervous system automatically provides postural orientation while performing a task.

3. *Perceptual process:* Basic structures involved in the perceptual process of postural control are the primary sensory cortex, association areas, putamen, limbic system, reticular formation, and the connections between these structures. Data provided by these structures form our anticipatory and adapted responses that significantly contribute to our postural control. As the difficulty and complexity of postural tasks increase, cognitive functioning and reaction time decrease. For instance, the risk of falling increases when walking on a slippery surface is combined with a dual cognitive task.

4. *Movement strategies:* To maintain balance in the upright position, four different movement strategies are involved as follows:
   (a) Postural oscillations: In a standing position, postural oscillations are commonly seen in the antero-posterior and less frequently in the lateral directions. The magnitude of the oscillations increases as the base of support gets smaller.
   (b) Ankle strategy: When the base of support is further narrowed and at the same time the person is pulled back slightly (i.e., center of gravity falls behind the body), ankle dorsiflexor and plantarflexor muscles are activated to keep the center of gravity within the base of support. The paraspinal muscles, hamstrings, and gastrocnemius contract in the forward oscillations of the ankle strategy, while the abdominal muscles, quadriceps, and tibialis anterior contract in the backward oscillations.
   (c) Hip strategy: In oscillations where the ankle strategy is insufficient to maintain balance, the hip and trunk muscles are activated, and the upper and lower body move in opposite directions. In case of an unpredicted backward shift of the center of gravity, the upper body quickly bends forward, and the pelvis moves backward. In the hip strategy, the abdominal muscles and quadriceps contract during the forward oscillation, while the paraspinal muscles and hamstrings contract during the posterior oscillation.
   (d) Stepping strategy: When balance disturbance exceeds the stability limits, stepping in a certain direction helps increase the base of support. Individuals with lower levels of stability (e.g., due to central nervous system damage) use the stepping strategy to compensate even the smallest loss of balance (Fig. 26.2).

5. *Biomechanical competence:* An individual's biomechanical features play a key role in the quality of their base of support. For instance, any limitation, pain, and loss of strength in the ankle joint affect balance. Controlling the center of gravity within the base of support requires optimal biomechanical competence. The ability to dynamically transfer the center of gravity without changing the base of support while maintaining balance defines the "Limits of Stability" and requires biomechanical competence.

6. *Control of dynamics:* During movements (e.g., walking or changing from one posture to another), controlling the center of gravity is quite complex, as such it often falls beyond the limits of the base of support. For instance, forward postural stability is maintained in gait, as the swinging leg is placed where the center of gravity falls. Lateral postural stability necessitates hip abductions to control lateral oscillations. It was reported that balance deficits are mainly caused by disorders in three systems, namely biomechanics, sensory organization, and motor coordination. While

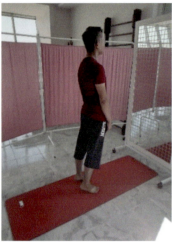 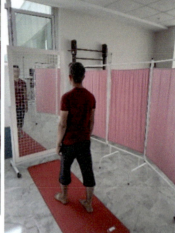 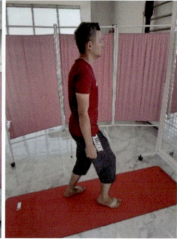

Fig. 26.2 Examples of movement strategies

any problem in each of these systems can cause balance disorders, a combined deficit can also lead to balance dysfunction. For example, maintaining an upright posture against external perturbations requires efficient collaboration between the sensory organization and motor coordination.

Types of postural control are as follows:

- Static postural control: When the center of gravity stays stable within the limits of the base of support.
- Reactive (compensatory) postural control: Regaining balance using body reactions when the center of gravity moves beyond or out of the limits of the base of support due to an unexpected perturbation.
- Proactive postural control: Involves predicting and activating necessary control strategies and motor movements based on previous experiences in a certain situation.
- Adaptive postural control: Preparation of motor and sensory systems in response to changing task requirements and environment.

26.1.1 Causes of Balance Dysfunction

The inability of the postural control systems in effectively responding to extrinsic stimuli, leads to balance deficits. According to dynamic and static balance theory, sensory and motor systems interact with each other to control balance. Any disturbance to this interaction hinders balance preservation. In order to know the factors causing balance dysfunction, it is necessary to know the functions of the vestibular system first, which consists of four parts:

1. Peripheral vestibular system
2. Vestibular nerve
3. Vestibular nuclei
4. Central vestibular tracts

The peripheral vestibular system is located within the petrous bone and is sensitive to head and neck movements. It transmits the straight and circular movements of the head to both the cerebellum and vestibular nuclei. Cupula and otolith membranes move on the tufts of cilia. The movement of hair bundles causes a polarization between the cell and the surrounding endolymph fluid. These polarizations are sensed by nerve fibers to which cells are attached and transmitted to the vestibular nuclei in the cerebellum via the vestibular nerve. While the cupula in the semicircular canals is sensitive to circular movements, the otoconial membranes in the macula are affected by linear movements due to their specific bulk density. Each of the semicircular canals (namely horizontal, posterior, and anterior canals) is placed at an angle of 90 degrees to the other two. The sensorial epithelium in the ampullae of the semicircular canals consists of two parts, the crista and the ampulla. The crista is on the bony labyrinth projection. On top of the crista is the cupula that waterproofs the edges of the ampulla and prevents the stimulation of hair bundles during antigravity movements. The sensorial epithelium of the otolith organs is called the macula. The sensorial epithelium in each macula has an otolith membrane and stereocilia. The vestibular nerve ganglion is located in the inner ear canal. While the nerve axons enter the vestibular sensory epithelium, the dendrites are connected to the central nervous system. The interstitial nucleus of the vestibular nerve receives signals originating from the cervical region, cerebellum, reticular formation, spinal cord, and contralateral vestibular nuclei. Among the central vestibular pathways, the most important is the vestibulo-ocular reflex (VOR), which fixes the straight gaze. An optokinetic system is needed to transmit head position movements to the brain. Three types of neurons are involved in the mechanism of the VOR: vestibular nerve, secondary vestibular neuron, and motor neuron. Secondary vestibular neurons form the connection between vestibular nuclei and oculomotor nuclei. Motor neurons, on the other hand, connect the oculomotor nuclei to the eye muscles. Three canals are associated with the VOR: (1) Horizontal canal: The stimulation of this canal leads to horizontal eye movement in the opposite direction of the stimulated canal. (2) Superior canal: Causes both eyes to move upward and to the opposite side. (3) Posterior canal: The stimulation of this canal leads to ipsilateral rotation downward tilt of the head movement to the same side.

26.1.1.1 Peripheral Sensory Disorders

The visual system (consisting of eyes, vision receptors, occipital located optic nerves, and muscles and nerves of the oculomotor system) plays a key role in postural control. While central vision determines our spatial position, peripheral vision combines data from head movements and postural oscillations to provide information about the environment. Vestibulo-ocular reflex is especially important in tracking moving objects. However, if the individual's head is in motion while following the moving object, the VOR is suppressed. In such cases, nystagmus occurs. Nystagmus is the side-to-side, up-and-down, or circular motion of the eyes in response to rotational movements of the environment or the head.

26.1.1.2 Central and Peripheral Vestibular Disorders

Vestibular diseases are diverse but can be classified into two main groups.

Disorders Associated with Diseases Such As Vestibular Neuritis and Labyrinthitis

Vestibular neuritis is characterized with severe dizziness, imbalance, nausea, and vomiting due to inflammation of the balance nerve, which carries signals from the balance organ in the inner ear to the brain. The most likely cause of vestibular neuritis seems to be a virus that causes inflammation in and around the nerve tissue. Symptoms are often with a sudden onset, very severe for the first few days, and exacerbated by head movements. Symptoms begin to relieve after a few days, but full recovery may take weeks or even months.

Labyrinthitis is an inner ear disorder. There are two vestibular nerves in the inner ear that send information to the brain about spatial navigation and balance control. Inflammation of any of these vestibular nerves leads to labyrinthitis. The symptoms are quite severe for several days before relieving. There is always the possibility of symptom relapse with sudden head movements.

Disorders Associated with Benign Paroxysmal Positional Vertigo (BPPV)

Similar to semicircular canal dysfunction, the BPPV is caused by the crystals that are detached from their original location and adhere to the cupula. In both cases, head movements cause vertigo. The vestibular system has four main tasks in balance control. These are perceiving one's own movements, adapting to vertical position, controlling body center of gravity, and stabilizing the head.

Perceiving one's own movements helps filtering inaccurate and uncoordinated information from other sensory systems. At this point, the vestibular system plays a key role in controlling antigravity muscles and generating an automatic postural response. Somatosensory receptors allow us to perceive, realize, and control our position in space. Especially receptors in the foot, ankle, knee, hip, back, and neck are important for static and dynamic balance. Diseases or traumas can damage peripheral sensory receptors and altered sensory nerve functions can lead to loss of balance.

26.1.1.3 Central Sensory Disorders

Visual, vestibular, and somatosensory data collected from the body are combined and processed in the central nervous system. Any deficit in processing the data can lead to inaccurate or false responses. If the data from the three systems are incompatible or discordant, generating the appropriate motor response becomes difficult. Since the parietal lobe is responsible for somatosensory data processing and motor learning, any damage to this lobe (as in patients with multiple sclerosis, cerebral palsy, stroke, and some types of brain tumors) may impair central sensory function.

26.1.1.4 Peripheral Motor Disorders

The peripheral motor system activates various strategies in case of balance disturbance. Although the most frequent strategies are upper extremity reactions, lower extremity strategies have been studied more in scientific sources.

26.1.2 Balance Assessment Methods

The assessment of balance is indicated in many patients, including those with neurological deficits, orthopedic problems, and vestibular disorders. Balance assessment methods in clinical or academic studies are categorized in two main groups.

26.1.2.1 Computerized Balance Assessment Methods

Static Posturography

This method consists of measuring body oscillations (i.e., displacement of the center of gravity) while standing on a fixed instrumented platform (force plate), both with eyes open and closed. Tiny oscillations of the body are detected by the sensitive detectors (force and movement transducers) of the platform. The device generates electrical waves proportional to the amount of pressure applied to the detectors. A special computer software integrates all the data and produces detailed graphics and reports. The device includes various protocols to measure static and dynamic balance parameters.

Dynamic Posturography

This method assesses an individual's ability to use or coordinate information from the visual, vestibular, and somatosensory systems. Computerized posturography systems used in evaluation and rehabilitation protocols include sensory, the VOR, automatic motor, voluntary motor, and functional limitations.

Balance Systems

It is a device that evaluates balance and the challenges of individuals as they struggle to control and move the center of gravity once on the device platform (Fig. 26.3).

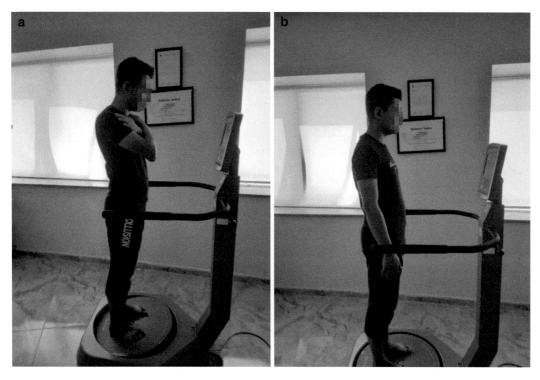

Fig. 26.3 (**a**) Dynamic balance assessment (picture on left); (**b**) Static balance assessment (picture on right)

26.1.2.2 Manual (Non-Computerized) Balance Assessment Tools

Some of the most common balance tests, which are frequently used in physiotherapy and rehabilitation clinics, are listed below and examples of balance exercises are shown in Fig. 26.4.

- Single leg stance test
- Romberg test
- Tandem walking test
- Timed up and go test
- Functional reach test
- Berg balance test
- Tinetti balance and gait scale
- Fall risk assessment tool
- Activity-specific balance-confidence scale
- Performance-oriented mobility assessment (POMA)
- Dynamic gait index
- Y-shaped balance test
- Star excursion balance test
- Four-frame stepping test
- Balance beam test
- Balanced beard test
- Flamingo balance test
- Stork stand test
- Stick lengthwise test
- Beam walk
- Bass test

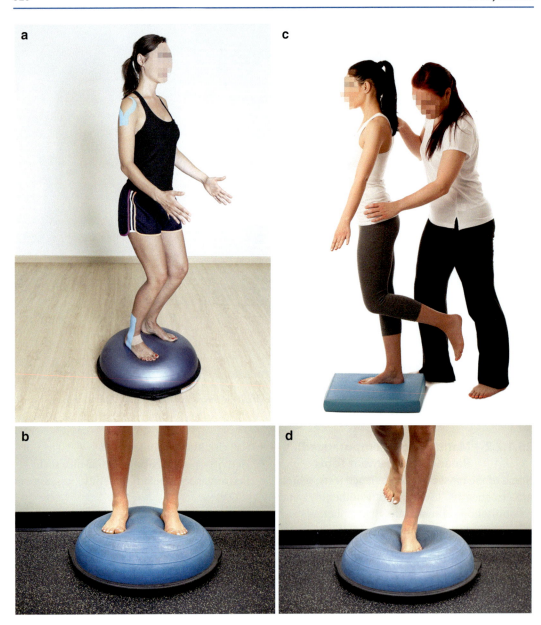

Fig. 26.4 (a–d) Balance exercises. (a) (Source: Adam Gregor/Shutterstock.com), (b) (Source: KBYC photography/Shutterstock.com), (c) (Source: Samo Trebizan/Shutterstock.com), (d) (Source: KBYC photogr/Shutterstock.com aphy)

26.2 Coordination

Coordination can be defined as the ability to make appropriate, controlled movements. Intact and high-level motor coordination is required when performing daily living activities such as walking and driving and when performing occupational tasks and fine motor skills. Coordinated movements require good balance and postural control, as well as the correct sequence and timing of synergistic and reciprocal muscle activity. Coordination, a complex motor skill, is closely related to skills such as balance, speed, reaction time, strength, endurance, and flexibility. Age,

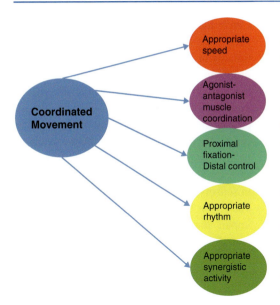

Fig. 26.5 Coordinated movement

height, body mass, balance, direction and distance of movement, muscle spasm tension, endurance, motor learning, and injury are some of the factors affecting coordination. Balance is very important for maintaining coordination. A high level of balance contributes significantly to smooth movements and regaining equilibrium when the balance is disturbed. The characteristics of balanced and coordinated movement are shown in Fig. 26.5.

26.2.1 Motor Coordination

Motor coordination is the ability to coordinate muscle activation in a sequence that maintains posture. Using muscle synergies in postural reactions and maintaining postural control in unstable conditions are examples of motor coordination. The muscles to be activated in a postural synergy are determined by the intended task and the environment. Muscle strength and tone and its ability to act against gravity are prerequisites for motor coordination. However, one of the most important components of coordination is central control. For a purposeful movement to occur, the central nervous system and the musculoskeletal system must work in harmony. The primary motor cortex, premotor areas, association areas, supplementary motor area, and somatosensory areas contribute to the coordinated movement, which is a common and complex function of cortical and subcortical structures. Cortical centers such as the basal ganglia and cerebellum directly or indirectly regulate motor neuron activity in the brain stem and spinal cord. The most active part of the central nervous system in this aspect is the cerebellum.

The theory of cerebellar function, suggesting that the cerebellum is directly and primarily involved in coordinating movement, gained importance when in the mid-eighteenth century Marie Jean Pierre Flourens observed that cerebellar ablation in rabbits leads to loss of motor coordination. Since then, most of the mechanistic theories supporting this hypothesis have suggested that the cerebellum is capable of modifying coordinated movement, underlying muscle activation patterns, and related synergies. In contrast, it was suggested that the cerebellar circuitry is not involved in the coordination of smooth movement, but instead coordinates the acquisition of sensory data on which motor systems and all other brain systems depend. The cerebellum is effective on sensory data collection through motor neurons with the effect of physical characteristics of the individual on different surfaces. The effect of the cerebellum on these motor neurons subtly controls the position of the sensory surfaces (e.g., retina in the case of VOR) and therefore influences the quality of the sensory data obtained (e.g., VOR minimizes retinal drift). The calculation of this control over sensory data acquisition is thought to have a direct impact on productivity and thus the processing power of other brain systems. For more than a century, the cerebellum was considered the only structure responsible for any deficit in the timing and pattern of axial movements. However, we now know that the motor cortex, basal ganglia, spinal cord, and muscle activation patterns are the main responsible structures and the cerebellum plays a secondary role. The idea that the cerebellum is a sensory data collection site, not a motor coordination device, arose as a result of experimenting with tactile stimuli to the lateral hemispheres of the rat cerebellum.

The sensory acquisition hypothesis introduces a new aspect to a few very basic cerebellar features:

1. To continuously assess the quality of sensory data, the cerebellum must receive direct and rapid projections from the sensory structures that collect movement-related data. Spinocerebellar proprioceptive and tactile pathways are the fastest transmitting pathways in the brain and provide extensive input to the cerebellum.
2. To coordinate sensory data acquisition, the cerebellar output must directly influence the transmission of sensory information in the earliest stages. Outputs from the cerebellum red nucleus have a direct impact on the fusimotor system, which is responsible for controlling sensory transduction in muscle spindles.
3. It is important to extensively examine the specific movement-related effects of any cerebellar lesion. For example, patients with cerebellar damage cannot respond to postural perturbations and exhibit specific deficits in sensory control prior to or during movement.
4. The sensory acquisition theory suggests that cerebellar deficiencies lead to impaired coordination and motor control in multi-joint multiplanar movements. Thus, as an adaptive strategy for coping with the lack of coordinated sensory data, patients with cerebellar deficits divide complex movements into a series of simpler movements. As this theory suggests, the cerebellum has an important role in maintaining and planning motor coordination.
5. In fact, the most important secret of cerebellar motor function is to work together with other structures responsible for motor coordination (e.g., cortex, basal ganglia, spinal cord) and organize all the collected data. Developing new strategies to cope with poorly coordinated sensory data at the expense of slower, less complex, and less efficient movements is a major motor coordination compensation mechanism for patients with cerebellar dysfunction.
6. Cerebellum receives projections from all sensory areas and is the only structure to functionally organize the collected data. Thus, any proposed theory of cerebellar function will eventually need to be extended to all sensory systems. Sensory data collection theory clearly meets this standard by predicting that cerebellar extraction or dysfunction leads to behavioral performance deficits in all sensory systems and can be attributed to impairments in sensory data collection control. It has been known for many years that cerebellar lesions impair the performance of visual systems, including VOR. As briefly mentioned above, VOR originates from the activation of the ocular motor muscles; however, cerebellar mechanisms are functionally responsible for improving overall visual acuity by fine-tuning the retina position. It has never been claimed that the cerebellum is involved in visual object recognition, as disruption of VOR causes decreased visual acuity. In summary, the key question is whether the cerebellum and its associated structures calculate how to perform smooth and coordinated movements and actuate motor neurons accordingly, or whether it controls all responses (including smooth and coordinated movements) together with other structures responsible for motor coordination. In conclusion, although the cerebellum is known to be one of the important structures of the cortical system for motor coordination, there is still a need for more research.

26.2.2 Coordination Assessment Methods

There are two main categories of coordination tests in the field of physiotherapy and rehabilitation, namely balanced and non-balanced coordination tests.

26.2.2.1 Balanced Coordination Tests

These are used to evaluate posture and gait coordination where multiple joint movements are involved. These tests evaluate not only balance, but also sequencing, timing, and movement graduation skills (e.g., dysmetria), all of which are essential components of coordination. Some examples of this category include bipedal stance, standing with feet together, unipedal stance, and performing upper extremity and trunk movements while standing. The Romberg test (examines the ability to stand with eyes closed) and the Sharpened Romberg test (examines the ability to stand in tandem with eyes closed) are two common tests of balanced coordination.

26.2.2.2 Non-Balanced Coordination Tests

These tests examine whether an individual can perform postural fixation and sequential or goal-directed activities in a coordinated manner. Some common examples of this category include:

- Postural fixation: Proximal stabilization is essential for distal coordination. The patient is observed for coordination as he/she lies down quickly from a sitting position.
- Finger-to-nose test: The patient first touches their own nose and then the therapist's fingertip.
- Finger-to-finger test: The patient first touches their own fingertip and then the therapist's fingertip.
- Finger opposition: The patient touches the tips of his/her fingers with the thumb of the same hand (opposition of the thumb).
- Object grasping: The patient is asked to grasp and release an object.
- Pronation/supination: Supination and pronation of the forearm is performed sequentially and rhythmically.
- Rebound test: The patient flexes his/her elbow against the therapist's resistance. When the resistance is suddenly released, the patient's forearm flies upward and may hit his/her face or shoulder. The test checks whether the antagonist muscle group can control the arm.
- Manual tempo: Rhythmically tapping on the knees.
- Tempo with the feet: Rhythmically tapping the forefoot on the ground.
- Alternating heel-knee, heel-toe: Touching the therapist's finger with the tip of the toe.
- Heel-tibia test: The patient follows the tibia line with the contralateral heel.
- Circle drawing: The patient performs circulatory movements with his/her upper or lower extremities on a chosen ground.

26.2.3 Coordination Exercises

All exercises should initially be performed consciously, and only in following stages automatization of movements should be targeted. Selected exercises should follow an order from simple to complex. Proximal stabilization should be achieved first, before moving on to the stabilization of other (and distal) segments. The treatment should be supported by a home program and sportive activities suitable for the individual. As an example, the following exercises can be used to improve coordination.

- Proprioceptive neuromuscular facilitation
- Frenkel coordination exercises
- Balance exercises
- Gait training (on different surfaces)
- Posture exercises (mirror and biofeedback)
- Plyometric exercises
- Cawthorne-Cooksey exercises

At more advanced levels, exercises such as sudden change of direction during fast movements, throwing and catching the ball while standing on flexible surfaces, target exercises, and rope jumping can be used to improve coordination.

26.3 Proprioception

Proprioception was first described as "muscle sensation" by Charles Bell in 1826. After this simple definition, Sherrington was the first to scientifically define proprioception as "the ability to perceive the positions and movements of our body segments in space (Kim 2001)." Several mechanoreceptors located in joints, muscles, tendons, and ligaments collect important data regarding the movement and position of our body in space. Proprioception, commonly considered the sixth sense, is divided into three main submodalities.

1. *Sense of movement (kinesthesia):* It is the ability to appreciate joint movement and give information about the movement characteristics such as duration, direction, speed, and amplitude. For example, in sit-to-stand transfer, the features of knee extension (start point [= forward movement in the sagittal plane], end point [= upright standing], duration, acceleration, timing, and direction of the movement in the knee joint) are realized by the sense of joint movement.
2. *Sense of joint position:* It detects the joint position at any point in its movement. In other words, it is the ability of an individual to perceive a presented joint angle and then, after the limb has been moved, to reproduce the same joint angle actively or passively.
3. *Sense of tension (resistance):* It is the ability to appreciate force generated within a joint. It enables us to produce the desired level of muscle force in a certain movement. For example, in 90° knee flexion, the person is asked to perform maximum isometric contraction against high resistance. Then the same person can reproduce 50% of the maximum force thanks to the sense of tension.

26.3.1 Proprioceptive Organs and Their Relationship with the Nervous System

Mechanoreceptors are located in the skin, cartilage, joint capsules, muscles, tendons, and ligaments. These receptors have specialized neurons perceiving mechanical events such as movement and positional changes and transmitting them to the central nervous system. When these receptors are stimulated, sudden acceleration or deceleration, control of movement, and reflex muscle contraction-response occur in the related joint and muscle. These mechanoreceptors include Pacini–Ruffini bodies, Meissner–Merkel bodies, and free nerve endings. Pacini corpuscle is known for its fast adaptation feature. Ruffini corpuscle is very sensitive to stimulus changes and contributes to the joint movement sensation. Ruffini corpuscles are specialized in detecting continuous stimulus with a slow adaptation feature. They are highly stimulated at certain joint angles and therefore play an important role in the sense of joint position. Meissner corpuscles are known for their rapid adaptation feature and sensitive to light touch and fine vibrations on the hairless skin (such as fingertips and lips). Merkel bodies are sensitive to touch and pressure stimuli and can perceive the surface structures such as curves, edges, and points.

Golgi tendon organ is the proprioceptive sensory receptor organ located at the muscle–tendon junction in the origin and insertions of skeletal muscles. This organ is activated by the stretching and active contraction of the muscle and perceives the muscle tension level. The most important task of the Golgi tendon organ is to prevent muscle injuries. When the muscle fibers are overstretched, it prevents further stretch by reflex inhibition and keeps the movement within physiological limits. Muscle spindles are proprioceptive sensory receptors located in the connective tissue of the muscle and detect changes in the muscle length. These receptors send information to the central nervous system about the muscle tension level and the movement speed, providing an endpoint message in cases where the muscle is overextended. Muscle spindles and Golgi tendon organs work in close relationship with each other.

The proprioceptive mechanism relies on the sensorimotor feedback provided by the muscle and joint receptors. The proprioceptive mechanism also creates a feedback and feedforward system by the activation of the abovementioned mechanoreceptors. The sensory stimulus from the mechanoreceptors is transferred from the peripheral nervous system to the central nervous system, which responds with a motor command that activates relevant muscles controlling the movement and position of the joint.

26.3.2 Factors Affecting Proprioception

Factors such as age, weight, body temperature, fatigue, joint degeneration, and level of physical activity have an impact on proprioception. For instance, a cold climate seems to be associated with a lower level of proprioception. Individuals with regular physical activity or exercise routines have a better sense of proprioception. Aging and joint degenerative diseases damage capsules, cartilage, and joint and ligament receptors, leading to a decrease in motor neuron activity and impairing proprioceptive function. The sensitivity of muscle receptors decreases as a result of fatigue, altering the precise sense of position. In addition, conditions such as joint surgeries, skin injuries, long-term immobilizations, and incorrect training techniques adversely affect proprioception.

26.3.3 Proprioception Assessment Methods

Evaluation of proprioception may vary depending on the component(s) of interest. The tools and measurement methods used in different fields are shown as follows:

To evaluate kinesthesia and sense of joint position:

- Isokinetic dynamometers
- Goniometers
- Inclinometers
- Motion analysis systems

To evaluate balance and postural control:

- Stability platforms (stabilometers)
- Force plates

To evaluate delay in muscle activation:

- Electromyography

Other methods:

- Contralateral joint position matching tests
- Jumping tests

The most frequently used methods in the field of physiotherapy and rehabilitation are summarized below.

Various methods have been described in the literature for the assessment of proprioception. The main evaluation tests focus on determining threshold, reproduction, and visual analog model tests. Reproduction tests evaluate the sense of joint position. In other words, these tests examine an individual's ability to actively and/or passively reproduce a given joint angle/position. First, the patient positions the intended joint in the given angle, holds the position for a short period to memorize it, moves the joint out of the position, and then tries to reproduce the initial position. The difference between the reproduced angle and the intended angle is recorded as the deviation angle. Threshold determination tests, on the other hand, evaluate the sense of joint movement (kinesthesia). To do so, the intended joint is subjected to continuous passive motion, which starts with low angular velocities such as 0.5–2.5°/s and gradually accelerates. The patient is asked to notify the tester the moment he/she feels the motion. To evaluate the sense of tension, the patient is asked to generate a predetermined level of muscle force. Then, the patient is asked to produce a specific proportion of the initial force (e.g., 70% or 40% of it). Different devices are used to evaluate proprioception. The most common and functional one is isokinetic dynamometers. In isokinetic devices, the speed, direction, force, and joint angle can be evaluated. Examples of isokinetic measurement are shown in Fig. 26.6.

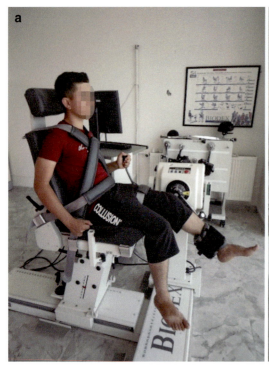 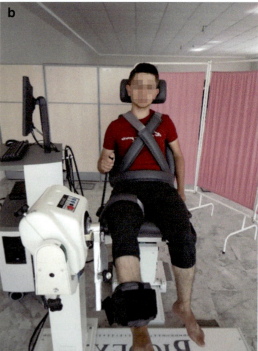

Fig. 26.6 (**a**, **b**) Isokinetic assessment of proprioception

26.4 Conclusion

Balance, coordination, and proprioception should be a part of the program for patients who need rehabilitation at all stages of treatment. A deficiency in one of these parameters causes the patient/person to not reach the previous daily life, sports, or wellness level. In each step of the early, middle, and late stages of rehabilitation, exercises and training that will develop balance, coordination, and proprioception at different levels of difficulty should be planned.

Further Readings

He M, Zhang HN, Tang ZC, Gao SG. Balance and coordination training for patients with genetic degenerative ataxia: a systematic review. J Neurol. 2021;268(10):3690–705.

Verbecque E, Johnson C, Rameckers E, Thijs A, van der Veer I, Meyns P, et al. Balance control in individuals with developmental coordination disorder: a systematic review and meta-analysis. Gait Posture. 2021;83:268–79.

McKeon PO, Hertel J. Systematic review of postural control and lateral ankle instability, part II: is balance training clinically effective? J Athl Train. 2008;43(3):305–15.

Surgent OJ, Dadalko OI, Pickett KA, Travers BG. Balance and the brain: a review of structural brain correlates of postural balance and balance training in humans. Gait Posture. 2019;71:245–52.

Kurt EE, Büyükturan B, Büyükturan Ö, Erdem HR, Tuncay F. Effects of Ai Chi on balance, quality of life, functional mobility, and motor impairment in patients with Parkinson's disease. Disabil Rehabil. 2018;40(7):791–7.

Rivera MJ, Winkelmann ZK, Powden CJ, Games KE. Proprioceptive training for the prevention of ankle sprains: an evidence-based review. J Athl Train. 2017;52(11):1065–7.

Kurt EE, Büyükturan Ö, Erdem HR, Tuncay F, Sezgin H. Short-term effects of kinesio tape on joint position sense, isokinetic measurements, and clinical parameters in patellofemoral pain syndrome. J Phys Ther Sci. 2016;28(7):2034–40.

Hillier S, Immink M, Thewlis D. Assessing proprioception: a systematic review of possibilities. Neurorehabil Neural Repair. 2015;29(10):933–49.

Barnett AL. Motor assessment in developmental coordination disorder: from identification to intervention. Int J Disabil Dev Educ. 2008;55(2):113–29.

Mancini M, Horak FB. The relevance of clinical balance assessment tools to differentiate balance deficits. Eur J Phys Rehabil Med. 2010;46(2):239.

Dijkstra BW, Bekkers EMJ, Gilat M, de Rond V, Hardwick RM, Nieuwboer A. Functional neuroimaging of human postural control: a systematic review with meta-analysis. Neurosci Biobehav Rev. 2020;115:351–62.

Lim JM, Cho JJ, Kim TY, Yoon BC. Isokinetic knee strength and proprioception before and after anterior cruciate ligament reconstruction: a comparison between home-based and supervised rehabilitation. J Back Musculoskelet Rehabil. 2019;32(3):421–9.

Jimsheleishvili S, Dididze M. Neuroanatomy, Cerebellum. In: StatPearls [Internet] 2021. StatPearls Publishing.

Kim OJ. Development of neurophysiology in the early twentieth century: Charles Scott Sherrington and The Integrative action of the nervous system. Uisahak. 2001;10(1):1–21.

Yu JJ, Burnett AF, Sit CH. Motor skill interventions in children with developmental coordination disorder: a systematic review and meta-Analysis. Arch Phys Med Rehabil. 2018;99(10):2076–99.

Cavalcante Neto JL, Steenbergen B, Tudella E. Motor intervention with and without Nintendo® Wii for children with developmental coordination disorder: protocol for a randomized clinical trial. Trials. 2019;20(1):794.

Movement and Nutrition Principles

27

Metin Guldas, Ozge Yesıldemır, Ozan Gurbuz, Seda Ozder, and Elif Yildiz

Abstract

Movement and nutrition play a very important role in maintaining health throughout life and preventing chronic diseases. Obesity and physical inactivity are among the leading causes of death at an early age, and factors that define an individual's lifestyle, such as exercise and healthy nutrition, can reduce the risk of developing many chronic diseases. Regular physical activity and a balanced diet not only prolong life but also improve the quality of life and lead to a healthy life. In this chapter, the effects of nutrition on musculoskeletal health will be considered.

27.1 Nutrition

Nutrition means taking the necessary nutrients for a person to grow, develop, and maintain his/her life and health. Balanced and adequate nutrition means that a person receives enough of the nutrients he/she needs to survive and maintain his/her health. Consumed foods have functions, such as providing the necessary energy for cells in human metabolism; restructuring, renewing, and repairing cells; and protecting the body and organs. The necessary energy from foods is provided by the conversion of the carbon atoms they contain into heat energy by burning them together with oxygen. In addition, foods provide cellular construction–repair with their components, especially bioactive components that cyclically ensure the continuity of the body and strengthen the immune system.

Today, health-related factors such as socio-economic problems, insufficient physical activity, and high body mass index have increased considerably. It is known that an unhealthy and unconsciously applied diet paves the way for many chronic diseases and shortens the lifespan. In particular, obesity is defined as a non-communicable public health problem.

The essential nutrients needed for a healthy life, growth, and development are carbohydrates, lipids, proteins, vitamins, minerals, and water. Proteins, carbohydrates, and lipids are energy-providing macronutrients (Table 27.1).

M. Guldas (✉) · O. Yesıldemır
Nutrition and Dietetics, Faculty of Health Sciences, Bursa Uludag University, Bursa, Turkey
e-mail: mguldas@uludag.edu.tr; ozgeyesildemir@uludag.edu.tr

O. Gurbuz
Food Engineering, Faculty of Agricultural, Bursa Uludag University, Bursa, Turkey
e-mail: ozang@uludag.edu.tr

S. Ozder
Nutrition and Dietetics, Okan University, Istanbul, Turkey

E. Yildiz
Food Processing, Keles Vocational School, Bursa Uludag University, Bursa, Turkey
e-mail: elifyildiz@uludag.edu.tr

Table 27.1 Energy values of protein, carbohydrate, and lipid

Nutrients	The energy produced by 1 g of nutrients
Protein	4 kcal = 17 kJ
Carbohydrate	4 kcal = 17 kJ
Lipid	9 kcal = 37 kJ

Acceptable macronutrient distribution range for carbohydrates, proteins, and lipids are 45–65%, 10–15%, and 25–30% of total daily calories, respectively.

27.1.1 Essential Nutrients

Carbohydrates, proteins, lipids, minerals, vitamins, and water are considered essential nutrients for living organisms.

27.1.1.1 Carbohydrates

Carbohydrates are the most abundant and energy-providing macronutrients in nature. It is found in the form of glucose in the blood and is used in the body in this form. It is stored in muscle glycogen stores to be used as energy in the muscles when necessary. The entry of glucose into cells is controlled by the insulin secreted from the pancreas.

27.1.1.2 Proteins

Proteins are complex organic compounds formed by chain linkage of amino acids and are the most abundant macromolecules in cells. It is effective in gene function, muscle contraction, the transmission of nerves, and embryo development. In the synthesis of hormones and enzymes, the regulation of body fluid balance and the control of many metabolic events have a regulatory function. Components such as protein and calcium are also the building blocks of our body, and calcium is present in the structure of bones and teeth.

Dietary proteins provide essential amino acids for building new muscle tissue. The essential amino acid supplements help minimize muscle loss in cases where the muscles are not actively exercised (at rest, etc.) during muscle injuries. Muscle wasting is due to decreased myofibrillar protein synthesis. The healing processes of muscle injuries depend on collagen and other protein syntheses. A low-protein diet can cause muscle loss.

27.1.1.3 Lipids

Lipids represent the major energy stores in the human body. It is also an important component in the structure of the cell membrane. In addition, it plays many regulatory roles in the body and hormones can be given as an example of this mechanism. In this respect, some hormones, such as testosterone and estrogen, are produced from fat and cholesterol.

27.1.1.4 Vitamins and Minerals

Vitamins and minerals, as the building blocks of the body, play an important role in the processes of construction and destruction. Vitamins A, D, E, and K, which are fat-soluble vitamins, support metabolism for increased muscle mass. B complex vitamins have an important role in the efficiency of energy metabolism.

27.1.1.5 Water

Water is an important aid in food digestion, maintaining body temperature, sustaining metabolic processes in the cell, and removing toxins. Maintaining body water balance is vital. Although it varies from person to person, it is recommended that an adult person should drink 2–2.5 L of water daily. The amount of water that should be consumed daily can be found by a simple calculation, according to body weight, as "35 mL" for every 1 kg. In addition, water requirements during exercise increase depending on the fluid loss from sweating.

27.2 Nutritional Principles Affecting Body Movement

A healthier diet and physical activity are necessary to lead a healthy life, and for prevention and treatment of chronic diseases. In order to increase physical activity, it is necessary to protect and support the musculoskeletal system. The musculoskeletal system consists of bones, joints, and muscles. All these tissues enable movement, active life, and maintaining body posture. Maintaining bone and muscle health is very important for general health and mobility.

A healthy diet and regular exercise are the keys to maintaining muscle and joint health, which must begin in adolescence and adulthood and continue throughout aging. Although it is accepted that a healthy diet is an important factor in the prevention and treatment of non-communicable diseases, the importance of maintaining an active lifestyle throughout life is unfortunately not held equally by all segments of society. The combination of a healthy, nutritious, balanced diet and exercise helps preserve muscle mass and function, prevent excessive fat accumulation in the body, and support the structural components of the joints. The World Health Organization (WHO) has recognized that physical inactivity is one of the leading global risk factors for morbidity and premature death. In addition, the United Nations accepts that physical activity is a basic building block in the fight against non-communicable diseases.

27.3 Energy Requirement

Although it is thought that the energy requirement decreases in bone and muscle injuries, energy consumption increases during the healing process in severe injuries. The energy requirement can increase between 15 and 50% depending on the type and severity of the injury. Insufficient energy intake is a factor that can delay recovery and cause serious muscle loss. Excessive energy intake causes undesirable conditions such as increased body fat. The daily energy expenditure is composed of resting metabolic rate, thermic effect of food, and energy cost of physical activity.

$$\text{Daily Energy Expenditure}(\text{kcal}) = \text{Resting metabolic rate} + \text{Thermic effect of food} + \text{Physical activity}$$

The balance between energy intake and energy expenditure ensures body weight maintenance. When energy intake exceeds energy expenditure, energy balance is positive and leads to weight gain. Excessive weight gain results in chronic diseases, especially obesity. Increasing body weight can cause musculoskeletal system disorders.

Each movement requires a certain amount of energy expenditure. Protein, fat, and carbohydrates, which are energy-providing sources, are used to provide the energy necessary for muscle contraction. Apart from daily activities, the energy sources required for exercise vary by exercise duration and intensity, the capacity of muscle glycogen stores, and the nutritional status of an individual. Creatine phosphate and adenosine triphosphate (ATP) are used in intense activities of less than one minute in the body. Carbohydrates are used in endurance exercises for up to eight minutes. In addition, carbohydrates and lipids are used together in long-term exercises. Fatigue occurs in the body as muscle glycogen stores are depleted in exercises that last longer than a few hours. As carbohydrate intake decreases, glycogen stores decrease and fatigue symptoms begin to appear in a shorter time.

The main energy source of the human body is carbohydrates. Glucose is synthesized from non-carbohydrate metabolites even when following a low-carbohydrate diet. Glucose is stored as storage energy, that is fat, when the body does not need energy. Therefore, in parallel with the increasing energy requirement, it is important to have a balanced diet in accordance with the basic rules. Nutrients are used as needed in the body, and the excess nutrients are stored in the body's energy store (fat). After high fat or protein and low carbohydrate intake, glucose is used as the body's energy source. In this case, the liver and kidney work harder to remove waste materials caused by gluconeogenesis.

27.4 Carbohydrate Selection

Carbohydrates are the main energy source of the human body. The brain and central nervous system use only glucose as an energy source. Adequate intake of the right carbohydrates prevents the use of proteins as an energy source and supports muscle building. In addition, it also aids weight loss by enabling the fat-burning mechanism to work.

It is necessary to choose complex carbohydrates for optimal health. Complex carbohydrates, which are digested more slowly, have a low glycemic index. Complex carbohydrates are foods that are high in fiber, more difficult to digest, and slow to digest, such as whole grain products, bulgur wheat, brown rice, vegetables, and legumes. The rate at which food raises blood glucose level is called the glycemic index. Foods with a high glycemic index raise blood glucose levels quickly. Rising blood glucose level causes the secretion of insulin. Excessive glucose in the blood is quickly transported to the muscle and other tissues, causing a sudden drop in blood glucose level. Foods with a low glycemic index, on the other hand, create a more balanced picture by slowly releasing glucose into the blood, and blood glucose level remains in balance thanks to the slower and controlled secretion of insulin.

A snack consisting of carbohydrates with a medium/high glycemic index can be consumed to quickly replenish the muscle glycogen stores that are empty after long-term exercises and to perform well before exercise. It has been seen that supplementing with some protein in addition to carbohydrates is an effective method in repairing muscles faster and preventing muscle loss.

27.5 Important Nutrients for a Healthy Musculoskeletal System

It is known that exercise benefits bone health for individuals of all ages and is an important factor in the prevention and treatment of bone disorders such as osteoporosis. Nutrition and exercise should be evaluated as a whole in this respect. Bone density and muscle mass decrease when following an unhealthy and inadequate diet. Many nutrients such as vitamin D, calcium, and potassium should be intaken in sufficient amounts to maintain musculoskeletal health (Table 27.2).

Table 27.2 Important nutrients and their functions for a healthy musculoskeletal system

Nutrients	Functions	Dietary reference intakes[a]
Protein	It is necessary for bone formation and collagen production.	0.66 g/kg/d
Calcium	It promotes bone formation and the proper functioning of the muscles. It plays a role in nerve conduction, fiber contraction, and heartbeat control.	800 mg/d
Vitamin C	It stimulates the synthesis of collagen, which is the most important component of the bone extracellular matrix, and the formation of osteoblasts, which are bone-forming cells. Its deficiency can lead to swelling and pain in the joints and weaken bone tissue.	90 mg/d for males
75 mg/d for females
Vitamin D	It provides calcium absorption, bone development, and bone remodeling. Its deficiency causes bone diseases such as rickets and osteomalacia.	10 µg/d
Magnesium	It contributes to the structure of bones and teeth. It plays a role in the activation of vitamin D.	350 mg/d for males[b]
265 mg/d for females[b]
Omega-3 fatty acid	It reduces the incidence and severity of inflammatory bone/joint diseases.	0.6–1.2% of energy
Potassium	It is important in maintaining the structure of bones.	4.7 g/d
Collagen	It is a protein found in connective tissues, muscles, and bones.	–
Glucosamine and chondroitin	They are used together in the treatment of disorders related to joints, articular cartilage, and synovial fluid.	–
Polyphenols	They help reduce joint inflammation and slow cartilage degeneration.	–
Sulforaphane	It blocks enzymes that destroy joint cartilage and helps reduce inflammation. It is effective in the treatment of osteoarthritis.	–
Diallyl disulfide	It blocks enzymes that destroy joint cartilage and delays the symptoms of osteoarthritis.	–

[a]This table includes the Recommended Dietary Allowance (RDA) recommendations for adults aged 19–50 years. Nutritional requirements differ during pregnancy, lactation, infancy, and childhood
[b]Magnesium requirements are for adults aged 31–50 years. For males and females, 19–30 years of age, magnesium requirements are 330 mg/day and 255 mg/day, respectively

There are some dietary supplements that are commonly taken to control these deficiencies of nutrients. Chondroprotective (cartilage protection) dietary supplements such as glucosamine, chondroitin, hyaluronic acid, and s-adenosylmethionine (SAMe) are used to help support healthy joints.

These protective components act as building blocks for joint cartilage and synovial fluid or provide a delayed effect on osteoarthritis. In addition, other supplements such as omega-3 fatty acids, antioxidant vitamins (A, C, and E), and some foods containing bioactive components such as fruits, vegetables, tea, spices, and nuts are used to support joint health and treat inflammatory arthritis. Extracts of *Boswellia serrata* can be used as herbal therapeutics in the treatment of osteoarthritis and rheumatoid arthritis. It is shown that evening primrose oil or blackcurrant oil containing gamma-linolenic acid (GLA) may reduce pain in patients with rheumatoid arthritis. A Cochrane systematic review found that GLA can reduce pain severity scores and health-related distress in rheumatoid arthritis. However, although dietary supplements are often used to relieve joint pain, modern medical management is primarily recommended for the treatment of arthritis.

27.5.1 Protein

Adequate protein intake is necessary for bone formation, bone maintenance, and collagen production. Protein-rich foods help increase the mineral content in bones and reduce the risk of bone breaking. Human milk and egg protein are assumed to be the most readily utilizable protein and given a biological value of 100. Good-quality protein sources are lean beef, chicken, turkey, seafood, and soy-based products. Legumes, which are medium-quality protein sources, create a better-quality protein source when consumed with whole grains. In addition, vitamin B6, which can be obtained from foods such as banana, prune, spinach, avocado, and sunflower seeds, supports muscle development, and increases protein intake and bioavailability.

27.5.2 Vitamin C

Vitamin C stimulates the synthesis of collagen, which is the most important component of the bone extracellular matrix, and the formation of osteoblasts, which are bone-forming cells. It is also thought to reduce oxidative stress as it scavenges free radicals that are harmful to bone health, thus preventing bone resorption and protecting against osteoporosis. It plays an important role in the musculoskeletal system by supporting collagen formation and helping to protect these tissues with its antioxidant properties. Vitamin C deficiency can cause break down of collagen, leading to joint pain or swelling and bone weakness. A healthy diet that includes adequate vitamin C is essential for optimum joint development and maintenance. The Recommended Dietary Allowance (RDA) for adults, 19 years and older, for vitamin C is set at 90 mg/day for males and 75 mg/day for females. Good sources of vitamin C include citrus fruits, kiwi, strawberries, rose hips, tomatoes, red peppers, parsley, and green leafy vegetables.

27.5.3 Calcium

About 99% of the calcium in the body is stored in the skeletal system, and the blood calcium level is decisive for bone health. Calcium is obtained from food as it cannot be produced by the body. When enough calcium cannot be taken from food and drink, the body removes calcium from bones. Therefore, it may weaken the bones and may even lead to osteoporosis. In fact, although bone density decreases with increasing age, adequate calcium intake has a protective effect against this process. It is also needed for nerve conduction, heartbeat control, and muscle contraction. Shortly, calcium is vital for the formation of strong bones and the proper functioning of the muscles. The WHO and Institute of Medicine (IOM) recommend 1000 mg of calcium per day for adults aged 19–50 years. The recommendation for calcium intake is 950–1000 mg per day for adults according to the Turkish Dietary Guideline. Milk and dairy products are among the best calcium sources, but green leafy vegetables are also a good source of calcium. Other calcium-rich foods include almonds, calcium-fortified dairy products, fruit juices, cereals, and vegetables such as broccoli and cabbage.

27.5.4 Vitamin D

7-Dehydrocholesterol is converted to vitamin D by the action of solar ultraviolet radiation on the skin. The main source of vitamin D is the sun, and it is predominantly stored in adipose tissues. Thus, vitamin D can be used from adipose tissues during the winter when the effect of sun rays decreases. Vitamin D provides calcium absorption, transportation of calcium from bone and kidney to the blood, and calcium resorption from the kidney when needed. Its deficiency causes bone diseases such as rickets and osteomalacia. It also takes longer to recover from knee joint discomfort and loss of functionality in patients with vitamin D deficiency. The current recommendations suggest consuming 10 μg of vitamin D per day. It has been recommended to meet the vitamin D requirement with diet and dietary supplements in recent years because cumulative sun exposure can cause skin cancer. Other foods, except fish liver, are very low in vitamin D. Foods such as milk, cheese, and fruit juice fortified with vitamin D are consumed in some countries. Other sources of vitamin D include fish liver, egg yolk, salmon, milk, and oily fish such as tuna, sardines, mackerel, and herring.

27.5.5 Magnesium

About 60% of magnesium is stored in the bones, and its deficiency causes osteoporosis. It is found together with calcium and phosphorus in the structure of bones and teeth. It plays a role with calcium in the muscle and nervous system functions. Calcium and magnesium play a role in regulating muscle contraction and relaxation, respectively. Magnesium also plays a role in the activation of vitamin D. The RDA for adults aged 19–50 years is 330–350 mg daily for males and 255–265 mg for females. Nuts, legumes, green leafy vegetables, and whole grains are good sources of magnesium. It is also in black beans, soybeans, quinoa, brown rice, spinach, chard, artichokes, prunes, and pumpkin seeds.

27.5.6 Potassium

Potassium is an essential component that maintains fluid and electrolyte balance in the body. It is also the third most abundant mineral in the body. It is essential for the functions of many organs including the heart, kidneys, brain, and muscle tissues. Potassium plays a role with sodium to support cellular function with the sodium–potassium pump. The sodium–potassium pump is the primary mechanism in maintaining water balance between the intracellular and extracellular fluid. The IOM recommends 4.7 g of potassium per day for adults aged 19–50 years. Bananas, green beans, cabbage, liver, coffee, parsley, and spinach are among the sources of potassium.

27.5.7 Omega-3 Fatty Acids

Joints are susceptible to inflammation. Swelling and tissue micro-injuries resulting from inflammation predispose to joint degeneration and pain. Omega-3 fatty acids also help control inflammation. They can improve the symptoms of some diseases that cause inflammation in the joints, such as rheumatoid arthritis, and can reduce the severity of pain by increasing joint flexibility. The omega-3 fatty acid recommendation is 0.6–1.2% of energy. Due to its high omega-3 fatty acid content, fish should be consumed by grilling, baking, and steaming at least two to three times per week (350–400 g/week). Also, marine fish have a higher omega-3 content compared to freshwater fish. Flaxseed, canola, soybeans, chia seeds, hemp seeds, walnuts, and algae are also plant sources of omega-3 fatty acids.

27.5.8 Collagen

Muscles, joints, and bones contain collagen, a structural protein. Collagen (type 1) constitutes the majority of the dry weight of tendons and ligaments. Strong collagen fibers act as a glue that holds the tissues together. Collagen, which prevents the bones from becoming brittle, strengthens the tendons that fix the bones to the skeleton and the ligaments that stabilize the joints. It also supports the structure of the cartilages in the joints.

The most common types of collagen and the tissues in which they are usually found are given below:

- Type 1 collagen: Bone, teeth, connective tissue, tendons, and skin
- Type 2 collagen: Cartilage and eyes
- Type 3 collagen: Connective tissue, muscle, blood tissues, and skin
- Type 4 collagen: Epithelial tissue
- Type 5 collagen: Hair and placenta

The most common types used in dietary supplements are type 1, type 2, and type 3. These bovine and marine collagens are generally recommended for the treatment of bone and connective tissue disorders. While minerals mainly ensure bone hardness, collagens provide skeletal strength. They determine the tissue shape, forming the skeleton for the attachment of cells and fixation of macromolecules. Collagen fibers in bone are arranged in concentric layers that provide maximum resistance to rotational and compressive stress. Collagen also supports intestinal health, provides skin elasticity, improves cardiovascular health, and contributes to hair and nail development.

27.5.9 Glucosamine and Chondroitin

Glucosamine is the main component of connective tissue. Chondroitin is found in the connective tissues as well as cartilages, tendons, and skin. It is shown that the use of glucosamine and chondroitin as a dietary supplement provides positive results in treating disorders related to the joints, cartilage, and synovial fluid.

27.5.10 Polyphenols

Polyphenols are antioxidants that help reduce joint inflammation and slow cartilage degeneration. They support bone structure and increase the body's immunity against infections. Anthocyanins, primarily found in red and purple fruits, reduce the level of C-reactive protein, which is an indicator of inflammation.

27.5.11 Sulforaphane

Sulforaphane is a bioactive component found in many cruciferous vegetables like broccoli, Brussels sprouts, cabbage, cauliflower, and kale. It has been determined that sulforaphane, known for its anti-carcinogenic effect, can block enzymes that destroy articular cartilage and help reduce inflammation. Therefore, patients with osteoarthritis should consume these foods regularly.

27.5.12 Diallyl Disulfide

It has been determined that diallyl disulfide, which is found in foods such as garlic, onions, and leeks from the Allium family, can block enzymes that destroy articular cartilage, just like sulforaphane. It can also delay the progression of osteoarthritis.

27.5.13 Eggshell Membrane Supplements

The eggshell membrane contains a significant amount of calcium. It is effective in the healing of wounds and bone formation by supporting collagen production (after regular use in as few as ten days). Many studies have reported that it is effective in reducing joint pain intensity. Usage of eggshell membrane supplements has increased significantly in recent years due to their affordable prices.

27.6 Conclusion

Physical activity and healthy nutrition are beneficial to musculoskeletal health. Balanced and adequate nutrition contributes to the prevention of muscle loss in muscle injuries and shortens the time of treatment. Nutrients are essential for the human body. They are needed for the functions of the complex and interactive organs, and there are also interactions between nutrients within these complex processes. In addition, it is necessary to provide adequate amounts of various nutrients to maintain health and well-being. Nutrient deficiencies result in serious health problems. A healthy diet plan that includes sufficient energy, protein, vitamins, and minerals is essential for the treatment of diseases to be effective. To protect and improve the musculoskeletal system health:

- Pay attention to adequate protein intake and balanced amino acid profile.
- Consume adequate amounts of carbohydrates, especially to avoid muscle loss before and after exercise.
- Consider speeding up the healing process with dietary supplements for bone and muscle damage.
- Maintain a balanced diet so as not to damage the musculoskeletal structures.
- Support the musculoskeletal system with regular exercise.
- Delay, control, or prevent musculoskeletal diseases with a healthy diet, although there is a predisposition to chronic and/or progressive diseases such as osteoporosis.

Further Reading

Baykara C, Cana H, Sarikabak M, Aydemir U. Overview of sports injuries. In: Herguner G, Hazer G, Ozdemir M, editors. Sports in all aspects. Güven Plus Group Consulting Inc. Publications; 2019. p. 101–28. E-ISBN: 978-605-7594-10-5.

Burke ML, Ross LM, Garvican-Lewis LA, Welvaert M, Heikura AI, Forbes GS, Mirtschin GJ, Cato EL, Strobel N, Sharma PA, Hawley AJ. Low carbohydrate, high fat diet impairs exercise economy and negates the performance benefit from intensified training in elite race walkers. J Physiol. 2017;595(9):2785–807.

Daneault A, Prawitt J, Fabien Soulé V, Coxam V, Wittrant Y. Biological effect of hydrolyzed collagen on bone metabolism. Crit Rev Food Sci Nutr. 2017;57(9):1922–37.

Eskici G. Protein and exercise: new approaches. Spormetre. 2020;18(3):1–13.

Food and Agriculture Organization of the United Nations. Dietary protein quality evaluation in human nutrition report of an FAO Expert Consultation Rome; 2013.

Goolsby MA, Boniquit N. Bone health in athletes: the role of exercise, nutrition, and hormones. Sports Health. 2017;9(2):108–17.

Hatting M, Tavares CD, Sharabi K, Rines AK, Puigserver P. Insulin regulation of gluconeogenesis. Ann N Y Acad Sci 2018;1411(1);21.

Henriksen K, Karsdal AM. Chapter 1: Type I collagen. In: Karsdal MA, editor. Biochemistry of collagens, laminins and elastin. Academic Press; 2016. p. 1–11. ISBN: 978-0-12-809847-9.

Howard EE, Margolis LM. Intramuscular mechanisms mediating adaptation to low-carbohydrate, high-fat diets during exercise training. Nutrients. 2020;12(9):2496.

Hutson MJ, O'Donnell E, Brooke-Wavell K, Sale C, Blagrove RC. Effects of low energy availability on bone health in endurance athletes and high-impact exercise as a potential countermeasure: a narrative review. Sports Med. 2020;1-13

Institute of Medicine. Dietary reference intakes for calcium, phosphorous, magnesium, vitamin D, and fluoride. Washington: National Academy of Science; 1997.

Institute of Medicine. Dietary reference intakes for vitamin C, vitamin E, selenium, and carotenoids. Washington: National Academy of Science; 2000.

Institute of Medicine. Dietary reference intakes for water, potassium, sodium, chloride, and sulfate. Washington: National Academy of Science; 2005.

Institute of Medicine. Dietary reference intakes for calcium and vitamin D. Washington: National Academy of Science; 2011.

Jia H, Hanate M, Aw W, Itoh H, Saito K, Kobayashi S, Hachimura S, Fukuda S, Tomita M, Hasebe Y, Kato H. Eggshell membrane powder ameliorates intestinal inflammation by facilitating the restitution of epithelial injury and alleviating microbial dysbiosis. Sci Rep. 2017;7(1):1–15.

Lange KW. Movement and nutrition in health and disease. Movement Nutr Health Dis. 2017:1–2.

Malmir H, Shab-Bidar S, Djafarian K. Vitamin C intake in relation to bone mineral density and risk of hip fracture and osteoporosis: a systematic review and meta-analysis of observational studies. Br J Nutr. 2018;119(8):847–58.

Owens DJ, Fraser WD, Close GL. Vitamin D and the athlete: Emerging insights. Eur J Sport Sci. 2015;15(1):73–84.

Sale C, Elliott-Sale KJ. Nutrition and athlete bone health. Sports Med. 2019;49:139–51.

Shams-White MM, Chung M, Du M, Fu Z, Insogna KL, Karlsen MC, Weaver CM. Dietary protein and bone health: a systematic review and meta-analysis from the National Osteoporosis Foundation. Am J Clin Nutr. 2017;105(6):1528–43.

Silvipriya KS, Kumar KK, Bhat AR, Kumar BD, John A, Lakshmanan P. Collagen: animal sources and biomedical application. J Appl Pharm Sci. 2015;5(3):123–7.

Suesca E, Dias AMA, Braga MEM, de Sousa HC, Fontanilla MR. Multifactor analysis on the effect of collagen concentration, cross-linking and fiber/pore orientation on chemical, microstructural, mechanical and biological properties of collagen type I scaffolds. Mater Sci Eng C. 2017;77:333–41.

Tipton KD. Nutritional support for exercise-induced injuries. Sports Med. 2015;45(1):93–104.

Turkey Dietary Guideline (TUBER). Ministry of Health Publications, Ankara, p. 20; 2019.

Nutritional Supplements for Musculoskeletal Health

Aysegul Birlik

28

Abstract

In order to supplement the normal diet, it is necessary to use concentrates or extracts of nutrients such as vitamins, minerals, proteins, carbohydrates, fibers, fatty acids, amino acids or other substances of plant and animal origin, bioactive substances, and similar substances that have nutritional or physiological effects. They are products for which daily intake dose is determined by preparing their own or mixtures in capsules, tablets, lozenges, disposable powder packs, liquid ampoules, and other similar forms. Nutritional supplements are not drugs. They are used to meet individual needs, not therapeutic, and they do not replace nutrition but eliminate nutritional deficiency. Nutritional supplements used in musculoskeletal health can affect the structure or functions of muscle, joint tissue, and bone. Considering deficiencies and needs of the body in people who exercise, supporting joint, bone, and muscle structures with appropriate nutritional supplements is required for: repair and restructuring of cartilage and connective tissues; prevention and/or relief of inflammation, pain, spasm, and cramp complaints; and improving recovery and healing process. In this section, natural building blocks from extracellular matrix molecules for healthy bone, articular cartilage, and peripheral synovium, glycosaminoglycans, chondroitin sulfate, hyaluronic acid, glycoproteins, and vitamin and mineral supplements will be explained.

28.1 Nutritional Supplements for Bone, Joint, and Connective Tissue Health

Supplements that affect bone health have effects on bone mass and integrity. These supplements can affect the strength and vulnerability of bones by acting as essential parts of bone, such as calcium. They may play a role in mineralization or prevent bone loss, such as vitamin K. Joint health supplements are effective on the structure and function of articular cartilage or joint pain and have significant effects on cartilage synthesis or low-grade inflammation, pain, swelling, and stiffness.

28.1.1 Supplements for Structural Content and Repairment

Extracellular matrix molecules, natural building blocks of joint cartilage, glycosaminoglycans (GAG), chondroitin sulfate and hyaluronic acid, and glucosamine, one of the glycoproteins, have

A. Birlik (✉)
Ayşegül Birlik Wellbeing & Healthcare Consultancy, Istanbul, Turkey

been used for many years as ingredients of supplements to support healthy joint cartilage and peripheral synovium.

Supplementation of *glucosamine sulfate* strengthens blood vessels, stimulates regeneration processes in tissues, stimulates the synthesis of enzymes, and relieves inflammation. There are studies that show that glucosamine sulfate can slow symptom progression in people with knee osteoarthritis, as well as cause a long-term reduction in symptoms and reduce the need for other pain medications and non-steroidal anti-inflammatory drugs (NSAIDs). However, although glucosamine helps some symptoms such as joint stiffness, there are studies showing that it is not effective for other symptoms, which still creates mixed data for glucosamine.

The effective supplement form of glucosamine sulfate has a general use of 900–1500 mg/day (three times a day, 300–500 mg each time), for three to six months. Higher doses impair the absorption and distribution of glucosamine sulfate, while lower doses proportionally decrease the glucosamine blood concentration with little physiological effect. Glucosamine sulfate supplementation can affect the way the body uses glucose. For this reason, it was stated that diabetic people and/or those with insulin resistance should be careful.

The effects of glucosamine on insulin and sugar metabolism have attracted the attention of researchers for many years. In 16 clinical studies, it was determined that it did not cause a remarkable change in blood sugar levels when administered to 854 volunteers for a long time period (average of 37 weeks). However, considering that the responses vary from person to person, it may be recommended that patients check their blood sugar and glycosylated hemoglobin (HbA1c) levels for a month after they start using glucosamine.

Chondroitin sulfate stimulates fluid production and prevents tissue destruction. Combined use with glucosamine has been reported to be more effective. It was found to be more effective than a placebo in controlling pain in the joints and improving the function of the joints. It is normally effective in reducing pain but is known to be a better option for long-term use in some cases, as fewer side effects have been reported compared to NSAIDs. It can be used for three to six months at doses of 900–1200 mg/day (three times a day, 300–400 mg each time). We should also pay attention to allergic side effects. Most of the glucosamine on the market comes from shellfish such as crab, lobster, and shrimp, and caution should be exercised in allergic individuals. Chondroitin has a blood-thinning effect, so the risk of bleeding should be considered, and it should be controlled while it is given with blood thinners. Large chondroitin molecules can cause possible gastrointestinal discomfort due to difficult digestion.

The joint health interventions have been dominated by glucosamine sulfate for about three decades, and chondroitin sulfate alone or in combination with glucosamine products began to appear about 15 years ago. While these two ingredients still make up the majority of joint health products, both appear to have significant shortcomings. High daily dosages, long duration of use for benefits, and problems with absorption are just some of the reasons why consumer preferences are changing. A meta-analysis with more than 3800 people with knee or hip osteoarthritis found that treatment with glucosamine, chondroitin, or the combination was no more effective than placebo. In general, glucosamine and chondroitin are considered safe but as with any medication, there are potential risks. In a recent study, people who had the glucosamine–chondroitin combination reported more frequent diarrhea and abdominal pain than those in the placebo group. Other reported side effects are painful burning sensation in the chest, drowsiness, headache, and allergic reactions.

In the multicenter clinical study of GAIT—Glucosamine/chondroitin Arthritis Intervention Trial—performed by the American National Institutes of Health (NIH) in 1583 knee arthritis patients for 6 months, it was noted that no significant response was obtained with glucosamine–chondroitin supplements in joint pain, and the effect was insufficient. European study GUIDE—Glucosamine Unum In Die—which included 318 patients, noted that no significant response was obtained against placebo in the 6 months.

Hyaluronic acid (hyaluronan) is a natural polymer that increases the viscosity and compressive strength of synovial fluid. It is suggested that its effect on osteoarthritis is exerted by suppressing the phagocytosis and oxidative stress of macrophages. Although there are conflicting data in the literature, recent studies show that hyaluronic acid has superior pain relief and functional gain effect over placebo in cases with osteoarthritis. It has moisturizing, lubricating, anti-inflammatory, and chondroprotective effects in terms of effectiveness. In tablet form, they are used in daily doses of 100–120 mg in the content of a combined supplement.

Body parts containing intense sulfur such as cartilage tissue need excessive sulfur during the repair process; in these cases *methylsulfonylmethane* (MSM) supplementation as the organic sulfur compound with the highest bioavailability is beneficial. Literature suggests that the ingredient helps the body maintain healthy connective tissues by promoting its sulfur content and support. While MSM supports the formation of connective tissue, it initiates regeneration processes in conjunction with glucosamine and chondroitin, provides nutrients and protection of cartilage tissue in bones, and increases joint mobility. There is evidence suggesting that it may be beneficial in aging knee arthritis, and patients with osteoarthritis who do long-term exercises and have persistent inflammation may benefit from using MSM. It has reducing effects on inflammation, joint pain, and oxidative stress. Extensive research has shown that MSM reduces joint pain, improves stiffness and swelling, and increases the range of motion and physical function of individuals with osteoarthritis. Reduction in joint pain has also been noted in healthy athletes. It is well tolerated in most people at normal doses, and it is recommended to use between 900 mg and 2 g per day for at least six weeks.

Collagen, which forms the backbone of the mechanical strength of the bones, is a vital structural protein for bones, consisting of the amino acids glycine, proline, and hydroxyproline. Around 80% of collagen is found in bones and other connective tissues. In bones, collagen is intertwined with minerals, including calcium apatite crystals. While there are at least 16 types of collagen, the dense types—type I, II, III collagens—also constitute the contents of the supplement products.

Type I: It gives structure to skin, bones, tendons, fibrous cartilage, connective tissues, and teeth. Approximately 95% of the collagen in bones is type I, while type II collagen is also present. Studies show that type I collagen synthesis promotes osteoblast growth and increases bone mineral density.

Type II: Up to 60% of joints are type II collagen, produced by the acellular cartilage matrix. Type II collagen, which helps cartilage formation in connective tissues, is very important for joint health. The use of additional supplements is effective in the treatment of age-related joint pain and various symptoms that occur accordingly. In addition, type X collagen is also found in articular cartilage, and is important for the formation of new bone and the development of articular cartilage.

Type III: All tendons are of this type. It supports the structure of muscles, organs, and arteries, and gives elasticity to the vessels and strength to the muscles.

Collagen sources hydrolyzed in private laboratories are available as supplements for the purpose of strengthening connective tissue and mobility support with collagen regeneration, supporting muscle building, and increasing bone density and strength. Cattle, pigs, poultry (chicken, etc.), and fish are sources of collagen. Since bovine collagen is abundant, it is cheaper, but allergic side effects have been shown in humans at a rate of 3%. Fish collagen hydrolysates are also known as important supplements that the body can use with their lower molecular weights. In recent years, a specially patented eggshell membrane has also been preferred as a source of collagen. Laboratory studies on preosteoblasts from mice also highlight the bone-protective effects of bovine collagen peptides by increasing the growth and proliferation of osteoblasts and promoting the formation of a mineralized bone matrix. These factors prove the importance of regenerating collagen in addition to key bone-supporting vitamins and minerals for maintaining bone health.

Nutritional supplements in the form of hydrolyzed collagen or non-denatured type II collagen have different dosing strategies and can be considered two different supplements, although their benefits may show some similarities. The hydrolysis and denaturation process breaks down the peptides into smaller peptide chains and ultimately the amino acids that form them. Most supplements are in the hydrolyzed form of collagen. The terms hydrolyzed collagen, collagen hydrolysate, hydrolyzed gelatin, and collagen peptides are essentially synonymous. Oral hydrolyzed collagen is digested in the gut and crosses the intestinal barrier. It is relatively well absorbed, enters the circulation, and has been found to reach target tissues in various researches. Hydrolyzed collagen, peptide collagen 2–2.5 g/day, and natural collagen powders 6–10 g/day can be used for supplementation purposes.

While the number of human studies evaluating the use of collagen for bone health is few, the results of the initial studies are promising. In literature, it was stated that supplementation with hydrolyzed collagen has a positive therapeutic role in conditions such as osteoporosis and osteoarthritis. A recent clinical study has shown that supplementation of specific collagen peptides in postmenopausal women increases bone formation, leading to a positive change in bone mineral density and markers of bone health.

Combined supplements of glycosaminoglycans with hydrolyzed collagen and hyaluronic acid reduce synovial effusion and pain, and facilitate joint movements, especially in problems such as arthritis, and meniscus tearing, which cause synovial effusion. Glycosaminoglycan, hydrolyzed collagen type 1, and vitamin C combination products that support regular fibril formation after all tendon discomforts and tendon surgery are also useful as additional supplements to the treatment. The synthesis of collagen, which is preferred as a nutritional supplement in injury prevention and rehabilitation, increases in the presence of sufficient vitamin C.

Eggshell membrane has been used as a supplement in recent years, with studies showing that its content supports connective tissue and joints. Natural eggshell membrane (NEM), a partially hydrolyzed eggshell membrane developed by a patented enzymatic process, is at the forefront of the development of these new supplements. Type I collagen and elastin are important in the content of the complex structure. The basic structural elements such as glucosamine, chondroitin, and hyaluronic acid, and the content of desmosine and isodesmosine, two lesser-known amino acids responsible for the elastic properties of elastin, are also important.

The natural eggshell membrane is already sufficiently predigested to digest its fibrous membrane and release its nutrient content. This "partially hydrolyzed structure" has two important consequences. First, the combination of partial digestion and the body's own digestive processes ensures that the bioactive components in NEM are optimally bioavailable for absorption through the intestinal wall and use in joint tissue. Second, predigestion releases peptides, specifically collagen peptides, that interact with the intestinal immune system to indirectly modulate the immune response to rheumatoid arthritis via oral tolerance. If the NEM had not been fully hydrolyzed or unhydrolyzed, this two-pronged operation would not have been possible. Literature shows that once daily use of 500 mg of the eggshell membrane provides rapid relief from exercise-induced joint pain (day 8) and stiffness (day 4), as well as significantly reducing discomfort from stiffness immediately after exercise (day 7). It also showed a significant chondroprotective effect by reducing the cartilage degradation biomarker C-Terminal Cross-Linking Telopeptide (CTX-II).

Calcium may be the first supplement that comes to mind in bone health, but it is increasingly understood that calcium supplementation alone cannot fully improve bone health or may be partially effective. *Vitamin D* and calcium are often studied together because vitamin D is the primary regulator of calcium absorption in the body. Adequate vitamin D levels are important in regulating calcium and phosphorus absorption in bone health, enzyme activation in muscle contraction, increase in muscle protein anabolism, decrease in muscle breakdown, regulation of anti-inflammatory reactions, and regulation of immune function.

In case of need, the Institute of Medicine (IOM) recommends vitamin D supplementation at a dose of 600 IU/day. The safe upper limit for vitamin D intake in adults is 4000 IU/day. Since the majority of our society is known to be deficient in vitamin D, daily supplemental doses of 1000–2500 IU may be appropriate. Sunlight intake and adequate levels of vitamin K2 and magnesium ensure the correct processing of vitamin D. Various studies show that vitamin D supplementation in the elderly reduces falls and fractures. The risk of falls (and subsequent rate of bone fractures) in the elderly is significantly reduced with daily supplementation of 700 IU or higher (cholecalciferol) vitamin D3. Although lower doses are not effective, it shows a greater protective effect with calcium (1000–1200 mg daily) and vitamin K supplements.

When it comes to supplements in bone health, *calcium* ingredients take the biggest share. Known to support healthy bones, calcium is one of the few nutritional components with a fully approved health claim and helps reduce the risk of osteoporosis. Calcium increases bone density and is required by the body for skeletal building, muscle contraction, nerve signaling, and other metabolic processes. It is recommended to supplement at a daily dose of 1000–2000 mg for low calcium levels and to combine it with vitamin K2, which can "improve functional balance in the cardiovascular and skeletal systems" to ensure proper use of calcium.

Vitamin K is known for its cofactor role in the blood clotting process and is one of the fat-soluble vitamins. K1 (phylloquinone) is the form commonly found in many fruits, vegetables, and oils. Additionally, K1 is mainly stored in the liver and plays a greater role in coagulation. K2 (menaquinone) is distributed throughout the body and has a greater systemic effect. In particular, menaquinones play a central role in bone and cardiovascular health due to their effect on calcium balance in the body. The role of vitamin K2 in bone health derives from its function of activating several vitamin K2-dependent proteins in a process known as gamma-carboxylation, the most important of which are osteocalcin and matrix Gla protein (MGP). Vitamin K2 prevents the risk of accumulation in the vessels (arterial calcification), and supports bone strength and circulatory health by keeping calcium in the bones.

There are also different subtypes of vitamin K2, including MK-4 (animal) and MK-7 (from beneficial bacteria). Human clinical trials using the most common vitamin K2 supplement known as MK-7 have recently shown promising results for a protective effect on healthy bone. According to clinical studies, the dose of vitamin K2 required to maintain bone and vascular health was found to be 50 mcg/day MK-7.

The combination of D3 and K2 vitamins works together in maintaining bone mineral density. This combination also protects vascular health and shows a proven synergistic effect. Vitamin D3 and K2 combinations should be considered for anyone at risk of decreased bone mineral density. It supports the treatment in the prevention of secondary osteoporosis in patients of all ages who have to use corticosteroid products due to allergic or autoimmune chronic diseases. It can be used alone or in support of other treatments to maintain bone mineral density and reduce loss in the postmenopausal period. There are also other minerals to consider in maintaining healthy bones.

Magnesium is an essential mineral that acts as a critical cofactor for hundreds of biochemical reactions in the body. About half of total body magnesium stores, the fourth most abundant mineral in the human body, are found in bone tissue. Laboratory studies have found that low extracellular magnesium levels increase the production of osteoclasts in bone tissue, the cells responsible for bone breakdown. At the same time, low magnesium levels interfere with the proliferation of osteoblasts, which are bone-forming cells. In general, this causes a decrease in bone strength. Laboratory and human studies also show that magnesium has a suppressive effect on parathyroid hormone (PTH) secretion when serum calcium levels are marginally low, allowing calcium to remain in bone tissue, resulting in a protective effect on bone.

A recent review shows that nearly all enzymes that metabolize vitamin D require magnesium as a cofactor. Thus, the relationship between magnesium and vitamin D is interconnected. While vitamin D improves intestinal magnesium absorption, magnesium is required as a cofactor for vitamin D-binding protein. In addition, activation of vitamin D metabolism in the liver and kidneys also requires magnesium. Therefore, vitamin D cannot be effective in affecting the growth of bone tissue by regulating the balance of calcium and phosphate without magnesium. It can be supplemented in adult doses of 300–400 mg daily if needed. Forms of magnesium malate and magnesium citrate are recommended for reducing muscle soreness and supporting muscular energy.

Zinc is the second most abundant trace mineral in the human body after iron and is necessary for the proper functioning of more than 300 different enzymes. It is mostly stored in muscle tissue (65%) in the body. The highest rate is in erythrocytes and leukocytes. Other high zinc-containing tissues are bone, skin, kidney, liver, pancreas, retina, and prostate. Zinc is effective in the formation of bone structure cells and prevents excessive fragmentation of bone. It is an important cofactor in enzymes involved in synthesizing various bone matrix cells and plays a role in bone deposition and resorption. It plays a structural role in the bone matrix itself. The hydroxyapatite crystals that make up the bone mineral contain a zinc-fluoride complex and zinc is required for osteoblastic (bone formation) activity. Zinc deficiency reduces the activity of matrix proteins, type 1 collagen, and alkaline phosphatase reduces calcium and phosphorus deposition. Therefore, zinc deficiency may be a risk factor for poor extracellular matrix calcification. The daily zinc requirement of adults is 15–30 mg.

Although *phosphorus* does not help with calcium intake, they work together in maintaining bone structure. When calcium levels are too high, the body absorbs less phosphorus and vice versa. Bone health requires the right amount of both calcium and phosphorus. Phosphorus also plays an important structural role in nucleic acids and cell membranes, and it is about the body's energy production. Vitamin D is needed for the effective absorption of phosphorus.

Iron deficiency (with or without anemia) is considered to adversely affect bone through different mechanisms. It is not known to what extent severe or mild iron deficiency affects bone. The protective effect of different hormones (Erythropoietin (EPO), hepcidin, etc.) and factors such as inflammation, acidosis, and hypoxia due to anemia or other causes are emphasized. After the blood levels of iron supplements are determined, it will be healthy to use with the recommendation of a specialist if necessary.

Potassium is known to reduce the acidity in the bloodstream and the amount of calcium lost in the urine.

Boron is a trace element that plays an important role in many biological functions, including calcium metabolism, growth, and maintenance of bone tissue. The possible role of boron supplementation in maintaining bone health and the amount of supplementation have not yet been determined.

Copper allows the body to form red blood cells with iron. It helps maintain healthy bones, blood vessels, nerves, and immune function, and contributes to iron absorption. Adequate copper in the diet can also help prevent cardiovascular disease and osteoporosis.

Reasonable amounts of zinc supplementation may be appropriate for vegetarians and the elderly. However, routine supplementation with zinc, manganese, copper, and other metals can be given with expert advice if needed, and excessive supplementation can also be harmful. There are no long-term studies that show that trace minerals such as phosphorus, copper, iron, and selenium reduce the risk of fractures when supplemented. It should be considered that these micro-level trace elements are taken with adequate nutrition rather than supplements.

28.1.2 Supplements for Inflammation and Pain Problems

28.1.2.1 Fatty Acids, Antioxidant Vitamins, and Others

Omega-3 and Omega-6 Fatty Acids

Fish oils are rich sources of omega-3 polyunsaturated fatty acids (PUFA). It has powerful anti-inflammatory properties. Omega-3 fatty acids, eicosapentaenoic acid (EPA), and docosahexaenoic acid (DHA) reduce inflammation by suppressing IL-1b and IL-6 by various mechanisms. Omega-3 fatty acids can also reduce the production of inflammatory prostaglandins.

Fish liver oil contains high levels of vitamins A and D. Vitamin A is a powerful antioxidant and can prevent cell damage by neutralizing harmful free radicals produced in cells. Vitamin D helps a healthy musculoskeletal system by playing an important role in the production of proteoglycan in cartilage. Studies on dogs with arthritis have shown that the DHA and EPA found in omega-3 stop cartilage degradation. People with higher omega-3 intakes and blood levels also tend to have better bone mineral density.

Evidence indicates that at therapeutic doses, fish oil (whole body and liver oil) is well tolerated and has no major adverse effects. Fish oil supplementation has good evidence for improving the symptoms of rheumatoid arthritis. It can also reduce daily NSAID use in addition to long-term treatment. Evidence for the efficacy of fish oil supplements in osteoarthritis is considered insufficient.

Omega-3 polyunsaturated fatty acids may be an alternative therapeutic agent for sarcopenia due to their anti-inflammatory properties. In addition, PUFAs have an anabolic effect on muscle through activation of mammalian target of rapamycin (mTOR) signaling and reduction of insulin resistance. Increasing evidence of a beneficial effect of omega-3 supplementation in the sarcopenic elderly indicates that a combination of exercise and/or protein supplementation may be beneficial. However, more research is needed for the precise dosage, frequency, and use (alone or combined) in the treatment and prevention of sarcopenia.

Fish oil is a direct source of EPA and DHA. It competitively inhibits cyclooxygenase-2 (COX-2) and reduces the long-term use of NSAIDs. Fish oil improves morning stiffness and causes less tenderness or swelling in the joints and less joint pain and fatigue. It also reduces serum markers of inflammation such as c-reactive protein (CRP), interleukin (IL), tumor necrosis factor (TNF), and leukotriene B4. Before its effects become apparent, fish oil should be consumed at a minimum daily dose of 3 g of combined EPA and DHA for at least 12 weeks. Fish oil may affect blood clotting, so care should be taken when taking it with anticoagulants. It has the potential to play a role in improving training adaptation, recovery after exercise, preventing of injury, and improving subsequent performance in athletes. While the literature is conflicting, some evidence suggests that omega-3 supplements may reduce muscle soreness and oxidative damage to muscle cells. For instance, a study of 11 healthy men and women given 3 g of omega-3 (2 g of EPA plus 1 g of DHA) for 1 week noted a reduction in severe, delayed muscle soreness following strenuous strength exercises. For athletes, focusing on increasing omega-3 fats, which are beneficial for reducing inflammation as well as omega-6 fat intake, will provide good support against cell damage caused by intense physical activity.

The International Olympic Committee (IOC) recommends a daily dose of approximately 2 g of omega-3 fatty acids from supplements or oily fish (but does not specify the amounts of DHA or EPA or the ratio of the two). Literature shows that at least two weeks of supplementation is needed for further entry of omega-3 into muscle cells, and the intake continues to increase after four weeks of supplementation. It may take more than four weeks of supplementation to maximize the muscle involvement of omega-3. Despite positive results in animal experiments on strength and endurance increases, more studies are needed to show the same results in humans. Omega-3 studies also provide strong evidence for improved respiratory function, reduced risk of upper respiratory tract infections, and reduced inflammation. Therefore, when we consider available evidence, the regular use of omega-3 may positively impact on the performance and overall health of athletes.

Borage Seed Oil

In addition to its tannin, oleic, and palmitic acid content, borage seed contains 25% gamma-linolenic acid (GLA) and linolenic acid as two types of polyunsaturated omega-6 essential fatty acids. It regulates the body's immune system and fights joint inflammation.

There is some evidence that taking borage seed oil along with traditional pain relief or anti-inflammatory medications may help reduce rheumatoid arthritis symptoms after six weeks of treatment. There was a reduction in the number and severity of tender and swollen joints in recovery. An adult dosage of 4.5–7 g daily orally can be used for up to 24 weeks.

Evening Primrose Oil

Evening primrose is rich in two types of polyunsaturated omega-6 fatty acids. It contains GLA and 70% linolenic acid. It helps to heal pain and inflammation. While its effectiveness in reducing joint pain in rheumatoid arthritis is uncertain, there is some evidence that it may improve morning stiffness. Taking evening primrose oil with fish oil and calcium appears to reduce bone loss and increase bone density in older people with osteoporosis. Oral doses of 500–1300 mg can be taken.

Gamma-linolenic acid (GLA) is an omega-6 fatty acid found in evening primrose oil and borage oil and is the precursor of 1-series anti-inflammatory prostaglandins. It is recommended to be taken at the same time as omega-3 fatty acids, especially for balance. An effective dose of GLA is 1.4 g/day. Recent literature showed statistically significant findings for GLA in pain and overall function, with results in favor of GLA even stronger than with fish oil.

Borage seed oil and evening primrose oil may interact with anti-inflammatory and anticoagulant medications. Expert supervision is recommended for oral use. It is safer to use in massage treatment oils in aromatherapy.

Antioxidant Vitamins (A, C, E)

Antioxidants help to protect cells from damage caused by free radicals. Free radicals are natural byproducts of the body that have a certain level of benefit. It is thought that if excessive free radicals form, they can cause bones to lose their strength. Vitamins A, C, and E have antioxidant activity, so they are theoretically thought to play a role in the treatment of arthritis-related conditions by preventing bone and joint cell damage. Current human studies show that antioxidant vitamins are not effective in the treatment of rheumatoid arthritis. While there are conflicting results in the efficacy of vitamin E in the treatment of osteoarthritis, promising results have been obtained in treatment with vitamin C.

Since free radicals will also be released along with the fracture, vitamin C supplementation, which increases the absorption of both antioxidants and collagen, and vitamin D, which is necessary for the production of collagen, will be beneficial in this process. It has been determined that the consumption of fish oil, parsley, blueberry, black tea, cocoa and peanuts, as well as some vegetables and fruits containing quercetin, and carrots and tomatoes containing lycopene are beneficial in the healing of fractures.

Vitamin C (ascorbic acid) is an important antioxidant and cofactor involved in the regulation of the development, function, and maintenance of various cell types in the body. Vitamin C deficiencies cause gingival, bone pain, and impaired wound healing and collagen synthesis. Analysis of several epidemiological studies and genetic mouse models of the effect of vitamin C showed a positive effect on bone health. Ascorbic acid has been shown to be a vital modulator of osteogenic and chondrogenic differentiation. Its impact on bone health is therefore vital and has been proven to be regulated by a number of complex interaction mechanisms. While there are some inconsistencies in human studies, the most common conclusion was that decreased serum vitamin C levels or intake may be associated with the development of osteoporosis and an increased risk of fractures. Besides its function as an antioxidant, it is important that it functions as a cofactor in gene regulation that can affect bone development and regeneration.

For vitamin A, 700–900 mcg per day is the requirement for adults. Vitamins A and E can accumulate in fatty tissue, and possible overdose with supplements should be avoided. In general, dietary intake should be considered. The recommended daily adult dose of vitamin C is 75 mg for women and 90 mg for men. However, these doses may be insufficient, especially for musculoskeletal problems. If necessary, a daily dose of 500–1000 mg can be given.

Vitamin B Complex (Non-Antioxidant) Vitamins

Vitamin B complexes contain water-soluble vitamins. Except for vitamin B12, which can be stored in the liver for up to four years, all are water-soluble and only stored in the body for a short time, then excreted in the urine. Therefore, water-soluble vitamins must be taken daily with food. In its deficiency, supplementary products should be used in cases where the need increases.

Evidence for vitamin B supplementation in osteoarthritis suggests that some of the vitamins B3 (niacinamide), B9 (folic acid), and B12 (cobalamin) may positively affect joint mobility and hand grip, in particular. B9 (folic acid) intake in patients with osteoarthritis was also found to be low. Vitamin B6 may reduce inflammatory marker levels in participants with rheumatoid arthritis, but there is insufficient evidence for clinical use. Several studies have found that vitamin B12 plays a role in regulating bone metabolism. The recommended effective and safe dose in the treatment of arthritis-related conditions has not been specified, but we see data of 3 g vitamin B3, 6400 μg vitamin B9, and 20 μg vitamin B12 daily in randomized controlled studies.

28.1.2.2 Medicinal Plant Extracts, Herbal Polyphenols

Current pharmacological treatment options are associated with variable efficacy and safety, particularly for the treatment of chronic pain and inflammation. Some herbal ingredients can be used as a complementary therapy to work with or reduce the need for pharmacological agents. Treatment with herbal remedies may also offer a safer alternative with equal or superior efficacy. Anti-arthritic mechanisms of plants include inhibition of proinflammatory and pro-catabolic mediators such as cytokines, prostaglandin E2 (PGE2), matrix metalloproteinases (MMPs), reactive oxygen species (ROS), and apoptotic proteins via signaling pathways (transcription factor nuclear factor-κB (NF-κB), receptor activator of nuclear factor kappa-B ligand (RANKL), and phosphatidylinositol 3-kinase/akt-(P13K/Akt). These activities can contribute to improvement in joint pain, inflammation, and swelling problems with minimal side effects in structure and function.

Bromelain

Bromelain, obtained from the *Ananas comosus* plant, shows its digestive effect by breaking down proteins into hydrolyzed oligopeptides and amino acids. It stimulates collagen production. It has an anti-inflammatory effect by inhibiting prostaglandin synthesis. Thus, it is widely used in soft tissue injuries. It can be preferred especially for the relief of pain and edema due to infection caused by sports injuries. It is also preferred in the treatment of joint swelling after trauma or surgery with its edema-relieving effect. Literature shows that bromelain increases the absorption of actives such as glucosamine and MSM. Supplements are available at doses of 500–1000 mg/day.

Capsaicin

The fruit of the *Capsicum* plant contains a chemical called capsaicin. It is most commonly used in osteoarthritis and other painful conditions. It has a reducing effect on "Substance P," which is a pain transmitter in nerves. It has been shown to be safe and effective in reducing pain and tenderness in the affected joints in the treatment of osteoarthritis. Available evidence supports the effectiveness of topical capsaicin in reducing osteoarthritis pain compared to placebo. Evidence of effectiveness for fibromyalgia is less. Supplements are mostly used in the form of gel, patch, and cream for topical use, and may be irritant and allergenic on sensitive skin.

Quercetin

It is a flavonoid found in abundance in fruits and vegetables. It has a wide range of biological activities, thus suggesting that it plays a role in disease prevention and health promotion. More recently, animal studies have found that the effect of quercetin on bone is largely protective. Quercetin, a bioactive substance with anti-inflammatory, immunosuppressive, and protective properties, is also a potential agent for the treatment of rheumatoid arthritis.

Quercetin supplementation has been reported to reduce pain and inflammation associated with arthritis. This dietary flavonoid inhibits knee joint mechanical hyperalgesia, edema, and leukocyte uptake in mice in a dose-dependent manner without adverse effects on other organs such as the liver, kidney, and stomach. Quercetin supplementation was found to be more effective than methotrexate alone or in combination with methotrexate in reducing rheumatoid arthritis and providing the highest protection in mice. In summary, quercetin is a promising natural compound for treating pain and inflammation associated with arthritis. It is effective in prolonging the life of collagen tissue and increasing its durability. It has low bioavailability in the body. It would be beneficial to prefer liposomal supplements in daily doses of 120 mg.

Curcumin

A key ingredient in joint health is the active ingredient in turmeric. Due to its anti-inflammatory properties, it has been shown to be effective in problems such as rheumatoid arthritis. Numerous animal tests demonstrated that cell culture and turmeric can be used effectively in the treatment of inflammatory diseases such as arthritis. In 2010, Buhrman et al. demonstrated that it slowed down the inflammatory process by inhibiting the formation of NF-κB in chondrocyte cells. Therefore, curcumin emerges as a potential therapeutic agent in osteoarthritis.

Known for its potential as a complementary component for healthy aging and cellular recovery, curcumin is considered to play a key role in supporting athletic health and muscle recovery. Because the antioxidant curcumin interacts with multiple inflammatory pathways, it can eliminate oxidative stress and inflammation, the two main causes of muscle damage. In a study of athletes, participants who had taken curcuminoid (the active ingredient in curcumin) experienced a significant reduction in creatine kinase levels following muscle-strengthening exercises compared to the placebo group. It was found that curcuminoids reduce muscle damage and improve muscle soreness in healthy young participants following a muscle-damaging exercise. As a result of faster recovery, improved adaptation speed and performance are provided within intense training.

The anti-inflammatory properties of curcumin help control inflammation by regulating transcription factors, cytokines, protein kinases, enzymes, and many other downstream processes and compounds involved in inflammation. There are also studies showing that curcumin can be as effective as an anti-inflammatory, if not more than ibuprofen or aspirin.

According to a 2015 animal study, curcumin consumed orally may help relieve pain caused by muscle damage and delay soreness that occurs after workouts. Curcumin targets a number of inflammatory molecules and enzymes at a biochemical level, all of which can contribute to pain, and its ability to hit all these pathways (COX and lipoxygenase (LOX), inhibition) simultaneously makes it so effective. Literature shows that the effect of curcumin reduces muscle breakdown, stress, and pain in endurance cyclists, and relieves pain and inflammation in people with arthritis. It was found that curcumin given 500 mg three times a day was as effective in relieving pain as diclofenac, an NSAID in knee osteoarthritis pain, and had fewer side effects.

However, an important detail is that the effect results shown in clinical studies are obtained only with the same standardized dose effect in the human body. For this, it is very important to prepare and administer curcumin in appropriate forms to increase its bioavailability. The rate of bioavailability in conventional curcumin supplements is an issue. Powdered turmeric is not enough to have an effect as it contains only about 3% by the weight of curcumin. Most of the tablet and capsule forms fail to deliver the effective dose of curcumin to the body.

Liposomal encapsulation is advantageous because it allows higher absorption of the liposome content than the plain drug or supplement equivalent. The liposomal formulation of curcuminoids (active compounds in curcumin) has higher bioavailability than other curcumin supplements. In particular, liposomal curcumin has been found to have promising effects not only in relieving the symptoms of osteoarthritis patients but also in preserving bone mass. Curcumin and *Boswellia* combination supplementation was found to be more effective than curcumin alone in the treatment of pain associated with osteoarthritis.

Boswellia serrata

Boswellia is a tree native to India, Africa, and Arabia. It is often used in the traditional Indian medicine Ayurveda and most commonly for osteoarthritis. Research shows that taking certain *Boswellia* extracts can moderately reduce pain and increase mobility in people with osteoarthritis. Based on available evidence, *Boswellia* and its extract boswellic acid may be an effective and safe treatment option for osteoarthritis patients, with varying doses of 100–1000 mg alone or in combination with other herbs for at least four weeks. *Boswellia* can make the immune system more active. Thus, it can worsen the symptoms of autoimmune diseases. The use of *Boswellia* is not recommended in problems such as rheumatoid arthritis, lupus, and so on.

Ginger

Ginger (*Zingiber officinale*) is a medicinal herb that contains chemicals that may reduce inflammation and nausea. Ginger has anti-inflammatory, antioxidant, and anticancer properties. Thus, it increases the overall immunity. Ginger contains anti-inflammatory compounds that function in the same way as COX-2 inhibitors (a group of drugs used to treat pain and inflammation). It is especially useful in arthritis problems with this effect. Most research shows that taking ginger by mouth can slightly reduce pain in some people with osteoarthritis. There is different effective doses of different plant extracts, oral or topical use. In the latest report published by Arthritis Research UK, *Boswellia* (boswellic acid) and ginger (ginger) are among the options with the highest efficacy and safety scores in the treatment of osteoarthritis. A 2016 study noted that ginger supplements effectively reduced inflammation and pain after knee surgery. According to the findings of a 2015 study, ginger extract nanoparticles can improve osteoarthritis in the knee when applied topically. Participants applied ginger extract 3 times a day for 12 weeks. During this time, they experienced a reduction in pain and other symptoms.

Harpagophytum procumbens

Also known as Devil's claw, it is a traditional herb that has been used for a wide variety of health conditions, including back pain and arthritis (both osteoarthritis and rheumatoid arthritis), indigestion, fever, and allergic reactions. Of the main compounds, *harpagoside* is most responsible for the therapeutic activity. In modern herbal medicine, Devil's claw is used to reduce pain and inflammation caused by degenerative joint diseases such as osteoarthritis. Devil's claw extract harpagoside for osteoarthritis is given 2–2.6 g in three divided doses daily for up to four months.

28.2 Nutritional Supplements for Muscle Health

Both protein and non-protein supplements can be used in muscle health, structuring, and post-injury recovery periods. In addition to rapidly digesting whey protein (whey) and slow digesting casein protein supplement, leucine amino acid support, especially with branched-chain amino acids (BCAA) (Leucine-Isoleucine-Valine amino acids) complex, is important in muscle mass building. Especially after exercise, complete protein supplementation is valuable for both anabolic and anti-catabolic effects.

Balanced free amino acid levels in the body increase muscle mass and reduce muscle pain, muscle and connective tissue damage, and cytokines that cause inflammation in the body. Especially (BCAA) leucine, creatine, and glutamine amino acid supplements are recommended. Glutamine amino acid supplementation should also be preferred, especially for muscle recovery after heavy exercise. Zinc, magnesium, selenium, vitamin D, and vitamins B6 and B12 play a role in protein synthesis, and their amounts in the body should be sufficient.

28.2.1 Recovery from Muscle Injuries

In addition to rehabilitation exercises, 0.3 g/kg of high-quality complete protein supplementation and creatine supplementation at each meal may be considered (e.g., creatine 10 g/day for three weeks, then 2 g/day). Energy balance must be observed. In the inactive state, more leucine amino acids will be required to increase anabolic sensitivity. Vitamin A, D, E, selenium, and zinc supplements directly affect the anabolic response in the muscles. Omega-3 supplementation (high EPA–DHA) for eight weeks supports muscle protein synthesis in adults of all ages.

28.2.2 Tendon and Connective Tissue Injuries

Protein and amino acid supplementation should be considered in muscle injuries. In addition, daily supplementation of at least 5 g of hydrolyzed collagen and vitamin C is recommended. Energy balance must be observed. The effectiveness of sour cherry juice in the healing and recovery of soft tissue injuries has been demonstrated by its valuable antioxidant polyphenol content. Vitamin A is an important support in tissue repair with collagenase modulation. Zinc and BCAA supplementation, which supports the growth, construction, and repair of muscle tissue in muscle and tendon injuries, accelerates healing in combination with tissue repair and protein synthesis.

28.3 Conclusion

It is important to evaluate and supplement the body's needs individually for a healthy life and healthy exercise. The first thing to consider should be to meet the body's needs from foods with daily nutrition. If the nutrition is disturbed, the use of quality nutritional supplements should be considered in cases where the need increases (sports, growth, injury, stress, etc.). The effects of nutritional supplements, especially herbal supplements, on liver cytochrome enzymes responsible for the metabolism of drugs are an important detail. The potential that the person may change the effects of concomitant medications, if any, should not be ignored, and it should be given in addition to the treatment by consulting a specialist. The use of supplements, especially in people with kidney, liver, or heart disease, those who use blood thinners, children, pregnant, and lactating, should only be under the permission and control of a medical doctor.

Further Reading

Aghajanian P, Hall S, Wongworawat MD, Mohan S. The roles and mechanisms of actions of vitamin C in bone: new developments. J Bone Miner Res. 2015;30(11):1945–55.

Amorndoljai P, Taneepanichskul S, Niempoog S, Nimmannit U. Improving of knee osteoarthritic symptom by the local application of ginger extract nanoparticles: a preliminary report with short term follow-up. J Med Assoc Thai. 2015;98(9):871–7.

Bowman S, Awad ME, Hamrick MW, Hunter M, Fulzele S. Recent advances in hyaluronic acid based therapy for osteoarthritis. Clin Transl Med. 2018;7(1):6.

Buddhachat K, Siengdee P, Chomdej S, Soontornvipart K, Nganvongpanit K. Effects of different omega-3 sources, fish oil, krill oil, and green-lipped mussel against cytokine-mediated canine cartilage degradation. In Vitro Cell Dev Biol Anim. 2017;53(5):448–57.

Dupont J, Dedeyne L, Dalle S, Koppo K, Gielen E. The role of omega-3 in the prevention and treatment of sarcopenia. Aging Clin Exp Res. 2019;31(6):825–36.

Haroyan A, et al. Efficacy and safety of curcumin and its combination with boswellic acid in osteoarthritis: a comparative, randomized, double-blind, placebo-controlled study. BMC Complement Altern Med. 2018;18(1):1–16.

Iolascon G, Gimigliano R, Bianco M, De Sire A, Moretti A, Giusti A, Malavolta N, Migliaccio S, Migliore A, Napoli N, Piscitelli P, Resmini G, Tarantino U,

Gimigliano F. Are dietary supplements and nutraceuticals effective for musculoskeletal health and cognitive function? A scoping review. J Nutr Health Aging. 2017;21(5):527–38.

Pizzorno JE, Murray MT, Joiner-Bey H. The clinician's handbook of natural medicine. 3rd ed. Churchill Livingstone; 2016. p. 875–93. https://doi.org/10.1016/B978-0-7020-5514-0.00079-8, ISBN: 978-0-7020-5514-0.

König D, Oesser S, Scharla S, Zdzieblik D, Gollhofer A. Specific collagen peptides improve bone mineral density and bone markers in postmenopausal women—a randomized controlled study. Nutrients. 2018;10(1):97.

Lindler BN, Long KE, Taylor NA, Lei W. Use of herbal medications for treatment of osteoarthritis and rheumatoid arthritis. Medicines (Basel). 2020;7(11):67.

Matsui Y, Takayanagi S, Ohira T, Watanabe M, Murano H, Furuhata Y, Miyakawa S. Effect of a leucine-enriched essential amino acids mixture on muscle recovery. J Phys Ther Sci. 2019;31(1):95–101.

Maughan RJ, Burke LM, Dvorak J, et al. IOC consensus statement: dietary supplements and the high-performance athlete. Br J Sports Med. 2018;52(7):439–55.

Menghini L, Recinella L, Leone S, Chiavaroli A, Cicala C, Brunetti L, Vladimir-Knežević S, Orlando G, Ferrante C. Devil's claw (Harpagophytum procumbens) and chronic inflammatory diseases: a concise overview on preclinical and clinical data. Phytother Res. 2019;33(9):2152–62.

Nahin RL, Boineau R, Khalsa PS, Stussman BJ, Weber WJ. Evidence-based evaluation of complementary health approaches for pain management in the United States. Mayo Clin Proc. 2016;91(9):1292–306.

Philpott JD, Witard OC, Galloway SDR. Applications of omega-3 polyunsaturated fatty acid supplementation for sport performance. Res Sports Med. 2019;27(2):219–37.

Qu X, He Z, Qiao H, Zhai Z, Mao Z, Yu Z, Dai K. Serum copper levels are associated with bone mineral density and total fracture. J Orthop Translat. 2018;14:34–44.

Ruff KJ, Morrison D, Duncan SA, Back M, Aydogan C, Theodosakis J. Beneficial effects of natural eggshell membrane versus placebo in exercise-induced joint pain, stiffness, and cartilage turnover in healthy, postmenopausal women. Clin Interv Aging. 2018;13:285–95.

Shep D, et al. Safety and efficacy of curcumin versus diclofenac in knee osteoarthritis: a randomized open-label parallel-arm study. Trials. 2019;20(1):1–11.

Tachtsis B, Camera D, Lacham-Kaplan O. Potential roles of n-3 PUFAs during skeletal muscle growth and regeneration. Nutrients. 2018;10(3):309.

Toxqui L, Vaquero MP. Chronic iron deficiency as an emerging risk factor for osteoporosis: a hypothesis. Nutrients. 2015;7(4):2324–44.

Vânia G, João Paulo C, Iva B. Topical capsaicin for pain in osteoarthritis: a literature review. Reumatologia Clinica. 2018;14(1):40–5.

Wong SK, Chin KY, Ima-Nirwana S. Quercetin as an agent for protecting the bone: a review of the current evidence. Int J Mol Sci. 2020;21(17):6448.

Yao P, Bennett D, Mafham M, Lin X, Chen Z, Armitage J, Clarke R. Vitamin D and calcium for the prevention of fracture: a systematic review and meta-analysis. JAMA Netw Open. 2019;2(12):e1917789.

Yu G, Xiang W, Zhang T, Zeng L, Yang K, Li J. Effectiveness of Boswellia and Boswellia extract for osteoarthritis patients: a systematic review and meta-analysis. BMC Complement Med Ther. 2020;20(1):225.

Zhu X, Sang L, Wu D, Rong J, Jiang L. Effectiveness and safety of glucosamine and chondroitin for the treatment of osteoarthritis: a meta-analysis of randomized controlled trials. J Orthop Surg Res. 2018;13(1):170.

Exercise-Induced Anaphylaxis

Nurhan Sayaca

Abstract

Anaphylaxis is an acute, systemic reaction with a potential risk of death. The annual incidence is between 50 and 112 per 100,000 and the prevalence varies between 0.3 and 5.1%. Many risk factors have been identified for anaphylaxis. Anaphylaxis is a sudden onset and life-threatening systemic hypersensitivity reaction due to mast cell and basophil-derived mediators. Common clinical symptoms of anaphylaxis are redness of the skin, pruritus, urticaria, angioedema, morbilliform rash, shortness of breath, chest tightness, deep coughing, wheezing/bronchospasm, itching, sneezing, congestion, discharge in the nose, chest pain, tachycardia, palpitations, bradycardia, dysrhythmia, hypotension, feeling faint, mental change, loss of sphincter control, shock, arrest, dizziness, throbbing headache, feeling of death, restlessness, and confusion. Anaphylaxis can be triggered by exercise or physical activity. Exercise-induced anaphylaxis (EIA) and food-dependent exercise-induced anaphylaxis (FDEIA) are defined in this context. Anaphylaxis can occur during exercise or appear soon after. If the occurrence of anaphylaxis is related to pre-exercise food intake (especially a food to which the patient is sensitive), the terminology of FDEIA is used. The frequency of attacks in both EIA and FDEIA is variable. Generally, attacks do not occur with every exercise. Although both types of anaphylaxis have been reported in all age groups, especially in the 4–74 age range, it is usually seen in adolescent and young adult patients. It is seen slightly more in men than women. It is usually sporadic, but familial cases have also been reported. FDEIA can be classified as specific FDEIA or non-specific FDEIA according to the identification of a culprit food allergen. Symptoms of both FDIEA and EIA can occur at any stage of the exercise, from ten minutes to four hours after food allergen ingestion. Most patients ingest the culprit allergen four to five hours before exercise and can exercise independently. With the cessation of exercise, the symptoms usually improve and may completely disappear in mild cases. In terms of follow-up and treatment, it is important to limit and control the physical activities that trigger the symptoms. Also, training about anaphylaxis action plans should be given to all patients and an adrenaline autoinjector should be prescribed.

N. Sayaca (✉)
Immunology and Allergy, Faculty of Medicine,
Manisa Celal Bayar University,
Manisa, Turkey
e-mail: nurhan.sayaca@cbu.edu.tr

29.1 Epidemiology of Anaphylaxis

The American Anaphylaxis Epidemiology Study Group reported that anaphylaxis prevalence is between 0.05 and 2.00%. Based on similar results in Europe, prevalence is estimated at 0.3%. Recent research studies report that the annual incidence is between 50 and 112 per 100,000 and the prevalence varies between 0.3 and 5.1%. Although it is observed that hospitalizations due to anaphylaxis are increasing in many countries, the mortality rate remains low. Mortality rates per year are estimated at 0.05–0.51 per million people for drug-induced anaphylaxis, 0.03–0.32 for food, and 0.09–0.13 for venom. This increase is probably related to many factors such as the increase in the global frequency of allergic diseases, better recognition of anaphylaxis, and the cumulative incidence of this condition.

29.2 Risk Factors for Anaphylaxis

Many risk factors have been identified for anaphylaxis (Table 29.1). The most important risk factors are asthma, the high severity of asthma, and the use of drugs such as beta-blockers and angiotensin-converting enzyme inhibitors (ACEI). These drugs may interfere with the effects of epinephrine on adrenergic receptors.

Some risk factors were also identified for fatal anaphylaxis such as age with more adults experiencing fatal anaphylaxis. Elder people are more susceptible to anaphylaxis. However, younger people suffer more from food-related fatal anaphylaxis. History of previous anaphylaxis is an important risk factor for fatal anaphylaxis, while the severity of a previous anaphylactic reaction is not. Medical conditions such as complex medical history, conditions requiring frequent antibiotic use, asthma, cardiovascular disease, and mast cell disorders are also risk factors for fatal anaphylaxis.

Table 29.1 Risk factors for anaphylaxis

Age-related factors
• **Pregnancy:** Intensive and various drug use (e.g., beta-lactam antibiotics) and the possibility of medical/surgical intervention (e.g., cesarean section) may pose a risk of anaphylaxis due to iatrogenic reasons such as perioperative and latex anaphylaxis
• **Infants:** Anaphylaxis may go undetected, especially if it is the first attack; the patient cannot describe the symptoms
• **Adolescents and young adults:** They may exhibit behaviors such as risk-taking and impassivity due to their age; also, they may not avoid known stimuli sufficiently or carry an adrenaline autoinjector
• **Elderly:** High risk of death due to comorbidities and medications
Comorbidities
• Asthma and other chronic respiratory diseases
• Allergic rhinitis and atopic dermatitis (eczema): Atopic diseases are risk factors for food, latex, and exercise-related anaphylaxis, but not for drug or venom-related anaphylaxis
• Cardiovascular diseases
• Psychiatric/psychological diseases: The patient's tendency to engage in risky behaviors
• Mastocytosis
Drugs
• Angiotensin-converting enzyme inhibitors (ACEI)
• Beta-adrenergic blockers
• Sedatives, antidepressants, narcotics, addictive/drugs, alcohol: The patient can not recognize stimuli or symptoms
Cofactors that exacerbate anaphylaxis
• Exercise: Food or drug (non-steroidal anti-inflammatory drugs [NSAIDs]) related or exercise only
• Fever
• Acute infections
• Emotional stress
• Premenstrual period
• Non-routine work: Travel

29.3 Pathophysiology of Anaphylaxis

Anaphylaxis is a sudden onset and life-threatening systemic hypersensitivity reaction due to mast cell and basophil-derived mediators. Anaphylaxis is mostly caused by immunological mechanisms triggered by allergens such as foods, drugs, and venom, but non-immunological mechanisms may also play a role in the development of anaphylaxis by causing mast cell and basophil degranulation. A significant portion of anaphylaxis is IgE-mediated, which occurs with immunological mechanisms (Fig. 29.1). IgG-mediated anaphylaxis has also been described in animal models. Non-immunological factors that cause anaphylaxis include exercise, cold, and various drugs (opiates, vancomycin, radiocontrast agent, cyclooxygenase [COX]-1 inhibitors).

29.4 Clinical Findings of Anaphylaxis

Common clinical symptoms of anaphylaxis are redness of the skin, pruritus, urticaria, angioedema, morbilliform rash, shortness of breath, chest tightness, deep coughing, wheezing/bronchospasm, itching, sneezing, congestion, discharge in the nose, chest pain, tachycardia, palpitations, bradycardia, dysrhythmia, hypotension, feeling faint, mental change, loss of sphincter control, shock, arrest, dizziness, throbbing headache, feeling of death, restlessness, and confusion (Fig. 29.2).

Anaphylaxis is diagnosed by widely accepted clinical criteria using patient (case) history and physical examination (Table 29.2). While evaluating the medical history, the patient should be questioned in detail on the time of the event, how

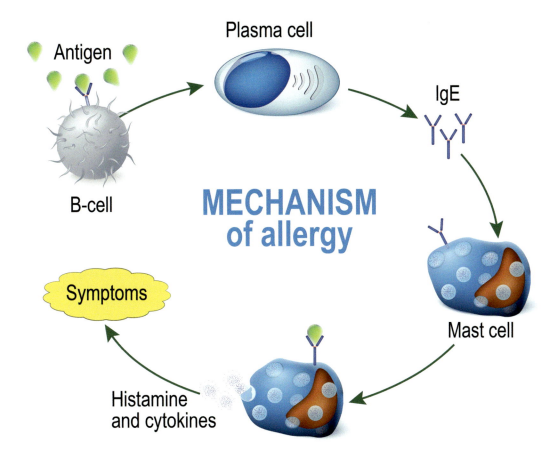

Fig. 29.1 IgE-mediated mechanisms of anaphylaxis (Designua/Shutterstock.com)

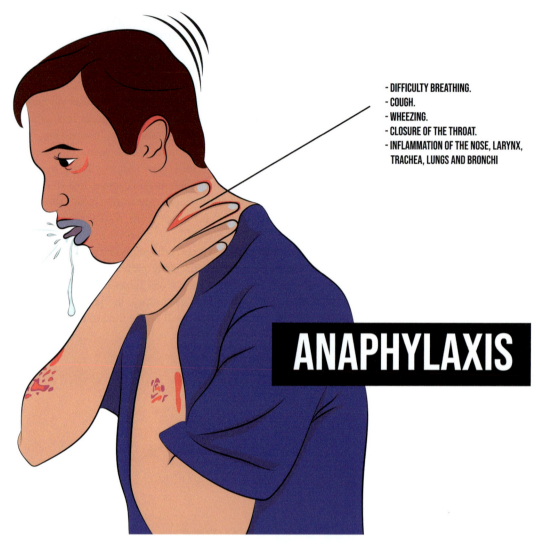

Fig. 29.2 Clinical findings of anaphylaxis (NEITPIX/Shutterstock.com)

long it lasted, whether any treatment was applied, and potential triggers. Anaphylaxis usually occurs within the first two hours after exposure to the first stimulus. Usually, at least two organ systems are involved in anaphylaxis, but, in some cases, the involvement of only one organ system (hypotension in the cardiovascular system [CVS]) may be considered sufficient for the diagnosis.

The clinical manifestations of anaphylaxis depend on the organ systems presented in Fig. 29.3. Among the symptoms of anaphylaxis, the most common are skin findings. However, skin manifestations may not occur or cannot be seen initially. Respiratory or CVS findings are the most important indicators for life-threatening anaphylaxis. Respiratory system findings are more common in children while CVS findings are more common in adults. The signs and symptoms of anaphylaxis according to the affected systems are summarized in Table 29.3. During the course of anaphylaxis, recurrence of the reaction may occur up to 72 h (average 6–8 h) after improvement

Table 29.2 Diagnostic criteria of anaphylaxis

The probability of anaphylaxis is very high if any of the following are met:

1. Acutely occurring signs in the involvement of the skin, mucous membranes, or both (within minutes to hours) (diffuse urticaria, itching, redness, swelling of the lips/tongue/uvula) and at least one of the following:
  (a) Symptoms associated with a decrease in blood pressure or impaired end-organ function (e.g., hypotonia [collapse], syncope, incontinence)
  (b) Respiratory distress (e.g., dyspnea, wheezing/bronchospasm, stridor, PEF decreased, hypoxemia)
2. Two or more of the following occur rapidly (within minutes to hours) after the patient is exposed to a possible allergen:
  (a) Involvement of skin, mucous membranes, or both (diffuse urticaria, itching, redness, swelling of lips/tongue/uvula)
  (b) Symptoms associated with a decrease in blood pressure or impaired end-organ function (e.g., hypotonia [collapse], syncope, incontinence)
  (c) Respiratory distress (e.g., dyspnea, wheezing/bronchospasm, stridor, PEF decreased, hypoxemia)
  (d) Persistent gastrointestinal symptoms (e.g., cramping abdominal pain, vomiting)
3. Reduction of blood pressure (within minutes to hours) after exposure to a known allergen for the patient:
  (a) Adults: Blood pressure <90 mmHg or >30% reduction from patient's baseline
  (b) Infants and children: Age-adjusted low systolic blood pressure or >30% reduction in systolic blood pressure

PEF Peak expiratory flow

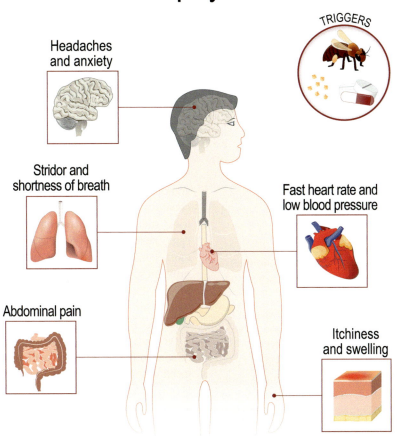

Fig. 29.3 Triggers and clinical findings of anaphylaxis according to the organ systems (Designua/Shutterstock.com)

Table 29.3 Signs and symptoms of anaphylaxis

Systems	Signs and symptoms	Occurrence (%)
Skin and mucous membranes	• Redness, pruritus, urticaria, angioedema, morbilliform rash • Itching and swelling of the lips, tongue, palate, and uvula • Conjunctival erythema, lacrimation	80–90
Respiratory	• Nose: itching, congestion, discharge, sneezing • Lung: shortness of breath, chest tightness, deep coughing, wheezing/bronchospasm (reduced PEF) • Larynx: pruritus, tightness, dysphonia, hoarseness, dry-hard cough, stridor, cyanosis	70
Gastrointestinal	• Dysphagia, nausea, vomiting, cramp-like abdominal pain, diarrhea	30–45
Cardiovascular	• Chest pain, tachycardia, palpitations, bradycardia, dysrhythmia, hypotension, feeling faint, mental change, loss of sphincter control, shock, arrest	10–45
Neurological	• Dizziness, throbbing headache, feeling of death, restlessness, confusion • Sudden behavioral changes in infants and young children (irritability, interrupting play, clinging to parents, etc.)	10–15
Other	• Metallic taste in the mouth, uterine contractions (postpubertal)	

of symptoms. This condition is called "biphasic anaphylaxis." The severity of biphasic anaphylaxis may be similar to the first reaction, or it may be milder or much more severe, or even fatal.

> **Clinical Information**
> **When Should We Think About Anaphylaxis?**
>
> 1. Skin findings: Pruritus, urticaria, angioedema, morbilliform rash
> 2. Upper respiratory system findings: Sneezing, nasal congestion, itching, and discharge in nose
> 3. Lower respiratory system findings: Shortness of breath, chest tightness, deep coughing, wheezing/bronchospasm
> 4. Cardiovascular system findings: Chest pain, tachycardia, palpitations, bradycardia, dysrhythmia, hypotension
> 5. Nervous system findings: Feeling faint, mental change, loss of sphincter control, shock, arrest, dizziness, throbbing headache, feeling of death, restlessness, confusion

29.5 Stimuli of Anaphylaxis

Age-related stimuli of anaphylaxis are generally considered to be similar. For children, adolescents, and young adults, foods are first; followed by venoms and drugs. Venoms and drugs are more common in adults and the elderly. Idiopathic anaphylaxis is also more common in adults and the elderly than in children.

While some of the food stimuli of anaphylaxis can be seen with similar frequencies all over the world, some of them may show geographical variability according to local dietary habits, preparation of foods, and exposure type. In developed countries (the USA and some European countries) and some Asian countries, cow's milk, eggs, peanuts, nuts, shellfish, and fish are the most common foods that cause anaphylaxis. Fruits in some European countries, sesame in the Middle East, beef in the Eastern Black Sea Region of Turkey, and buckwheat, rice, and chickpeas in Asia are more common causes.

Venom sources causing anaphylaxis also show regional differences. The most frequently investigated venoms are insect venoms belonging to the Hymenoptera family (honey and wasps, fire ants). Venom anaphylaxis due to bee stings is seen in Turkey and anaphylaxis due to honeybee venom is the most common.

Anaphylaxis can develop with all drugs, and antibiotics are the leading cause. Among antibiotics, the beta-lactam group takes the first place. Non-steroidal anti-inflammatory drugs (NSAIDs), ACEIs, chemotherapy drugs (asparaginases, carboplatin, doxorubicin), and biological agents (monoclonal antibodies such as cetuximab, rituximab, infliximab, and rarely omalizumab) can be counted among the leading causes of drug anaphylaxis. Among the agents used for diagnostic procedures, the most known causes are radiocontrast agents. Anaphylaxis in the perioperative period may occur because of neuromuscular blockers (suxamethonium, rocuronium), hypnotics (thiopental, propofol), opioids, antimicrobial drugs, protamine, chlorhexidine, latex, and colloid plasma expanders such as dextran. Anaphylaxis may also develop during skin tests, especially intradermal tests, food and drug provocation tests, allergen-specific immunotherapy, and drug desensitization.

Latex (rubber), which is used in almost every area of daily life from toys to medical devices, should also be counted as an important cause of anaphylaxis. Latex is among the main reasons for occupational allergies.

The definition of idiopathic anaphylaxis should be used after all possible reasons for anaphylaxis have been excluded. Therefore, a detailed history, skin tests with obvious and hidden possible allergens and serum-specific IgE measurements, and provocation tests in selected patients may be required. During the etiological diagnostic tests for idiopathic anaphylaxis, unexpected stimuli such as galactose alpha-1,3 galactose (alpha-gal) can be detected, as well as conditions such as mastocytosis and clonal mast cell diseases.

> **Clinical Information**
> **Triggers of Anaphylaxis:**
>
> - Foods
> - Venoms
> - Drugs
> - Exercise
> - Idiopathic

29.6 Exercise-Induced Anaphylaxis

Anaphylaxis can be triggered by exercise or physical activity. Exercise-induced anaphylaxis (EIA) and food-dependent exercise-induced anaphylaxis (FDEIA) are defined in this context. The diagnosis of both diseases is mainly based on medical history and clinical findings. Because of similar clinical conditions, a careful differential diagnosis should be performed.

Exercise is an uncommon trigger of anaphylaxis. Wood et al. reported that exercise accounts for 1.5% of all cases of anaphylaxis. The prevalence of EIA was estimated at 0.03% in Japanese junior-high children. The same scientists reported the prevalence of FDEIA to be 0.005% in elementary school children and 0.02% in junior-high-aged children.

Anaphylaxis can occur during exercise or appear soon after. If the occurrence of anaphylaxis is related to pre-exercise food intake (especially a food to which the patient is sensitive), the terminology of FDEIA is used. The frequency of attacks in both EIA and FDEIA is variable. Generally, attacks do not occur with every exercise. However, there are also patients who experience symptoms after each exercise. It can be seen at any exercise intensity, but it is more common at challenging levels.

Maulitz reported EIA firstly in 1979. He presented a recurrent anaphylaxis case induced by jogging after consuming shellfish, in a 31-year-old male. Before this case, this patient had no anaphylactic reaction after exercise and could eat shellfish without any symptoms. However, when consuming shellfish before the exercise he had sudden onset symptoms. Maulitz showed evidence of IgE-mediated sensitivity by skin prick test. After this description of EIA or more correctly FDEIA, scientific studies progressed.

Recent literature supports Maulitz and suggests that FDEIA is a primary IgE-mediated food allergy that is induced by several cofactors. The symptoms can appear via cofactors such as NSAIDs, exercise, and alcohol. These cofactors increase intestinal permeability and allow increased antigen uptake.

Although both types of anaphylaxis have been reported in all age groups, especially in the 4–74 age range, it is usually seen in adolescent and young adult patients. It is seen slightly more in men than women. It is usually sporadic, but familial cases have also been reported. EIA can affect all people who do optional exercise as well as athletes but it is seen more frequently among atopic people.

29.6.1 Food-Dependent Exercise-Induced Anaphylaxis

FDEIA can be classified as specific FDEIA or non-specific FDEIA according to the identification of a culprit food allergen. Most commonly reported foods related to FDEIA reactions can be both plant and animal proteins. Mostly reported food allergens are wheat, in particular omega-5-gliadin, nuts, and shellfish. However, there are a lot of other foods, including seafood (e.g., finfish, shellfish, mollusks), other grains/cereals (oats, barley, rye, rice, buckwheat), cow's milk, fruit and vegetables (tomato, onion, orange, grape, celery), meat (e.g., wild boar meat, pork, beef), snails, wine, red bean, taro, mushroom, and foods contaminated with aeroallergens (house-dust mite, *Penicillium* mold). Potential food allergen exposure, particularly associated with exercise, should also be considered, such as energy drinks that may contain soya or animal-derived gelatin. Allergens such as maize, omega-5-gliadin, rice, or concentrated fruit puree can be found in "energy-boosting" carbohydrate meals. The allergenic potential of the IgE-binding epitopes of the food proteins, and their resistance to heat, digestion, and processing, can have an important role in eliciting FDEIA.

29.6.2 Pathophysiology of Exercise-Induced Anaphylaxis

The pathogenesis of this group of anaphylaxis has not been fully understood. Investigations about the mechanisms of both FDIEA and EIA are still ongoing. Exercise reduces the mast cell degranulation threshold and causes the release of bioactive mediators such as arachidonic acid metabolites (leukotrienes, prostaglandins, and platelet-activating factor), histamine, and tryptase associated with an allergic reaction. Histamine has pleiotropic effects including flushing, urticaria, bronchoconstriction, and tachycardia. Arachidonic acid metabolites can cause vasodilation, bronchoconstriction, and increased vascular permeability. Tryptase is a serine protease and activates the cascade and complement pathways.

During the non-exercise period, if the food is ingested, the gut mast cell degranulation is not induced by the allergenic peptides; so anaphylaxis does not elicit. However, during exercise, the redistribution of blood flow occurs away from the visceral organs (primarily the kidneys, liver, stomach, and intestine) to supply the skeletal muscle, heart, and skin instead, where mast cells with different phenotypes are found. EIA may occur as a result of the interaction between the unique mast cells in these tissues with these food allergen peptides. Also, the blood pH and osmolarity can take a role in the pathophysiology of EIA. However, this theory can be refuted, because generally non-maximal intensity exercise causes EIA, where alterations in blood pH and osmolarity would not be affected.

However, it is suggested by exercise physiology studies that regular exercise intensities can unlikely alter gastrointestinal permeability. Indeed, only moderate activity can trigger EIA. It should be considered that the gastrointestinal barrier can be altered by other cofactors such as NSAIDs or alcohol.

29.6.3 Clinical Findings of Exercise-Induced Anaphylaxis

Symptoms of EIA consist of pruritus, hives, wheezing, shortness of breath, chest tightness, profuse sweating, headache, flushing, nausea, dysphagia, abdominal pain, and diarrhea, including more severe symptoms, especially if physical activity is persisted, such as laryngeal edema, choking, hoarseness, throat constriction, angioedema, hypotension, cardiovascular collapse, or shock resulting in life-threatening anaphylaxis.

Symptoms of both FDIEA and EIA can occur at any stage of the exercise, from ten minutes to four hours after food allergen ingestion. The frequency of anaphylactic biphasic reactions in FDEIA is not known. Most patients ingest the culprit allergen four to five hours before the exercise and can exercise independently.

With the cessation of exercise, the symptoms usually improve and sometimes (in mild cases) disappear completely. Therefore, it is important to stop exercising as soon as the initial symptoms appear, stay where you are, and not move even to seek help or try to get to the hospital.

Mortality is rare and only described in adults. However, in such fatal cases, the cause of mortality is often associated with other factors, such as cardiac events, rather than anaphylaxis, and the true diagnosis is overlooked.

Wheat is the most commonly reported food trigger for FDIEA. Four wheat protein categories are classified: alcohol-soluble gliadins, salt-soluble globulins, water-soluble albumins, and insoluble glutenins. In FDEIA, grains and shellfish are the main factors besides wheat. However, many foods associated with FDEIA have been reported in the literature (vegetables, fruits, legumes, meat, cow's milk, and eggs). Most frequently same foods cause symptoms, but there are some exceptions. It has even been reported that in some patients, symptoms only occur when different foods are taken together, even if the food is raw or cooked, and the way of cooking has been associated with the onset of symptoms. There may also be factors that affect the onset of symptoms in EIA and FDEIA. Drinking alcoholic beverages, exercising during the pollen season for pollen-sensitive patients, exercising at very hot or cold temperatures, or taking NSAIDs may cause anaphylaxis to start more easily.

29.6.4 Diagnosis of Exercise-Induced Anaphylaxis

In order to diagnose EIA, a very meticulous evaluation is required. It is essential to take a very detailed anamnesis before, during, and after the attack:

- It is important to determine whether the attacks occur at a certain stage of the exercise or at any stage. Because, a safe exercise level can be recommended to the patient in the future.
- Before making the diagnosis of FDEIA, the relationship between the symptoms of food intake and exercise should be questioned in detail, and the presence of a primary food allergy that is exacerbated by exercise should not be unnoticed. The clinicians must focus on the foods potentially triggering the reaction, route of exposure, the quantity, time relationship between the reaction and the ingestion of the food, symptoms, relationship with physical exercise, and the presence of cofactors.
- It should be well questioned whether the symptoms decrease with the termination of exercise.
- Apart from exercise, it should be questioned whether symptoms occur in other situations that cause an increase in body temperature (most importantly, hot bath) and it should be differentiated from cholinergic urticaria attacks.
- It should be questioned whether there are conditions known as facilitating factors (drugs, alcohol intake, etc.) in EIA and FDEIA.
- It should be learned whether the exercise was performed in outdoor or indoor (relationship with weather conditions, presence of specific allergens in the environment, etc.).
- It should be known whether the patient has an allergic disease associated with the respiratory tract or whether there is a history of physical urticaria.
- It should be learned whether the food presumed to be responsible for FDEIA is tolerated without exercise.
- In patients with pollen allergy, food-related symptoms should be differentiated from oral allergy syndrome.
- While investigating the responsible food in FDEIA, it should be learned whether there are supportive products taken before exercise, which is often unnoticed.

In general, clinical findings in EIA should be compatible with anaphylaxis and there should be no other reasons to explain the clinical picture. There is no accepted provocation test, and a negative provocation test cannot exclude the diagnosis. For this reason, it is not very meaningful to perform a provocation test in EIA.

In FDEIA, however, the clinical findings that appeared should be compatible with anaphylaxis, there should be no other reasons to explain the clinical picture, and there should be food intake before exercise. If a certain food is thought to be responsible, the presence of sensitivity to that food (presence of specific IgE) should be demonstrated. The same is true for provocation tests; the lack of a standardized test protocol and the fact that negative results do not exclude the diagnosis make provocation tests unnecessary in FDEIA.

Before diagnosing the EIA and FDEIA, some situations should be considered in the differential diagnosis:

- Sudden fatigue, dyspnea, or hypotension during exercise may be due to cardiac events. Distinguishing features: no findings such as pruritus, urticaria, angioedema, or laryngeal edema.
- Exercise-induced bronchospasm. Distinguishing feature: symptoms are limited to the airways.
- Reflux caused by exercise can cause symptoms such as burning in the throat, retrosternal burning, or coughing. The distinguishing feature: the symptoms are not progressive and there are no signs such as pruritus, urticaria, angioedema, or laryngeal edema.
- Cold urticaria/anaphylaxis is a diagnosis that should be considered only if symptoms occur during exercise in a cold environment.
- Cholinergic urticaria can cause both skin symptoms and systemic symptoms if massive mast cell degranulation has occurred. Distinguishing features: lesions on the skin are itchy plaques in the form of small dots. The exercise is not necessary for its occurrence; it also occurs when the body temperature rises passively.
- It is difficult to distinguish mast cell diseases from EIA, either clinically or by history. Continuously elevated serum mast cell mediator levels during an anaphylaxis attack and in the asymptomatic period are required for diagnosis.
- Reactions due to food allergies may worsen during exercise. It is possible to confuse this situation with FDEIA.

Some important points that should be emphasized in this group of anaphylaxis:

1. The patient and/or family should be informed about the characteristics of the attacks, the triggers of the attacks (if detected), and the factors that facilitate/worsen the attacks.
2. The prodromal signs of the attacks should be known by the patient and the exercise should be stopped as soon as they occur.
3. If necessary, adrenaline should be administered by the emergency treatment plan.
4. If the food responsible for FDEIA has been determined, it should not be taken four hours before or one hour after exercise.

Although some prophylactic treatments have been recommended, there is insufficient evidence for their routine use.

29.7 Treatment of Anaphylaxis

Since anaphylaxis is a life-threatening emergency clinical case, it should be promptly treated after diagnosis. The first intervention and treatment must be performed immediately after the place of diagnosis. The steps of treatment that should be performed after calling the emergency medical service are as follows:

1. The patient should be placed on his back with the legs above the level of the trunk and breathing should be provided by keeping the airway open.
2. Adrenaline should be administered immediately. The dose of adrenaline is 0.5 mg in adults and 0.01 mg/kg (maximum 0.3 mg) in

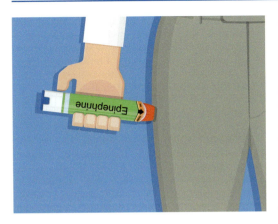

Fig. 29.4 Adrenaline autoinjector (Pepermpron/Shutterstock.com)

children. It should be given intramuscularly from the anterior-lateral side of the thigh (Fig. 29.4). If there is no improvement, adrenaline should be continued at the same dose with an interval of 5–15 min.

3. The patient's contact with the antigen should be discontinued. For example, if there is a bee sting, the bee's sting should be removed before it breaks. In food-related anaphylaxis, the inside of the mouth should be cleaned by washing.
4. Diphenhydramine should be given intramuscularly or intravenously with a dose of 50 mg to adults, and 1 mg/kg to children.
5. If possible, vascular access should be obtained and the infusion of physiological saline should be started.
6. Methylprednisolone 2 mg/kg (50 mg maximum) (or an equivalent corticosteroid) should be given orally, intramuscularly, or intravenously.
7. The patient should be immediately referred to a professional healthcare facility.

29.8 Conclusion

In terms of follow-up and treatment, it is important to limit and control the physical activities that trigger the symptoms. Also, training about anaphylaxis action plans should be given to all patients and an adrenaline autoinjector should be prescribed. They must always carry the adrenaline autoinjector with them. Adrenaline is a banned substance in professional sports competitions. However, the use and possession of adrenaline are possible with certain rules. Drugs such as omalizumab, cromolyn sodium, and misoprostol, which are successful in preventing the disease in a limited number of studies, are not yet included in routine treatment.

Further Reading

Tanno LK, Bierrenbach AL, Simons FER, Cardona V, Thong BY, Molinari N, et al. Critical view of anaphylaxis epidemiology: open questions and new perspectives. Allergy Asthma Clin Immunol. 2018;14(1):1–11. https://doi.org/10.1186/s13223-018-0234-0.

Turner PJ, Campbell DE, Motosue MS, Campbell RL. Global trends in anaphylaxis epidemiology and clinical implications. J Allergy Clin Immunol Pract. 2020;8(4):1169–76. https://doi.org/10.1016/j.jaip.2019.11.027.

Tanno LK, Demoly P. Epidemiology of anaphylaxis. Curr Opin Allergy Clin Immunol. 2021;21(2):168–74. https://doi.org/10.1097/ACI.0000000000000722.

Orhan F, Civelek E, Şahiner Ü, Arga M, Can M, Çalıkaner D, et al. Anaphylaxis: Turkish national guideline 2018. Asthma. 2018;16: Ek Sayı/Supplement:1:1–62.

Lee S, Hess EP, Nestler DM, Athmaram VRB, Bellolio MF, Decker WW, et al. Antihypertensive medication use is associated with increased organ system involvement and hospitalization in emergency department patients with anaphylaxis. J Allergy Clin Immunol. 2013;131(4):1103–8. https://doi.org/10.1016/j.jaci.2013.01.011. Epub 2013 Feb 27.

Greenberger PA. Fatal and near-fatal anaphylaxis: Factors that can worsen or contribute to fatal outcomes. Immunol Allergy Clin North Am. 2015;35(2):375–86. https://doi.org/10.1016/j.iac.2015.01.001. Epub 2015 Feb 27.

Jerschow E, Lin RY, Scaperotti MM, McGinn AP. Fatal anaphylaxis in the United States, 1999-2010: Temporal patterns and demographic associations. J Allergy Clin Immunol. 2014;134(6):1318–1328.e7. https://doi.org/10.1016/j.jaci.2014.08.018. Epub 2014 Sep 30.

Golden DBK. Anaphylaxis: recognizing risk and targeting treatment. J Allergy Clin Immunol Pract. 2017;5(5):1224–6. https://doi.org/10.1016/j.jaip.2017.06.028.

Mikhail I, Stukus DR, Prince BT. Fatal anaphylaxis: epidemiology and risk factors. Curr Allergy Asthma Rep. 2021;21(4):1–10. https://doi.org/10.1007/s11882-021-01006-x.

Turner PJ, Gowland MH, Sharma V, Ierodiakonou D, Harper N, Garcez T, et al. Increase in anaphylaxis-related hospitalizations but no increase in fatalities: an analysis of United Kingdom national anaphylaxis data, 1992-2012. J Allergy Clin Immunol. 2015;135(4):956–963.e1. https://doi.org/10.1016/j.jaci.2014.10.021. Epub 2014 Nov 25.

Gülen T, Ljung C, Nilsson G, Akin C. Risk factor analysis of anaphylactic reactions in patients with systemic mastocytosis. J Allergy Clin Immunol Pract. 2017;5(5):1248–55. https://doi.org/10.1016/j.jaip.2017.02.008. Epub 2017 Mar 25.

Kemp SF, Lockey RF. Anaphylaxis: a review of causes and mechanisms. J Allergy Clin Immunol. 2002;110(3):341–8. https://doi.org/10.1067/mai.2002.126811.

Simons FER, Ebisawa M, Sanchez-Borges M, Thong BY, Worm M, Tanno LK, et al. 2015 update of the evidence base: World Allergy Organization anaphylaxis guidelines. World Allergy Organ J. 2015;8(1):1–16. https://doi.org/10.1186/s40413-015-0080-1.

Lee S, Bellolio MF, Hess EP, Erwin P, Murad MH, Campbell RL. Time of onset and predictors of biphasic anaphylactic reactions: a systematic review and meta-analysis. J Allergy Clin Immunol Pract. 2015;3(3):408–16.e1-2. https://doi.org/10.1016/j.jaip.2014.12.010. Epub 2015 Feb 11.

Giannetti MP. Exercise-induced anaphylaxis: literature review and recent updates. Curr Allergy Asthma Rep. 2018;18(12):1–8. https://doi.org/10.1007/s11882-018-0830-6.

Wood RA, Camargo CA, Lieberman P, Sampson HA, Schwartz LB, Zitt M, et al. Anaphylaxis in America: the prevalence and characteristics of anaphylaxis in the United States. J Allergy Clin Immunol. 2014;133(2):461–7. https://doi.org/10.1016/J.JACI.2013.08.016.

Foong RX, Giovannini M, du Toit G. Food-dependent exercise-induced anaphylaxis. Curr Opin Allergy Clin Immunol. 2019;19(3):224–8. https://doi.org/10.1097/ACI.0000000000000531.

Printed by Printforce, the Netherlands